The Anatomical Basis of Dentistry

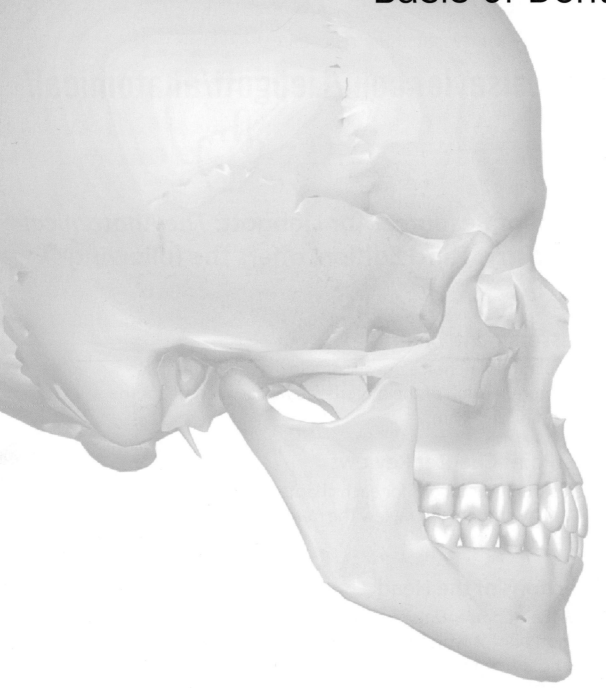

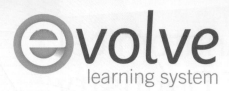

To access your Student Resources, visit the web address below:

http://evolve.elsevier.com/Liebgott/anatomical/

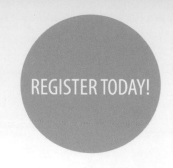

Evolve®Student Resources for Liebgott: *The Anatomical Basis of Dentistry*, **Third Edition, offers the following features:**

- ## Self-assessment Exam

  Over 170 multiple-choice questions allow students to test their comprehension of the material as well as prepare for the NBDE and future exams.

- ## PowerPoint Chapter Reviews

  PowerPoint presentations for each chapter provide a quick and easy way for students to review the material presented in each chapter.

- ## Dissections of the Head

  A PowerPoint presentation containing full-color cadaver dissection photos which clearly depicts the location of anatomic structures. These photos allow students to see anatomical details impossible to view in clinical examination.

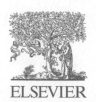

ELSEVIER

THIRD EDITION

The Anatomical Basis of Dentistry

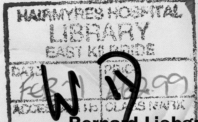
Bernard Liebgott, DDS, MScD, PhD
Professor Emeritus, Department of Surgery
Division of Anatomy
Faculty of Medicine
Faculty of Dentistry
University of Toronto
Toronto, Ontario
Canada

MOSBY
ELSEVIER

3251 Riverport Lane
Maryland Heights, Missouri 63043

ISBN: 978-0-323-06807-9

Vice President and Publisher: Linda Duncan
Executive Editor: John Dolan
Senior Developmental Editor: Courtney Sprehe
Publishing Services Manager: Julie Eddy
Project Manager: Marquita Parker
Designer: Jessica Williams

Printed in China

Last digit is the print number: 9   8   7   6   5   4   3   2

DEDICATION

To Dorion, my wife and life companion, who fully supported and encouraged my move to academia and teaching.

To all my students, who made my chosen career in teaching fulfilling and rewarding.

Preface

The third edition of *The Anatomical Basis of Dentistry* continues to fulfill the need for a textbook of gross anatomy specifically written for the dental profession. Yet another edition, however, begs the question, "How has the study of anatomy changed since the last version of the book?" Human gross anatomy has not changed greatly over the centuries, but the methods of describing, illustrating, and presenting the material have changed considerably and continue to change. In addition, the introduction of clinical relevance has transformed the study of anatomy from an insufferable mandatory first-year hurdle to a meaningful experience on which to build a successful career in the practice of dentistry.

Another question that is posed to virtually all students of dentistry is, "Why are dentists required to study the complete body and not just the head and neck?" The answer is that, as dental professionals, we are licensed to write prescriptions, take and interpret radiographs, administer anesthesia (local and general), and perform orofacial surgical procedures. Treatment, however, cannot be administered until an evaluation of the patient's health is undertaken through a medical history, which may reveal existing medical conditions that may modify or even preclude some procedures. Furthermore, despite medical histories and necessary precautions, complications can arise during routine treatment. Prevention and treatment of complications require sound background knowledge (of the form and function) of the human body that transcends a basic knowledge of the dental arches.

ORGANIZATION

As in previous editions, *The Anatomical Basis of Dentistry* features an introductory Chapter 1 that introduces the student to terminology and provides a general description of the body systems in preparation for the regional anatomy that follows. It is highly recommended that the student read this chapter initially and then reread it from time to time throughout the course. Chapters 2 through 5 deal with the regions of the trunk of the body (back, thorax, abdomen, and neck). Chapter 6 is devoted entirely to the study of the skull and the bones that comprise it as an introduction to a thorough study of the craniofacial complex. The head is presented in detail in Chapter 7 and then reviewed by systems in Chapter 8. Chapters 9 and 10 provide an overview of the upper and lower limbs to complete the study of the human body and to familiarize the student with sites of intravenous and intramuscular injections and surrounding anatomical structures that may compromise these procedures.

Clinical applications are featured throughout the book, and Chapter 11 remains devoted to applied or clinical anatomy, which is fundamental to the practice of dentistry. These sections have been updated to reflect advances that have developed in the past decade, such as treatments, imaging, and dental implants. No pretense is made to teach clinical dentistry, but rather the applied anatomy is presented to instill a keener interest in the anatomical structures involved and lay the foundations for upcoming clinical courses and eventual dental practice.

NEW TO THIS EDITION

The third edition maintains the principles and scope of previous editions but features several changes and improvements.

- Full-color anatomical artwork is now featured throughout the entire textbook.
- New artwork has been added to further complement the accompanying text.
- New information is introduced on the surface of the back, movements of spine, and back strain in Chapter 2; the movements of the head and neck and the muscles responsible in Chapter 5; and cone beam computed tomography (CBCT) and additional illustrations of the temporomandibular joint in Chapter 11.

- A companion Web site (*Evolve*) has been created to provide both student and instructor with materials such as:
  - PowerPoint teaching presentations, the complete image collection, and a 300 question test bank for instructors;
  - PowerPoint chapter reviews and a self-assessment exam for students; and
  - A PowerPoint presentation showing dissections of the head.

OBJECTIVE

Much thought has been given to the scope and amount of material presented in this book. It is the culmination of many years spent in the classroom, in the laboratory, and in the clinical practice of general dentistry. The book certainly is not intended to be an exhaustive, all-inclusive anatomical work replete with long lists of references; several excellent reference books are available for further study or clarification. Conversely, this book is not intended as a brief synopsis or a basic textbook of anatomy. It contains ample material to meet the requirements of a gross anatomy course for undergraduate dental students. At the same time, it is hoped that this book will maintain its usefulness and prove valuable throughout the undergraduate clinical years and eventually take its place on the desk of the practicing dentist and dental specialist.

Bernard Liebgott

Acknowledgments

I am extremely grateful to the following individuals who contributed to the third edition of this book:

Medical illustrators Raza Skudra, BScAAM, who created most of the original line drawings and artwork for the first edition that were subsequently digitized and colored for the second and third editions; David Mazierski, BScAAM; Brett Clayton, BSc, MScBMC; and Kevin Millar, BSc, MScBMC, who provided additional illustrations for the second and third editions.

Medical photographers Paul Schwartz, BA, and Bill Bolychuk, who provided the photographs used to illustrate the fine osseous details of the individual bones of the body, and Rita Bauer, who provided the intraoral photographs in Chapter 7.

Oral and maxillofacial surgeons Bohdan Kryshtalskyj, BSc, DDS, Dip Oral Surg, MRCD(C), FICD, who helped rewrite and provided clinical slides for the section dealing with the temporomandibular joint in Chapter 7; Simon Weinberg, DDS, Dip Oral Surg, DIP ABOMS, FRCD(C), FICD; Bruce R. Pynn, DDS, MSc, Dip Oral and Maxillofacial Surg; and Marco F. Caminiti, DDS, BSc, Dip Oral and Maxillofacial Surg, who rewrote and provided clinical slides for the section dealing with the spread of dental infections in Chapter 11.

Oral radiologists Sidney Fireman, DDS, Dip Oral Radiology, who generously provided the radiographs and CT scans for the section dealing with medical imaging in Chapter 11, and Michael Pharoah, DDS, BSc, MSc, FRDC(C), who provided the MRI scans for Chapter 11.

I am indebted to all those at Elsevier Inc. who have contributed toward this third edition. I am particularly grateful to John Dolan, Executive Editor, for his support and encouragement, and to Courtney Sprehe, Senior Developmental Editor, for her ongoing and greatly appreciated help in the planning, development, and design of *The Anatomical Basis of Dentistry*, third edition.

Contents

1 General Concepts

The Study of Anatomy 1
Terminology 2
Skeleton 4
Joints 8
Muscular System 12
Cardiovascular System 15
Nervous System 20
Body Coverings, Body Cavities, and Fascia.............31

2 The Back

Skeletal Parts 37
Surface Features of the Back 43
Spinal Cord...43
Muscles of the Back...47

3 The Thorax

Skeleton and Divisions 54
The Thoracic or Chest Wall..................................58
The Pleural Cavities and Lungs 63
The Mediastinum 68

4 The Abdomen, Pelvis, and Perineum

Skeleton and Subdivisions 87
The Abdominal Walls 89
Peritoneum and the Peritoneal Cavity 99
Blood and Nerve Supply to the Abdomen.............101
The Abdominal Viscera 104

5 The Neck

Skeleton and Surface Anatomy...........................133
Coverings and Regions 136
The Anterior Triangle 140
The Posterior Triangle 150
The Root..155
The Suboccipital Region...................................159
The Prevertebral Region....................................163

6 The Skull

Introduction 167
Views 167
Bones 184
Postnatal Development.....................................213

7 The Head by Regions

The Face and Scalp 221
The Contents of the Neurocranium 239
The Orbital Cavity 256
The Parotid Region 265
The Masticator Region......................................269
The Pterygopalatine Fossa 291
The Nasal Cavity and Paranasal Air Sinuses 297
The Oral Cavity...308
Structures and Areas of the Oral Cavity................314
The Pharynx 333
The Larynx 340
The Ear..349

8 Systemic Anatomy of the Head and Neck

Arteries 358
Veins...358
Lymphatics and Lymph Nodes 358
Cranial Nerves and Cranial Autonomics...............368

9 The Upper Limb

Skeleton...388
Joints, Movements, and Muscles.......................394
Muscles 401
Axilla 414
Nerve Supply: The Brachial Plexus 415
Arterial Supply 418
Venous Return 420
Lymphatic Drainage 422

10 The Lower Limb

Skeleton...425
Joints..429
Muscles 437
Nerve Supply: The Lumbar and Sacral Plexuses.....444
Arterial Supply 450
Venous Return 453
Lymphatics 454

11 Applied Anatomy

Anatomy of Local Anesthesia 457
Imaging 466
Fractures of the Face 473
Spread of Dental Infections............................480

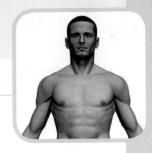

Chapter 1

General Concepts

1. The Study of Anatomy 1

2. Terminology 2

3. Skeleton 4

4. Joints 8

5. Muscular System 12

6. Cardiovascular System 15

7. Nervous System 20

8. Body Coverings, Body Cavities, and Fascia 31

1.   The Study of Anatomy

The word anatomy was coined from two Greek root words that mean "to cut up." This is precisely the way in which the early anatomists studied the structure of once living things—by dissecting animal or human remains, observing structures, and then speculating as to what function these structures might perform. The scope of anatomy has broadened considerably. Human anatomy is now the study of the structure of the human body through a variety of approaches, and these approaches have given rise to specialized subfields of human anatomy.

GROSS ANATOMY

Gross anatomy is concerned with the study of human form and structure as seen with the naked eye. When applicable, **applied** or **clinical anatomy** is introduced to illustrate the connection with everyday clinical problems in the health sciences. There are two classic approaches to the study of gross anatomy, both of which are used in this book.

A **systemic approach** is one in which the various systems of the body are studied as separate entities. This system of study is favored by college anatomy courses that do not include laboratory dissections.

A **regional approach** divides the body into a number of regions, which are then studied in turn. All the structures belonging to various systems are considered within the region being studied. This system of study follows the sequence of events encountered in a dissection and is favored in anatomy courses that include a dissecting laboratory component or a program that uses prosected specimens (specimens that were previously dissected).

This textbook largely follows a regional approach, because most dental school anatomy programs include a laboratory component. Bones, joints, muscles, blood vessels, nerves, fascia, and skin are found in every region of the body. For this reason a brief overview of the systems that give rise to these elements is presented in this chapter.

HISTOLOGY

Histology is the study of smaller details of structure as seen through a microscope. It is the study of human tissues and ranges from basic tissue and cell architecture, with use of light and confocal microscopes, to ultrastructural elements of tissues and cells, with use of the electron microscope. Biochemical techniques combined with histological techniques have given rise to applied disciplines of histochemistry and immunocytochemistry.

NEUROANATOMY

Neuroanatomy is the study of the central nervous system (CNS), meaning the brain and spinal cord, as viewed in gross dissection and histological preparations, as well as the study of pathways through immunocytochemical tracers.

DEVELOPMENTAL ANATOMY

Developmental anatomy is the study of age-related changes in size, complexity, shape, and ability to function. **Prenatal development** follows the development of the individual from the time of conception to birth. *Embryology* is particularly concerned with the first 2 months of life in utero, during which the organ systems are formed. **Postnatal development** traces the various changes in form and function after birth, and through infancy, childhood, adolescence, and adulthood.

SURFACE ANATOMY

Surface anatomy (living anatomy) deals with the surface or topography of the living person. Superficial structures can be readily located and deeper structures can be located and envisioned based on surface landmarks.

IMAGING ANATOMY

Imaging anatomy is the noninvasive study of living or dead subjects as revealed by conventional radiography, magnetic resonance imaging (MRI), and ultrasonography.

The use of serialized radiographs taken at ever-increasing depths through the body (computed tomography [CT]) and MRI has rekindled interest in sectional anatomy (i.e., the study of structures as they appear on the surface of cross-sectional or longitudinal sections through a cadaver).

2. Terminology

The basis for all communication in human gross anatomy and related basic and clinical sciences is standardized and universally accepted. A precise terminology enables us to name structures to distinguish them from all other structures and to relate the position of these named structures to the rest of the body so they can be located with consistency and precision.

THE ANATOMICAL POSITION

In the dissecting laboratory, we assume, by convention, that our subject is standing in the anatomical position (*Figure 1-1*): that is, standing erect with (1) the toes pointed forward, (2) the eyes directed to the horizon,

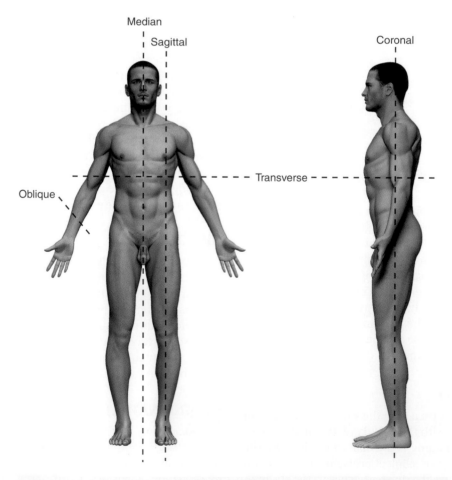

Figure 1-1 Anatomical position and planes of section.

(3) the arms by the sides, and (4) the palms of the hands facing forward.

From this basic position, we can divide the subject according to four different planes and introduce terminology that relates to these planes.

ANATOMICAL CUTS AND PLANES

There are two basic ways to visualize deep structures of the human body. One is to dissect down to the area of interest; the other is to cut through the cadaver in defined planes (see *Figure 1-1*). Sections also can be obtained from a living patient with CT or MRI.

1. A cut through the **median plane** divides the body into equal right and left halves.
2. A **sagittal plane** is any one of an infinite number of planes parallel to the midsagittal plane that divide the body into unequal right and left parts.
3. The **coronal plane** is any one of an infinite number of planes that are at right angles to the midsagittal plane.

A coronal cut will divide the body into anterior and posterior parts.

4. The **transverse,** or **horizontal, plane** is a plane that cuts across the body at right angles to the coronal and median planes, dividing the body into superior and inferior parts.
5. An **oblique plane** is, by default, any plane that deviates from the four aforementioned planes.
6. A **cross section** is any one of an infinite number of possible cuts across the body or one of its limbs at right angles to its long axis.
7. A **longitudinal section** is any one of an infinite number of possible cuts that parallel the long axis of the body or its components.

TERMS OF RELATIONSHIP

The following terms are presented in pairs because each term has an opposite (*Figure 1-2*). Again, the assumption is that our subject is in the anatomical position.

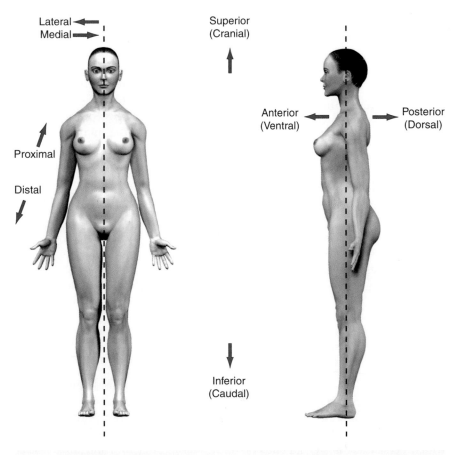

Figure 1-2 Terms of relationship.

3

Term	Definition
Anterior (ventral)	Toward the front of the body
Posterior (dorsal)	Toward the back of the body
Superior (cranial)	Toward the top of the head
Inferior (caudal)	Toward the soles of the feet
Medial	Toward the median plane
Lateral	Away from the median plane
Proximal (central)	Toward the trunk
Distal (peripheral)	Away from the trunk
Superficial	Toward the skin or body surface
Deep	Toward the interior of the body
Ipsilateral (homolateral)	On the same side
Contralateral	On the opposite side
Palmar surface of hand	Anterior surface of hand
Dorsal surface of hand	Posterior surface of hand
Plantar surface of foot	Inferior surface of foot
Dorsal surface of foot	Superior surface of foot

3. Skeleton

CARTILAGE

Cartilage is a specialized supporting connective tissue. It consists of cells (**chondroblasts,** which give rise to **chondrocytes**) contained within a ground substance in the form of a rigid gel. There are no neurovascular elements within cartilage; instead, nutrients diffuse through the ground substance to the enclosed chondrocytes. No calcium salts are present; therefore cartilage does not appear on radiographs.

During early development, most of the fetal skeleton is present as cartilage, and most of this cartilage is subsequently replaced by bone during fetal and postnatal development.

Types

Hyaline (from the Greek word *hyalos*, meaning "glass") **cartilage** is a bluish-white, translucent structure. Nearly all of the fetal skeleton is hyaline cartilage. In the adult, its remnants are:

1. Articular cartilage, which is smooth and slippery and persists at the ends of cartilaginous bones to line articular surfaces of movable joints
2. Costal cartilages, which persist at the sternal ends of the ribs

3. Respiratory cartilages, consisting of the movable external nose and septum, larynx, trachea, and bronchial tree
4. Auditory cartilages, which include the external auditory meatus and the cartilaginous portion of the auditory (pharyngotympanic) tube

Elastic cartilage is pliable and yellowish in color because of the presence of elastin fibers. It is found in the external ear and in the epiglottis.

Fibrocartilage contains proportionately more collagen fibers, which are arranged in a parallel fashion for high tensile strength. It is found in tendon insertions and intervertebral discs (not including the pulpal nucleus).

Growth

Although cartilage is a rigid tissue, its unique structure allows it to grow as most soft tissues do. Cartilage can increase in size in two ways: (1) by *internal growth,* in which young chondrocytes proliferate within the cartilage, and (2) by *appositional growth,* in which a surface perichondrium consisting of a fibrous outer layer and a chondroblastic inner layer lay down surface cartilage.

BONE

Bone, like cartilage, is a living tissue consisting of cells or osteoblasts, which give rise to osteocytes within an organic framework or matrix.

Bone is unlike cartilage in that the intercellular matrix becomes calcified for greater rigidity and strength. Calcification, however, prevents diffusion of nutrients, and each cell within the matrix must therefore have a direct vascular supply.

Because of its rigid structure, interstitial growth is not possible. Appositional growth takes place only below the covering periosteal layer of bone. Periosteum consists of a fibrous outer layer and a cellular inner layer of osteoblasts, which form the bony matrix.

Functions

Bone has the following functions:

1. Support. Bones provide a rigid framework for the body.
2. Movement. Bones act as levers for muscles. Muscle usually attaches to approximating bones, and these attachments are able to move one bone in relation to another.
3. Protection. The brain and the thoracic viscera are protected by bone.
4. Hemopoiesis. The principal blood cells are formed in the marrow space of bone.
5. Storage. Calcium and phosphorus are stored in bone as body reserves.

Classification

By Region. The adult skeleton is divided into an axial and an appendicular skeleton. The **axial skeleton** comprises the skull, the vertebral or spinal column, the ribs, and the sternum. The **appendicular skeleton** includes the bones of the upper and lower limbs. The individual bones and their numbers are illustrated in *Figure 1-3*.

By Shape. **Long bones** are hollow tubes, shafts, or *diaphyses* that are capped at both ends by knoblike epiphyses. A section through a long bone (*Figure 1-4*) reveals (1) an outer compact layer for rigidity, (2) an inner cancellous or spongy layer consisting of trabeculated bone for inner support, and (3) a marrow space containing blood cell–forming tissues in active red marrow or just plain fat in inactive yellow marrow.

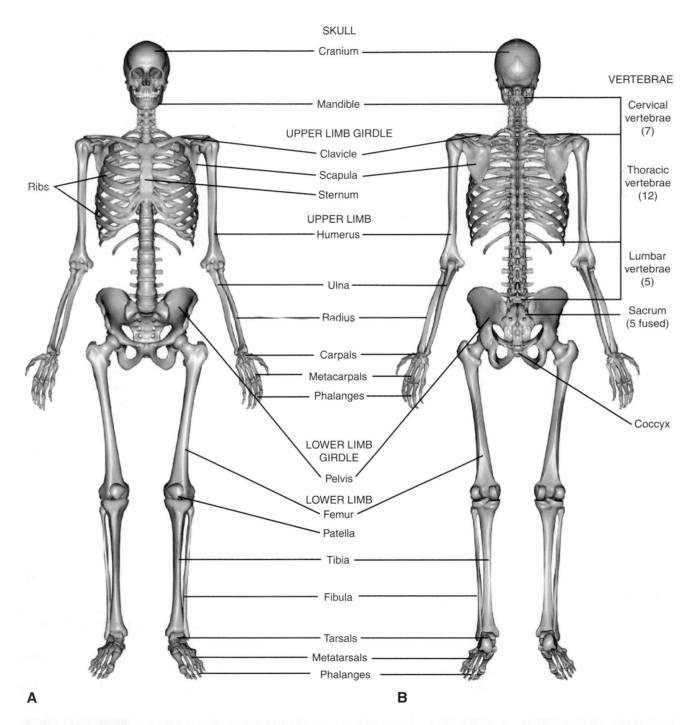

Figure 1-3 Skeleton. **A**, Anterior. **B**, Posterior.

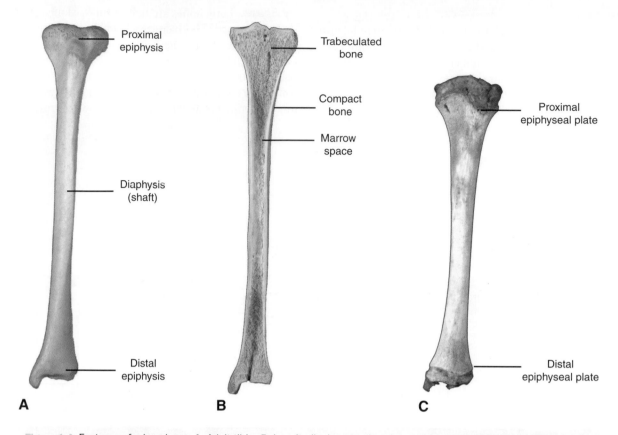

Figure 1-4 Features of a long bone. **A,** Adult tibia. **B,** Longitudinal cut to show internal features. **C,** Tibia of a child.

The blood supply to long bones (*Figure 1-5*) is from the following three different sources: (1) nutrient arteries pierce the shaft and supply all layers to the marrow cavity within, (2) periosteal arteries supply periosteum and some adjacent compact bone, and (3) epiphyseal arteries supply the epiphyses and the adjacent joint structures.

Short bones are similar to long bones, except they are cuboidal rather than tubular in shape and lack the shaft of long bones. They are usually six-sided, with cartilage covering the articular surfaces. Short bones consist of the same layered structures as long bones but have no epiphyses. The carpal bones of the wrist and the tarsal bones of the ankle are short bones.

Flat bones are thin and flat and are found in the vault of the skull and the scapula. They consist of a sandwich: two layers of compact bone encasing a cancellous layer called the *diploë.* The diploic layer contains red bone marrow.

Irregular bones are bones that fit none of the previous descriptions. Some irregular bones are mainly cancellous bone covered with only thin layers of compact bone. Others, such as the lacrimal bone (a small delicate bone of the orbit), consist only of a single compact layer. Still others, such as the maxilla (upper jaw), are invaded and hollowed by nasal mucosa during development, resulting in pneumatic bones. Pneumatic bones consist of thin compact bone surrounding an air-filled cavity or sinus.

Sesamoid bones (from the Greek word *sesamon,* meaning "like a seed") are not actually part of the skeleton. They occur rather in some tendons of the hands, feet, and knee where the tendon rubs against bone. The patella (knee cap) is a smooth, rounded, sesamoid bone found within the tendon of the quadriceps femoris muscle. Articular cartilage covers the areas in contact with bone.

Surface Features

The surface of individual bones is marked by several features that reflect (1) attachments of muscles and ligaments, producing raised areas; (2) passage of nerves and vessels through or over the bone, producing openings and depressions; and (3) articulations with other bones, producing joint surfaces that are raised or depressed. Some terms are self-descriptive, but most are not intuitive without a background in Latin and Greek.

Following is a list of bony features that will be encountered in the study of bones as they are presented throughout the book.

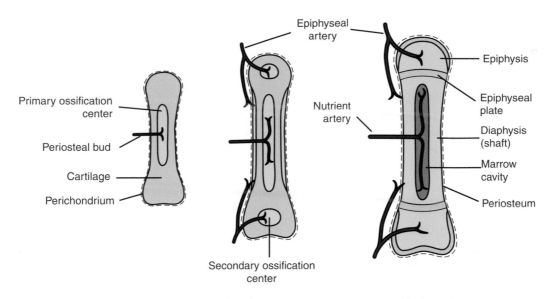

Figure 1-5 Three stages in development of a long bone.

Raised Markings or Elevations

Condyle. (From the Greek, meaning "knuckle") The rounded or widened end of a bone with a smooth articular surface covered by cartilage (e.g., medial and lateral condyles of the femur and the condyles of the mandible)

Epicondyle. A ridge of bone immediately above the condyle that provides muscle attachment (e.g., the medial and lateral epicondyles of the humerus)

Process. A projection of bone for the attachment of muscles (e.g., the spinous and transverse processes of vertebrae and the coronoid process of the mandible)

Plate. A flattened process that provides muscular attachment (e.g., the lateral pterygoid plate of the sphenoid bone of the skull)

Tubercle. A small rounded elevation on a bone for muscle attachment (e.g., the adductor tubercle of the femur and the pharyngeal tubercle at the base of the skull)

Tuberosity. A rounded prominence of bone (e.g., the ischial tuberosities of the os coxae on which we sit and the maxillary tuberosity forming the rounded posterior wall of the maxilla)

Trochanter. Large bony traction processes found only on the superior end of the femur (e.g., the greater and lesser trochanter of the femur, which provide attachment for large, powerful muscles of the lower limb)

Malleolus. Two bony prominences found only on bones of the leg that serve to bind the lower leg to the ankle below (e.g., the medial malleolus on the inferior end of the tibia and the lateral malleolus on the inferior end of the fibula)

Crest. An elongated raised process or ridge of bone produced by muscle attachment (e.g., the iliac crest of the os coxae and the infratemporal crest at the base of the skull)

Linea, or Line. A slightly raised ridge of bone produced by muscle attachment (e.g., the linea aspera of the femur and the superior nuchal line of the skull)

Spine. Yet another raised area of bone (e.g., the spine of the scapula, which is an elongated extension providing attachment for muscles, and the spine of the sphenoid bone in the skull, which provides attachment for a ligament)

Depressions and Openings

Fossa. A gently rounded depression that in some cases provides space for the muscles (e.g., supraspinous and infraspinous fossae of the scapula) and in other cases denotes the smooth concave area for joint surfaces (e.g., the glenoid fossa of the scapula and the mandibular fossa of the skull)

Groove, or Sulcus. Linear bony depressions that accommodate cylindrical or tubular structures (e.g., the bicipital or intertubercular groove of the humerus accommodates a tendon of the biceps muscle, and the superior sagittal sulcus accommodates the superior sagittal venous sinus within the skull)

Foramen. A hole that allows structures (usually nerves and vessels) to pass through the bone (e.g., the foramen ovale [round hole] and the foramen magnum [large hole] in the skull)

Canal. An opening that has length through bone; when a canal emerges onto the surface of the bone, that surface opening is sometimes referred to as a *foramen* (e.g., the infraorbital canal exits onto the face as the infraorbital foramen)

Notch. A "bite" from the edge of the bone that transmits vessels and nerves, like an incomplete foramen (e.g., the suprascapular notch of the scapula and the mandibular notch of the mandible)

Fissure. An elongated space between two bones of the skull (e.g., the superior and inferior orbital fissures)

Development

Bone develops from embryonic mesenchyme by one of two mechanisms—intramembranous ossification or endochondral ossification. Once bone is formed, however, there is no difference in appearance or properties between intramembranous and endochondral bone. The former replaces membrane; the latter replaces cartilage.

Intramembranous Ossification. During embryonic skeletal development, mesenchymal cells condense as a membrane in the area of the future bone. Osteoblasts differentiate from the mesenchymal cells and lay down a bone matrix at multiple sites that gradually coalesce to form a single bone. Bones of the skull vault and face develop in this fashion and are separated by fibrous sutures that are remnants of the bone precursor membrane. The clavicle develops in this fashion.

Endochondral Ossification. The remainder of the skeleton undergoes a slightly more complicated process of endochondral ossification (see *Figure 1-5*). Each of these bones is preformed in cartilage during early embryonic development. During the sixth to eighth weeks of embryonic development, cartilage within the center of the future bone shaft dies and is replaced by invading osteoblasts that form the **primary center of ossification.** The perichondrium surrounding the shaft becomes periosteum and it lays down an intramembranous collar of bone around the primary center. All the primary centers develop before birth. Invading vascular tissue hollows the shaft to form the medullary cavity that contains red bone marrow.

At birth, **secondary centers of ossification** develop in the epiphyses, or ends, of the long bones and increase in size until they ultimately fuse with the primary centers to form a complete bone. Up until maturation after puberty, a plate of remaining cartilage, the **epiphyseal plate,** separates the epiphyses from the shaft. Short bones do not have a shaft and develop in the same manner as secondary centers of ossification.

Postnatal Growth. The cartilage of the epiphyseal plate continues to proliferate at these sites and contributes to the increase in length of the entire bone. The shape of the bone is maintained by selective apposition and resorption (**bone remodeling**). During adolescence, two competing phenomena occur. The growth rate of long bones accelerates, and at the same time, hormonal changes cause gradual ossification of the epiphyseal plates (**synostosis**). Thus complete ossification of long bones results in

cessation of growth in the adult. Cartilage remains at both ends, covering the epiphyses as articular cartilage.

Mineralized bone appears on radiographs, but cartilage does not. Secondary centers and short bones begin to ossify and mineralize after birth in a more or less predictable sequence as the child grows. Knowing when these various centers ossify enables us to determine **bone** or **skeletal ages** of children.

4. Joints

A joint is an articulation or union between two or more bones. Joints may be classified according to the degree of possible movement and by the tissues that bind the bones together.

BY DEGREE OF MOVEMENT

Synarthrodial joints allow no movement between the bones they unite. A good example is the flat bones of the skull, which are bound together as a rigid entity. **Amphiarthrodial joints** are partially movable, and **diarthrodial joints** are freely movable.

BY JOINT TISSUES

Joints between bones may be composed of fibrous connective tissue, cartilage, a combination of connective tissue and cartilage, or cartilage and a joint cavity.

Fibrous Joints

There are three types of fibrous joints: (1) suture, (2) syndesmosis, and (3) gomphosis.

Sutures are found only between the bones of the skull (*Figure 1-6*). In the fetal skull the sutures are wide, and the bones present smooth opposing surfaces. This spacing between the flat bones of the skull allows a slight degree of movement between the skull bones during passage of the head through the birth canal (birth molding).

After birth, the sutures become quite rigid (synarthrodial) during infancy and early childhood, allowing no movement between skull bones. The developing sutures

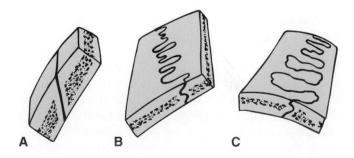

Figure 1-6 Sutures. **A,** Squamous. **B,** Serrated. **C,** Denticulate.

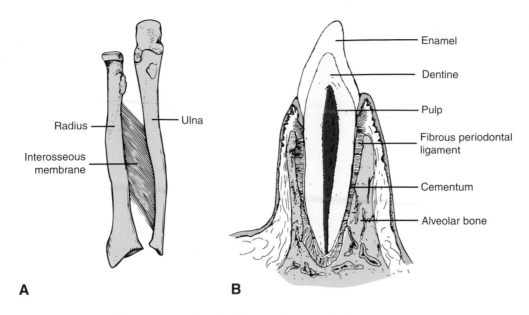

Figure 1-7 Other examples of fibrous joints. **A**, Syndesmosis. **B**, Gomphosis.

differentiate into one of three types (see *Figure 1-6*): (1) a *squamous suture* in which the bones simply overlap obliquely but are rendered immobile by intervening fibrous tissue; (2) a *serrated suture*, which develops sawtoothed interdigitating projections from the opposing bones; and (3) a *denticulate suture*, which features interlocking dovetailed surfaces.

A **syndesmosis**, unlike other fibrous joints, is partially movable (amphiarthrodial) and is a joint in which the two bony components are farther apart, united by a fibrous interosseous membrane (*Figure 1-7, A*). Examples are the joint between the two bones of the forearm (radius and ulna) and the joint between the bones of the leg (fibula and tibia). Syndesmoses also are found between the laminae of the vertebrae.

A **gomphosis** is a unique joint in the form of a peg-and-socket articulation between the roots of the teeth and the maxillary and mandibular aleveolar processes (*Figure 1-7, B*). Fibrous tissue organized as the periodontal ligament anchors the tooth securely in the socket. Mobility of this joint indicates a pathological state affecting the supporting structures of the tooth.

Primary Cartilaginous Joints (Synchondroses)

Primary cartilaginous joints develop between two bones of **endochondral** origin. They are characterized by a solid plate of hyaline cartilage between apposing surfaces (*Figure 1-8, A*). The cartilage plate functions in exactly the same manner as the epiphyseal plate between primary and secondary centers of long bones and provides an area of

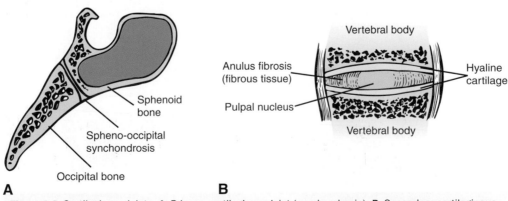

Figure 1-8 Cartilaginous joints. **A**, Primary cartilaginous joint (synchondrosis). **B**, Secondary cartilaginous joint (symphysis).

growth between bones. An example is the sphenooccipital synchondrosis in the young skull between the sphenoid bone and the occipital bone of the skull. This joint fuses after adolescence.

Secondary Cartilaginous Joints (Symphyses)

A secondary cartilaginous joint, or **symphysis,** is a partially movable (amphiarthrodial) joint in which the apposing bony surfaces are covered with cartilage but separated by intervening fibrous tissue or fibrocartilage (*Figure 1-8, B*). Symphyses are found in the midline of the body and include the joints between vertebral bodies (intervertebral discs), between right and left pubic bones (symphysis pubis), and in the newborn skull between the right and left halves of the mandible (symphysis menti). The symphysis menti starts to fuse during the first year of life to form a single bone, the mandible.

SYNOVIAL JOINTS

A synovial joint is freely movable (diarthrodial) and is typical of nearly all the joints of the upper and lower limbs. Synovial joints have a number of characteristic features (*Figure 1-9, A*).

Articular cartilage coats the surfaces of the apposing bones. The cartilage may be hyaline (where bones of endochondral origin articulate) or may be *fibrocartilage* (where bones of intramembranous origin articulate). Typical of cartilage, this layer contains no blood vessels or nerves but must instead be nourished from the epiphyseal vessels of the bone and derives nourishment from the synovial lubricating fluid within the joint. A joint cavity exists between the articular surfaces of the apposing bones. The **joint cavity** is not large but contains enough space to allow a thin intervening film of synovial fluid. A **capsular ligament** surrounds the joint like a fibrous sleeve and attaches to the circumference of both bones to completely enclose the joint cavity.

A synovial membrane consisting of loose areolar tissue contains a rich supply of capillaries. This membrane lines the inner aspect of the capsular ligament but does not line the articular surfaces of the cartilage. The **synovial membrane** secretes a lubricating synovial fluid, or synovium, into the joint cavity. Some joints contain **discs** interposed between the articular surfaces (*Figure 1-9, B*). A disc or meniscus is a fibrocartilaginous or sometimes condensed fibrous structure found within some joint cavities. These padlike structures divide the joint cavity into two compartments allowing for two types of movements, one for each subdivided joint compartment. The temporomandibular, or jaw, joint is an example of a synovial joint containing a disc.

Blood and Nerve Supply

Epiphyseal arteries that supply the epiphyses of long bones also supply the synovial joints between the long bones. Hilton's law states that the nerves that supply the muscles that move a synovial joint send sensory branches to supply the joint. There are two types of sensory nerve endings that convey two kinds of messages to the CNS. **Proprioceptive endings,** or *Ruffini corpuscles*, in the capsular ligament convey a sense of position and degree of movement of a joint. **Pain receptors** in the synovial membrane indicate whether the allowable degree of movement is being overtaxed.

Classification

Freely movable synovial joints may be classified in different ways (*Figure 1-10*). One classification is based on the number of axes in which a joint can be moved (i.e., uniaxial, biaxial, or multiaxial). The shape or form of the opposing bony surfaces determines the degree of movement.

Multiaxial Joints. Multiaxial joints provide the greatest degree of movement in three planes. There are two types of multiaxial joints.

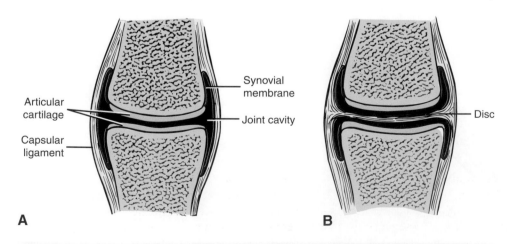

Figure 1-9 Synovial joint. **A,** Typical. **B,** With articular disc.

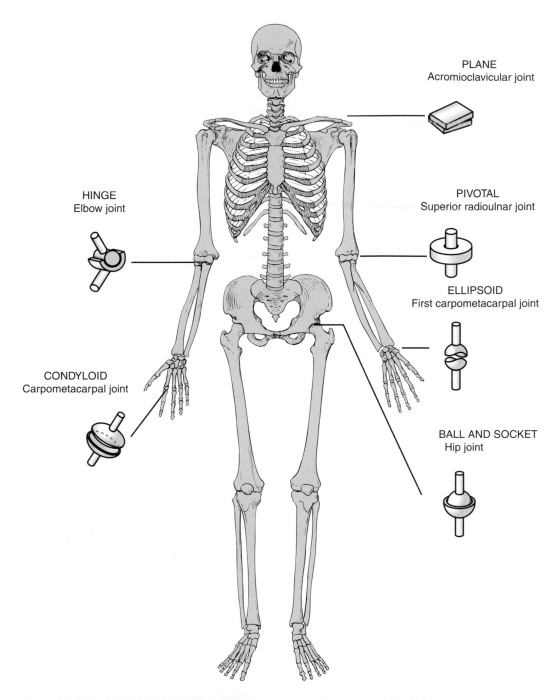

PLANE
Acromioclavicular joint

PIVOTAL
Superior radioulnar joint

HINGE
Elbow joint

ELLIPSOID
First carpometacarpal joint

CONDYLOID
Carpometacarpal joint

BALL AND SOCKET
Hip joint

Figure 1-10 Classification of synovial joints.

Ball-and-Socket Joint. One apposing bony surface is ball-shaped, and the other is a reciprocal socket allowing movement in all planes (multiaxial). An example is the freely moveable shoulder joint.

Saddle or Ellipsoid Joint. The apposing bony surfaces are reciprocally saddle-shaped, allowing a fair degree of movement in two planes and limited movement in the third plane. An example is the carpometacarpal joint of the thumb.

Biaxial Joints. A biaxial joint allows movement in two planes. The shape of the joint surfaces prevents rotation around a vertical axis (the third plane of movement). There is only one type of biaxial joint.

Condyloid Joint. One apposing bony surface is an ellipse; the other is an elliptical socket. Movements are in two planes at mutual right angles. Examples are the metacarpophalangeal joints of the fingers.

11

Uniaxial Joints. Uniaxial joints allow movements in one plane only. There are three types of uniaxial joints.

Plane Joint. The apposing surfaces of bone are almost flat and generally allow movement in one plane only. Examples are the intercarpal, intertarsal, and acromioclavicular joints.

Hinge (Ginglymus) Joint. One apposing bony surface is cylindrical, the other is reciprocally concave, and the joint allows movement in one plane. An example is the humeroulnar (elbow) joint that allows only flexion and extension.

Pivot Joint. One of the apposing bones is encircled at the joint end by a fibrous ring or cuff, enabling the bone within the cuff to rotate about the vertical axis. An example is the head of the radius rotating as the forearm is pronated and supinated (see Chapter 9).

5. Muscular System

Muscle is a specialized tissue that has the ability to contract and produce movement. The three kinds of muscle tissue within the body differ from each other in their histological appearances and in their ability to be controlled voluntarily. These tissues are (1) *skeletal muscle*, (2) *smooth muscle*, and (3) *cardiac muscle*.

SKELETAL MUSCLE

Skeletal muscle is so named because of its attachment to bones. Because muscles span joints, they have the ability to move one bone in relation to another; for example, the brachialis muscle flexes the elbow or the masseter muscle elevates the mandible. Contraction of all skeletal muscle is under voluntary control. Though operation of some skeletal muscles is "automatic," such as that of the muscles of respiration, which continue to work during sleep, we can still voluntarily override them, such as in holding one's breath. Skeletal muscle is also known as *striated muscle* because it appears striped in histological sections.

Nomenclature

The names of muscles are generally descriptive and give us either an indication of (1) shape (e.g., trapezius muscle), (2) number of origins (e.g., triceps, biceps), (3) location (e.g., temporalis), (4) number of bellies (e.g., digastric), (5) function (e.g., levator veli palatini), or (6) origin and insertion (e.g., thyrohyoid).

Parts

Skeletal muscle consists of a fleshy portion and a fibrous or tendinous portion.

Fleshy Portion. Muscle fibers are the basic functional and anatomical units of muscle. Fibers are actually elongated muscle cells, ranging in length from several millimeters to several centimeters and contain several nuclei, specialized protoplasm or *sarcoplasm*, and myofibrils within the sarcoplasm. The cell membrane, or *sarcolemma*, encases the cell.

The cells derive their individual blood and nerve supply via sheets of fibrous connective tissue membranes through which the vessels and nerves run. Surrounding the individual muscle cells is a fibrous sheet of *endomysium*. Surrounding a bundle of several fibers (fasciculus) is a fibrous sheet of *perimysium*. Finally, surrounding several bundles, there is an overall fibrous coating of *epimysium* covering the entire muscle. Each of the three levels of surrounding membranes is interconnected, allowing vessels and nerves entering the outer layer eventually to reach individual fibers (*Figure 1-11*).

Groups of muscles in the limbs can be bound into compartments by intermuscular septa, which separate various groups of muscles. An example is the anterior compartment of the arm containing flexor muscles and the posterior compartment of the arm containing extensor muscles (see Chapter 9).

Fibrous or Tendinous Portion. Most sites of muscular attachment are to bone. The muscle fibers do not attach directly but rather through specialized extensions of the fibrous tissue coverings in the form of tendons. The tendons may take various forms.

Cylindrical Tendons. The fibers composing the tendon may be closely packed together in a cylindrical form, and their attachments to bone usually produce an elevation, or tubercle.

Linear Tendons. Some muscles exhibit broad, fleshy attachments, such as the origin of the temporalis muscle. The attachment to bone generally produces a linear ridge.

Aponeurosis. This is a flattened, broad tendon that takes the form of a fibrous membranous sheet.

Common Tendons. Occasionally a tendon may serve as a common attachment for two muscles. This type of tendon may take three forms. First, an *intermediate tendon* is a cylindrical type of tendon that is common to two

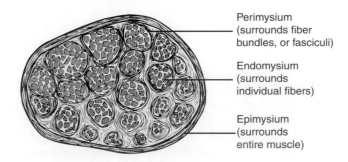

Perimysium (surrounds fiber bundles, or fasciculi)

Endomysium (surrounds individual fibers)

Epimysium (surrounds entire muscle)

Figure 1-11 Cross section of skeletal muscle.

fleshy bellies (e.g., the anterior and posterior bellies of the digastric muscles are united by an intermediate tendon). Second, a raphé occurs when two flat muscles share a common attachment. The fleshy fibers interdigitate and are separated by only a thin fibrous band or *raphé*. A raphé exists between the buccinator muscle and the superior constrictor muscle. The third form is an *aponeurosis*. Often an aponeurosis can serve as a common attachment for two muscles, such as the aponeurosis between the occipitalis and frontalis muscles.

Origins and Insertions

Traditionally the proximal end of a muscle is called the *origin* and the distal end is the *insertion*. In movements to or from the anatomical position, the insertion moves toward the stationary origin as the muscle contracts. Not all movements are made from the anatomical position, and technically origins and insertions can be interchanged because muscle movements can occur at either attachment, depending on which end is fixed and which end is movable. An example is flexing the forearm toward the fixed body in the anatomical position and flexing the body toward the forearm at the elbow while doing a chin-up on an overhead bar. Some texts get around this quandary by describing proximal and distal attachments of limb muscles, but this type of designation does not work well in describing attachments of head and neck muscles. The best advice is to think in terms of the most common movement of the muscle in question and consider the fixed end as the origin and the movable end as the insertion. For example, the muscles of mastication of the skull originate from the fixed skull and their insertions are into the movable lower jaw or mandible.

Architecture

Muscles can be classified according to the *arrangement* of the muscle fiber bundles, or fasciculi.

Parallel and Converging Fibers. Some muscles contain fiber bundles arranged in a parallel fashion along the long axis of the muscle. This arrangement gives the muscle a *great range of movement*, and such a muscle is capable of contracting from about one third to one half of its original length. Examples of this type are *rectangular* or *strap muscles* (*Figure 1-12, A*). Some fibers that have a linear origin and converge to a narrow insertion are triangular or fan-shaped muscles (*Figure 1-12, C*). In other muscles, fibers converge at both origin and insertion, with a wider intervening fleshy belly. These are fusiform muscles (*Figure 1-12, B*). In each case, however, the muscle bundles, or fasciculi, run uninterrupted from origin to insertion.

Pennate Muscles. This type of muscle is built for power rather than range of movement. The name means feather-like, and in this arrangement a central tendon extends well into the fleshy belly. Attaching to the tendon are obliquely arranged muscle bundles in a unipennate, bipennate, or multipennate form (*Figure 1-12, D*).

Sphincter Muscles. These circular muscles encircle openings, such as the eye and mouth (*Figure 1-12, E*). The muscle fibers are arranged in concentric fashion around the opening they encircle and can contract to close the opening.

Actions

Types of Contraction. Skeletal muscle can undergo two types of contraction: isotonic and isometric. **Isotonic contractions** of skeletal muscles produce actual movements around a joint. **Isometric contractions** of skeletal muscles contract or tense the muscles but produce no movements. Examples are tensing the abdominal muscles or tensing the muscles of mastication by clenching the teeth. Even at rest, muscles are in a midrange state of contraction, exhibiting tension and a resistance to passive stretching.

Actions of Muscle Groups. For each of the possible movements contracting muscles can produce, groups of muscles have specific roles.

Prime movers are muscles that are called upon by the brain via the pyramidal tract to initiate a particular movement. **Antagonists** are muscles that can produce movement in the opposite direction of the prime movers. The roles of antagonists and prime movers are interchanged. For example, the brachialis is a prime mover in flexing (bending) the elbow and contracts as the triceps brachii muscle of the arm relaxes. To extend (straighten) the elbow, the triceps (now the prime mover) contracts as the brachialis (now the antagonist) relaxes. **Synergists** are groups of muscles that are controlled by the extrapyramidal system of the CNS. This system controls and refines any undesirable movements after the prime movers have initiated a particular movement so that the desired movement takes place in a smooth, coordinated fashion. **Fixators** are muscles that play no direct part in the actual movement. Rather they "fix" the body (through isometric contractions) in the most advantageous position for that particular movement. Other muscles, responding to gravity's pull, maintain posture. Once a prime mover is called into play by the motor area of the cerebral cortex, a secondary complex coordination and fine adjustment of this movement is performed by synergists and fixators.

Synovial Bursae and Sheaths

A **bursa** is a sac of synovial membrane that separates a moving tendon from underlying bone or muscle or overlying skin to reduce friction. **Synovial sheaths** (*Figure 1-13*) are like elongated bursae or tunnels of synovial membrane, which surround and lubricate the long tendons of the hand and foot.

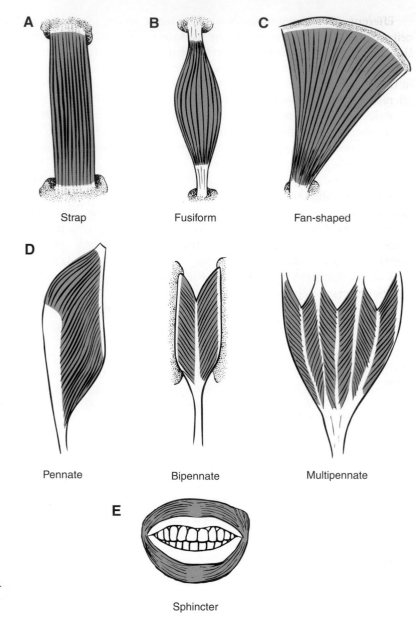

A Strap

B Fusiform

C Fan-shaped

D Pennate

Bipennate

Multipennate

E Sphincter

Figure 1-12 Classification of skeletal muscle by fiber arrangement.

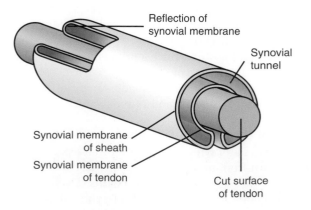

Reflection of synovial membrane

Synovial tunnel

Synovial membrane of sheath

Synovial membrane of tendon

Cut surface of tendon

Figure 1-13 Synovial sheath.

Blood and Nerve Supply

Vessels and nerves enter muscles as a neurovascular bundle and are conducted through the three fibrous tissue layers (see *Figure 1-11*) to eventually reach each muscle cell. The arterial supply forms an internal anastomosing (interconnected) network. The draining veins have valves, and venous return depends on the massaging effect of the muscle as it contracts and relaxes.

Although muscles are said to be supplied by motor nerves, the nerves actually contain mixed fibers. Approximately three fifths of a so-called motor nerve is composed of *motor* (*efferent*) fibers, and two fifths is composed of *sensory* (*afferent*) fibers.

Efferent fibers eventually reach individual muscle cells, and the nerve fibers terminate as branches beneath the sarcolemma or cell membrane as motor end plates. Acetylcholine, released by the nerve endings, plays a role in the contraction of the muscle fibers, and therefore the efferent nerve supply to voluntary muscle is cholinergic.

Afferent fibers originate as specialized receptors on the muscle cell itself, on the fibrous connective tissue sheath, from muscle spindles within the muscles, and from tendon spindles located at the junction of muscle and tendon. These endings carry *proprioceptive* information back to the CNS. This information, along with proprioceptive information from joints, gives us an awareness of the position of various parts of our body in space. For example, we know when the mandible is in the wide-open position without having to look in a mirror.

SMOOTH MUSCLE

Whereas skeletal muscle generally spans joints to produce movements around a joint, smooth muscle helps form the *walls* of *hollow viscera* and *tubes*. On contraction, smooth muscles expel contents of hollow structures or narrow the lumen of tubes, such as blood vessels. Smooth muscle contraction is under the control of the involuntary visceral (*autonomic*) *nervous system*.

Smooth muscle is so named because it lacks the striations of skeletal muscle in histological preparations. Smooth muscle cells are long, tapered cells that overlap neighboring cells. Cells are bound to each other by delicate connective tissue that transmits the neurovascular supply to individual cells. The cells are arranged in sheets around tubes (e.g., the blood vessels, ureters, gut) or hollow organs (e.g., the gallbladder, urinary bladder, uterus). A **circular** arrangement of fibers *decreases lumen size* on contraction. **Longitudinally** arranged fibers cause a *shortening* in *tubal length*.

CARDIAC MUSCLE

Cardiac muscle is similar in function to smooth muscle. Its rate of contraction is involuntarily controlled by the visceral (autonomic) nervous system and is found only in the heart, where it functions to expel blood from the various heart chambers. Histological sections of cardiac muscle, unlike those of smooth muscle, appear striated because of the presence of intercalated discs.

VOLUNTARY VERSUS INVOLUNTARY MUSCLE (EXCEPTIONS)

There is, unfortunately, no sharp distinction between voluntary and involuntary muscle control. Some skeletal muscle, such as the upper end of the esophagus, is involuntarily controlled and some smooth muscle, such as that in the urinary bladder, is under voluntary control. There is a definite distinction, however, in the type of contraction produced by both types of muscle. Skeletal muscle is capable of *rapid, powerful contractions* but becomes fatigued relatively quickly. Smooth muscle and cardiac muscle, on the other hand, are capable of *slow, sustained contractions* with no fatigue.

6. Cardiovascular System

The cardiovascular system consists of a quantity of fluid, a pump, and a series of tubes that contains the fluid (*Figure 1-14*). *Blood* carries respiratory gases and metabolites to and from the tissues. The heart pumps the blood through an enclosed system. *Blood vessels* transport the blood to capillaries where gases, metabolites, and fluid are exchanged at the tissue level. The *lymphatic system* conveys excess tissue fluid back to the circulation.

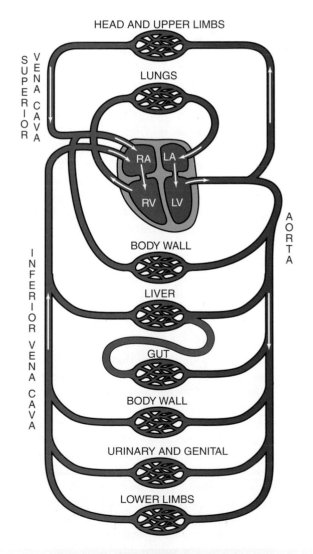

Figure 1-14 Scheme of cardiovascular system.

BLOOD

Approximately 5.5 L in volume, blood is composed of liquid (plasma) and cells. **Plasma** is primarily water (91%); the remainder consists of salts, metabolites, respiratory gases, proteins, and enzymes. The **cells** are *erythrocytes* (red blood cells), which transport respiratory gases, and *leukocytes* (white blood cells), which leave the blood vascular system to act as phagocytes or scavengers of debris. Some leukocytes (lymphocytes) take part in the body's immune mechanism. Bits of cytoplasm (*blood platelets*) are found along with the cells and take part in the blood clotting mechanism.

THE HEART

The heart is described only generally at this time. It is described in detail in Chapter 3. The heart is a four-chambered, muscular pump and can be divided into two sides based on function. The right side pumps blood through the lungs for oxygenation, constituting the *pulmonary*, or *lesser*, *circuit*. The left side pumps the oxygenated blood to the body tissues and constitutes the *systemic*, or *greater*, *circuit* (see *Figure 1-14*). Clinicians generally refer to the *right heart* (pulmonary) and the *left heart* (systemic).

The heart consists of two receiving chambers (**atria**) and two pumping chambers (**ventricles**). Each chamber holds roughly 60 to 70 mL of blood. Connecting each atrium to its respective ventricle is an **atrioventricular orifice**, which is guarded by **atrioventricular valves** to prevent the backflow of blood from ventricle to atrium.

The thickness of the chamber walls is a reflection of their functions. The atria are thin walled because they need only empty their contents into the ventricle below. The ventricles are thick-walled, with the left ventricle considerably thicker than the right, because high pressures are required to pump blood through the pulmonary circuit and still higher pressures are required to pump blood through the systemic circuit.

BLOOD VESSELS

Blood vessels are hollow tubes that conduct blood either *away from the heart* (arteries) or *to the heart* (veins). These definitions of *artery* and *vein* hold true for both systemic and pulmonary circuits.

Most blood vessels consist of three coats, or tunics, similar to those of the heart (*Figure 1-15*). The **tunica intima** is the *innermost coat*, which lines the lumen of the vessels and consists of a layer of flattened endothelial cells over a layer of collagen fibers. The **tunica media** is a *middle coat*, consisting of elastic fibers and smooth muscle cells, both disposed in a circular fashion. Depending on the size and type of vessel, there may be a predominance of elastic fibers or smooth muscle. The **tunica adventitia** is an *outer layer* of connective tissue arranged more or less in longitudinal

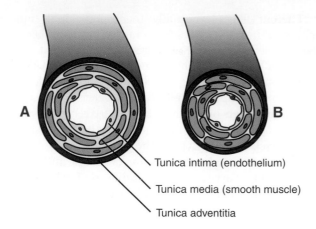

Tunica intima (endothelium)

Tunica media (smooth muscle)

Tunica adventitia

Figure 1-15 Walls of a blood vessel. **A**, Dilated. **B**, Constricted.

fashion. Through this layer run small vessels and nerves that supply the walls of larger vessels. In some vessels, longitudinal smooth muscle also may be found in this layer.

In general, arteries have thicker walls than their companion veins. The lumens of the veins, however, are larger than those of companion arteries.

Arteries

After leaving the heart, arteries become progressively smaller as they branch and rebranch on their way to supplying the tissues of the body. The structure of the arterial walls changes correspondingly to accommodate different functions and sizes.

Elastic arteries are large vessels (30 mm in diameter) that arise from the right and left ventricles as the pulmonary artery and aorta, respectively (*Figure 1-16*). The media consists primarily of circumferentially arranged elastic fibers, which are designed to stretch and recoil to accommodate successive spurts of blood expelled from the ventricles. **Distributing** or **muscular arteries** arise from the aorta and branch and rebranch, becoming progressively smaller (ranging from several millimeters in width to less than half a millimeter). The tunica media consists mainly of circular smooth muscle cells under the control of the visceral (autonomic) nervous system, which can increase or diminish the blood flow to specific areas.

Arterioles are still smaller branches (about 100 μm in diameter) in which the intima consists of only a single cell layer of endothelium. The media consists of only a few layers of smooth muscle cells disposed in a circular or spiral fashion around the endothelium. As the arterioles become progressively smaller, only a single muscle layer is left, and the vessel becomes a *terminal arteriole*. Occasionally, terminal arterioles display thicker, sphincterlike arrangements of muscle cells, termed *precapillary sphincters*. Arterioles

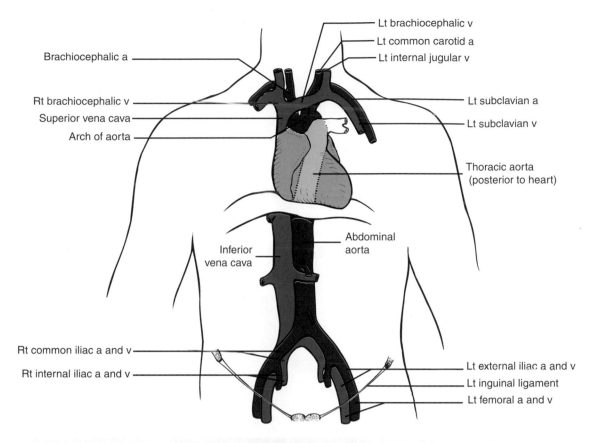

Brachiocephalic a

Rt brachiocephalic v
Superior vena cava
Arch of aorta

Lt brachiocephalic v
Lt common carotid a
Lt internal jugular v

Lt subclavian a
Lt subclavian v

Thoracic aorta
(posterior to heart)

Inferior
vena cava

Abdominal
aorta

Rt common iliac a and v
Rt internal iliac a and v

Lt external iliac a and v
Lt inguinal ligament
Lt femoral a and v

Figure 1-16 Major blood vessels.

and precapillary sphincters have the ability to turn on and off the blood flow to specific areas and directly affect arterial blood pressure levels.

Capillaries

The walls of the true capillary are reduced to a single layer of endothelial cells, which encircle a lumen of about 7 to 10 μm, large enough to accommodate erythrocytes one at a time or in single file. Capillaries form vast anastomosing networks, and it is here, through the endothelial barrier, that an exchange of gases and metabolites takes place. Capillary networks can accommodate large volumes of blood. The capillaries of certain tissues, such as spleen, liver, bone marrow, and certain glands, are somewhat wider and irregular and are termed *sinusoids*.

Veins

As the blood leaves the capillary beds, the vessels regroup as veins, which return blood to the heart.

Venules are small-caliber veins that drain the venous side of the capillary beds. These venules gradually coalesce with one another to form larger channels or veins of increasing diameter.

Veins generally accompany arteries but in a few instances are found without companion arteries. Superficial veins of the limbs course independently of

accompanying arteries. In addition, certain areas possess a venous drainage totally unlike the arterial supply. These include the portal vein, which drains the gut; azygous veins, which drain the thoracic and abdominal walls; and the vertebral plexus of veins, which drains the vertebral column and spinal cord. No corresponding arteries accompany these veins.

Arteriovenous Anastomoses

Occasionally, in various tissues of the body, direct communications exist between arteries and veins. These communications are able to shunt large volumes of blood quickly through a tissue while bypassing the capillary bed. Arteriovenous anastomoses are found in the skin (e.g., hands, feet, nose, ear, lips), mucosa (e.g., nasal, gut), organs, and glands (genitalia, erectile tissue, thyroid gland).

Arterial Anastomoses and Collateral Circulation

Many tissues are richly supplied with several arteries whose branches join and communicate directly. These communications are termed **anastomoses** and allow constant uninterrupted flows to the areas they eventually supply. They also provide alternative channels when one usual channel is blocked. Alternative flow to a blocked area is termed **collateral circulation.**

End Arteries

Some arteries do not anastomose with neighboring arteries, and, if blocked, no collateral circulation develops to help supply the affected area. The result is that the area not supplied dies. The classic example is the central artery of the retina. It is the sole source of arterial supply to the retina, and, if it is occluded, the retina degenerates and blindness results.

FETAL CIRCULATION

During fetal development, the lungs of course are not functioning. There is therefore no reason for the fetal heart to send all its blood to the lungs for gas exchanges because CO_2/O_2 exchange takes place at the placenta. A number of shunts help deflect blood away from the pulmonary circulation to enable oxygenated blood to reach the tissues quickly (*Figure 1-17*).

Blood is oxygenated at the placenta and enters the fetus via the **umbilical vein.** The umbilical vein ascends within the anterior abdominal wall to the liver but bypasses the liver via the **ductus venosus,** which shunts the blood to the inferior vena cava. From here the oxygenated blood ascends to the **right atrium** of the heart, where some of the blood passes through the foramen ovale (a hole in the interatrial septum) directly to the left atrium and then the **left ventricle.** The blood that remains in the right atrium passes to the right ventricle, and on contraction of the ventricle, blood is forced out of the pulmonary trunk. Blood in the pulmonary trunk is deflected by another fetal

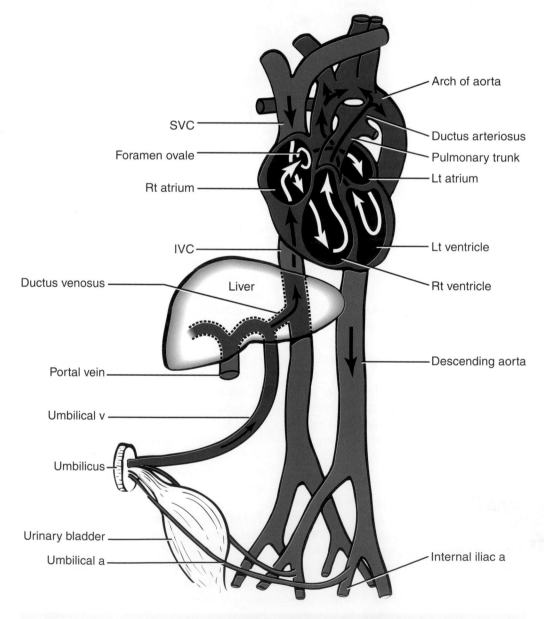

Figure 1-17 Scheme of fetal circulation. *SVC,* Superior vena cava; *IVC,* inferior vena cava.

shunt joining the pulmonary trunk and the aorta, termed the ***ductus arteriosus.*** The left ventricle then pumps the blood out to the system via the aorta.

Return of deoxygenated blood to the placenta is through the **umbilical arteries,** which arise from the internal iliac arteries and ascend along the inside of the anterior abdominal wall to the umbilicus and then via the umbilical cord to the placenta.

CHANGES IN CIRCULATION AT BIRTH

With the first breath of life, the lungs expand and begin to function. Pressure in the left atrium increases and closes the flaplike foramen ovale, which becomes fused after time. Spontaneously the ductus arteriosus closes and eventually undergoes fibrosis. Similarly the ductus venosus is obliterated, thus closing off the three major fetal shunts between arterial and venous circuits.

With the cutting and clamping of the umbilical cord, the umbilical vein becomes thrombosed, then fibrosed. The umbilical arteries are obliterated in the same way.

Each of the obliterated structures remains throughout postnatal life as a vestige of the fetal shunt but acquires a new name.

1. The foramen ovale becomes the fossa ovalis.
2. The ductus arteriosus becomes the ligamentum arteriosum.
3. The ductus venosus becomes the ligamentum venosum.
4. The umbilical vein becomes the ligamentum teres, or round ligament of the liver.
5. The umbilical arteries are simply referred to as the *obliterated umbilical arteries.*

LYMPHATIC SYSTEM

The lymphatic system consists of a series of *tubes* and *filters* that conveys excess tissue fluid from the extravascular tissue spaces back to the blood circulatory system. Unlike the blood vascular system, there is no heart pump to move the fluid through the lymph channels.

Lymph

As blood passes through the capillaries, fluid similar in composition to the blood plasma leaks across the semipermeable capillary walls to enter the tissue spaces (*Figure 1-18*). At this level the individual cells receive nourishment from and discard waste materials to the tissue fluid. Most of the fluid and suspended colloidal protein moves back across the capillary wall to reenter the blood vascular system. The remainder of this fluid drains to the lymphatic system as lymph.

Lymph also contains two types of lymphocytes that are produced by the bone marrow but mature in different sites. **B cells** mature in the bone marrow and are then carried by the blood circulation to lymph nodes and other lymphoid tissues described later. **T cells**, on the other hand, mature in the thymus gland and on maturation leave through the circulation to populate lymphoid tissues. Lymphocytes leave the lymphoid tissue periodically to circulate through the lymphatic system and blood circulatory systems.

Lymph Capillaries

Lymphatic channels begin as blind-ended capillaries alongside blood capillaries. Excess tissue fluid moves across the semipermeable membrane of the lymph capillary to form a clear, almost colorless fluid called *lymph*. Lymphatics

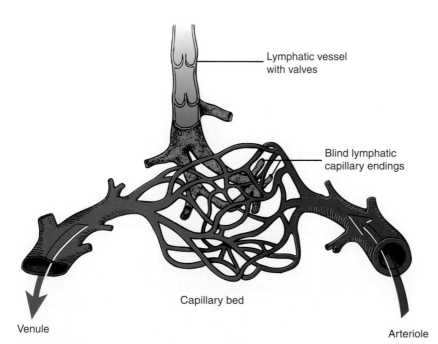

Lymphatic vessel with valves

Blind lymphatic capillary endings

Capillary bed

Venule

Arteriole

Figure 1-18 Collection of lymph from capillary bed.

returning from the gut contain absorbed fat, which gives the lymph a milky appearance (*chyle*).

Lymph Vessels

Lymph capillaries form vast networks, which eventually drain to larger channels or vessels. These lymphatic vessels are thin walled, contain many one-way valves, and generally accompany veins.

Lymph Nodes (Glands)

Lymph vessels pass through a series of enlarged filters or lymph nodes as they convey lymph back toward the blood vascular system (*Figure 1-19*). The glands are somewhat flattened and vary in size from less than a millimeter to several centimeters in diameter. Within, they consist of a number of compartments separated by fibrous tissue septa. Each compartment contains spherical lymphoid follicles consisting of a germinal center and a surrounding cluster of lymphocytes.

Lymph nodes are found in groups throughout the body and in two particularly large groupings in the axilla (**axillary nodes**) and in the groin (**inguinal nodes**). Lymph nodes are palpable under certain pathological conditions. Within the nodes, foreign particulate matter is filtered out by phagocytic cells as the lymph passes through a fine network of capillaries.

Large Lymphatic Vessels

Lymphatics drain to larger lymph trunks that drain various regions of the body (*Figure 1-20*).

1. The thoracic duct drains the lower limbs, abdomen, and chest wall.
2. The bronchomediastinal trunk drains the viscera of the thorax.
3. The subclavian trunks drain the upper limbs.
4. The jugular trunks drain the head and neck.

The thoracic duct empties its contents into the confluence of the subclavian and internal jugular veins on the left side only. The others drain into the same area on both the right and left sides.

Lymph Flow

Because lymph is not pumped through the system by the heart, lymph flow tends to be comparatively sluggish. Its flow is aided by (1) passage from the positive pressure abdominal cavity to the negative pressure thoracic cavity; (2) rhythmical contraction of the lymph vessels; (3) valves, which permit one-way flow only; and (4) massaging or milking of lymph vessels by neighboring active muscles of the upper and lower limbs.

Functions

The lymphatic system permits (1) drainage of tissue fluid and protein back to the blood venous system from the tissues, (2) conduction of fat from the intestines to the blood venous system, and (3) manufacture of antibodies and proliferation and circulation of lymphocytes that are active in an immune mechanism against foreign tissues within the body.

Lymphoid Tissues

The lymph nodes mentioned previously are examples of lymphoid tissues. There are other structures that contain lymphoid tissues.

Tonsils. The tonsils (see Chapter 7) include the **palatine tonsils, pharyngeal tonsils** (adenoids), and the **lingual tonsils.** Tonsils are clusters of lymphoid follicles that are buried below oral mucosa.

Spleen. The spleen (see Chapter 4) is a large abdominal organ containing lymphoid follicles and is characterized by small arterioles that pass through the follicles.

Thymus Gland. The thymus gland differs from the other lymphoid tissues in two ways. The thymus gland possesses no organized follicles. Instead, the lymphoid tissue is continuous throughout the cortex of the gland. In addition, T cells mature only in the thymus gland.

Lymphoid Tissue of the Gut. Lymphoid follicles are found throughout the mucosa of the gut. In the jejunum (distal portion of the small intestine) there are larger aggregations of follicles called *Peyer's patches*.

7. Nervous System

The human nervous system is a highly complex and specialized system that reacts to the external and internal environment by integrating and interpreting incoming stimuli and then directing the body to respond in the appropriate manner. Appreciation of and response to

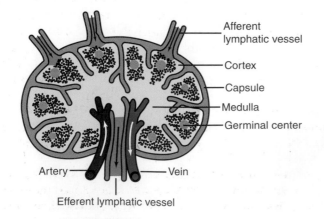

Afferent lymphatic vessel

Cortex

Capsule

Medulla

Germinal center

Artery — — Vein

Efferent lymphatic vessel

Figure 1-19 Lymph node.

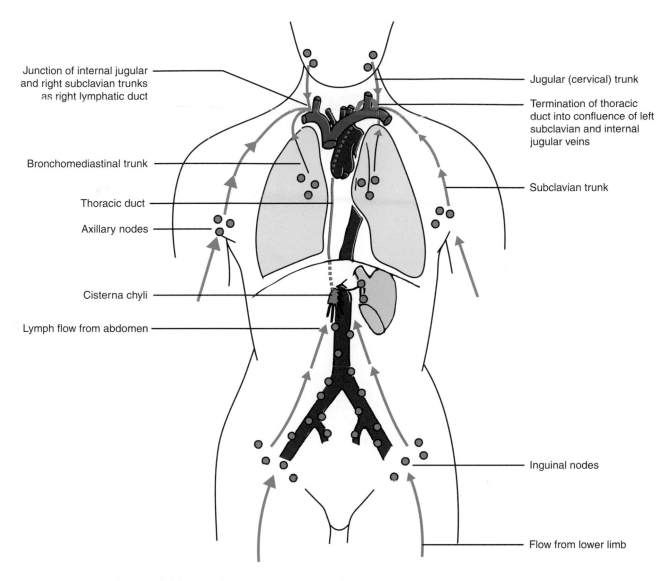

Junction of internal jugular
and right subclavian trunks
as right lymphatic duct

Jugular (cervical) trunk

Termination of thoracic
duct into confluence of left
subclavian and internal
jugular veins

Bronchomediastinal trunk

Subclavian trunk

Thoracic duct

Axillary nodes

Cisterna chyli

Lymph flow from abdomen

Inguinal nodes

Flow from lower limb

Figure 1-20 Scheme of lymphatic circulation.

environmental stimuli are either at a *conscious* or at an *unconscious* level. The nervous system is populated by two types of cells: (1) **neuroglia** that perform *supportive functions*, and (2) **neurons**, which are *reactive* cells that respond to stimuli.

THE NEURON

The neuron is the basic functional unit of the nervous system and responds to either excitation or inhibition. Like all cells, neurons consist of a plasma membrane encasing a mass of cytoplasm and a nucleus. Neurons differ in that they can conduct electrical impulses and communicate with each other through long cellular extensions and **synapses**. Neurons exist in a great variety of shapes and sizes, but only two types—motor and sensory—are described.

Motor Neuron

Motor neurons (*Figure 1-21, A*) consist of a **cell body** (**soma**) that contains a nucleus and cellular extensions, either *dendrites* or *axons*. **Dendrites** are short, branching cellular extensions that conduct impulses toward the cell body. **Axons** are long cellular extensions that conduct impulses away from the cell body. Near its termination the axon branches, with each branch ending as a bulbous **axon terminal** or **bouton**. Axon terminals synapse with muscle cells. Motor neurons are classified as being **multipolar** because several extensions arise from the cell body.

Sensory Neuron

The body of a sensory neuron (*Figure 1-21, B*) has only one cellular extension, or process, and is therefore classified as **unipolar**. The single process is short and divides into two **axons**. One axon continues to the periphery as

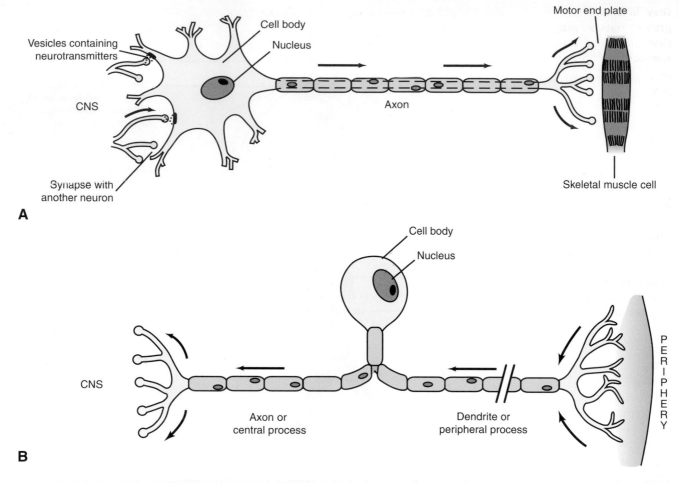

Figure 1-21 **A,** Multipolar motor neuron. **B,** Unipolar sensory neuron.

the **peripheral process** and ends as several branches. Each branch is either a sensory receptor or synapses with sensory receptors. Some authors refer to the branching component as *dendrites.* The other axon extends into the CNS as the **central process.**

Synapses

Synapses (see *Figure 1-21*) occur at the intercellular junctions of nerve processes or between nerve processes and cells of effector organs. Between the approximating cell surfaces is a **synaptic cleft** separating the *presynaptic cell membrane* from the *postsynaptic cell membrane.* Electrical impulses travel along an axon and at its terminus cause the release of chemical **neurotransmitters,** which diffuse across the cleft to receptor sites on the postsynaptic side. The neurotransmitter may be either *excitatory,* initiating an impulse on the postsynaptic side, or *inhibitory,* stopping the impulse at that point. Excitatory transmitters depolarize the postsynaptic membrane; an inhibitory transmitter hyperpolarizes the postsynaptic membrane. Target neurons receive from only a few to more than 1000

synapses with other neurons, some of which are inhibitory and some of which are excitatory. The target neuron may or may not propagate the impulse, depending on the net depolarization of its membrane. *Figure 1-21, A,* shows a presynaptic neuron synapsing with a typical multipolar motor neuron, which synapses with a muscle cell.

Neuroglia

Neuroglia are nonreactive nerve cells that fulfill a *supportive* role. They function to (1) maintain homeostasis in the extracellular environment, (2) electrically insulate nerve processes from each other, and (3) provide nutrition for the neurons. There are six classes of neuroglia, and their names and specific functions are covered in standard textbooks of neuroanatomy.

DEFINITIONS AND TERMS

Aggregations of cell bodies and their axonal processes ensheathed in myelin have distinct appearances and give rise to the following terms and definitions:

Gray Matter. Neuronal bodies grouped together appear gray or pinkish gray and are referred to as *gray matter.* Gray matter is found in the central part of the spinal cord surrounding the central canal, on the surfaces of the cerebral and cerebellar hemispheres (cortex), and scattered throughout the CNS as discrete, internal patches or nuclei.

White Matter. Myelin has a shiny white appearance and imparts this color to grouped bundles of myelinated axons within the CNS.

Peripheral Nerve. A bundle of myelinated axons that travel outside the CNS is called a *(peripheral) nerve.* Nerves arise from the brain as cranial nerves and from the spinal cord as spinal nerves. Nerves (with some cranial nerve exceptions) contain both motor (efferent) and sensory (afferent) axons.

Tract. A group of myelinated axons that travel together within the CNS and share a common origin, destination, and function are called a *tract.* Tracts are similar to nerves, but they run entirely within the brain and spinal cord.

Nucleus. Within the CNS, a group of neuronal cell bodies located in the same area and sharing the same function is called a *nucleus.* The *dorsal horns* of the spinal cord are elongated sensory nuclei; the *ventral horns* of the spinal cord are elongated motor nuclei.

Ganglion. Ganglia are similar to nuclei in that they are also collections of neuronal cell bodies with the same functions. A ganglion, however, sits outside the CNS as a discrete swelling. Examples are dorsal root ganglia and autonomic ganglia. There is one glaring exception to this definition. The basal ganglia of the cerebral hemispheres encountered in neuroanatomy are by definition nuclei.

Afferent Fibers. Afferent fibers are axons that carry impulses *toward* the CNS or toward higher centers. They are also referred to as *sensory* or *ascending fibers.*

Efferent Fibers. Efferent fibers are axons that carry impulses *away* from the CNS to muscles and glands. They are also referred to as *motor* or *descending fibers.*

The nervous system is conveniently divided into components based on *location* (central and peripheral nervous systems) and *function* (somatic and autonomic nervous systems).

DIVISION BASED ON LOCATION
Central Nervous System
The central nervous system (CNS) includes the **brain**, contained within the skull, and the **spinal cord**, contained within the vertebral canal. Functionally the CNS consists of (1) a *sensory component*, in which incoming data are received at a conscious or unconscious level; (2) a *motor component*, from which outgoing commands originate; and (3) an *association component*, which connects and coordinates the various CNS centers. The brain is not discussed in detail in this textbook.

Peripheral Nervous System
There are **31 pairs of spinal nerves** that arise from the spinal cord, and **12 pairs of cranial nerves** that arise from the brain. Peripheral nerves consist of bundles of axons that convey information to and from the CNS. Peripheral nerves are described in greater detail later.

DIVISION BASED ON FUNCTION
Somatic Nervous System
The somatic nervous system controls the body's **voluntary** and **reflex activities** through *somatic sensory* and *somatic motor* components of both the central and peripheral nervous systems.

Visceral (Autonomic) Nervous System
The visceral nervous system is that portion of both the CNS and the peripheral nervous system that controls **involuntary** smooth muscle, cardiac muscle, or glandular tissue. It has a *motor component* that is capable of controlling smooth muscle contractions of viscera and blood vessels and the secretions of glands. An *autonomic sensory component* provides feedback for CNS control of viscera, vessels, and glands.

The autonomic nervous system is further divided into the *parasympathetic division* and the *sympathetic division.*

Parasympathetic Division. The parasympathetic division is *necessary to sustain life* and is concerned with minute-to-minute vegetative functional activities of the viscera and glands. For example, it slows the heart, increases peristalsis and glandular secretions, and opens gut sphincters.

Sympathetic Division. The sympathetic division in contrast is *expendable* and may be cut with no loss to life. It is antagonistic to the parasympathetic division, and its effects are obvious during periods of stress or emergency. For example, in emergency situations the hair stands on end, the pupils dilate to allow more light to reach the retina, the heart beats faster to supply more blood to skeletal muscles for "fight or flight," respiration is increased, and the bronchioles dilate to oxygenate the increased blood flow.

Functions controlled by the parasympathetic division that are not necessary at this time of emergency slow down. Salivary secretions decrease, peristalsis of the gut decreases, and the urinary bladder relaxes.

PERIPHERAL NERVES
Structure
The basic unit of a peripheral nerve is the axon (*Figure 1-22*). Each individual axonal process is wrapped by myelin-containing **neurilemma (Schwann) cells** that act as insulators separating the axons from each other. Surrounding each process and its coatings is an outer

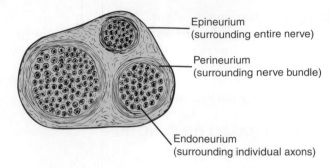

Epineurium
(surrounding entire nerve)

Perineurium
(surrounding nerve bundle)

Endoneurium
(surrounding individual axons)

Figure 1-22 Cross section through a peripheral nerve.

fibrous layer called *endoneurium.* Surrounding bundles of processes is a fibrous layer of **perineurium,** surrounding several bundles, which make up the entire peripheral nerve, is a final coating of epineurium. The **epineurium** in turn is in contact with surrounding areolar tissue, through which passes the blood supply to the nerve and eventually to each individual nerve cell via the interconnecting septa of fibrous connective tissue sheaths.

Function

During embryonic development, mesoderm gives rise to both an external body (**soma**) covered with skin and an internal tube lined with mucosa that forms the gut and its associated glands (**viscera**). In addition, viscera of the cardiovascular, genitourinary, and respiratory systems develop concurrently with the gastrointestinal viscera. Skeletal muscles develop within the body for movement and locomotion, and smooth muscle develops within the viscera for peristalsis and emptying of contents. These two basic body areas are controlled by **motor** (**efferent**) and **sensory** (**afferent**) **nerves.**

In this scheme there are four modalities: (1) **somatic efferent** to voluntary, skeletal muscles; (2) **somatic afferent** (touch, pain, temperature, pressure, and vibration) from skin and proprioception from endings in muscles, tendons, and joints; (3) **visceral efferent** (**autonomic**) to visceral smooth muscles and glands; and (4) **visceral afferent** providing sensory feedback from the organs and glands. These four modalities are found in all spinal nerves.

In the head region, two more modalities are added: (5) **special sensory** to accommodate the special senses of smell, vision, taste, hearing, and balance and (6) **branchial efferent** to supply those skeletal muscles of the head and neck that are derived from branchial arches.

To complicate matters considerably, developmental neuroanatomists have burdened us with extremely cumbersome and sometimes confusing classifications. The classic classification is presented as a footnote solely for reference and not for learning purposes.*

Central Nervous System Origins of Somatic Peripheral Nerves

Voluntary Motor (Somatic and Branchial Efferent) Components. Motor pathways comprise two groups of neurons—upper and lower motor neurons (*Figures 1-23* and *1-24*). The **upper motor neurons** reside in the *motor cortex of the cerebrum.* Axons of these neurons descend in bundles called *tracts* that cross the midline (decussate) at some point during their descent. They descend to synapse with **lower motor neurons** that give rise to motor components of peripheral nerves.

Cranial Nerves. In the brain stem, the lower motor neurons are located in cranial nerve motor nuclei. Bundles of their axons pass out of the brain stem as motor components of cranial nerves. Cranial nerves III, IV, VI, and XII carry **somatic efferent fibers** that innervate skeletal muscles of the head derived from somites.

Cranial nerves V, VII, IX, and X carry **branchial efferent fibers** to supply cranial muscles of branchial arch origin, but they follow the same scheme as somatic efferent pathways.

Spinal Nerves. In the spinal cord the lower motor neurons are located in the ventral (anterior) horn, an elongated motor nucleus that extends the length of the spinal cord. Axons of these neurons leave the spinal cord as ventral (anterior) roots that form the motor component of each of the 31 pairs of spinal nerves. These motor nerves supply all the skeletal muscles of the trunk and limbs.

General Sensory (Somatic Sensory) Components. General sensory pathways feature three sets of neurons (primary, secondary, and tertiary), which ultimately synapse with neurons in the sensory cortex of the brain.

Cranial Nerves. The cell bodies of the **primary neurons** of cranial nerves are located near the brainstem within *sensory ganglia,* swellings on cranial nerves that have a sensory component (cranial nerves V, VII, IX, and X). Peripheral

---

*Classification of Functional Components Based on Tissue Origins

Structures of the body supplied by afferent and efferent nerves fall into three main categories based on derivation. **Somatic structures** are derived from embryonic paraxial somites. **Visceral structures** include all structures derived from the gut or the genitourinary, cardiovascular, and respiratory systems, including associated glands. **Branchial structures** develop from the branchial arches. Modalities of spinal nerves are said to be *general*; those of cranial nerves are said to be *special*.

In this scheme there are seven modalities: (1) **general somatic afferent** (exteroceptive and proprioceptive sensation from structures of somatic origin); (2) **general visceral afferent** (interoceptive sensation from involuntary muscles and glands); (3) **special somatic afferent** (vision, hearing, and equilibrium); (4) **special visceral afferent** (smell and taste); (5) **general somatic efferent** (to skeletal muscles of somatic origin); (6) **general visceral efferent** (autonomic to smooth and cardiac muscle, and glands); and (7) **special visceral efferent** (to skeletal muscles of branchial arch origin).

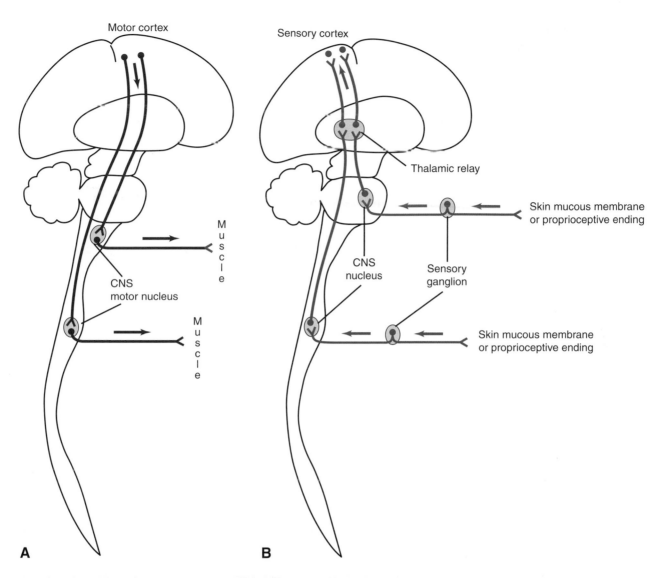

Figure 1-23 **A,** General scheme of voluntary efferent (motor) cranial and spinal nerve components. **B,** General scheme of afferent (sensory) cranial and spinal nerve components. Not obvious from this lateral view is that sensory and motor tracts cross over (decussate) within the CNS so each side of the brain controls the opposite side of the body.

processes pick up stimuli from various regions of the head (e.g., the skin of the face, mucosa of the oral and nasal cavity, pulps of teeth) and carry the stimuli past the ganglia and through central processes to *sensory nuclei* containing **secondary neurons** within the brain stem. Their axons decussate and rise to synapse with **tertiary neurons** in the *thalamus*, and these in turn send axons up to the *sensory cortex*.

Spinal Nerves. The cell bodies of the **primary neurons** of spinal nerves are contained in the *dorsal root ganglia* adjacent to the spinal cord. Their peripheral processes transmit impulses from sensory receptors in the skin or proprioceptive receptors in muscles, tendons, and joints. Central processes pass into the CNS through dorsal roots to synapse with **secondary neurons** contained within the *dorsal (posterior) horn*, which is a long sensory nucleus that runs the length of the spinal cord. Axons of these neurons cross the midline (decussate) and ascend to

synapse with **tertiary neurons** located in the thalamus of the brain. These neurons send axons up to synapse with the final set of neurons located in the **sensory cortex** of the brain, where sensations are ultimately perceived.

Central Nervous System Origins of Autonomic (Visceral) Nerves

Autonomic Motor (Visceral Efferent) Components. The visceral efferent or autonomic pathways consist of a two-neuron chain. The first neurons reside in *autonomic motor nuclei* within the CNS. They send axons outside the CNS that ultimately synapse with a second set of neurons within an *autonomic ganglion* outside the CNS. The second neurons send out axons (postsynaptic fibers) to the smooth muscle and glands of the viscera. As mentioned previously there are two divisions: parasympathetic and sympathetic.

25

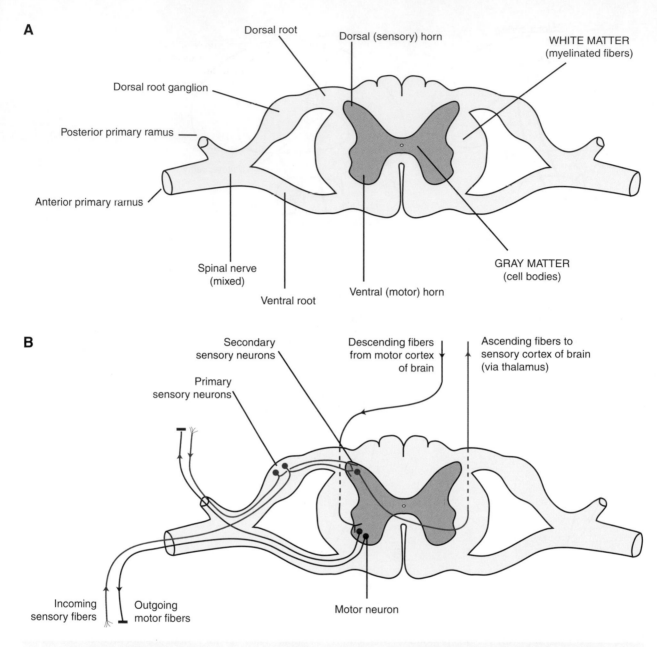

A

Dorsal root

Dorsal (sensory) horn

WHITE MATTER
(myelinated fibers)

Dorsal root ganglion

Posterior primary ramus

Anterior primary ramus

Spinal nerve
(mixed)

Ventral root

Ventral (motor) horn

GRAY MATTER
(cell bodies)

B

Secondary
sensory neurons

Descending fibers
from motor cortex
of brain

Ascending fibers to
sensory cortex of brain
(via thalamus)

Primary
sensory neurons

Incoming
sensory fibers

Outgoing
motor fibers

Motor neuron

Figure 1-24 Cross section through spinal cord to show origins of spinal nerves. **A,** Features seen in a typical cross section. **B,** Pathways of sensory and motor components. NOTE: These pathways are bilateral. Both ascending and descending pathways cross midline so that sensations and muscle movements on one side are perceived and controlled on opposite side of brain.

Parasympathetic Division. This division (*Figure 1-25*) originates from the brain and from the sacral region of the spinal cord (**craniosacral outflow**). The first neuron lies within parasympathetic motor nuclei in either the brain or sacral portion of the spinal cord.

Cranial preganglionic fibers arise from parasympathetic motor nuclei within the brain stem and leave as components of cranial nerves III, VII, IX, and X. The parasympathetic components of cranial nerves III, VII, and IX supply cranial visceral elements (mainly glands). The parasympathetic supply of cranial nerve X is far more

extensive. It supplies the respiratory system, cardiac system, and most of the gut and associated glands up to the left colic flexure (foregut and midgut derivatives).

Sacral preganglionic fibers arise from parasympathetic motor nuclei in the ventral horns of the spinal cord at levels S2, S3, and S4 and leave through the ventral roots of pelvic spinal nerves. They then form discrete pelvic splanchnic nerves that supply the distal portion of the gut (hindgut derivatives) and pelvic viscera. They synapse in parasympathetic ganglia that are close to or within the pelvic viscera they ultimately supply.

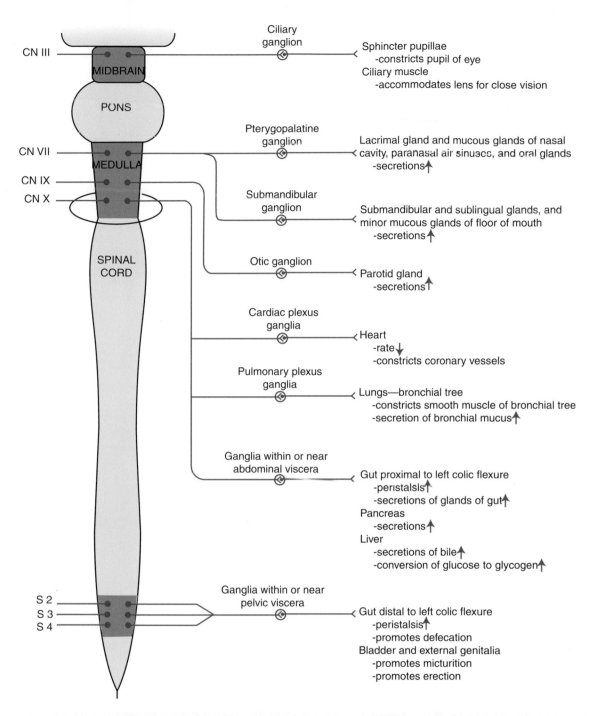

Figure 1-25 Scheme of parasympathetic division origins and distributions.

Sympathetic Division. Sympathetic outflow originates from the spinal cord at levels T1 to L2 (*Figures 1-26* and *1-27*). The first neurons lie within the **intermediolateral horns,** found only in this region of the spinal cord. Preganglionic fibers leave the spinal cord along with the anterior spinal nerve roots (see *Figure 1-27*). On leaving the vertebral canal and the intervertebral foramen, the fibers leave the spinal nerve as myelinated **white communicating rami.**

On either side of the vertebral column are a right and a left chain of sympathetic (*paravertebral*) ganglia. These are the **sympathetic trunks,** and they run the entire length of the vertebral column. There is a sympathetic ganglion at each vertebral level. In the cervical region the ganglia at levels C1 to C4 fuse to form the *superior cervical ganglion.* The ganglia at levels C5 and C6 fuse to form the *middle cervical ganglion,* and the ganglia at levels C7 and C8 fuse to form the *inferior cervical ganglion.*

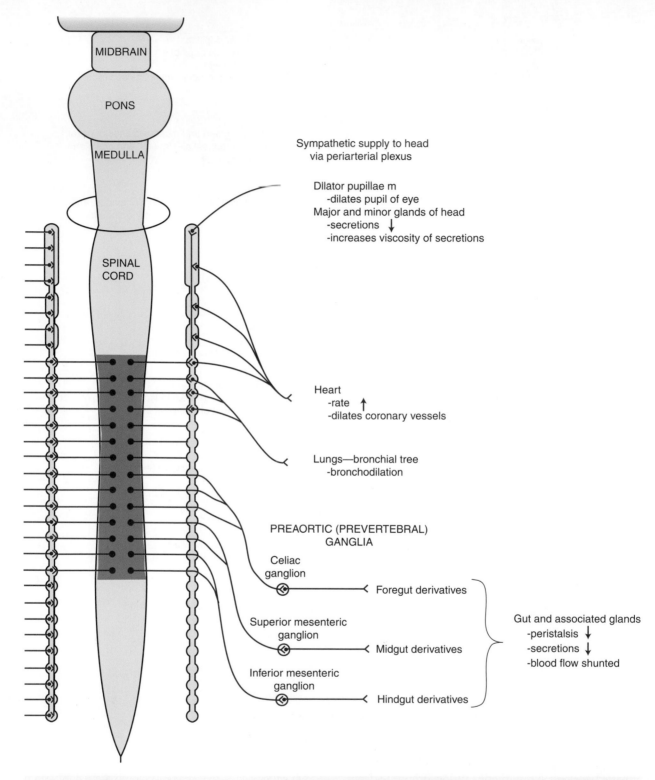

MIDBRAIN

PONS

MEDULLA

SPINAL CORD

Sympathetic supply to head
via periarterial plexus

Dilator pupillae m
-dilates pupil of eye
Major and minor glands of head
-secretions ↓
-increases viscosity of secretions

Heart
-rate ↑
-dilates coronary vessels

Lungs—bronchial tree
-bronchodilation

PREAORTIC (PREVERTEBRAL) GANGLIA

Celiac ganglion

Foregut derivatives

Superior mesenteric ganglion

Midgut derivatives

Gut and associated glands
-peristalsis ↓
-secretions ↓
-blood flow shunted

Inferior mesenteric ganglion

Hindgut derivatives

Figure 1-26 Scheme of sympathetic division origins and distributions. NOTE: To simplify scheme, sympathetic contributions are shown on right side and sympathetic innervation to head and viscera is shown on left side. Both sets of fibers are bilateral.

Running to the sympathetic trunk from spinal cord levels T1 to L2 are the **white communicating rami**, which enter the adjacent sympathetic ganglia. Within the sympathetic trunk, preganglionic fibers may (1) synapse with the neurons of the ganglion at that level; (2) travel up or down the sympathetic trunk to synapse in a ganglion at a higher or lower level; or (3) leave the sympathetic trunk as **splanchnic nerves**, which stream down into the abdomen to synapse

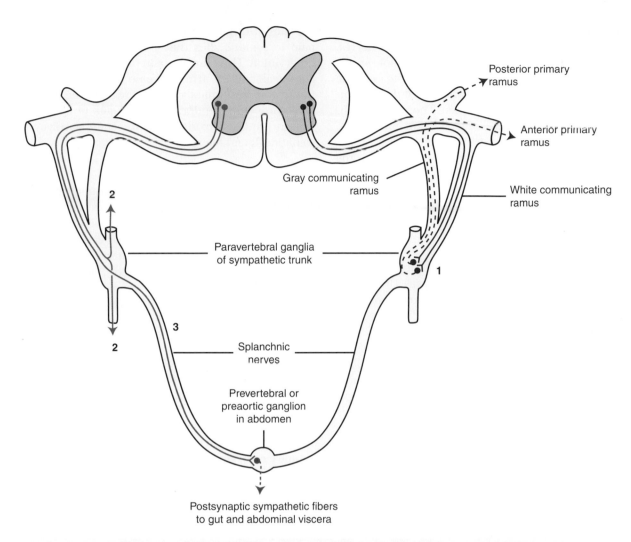

Figure 1-27 Cross section through thoracic spinal cord to demonstrate origin and distribution of sympathetic nerves. All sympathetic nerves originate in lateral horn of thoracic cord (T1-L2, and their outgoing fibers can synapse at three different sites). *1,* Some fibers synapse at their own level and join spinal nerves. *2,* Other fibers pass up or down sympathetic trunk to synapse at a higher or a lower level and join spinal nerves at that level. *3,* Some fibers leave as discrete splanchnic nerves that travel to abdomen to synapse in remote prevertebral ganglia.

in remote *prevertebral ganglia.* The postganglionic fibers in the first and second categories rejoin the spinal nerves as unmyelinated **gray communicating rami** and are distributed along with the spinal nerves.

There are only 14 pairs of white communicating rami arising from spinal levels T1 to L2. Leaving the sympathetic trunk to join the spinal nerves, however, are 31 pairs of gray rami.

Distribution of Postganglionic Sympathetic Fibers

Trunk and Limbs. Gray rami leave the sympathetic trunk at each spinal cord level to join each pair of spinal nerves. They are then distributed by the spinal nerves to the trunk and limbs where they supply smooth muscle of blood vessels. In addition, sympathetic fibers pass to the skin to supply sweat glands and *arrector pili muscles* that produce goose bumps and cause hair to stand on end.

Head and Neck. Preganglionic fibers of the sympathetic trunk rise to the *superior cervical ganglion.* Within the superior cervical ganglion, the preganglionic fibers synapse with the second set of neurons. Postganglionic fibers leave the ganglion to join the nearby carotid arteries as the **carotid periarterial plexus,** an external nerve plexus surrounding the vessel. The sympathetic postganglionic fibers are then distributed to the visceral effector organs of the head by the various branches of the external and internal carotid arteries.

Thorax. Postganglionic fibers of the three cervical sympathetic ganglia stream down to the thorax to form the *cardiac* and *pulmonary plexuses,* which supply the heart and smooth muscle of the bronchial tree.

Abdominal and Pelvic Viscera. Preganglionic fibers leave the sympathetic trunk in the thorax as **splanchnic nerves,** which then enter the abdomen to synapse in remote *prevertebral ganglia* (celiac and preaortic ganglia). Postganglionic fibers from these ganglia travel via branches of the abdominal aorta to the viscera of the abdomen. Thoracic splanchnic nerves supply the derivatives of the foregut and midgut. Hindgut derivatives and urogenital pelvic viscera are supplied from **lumbar splanchnic nerves** arising from the sympathetic trunk of the lumbar region.

Autonomic Sensory (Visceral Afferent) Components. Visceral receptors monitor smooth muscle tone in viscera and vessels, blood chemistry (chemoreceptors), blood pressure (baroreceptors), and the content volume in hollow organs. This information is conveyed back to the CNS via sensory components of autonomic nerves. Unlike general sensations (e.g., pain, temperature, touch) conveyed by somatic afferent nerves, we are generally unaware of visceral sensations. There are, however, exceptions.

We are aware of a sense of fullness of the stomach, rectum, and bladder. We are also aware of hunger and, when things go wrong, nausea. Afferent impulses that convey these conditions travel back to the CNS along *parasympathetic nerves.* The primary cell bodies of spinal nerves reside in the same ganglia (dorsal root ganglia) occupied by somatic afferent nerves, and the primary cell bodies of cranial nerves reside in sensory cranial ganglia for cranial nerves. The pathways for visceral or autonomic sensation within the CNS are the same as those for the somatic afferent nerve fibers.

Feelings of pain or cramps, however, travel back to the CNS along *sympathetic nerves.* The brain does not localize the sites of origin of visceral pain and instead refers the pain to somatic sites that share the same spinal nerve innervation. Thus cardiac pain (angina) is localized to the chest wall and left arm, and pain from appendicitis is felt in the umbilical (midabdominal) region. The primary cell bodies are found in dorsal root ganglia of spinal nerves. Within the CNS, axons follow the same pathway as the somatic afferent fibers.

Nomenclature and Summary

Cranial Nerves. There are 12 pairs of cranial nerves, which originate from the brain. They are individually named and by convention assigned Roman numerals (*Table 1-1*). Note the functional components listed for each cranial nerve. Some nerves, such as the trochlear nerve (cranial nerve IV), contain only one component (motor); other nerves, such as the glossopharyngeal nerve (cranial nerve IX), contain five functional components. The distributions and structures supplied by the cranial nerves are described in detail in Chapter 7 and reviewed as a group in Chapter 8.

Spinal Nerves. The formation of a typical spinal nerve is illustrated in *Figure 1-24*. The dorsal (sensory) root and the ventral (motor) root combine to form a mixed sensory and motor spinal nerve. Spinal nerves exit through intervertebral foramina and immediately break up into two main branches (*rami*; singular, *ramus*). The **posterior primary rami** supply mixed sensory and motor nerves to the structures of the back, the back of the neck, and the back of the head. The **anterior rami** supply mixed sensory and motor fibers to the lateral and anterior aspects of the trunk and all of the upper and lower limbs.

TABLE 1-1

The Cranial Nerves and Their Functional Components

Number	Name	Functional Components
I	Olfactory nerve	Special afferent (smell)
II	Optic nerve	Special afferent (sight)
III	Oculomotor nerve	Somatic motor, visceral efferent
IV	Trochlear nerve	Somatic motor
V	Trigeminal nerve	Somatic afferent, branchial motor
VI	Abducens nerve	Somatic efferent
VII	Facial nerve	Somatic afferent, branchial efferent, visceral efferent, special afferent (taste)
VIII	Vestibulocochlear nerve	Special afferent (hearing and balance)
IX	Glossopharyngeal nerve	Somatic afferent, branchial efferent, visceral efferent, visceral afferent, special afferent (taste)
X	Vagus nerve	Somatic afferent, branchial efferent, visceral efferent, visceral afferent, special afferent (taste)
XI	Spinal accessory nerve	Branchial efferent
XII	Hypoglossal nerve	Somatic efferent

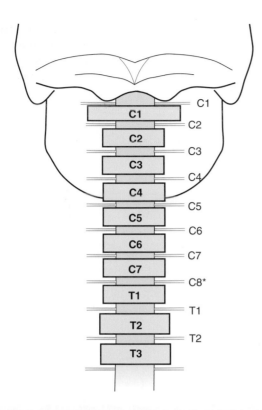

Figure 1-28 Nomenclature of spinal nerves. From vertebral levels C1-C7, spinal nerves arise above their respective vertebrae. From vertebral levels T1 downward, spinal nerves arise below their respective vertebrae. Spinal nerve C8 arises between C7-T1. (NOTE: There is a spinal nerve C8, but there is no vertebra C8.)

Spinal nerves derive their names from the vertebrae between which they arise (*Figure 1-28*). By convention, spinal nerves C1 to C7 take their names **from the vertebrae below.** For example, spinal nerve C1 arises between the skull and vertebra C1. Similarly, C2 exits between vertebrae C1 and C2 and so on. There are only seven cervical vertebrae, but there are eight cervical nerves. Spinal nerve C8 arises between the seventh cervical and first thoracic vertebrae. From vertebral level T1 downward, each spinal nerve derives its name **from the vertebra above,** so that spinal nerve T1 emerges between vertebrae T1 and T2, and so on.

Nerve Plexuses. In certain regions of the spinal cord, anterior rami tend to join and divide in complex patterns called *nerve plexuses* (*Figure 1-29*). The **cervical plexus** is formed by the anterior rami of spinal nerves C1 to C4. It supplies structures in the anterior and lateral regions of the neck. The **brachial plexus** is formed from the anterior rami of spinal nerves C5 to T1. It supplies all of the structures of the upper limb. The **lumbar plexus** is formed by the anterior rami of spinal nerves L1 to L4 and supplies the pelvis and the entire lower limb. The **sacral plexus** is formed by the anterior rami of spinal nerves L4 to S4 and supplies the perineum and lower limb. The **coccygeal**

plexus is formed by the anterior rami of spinal nerves S4 to Co1 and supplies skin of the coccygeal area.

Cutaneous Distribution

The sensory distribution from the skin of the body is shown in *Figure 1-30*. Most of the body is innervated by spinal nerves. However, the face and anterior scalp are innervated largely by cranial nerve V (trigeminal nerve).

8. Body Coverings, Body Cavities, and Fascia

The body is lined within and without by epithelial coverings, which are supported by underlying connective tissue layers (*Figure 1-31*). Externally the lining is **skin;** internally the linings of the gut and respiratory and genitourinary tracts are **mucous membrane,** which is red and kept moist by mucous glands. Areas of transition from skin to mucous membrane are found at both ends of the alimentary canal, at the nose, and on the external genitalia.

Invaginations of epithelium invade the underlying connective tissue to form (1) glands, teeth, and digestive organs, such as liver and pancreas *from mucous membrane*; and (2) hair follicles, nail beds, sebaceous glands, and sweat glands *from skin*.

MUCOUS MEMBRANE

The morphology of mucous membrane depends on its primary function. It can be (1) *mechanically protective*, as in the esophagus; (2) *secretory*, as in the stomach; (3) *absorptive*, as in the intestines, and (4) *protective* against foreign material, as in respiratory mucosa containing cilia. Mucous membrane is considered in greater detail in the chapters dealing with the study of the gastrointestinal, genitourinary, and respiratory systems.

SKIN

There are two types of skin. **Thick skin** covers the *palmar* and *plantar* surfaces of the hands and feet. Thick skin is completely devoid of hair, and its surface is heavily ridged for protection against wear and for grip (hands) and traction (feet). **Thin skin** covers the remainder of the body and is covered with hair or at least some fuzz. The skin covering the posterior aspect of the body is somewhat thicker than the skin of the anterior region.

Skin color can vary among individuals and ranges from pale to dark, depending on the amount of melanin, a brown pigment found in the skin. In addition, exposure to sunlight increases the production of melanin and deepens the color. In fair-skinned people, underlying vessels contribute to skin coloring. Diminished blood flow beneath the skin causes pallor; increased flow causes flushing.

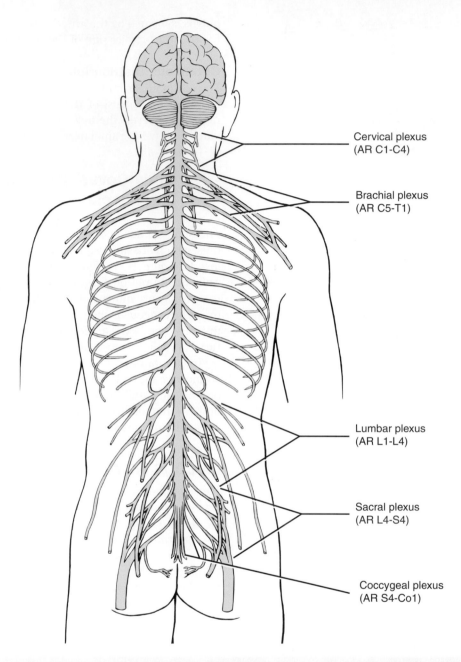

Figure 1-29 Examples of nerve plexuses. Anterior rami (*AR*) of spinal nerves in cervical, upper thoracic, and lumbar and sacral regions form nerve plexuses. Cervical plexus supplies some anterior and lateral structures of neck; brachial plexus supplies upper limb; lumbosacral plexus supplies lower limb.

Two components make up the total layer of skin. **Epidermis** is an outer epithelial layer, and **dermis** is an underlying connective tissue layer.

Epidermis

The epidermis consists of four layers and is classified as *stratified squamous epithelium* (*Figure 1-32*). The deepest layer proliferates to produce cells, which then migrate upward through four different levels, changing from columnar cells at the base to flattened, scalelike squamous cells near the surface. As the cells rise to the surface, they produce keratin within the cytoplasm and undergo cell degeneration with loss of the nuclei. The flat, keratinized cells at the surface are dead and are constantly being sloughed off as new cells rise from below as replacements.

Dermis

The junction between the epidermis and dermis is ridged (see *Figure 1-32*). The dermis is a layer of connective tissue consisting of cells in a matrix of relatively dense collagenous and elastic fibers. Scattered throughout this layer are deposits of *fat cells*, or *adipose tissue*. Running through

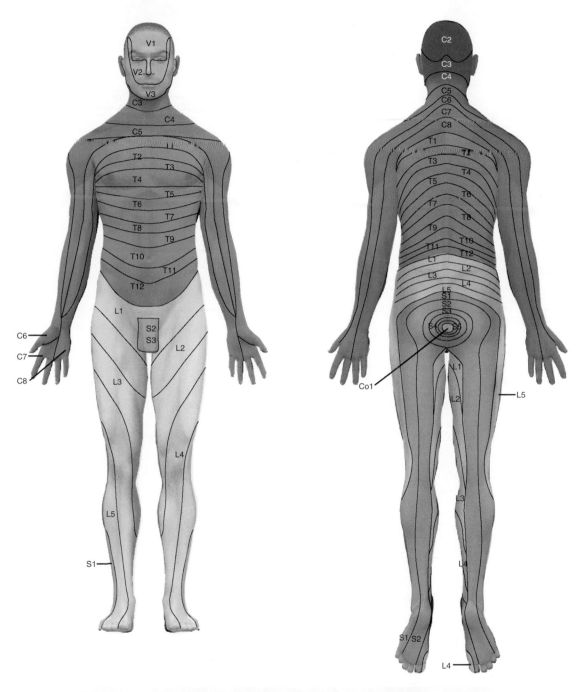

Figure 1-30 Cutaneous distribution (dermatomes) of spinal nerves and the trigeminal nerve (*CN V*).

the dermis from deeper layers are cutaneous branches of veins, arteries, and nerves, which supply but do not invade the overlying epithelial epidermis.

Functions

Mechanical Envelope. The skin acts as a physical barrier, preventing physical damage to and evaporation of underlying tissues.

Organ. *Vitamin D production* takes place in the skin when it is exposed to sunlight. *Heat regulation* of the body is a result of the

constriction or dilation of underlying blood vessels of the skin. Secretions of the sweat glands cool the body upon evaporation. Water, salts, and some urea are *excreted* through the skin glands. Sensations of touch, temperature, and pain are transmitted via cutaneous nerve receptors within the skin.

FASCIA

Deep to the dermal portion of the skin lies another layer of connective tissue, called *fascia*. It contains collagenous and elastic fibers, which are continuous with those of the dermis above (see *Figure 1-32*). There is no clear demarcation,

33

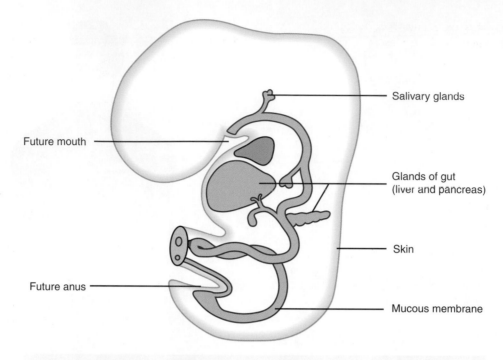

Figure 1-31 Longitudinal section through embryo at 35 days' gestation shows development of external body (covering skin) and internal gut lining (mucosa). Note that two coverings approach each other at sites of future mouth and future anus.

Future mouth

Salivary glands

Glands of gut (liver and pancreas)

Skin

Future anus

Mucous membrane

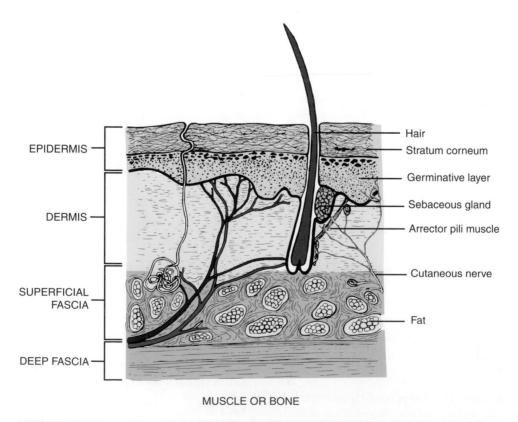

EPIDERMIS

DERMIS

SUPERFICIAL FASCIA

DEEP FASCIA

Hair

Stratum corneum

Germinative layer

Sebaceous gland

Arrector pili muscle

Cutaneous nerve

Fat

MUSCLE OR BONE

Figure 1-32 Skin and fascia.

however, between fascia and dermis. The two basic layers of fascia are superficial and deep fascia.

Superficial Fascia (Tela Subcutanea)

Because this layer is found immediately deep to the dermis, it is also called *subcutaneous tissue*. It contains collagenous and elastic fibers and considerably more fat. The superficial fascia of the ear, eyelid, and penis contains no fat.

Functions. Superficial fascia acts as a **storage depot.** Superficial fascia can contain considerable deposits of both water and fat. **Conduction** is another function. Superficial fascia contains nerves and blood vessels, which are transported to and from the skin above. Superficial fascia provides a **protective cushion.** Stored fat and water provide protection against mechanical shock. The layer of fat and water provides **thermal insulation** against rapid loss of body heat.

Superficial Muscles. Thin sheets of skeletal muscles are found within the superficial fascia of certain areas of the head and neck. In the face they are known collectively as *muscles of facial expression.* Because their insertions are into the skin of the face, the muscles are therefore able to move the skin into various positions or expressions.

Deep Fascia

Deep fascia forms a connective tissue covering or sheath for structures (muscles, vessels, and nerves) deep to the superficial fascia (see *Figure 1-32*). The collagenous fibers are more organized and run in parallel fashion, unlike the unorganized arrangement in the superficial fascia. Deep fascia generally contains little or no fat.

Functions. Deep fascia has three functions. The first function is **conduction.** Blood vessels and nerves are transported by means of the deep fascia to deep underlying structures, such as muscles and organs. Its second function is to facilitate the **movement of muscle.** Muscles wrapped in deep fascia are able to slide over one another. Last, the deep fascia serves as an **attachment for some muscles.** Some muscles, such as the temporalis muscle, gain partial attachment from deep fascia.

Fascial Planes. Areas between layers of deep fascia are termed *fascial clefts,* or *planes.* These sites are possible routes of infection; consequently an understanding of fascial architecture is necessary for the diagnosis and treatment of spread of infection.

SEROUS BODY CAVITIES

During embryonic development, a split occurs in the embryonic mesodermal layer, producing an intraembryonic coelom, or hollow cavity. This cavity develops into four serous membrane–lined body spaces: right and left pleural cavities housing the right and left lungs, the pericardial sac housing the heart, and the peritoneal cavity housing the gut and its associated glands (*Figure 1-33*). Each of these organs initially invades the spaces it ultimately occupies and in doing so assumes the serous membrane coverings of the cavities it invades. In general the serous membrane lining the body cavity is referred to as the ***parietal layer,*** and the serous membrane that covers the visceral organs is termed the ***visceral layer.*** Each of these body cavities is described in greater detail in the appropriate chapters (the pleural and pericardial cavities in Chapter 3 and the peritoneal cavity in Chapter 4).

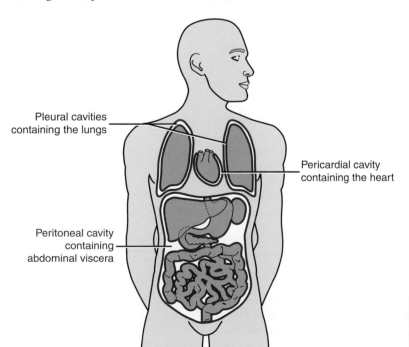

Pleural cavities containing the lungs

Pericardial cavity containing the heart

Peritoneal cavity containing abdominal viscera

Figure 1-33 Scheme of body cavities that are lined with parietal serous membranes. Each contains organs that are covered with visceral serous membranes.

Review Questions

1. The coronal plane _____.
   a. divides the body into equal right and left halves
   b. divides the body into anterior and posterior components
   c. divides the body into superior and inferior components
   d. is parallel to the sagittal plane
   e. is parallel to the transverse plane

2. All of the following structures contain hyaline cartilage EXCEPT _____.
   a. the auricle
   b. apposing surfaces of synovial joints
   c. the nasal septum
   d. the bronchial tree
   e. the larynx

3. An opening or a hole through a bone is termed a _____.
   a. *sulcus*
   b. *fissure*
   c. *foramen*
   d. *fossa*
   e. *tubercle*

4. Which of the following statements concerning joints is FALSE?
   a. The elbow is an example of a hinge or ginglymus synovial joint.
   b. Sutures are synarthrodial joints allowing no movement between the bones they unite.
   c. The joints between vertebral bodies are symphyses.
   d. Synchondroses permit growth between apposing bones.
   e. Proprioceptive nerve endings or Ruffini corpuscles in the capsular ligament of a synovial joint convey a sense of pain.

5. Muscle fibers arranged for power rather than ranges of movement are found in _____.
   a. parallel muscles
   b. converging muscles
   c. sphincter muscles
   d. digastric muscles
   e. pennate muscles

6. Which of the following statements regarding characteristics of smooth muscle is FALSE?
   a. Smooth muscle is capable of rapid, powerful contractions and fatigues quickly.
   b. Smooth muscle has no bony origin or insertion.
   c. Most smooth muscle is controlled by autonomic efferent nerves.
   d. Smooth muscle is nonstriated.
   e. Smooth muscle, in hollow organs or tubes, contracts to expel contents.

7. Which of the following statements concerning blood vessels is FALSE?
   a. A capillary wall consists of a single cell layer of endothelial cells.
   b. The tunica media of a terminal arteriole consists of a single muscle cell layer.
   c. The tunica media of the aorta contains elastic tissue but no smooth muscle.
   d. The retina of the eye receives good collateral circulation.
   e. An arteriovenous anastomosis shunts blood across the capillary bed.

8. Which of the following statements concerning the lymphatic system is FALSE?
   a. Lymph is propelled through the lymphatic vessels by the heart.
   b. Lymphocytes are produced in the bone marrow.
   c. Lymph nodes filter out bacteria, viruses, and cancer cells.
   d. Lymphatic vessels returning from the gut contain relatively high amounts of fat.
   e. The thoracic duct drains the lower limbs, abdomen, and chest wall.

9. The connective tissue sheath that intimately surrounds a peripheral nerve is termed the _____.
   a. *sarcolemma*
   b. *endoneurium*
   c. *perineurium*
   d. *deep investing fascia*
   e. *epineurium*

10. The parasympathetic nervous system _____.
    a. speeds up the heart
    b. decreases peristalsis
    c. closes gut sphincters
    d. is necessary to life
    e. decreases glandular secretions

11. Internal epithelial (mucous membrane) linings give rise to the _____.
    a. teeth
    b. liver
    c. pancreas
    d. mucous glands
    e. all of the above

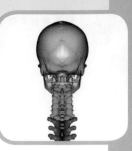

Chapter 2

The Back

1. Skeletal Parts 37

2. Surface Features of the Back 43

3. Spinal Cord... 43

4. Muscles of the Back.. 47

The skeleton of the back is presented in *Figure 2-1*. It consists of the skull, the vertebral column, and the ribs, which are appendages of the thoracic component of the vertebral column.

1. Skeletal Parts

POSTERIOR ASPECT OF THE SKULL

The various views and bones of the skull are considered in Chapter 6. Only the posterior aspect of the skull is described here. The posterior surface of the skull is convex and is commonly called the *occiput.* The **external occipital crest** is a midline ridge running superiorly from the foramen magnum. Arising from this crest are two transverse lines, the **inferior nuchal line** and above it the **superior nuchal line.** The external occipital crest ends at the midpoint of the superior nuchal line as a lump called the *inion,* or *external occipital protuberance.* Some muscles of the back extend up to this area of the skull and insert into these features.

VERTEBRAL COLUMN

The vertebral column, or spine, consists of 33 vertebrae: 7 cervical, 12 thoracic, 5 lumbar, 5 sacral (fused), and 4 coccygeal (fused); and the joints between the stacked components.

Vertebrae: Typical Features

All vertebrae have certain features in common. Learning these features and then noting regional differences makes the study of vertebrae far less difficult. A midthoracic vertebra is generally chosen as exhibiting features common to most other vertebrae (*Figure 2-2, A*).

The **body** is a spool-shaped mass of bone that provides support. All vertebrae (except C1) have a body. A vertebral arch is fastened to the posterior aspect of the body. The arch has two components: a *pedicle,* or short bony root, which fastens the arch to the body; and a *flattened lamina,* which forms the roof of the arch and body. The vertebral arch and body form the *vertebral foramen,* which encloses and protects the delicate spinal cord within. The arches in an articulated *vertebral column* form the vertebral canal, which houses the entire spinal cord.

Bilateral **superior** and **inferior articulating processes** are situated between the pedicle and lamina. They are bilateral articulating facets that are covered with hyaline cartilage and allow the vertebra above to articulate with the vertebra below (*Figure 2-2, B*).

Bilateral **superior** and **inferior vertebral notches** are found on the superior and inferior aspects of the pedicles. In the articulated spinal column the superior and inferior notches form the **intervertebral foramina**, which *transmit the spinal nerves.*

Attached to the vertebral arch are three processes that provide attachment for muscles of the back and therefore *act as levers in response to muscle contractions.* A single **spinous process** extends posteriorly and inferiorly from the top of the vertebral arch. Arising laterally from the arch are two **transverse processes.**

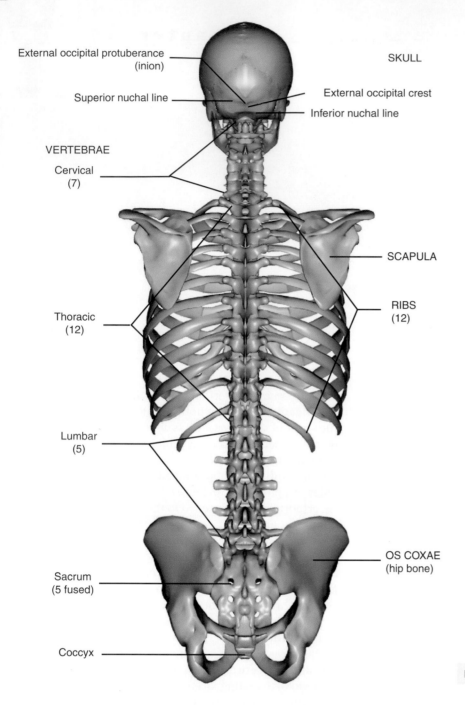

External occipital protuberance (inion)

SKULL

Superior nuchal line

External occipital crest

Inferior nuchal line

VERTEBRAE

Cervical (7)

SCAPULA

RIBS (12)

Thoracic (12)

Lumbar (5)

OS COXAE (hip bone)

Sacrum (5 fused)

Coccyx

Figure 2-1 Skeleton of back.

Cervical Vertebrae

Of the seven cervical vertebrae, C3 to C6 are considered typical of the cervical region in that they exhibit all of the features of vertebrae in general. They also display certain features that distinguish them as cervical vertebrae.

Typical Features. In addition to the general features, cervical vertebrae exhibit (1) a **transverse foramen,** a hole through the transverse processes to transmit the vertebral artery and vein; (2) a **bifid spinous process;** and

(3) a transverse process, which ends laterally as an **anterior** and a **posterior tubercle** for attachment of cervical muscles (*Figure 2-3, C*).

Atypical Features

Atlas (C1). The first cervical vertebra (*Figure 2-3, A*) differs from the remaining cervical vertebrae in the following ways: (1) the concave superior articulating facet is *bean-shaped* to accommodate the reciprocally shaped occipital condyles of the skull; (2) the body of the atlas is lost early in development and becomes fused to the

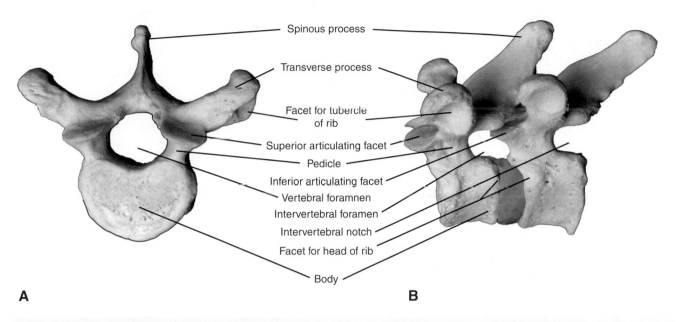

Figure 2-2 **A,** Superior view of a typical vertebra. **B,** Left lateral view of two articulated vertebrae.

body of the axis below, leaving only an anterior arch in its place; (3) there is no anterior tubercle on the transverse process; and (4) it exhibits two grooves for the vertebral arteries just posterior to the superior articulating facets.

The atlas consists of four segments: an **anterior** and **posterior arch**, and two lateral masses from which the transverse processes project laterally. The atlas has no spine but has a small elevation on the posterior arch termed the *posterior tubercle* (not to be confused with the posterior tubercle of the transverse processes).

Axis (C2). This vertebra (*Figure 2-3, B*) differs from the typical vertebrae of the cervical region in two respects: (1) the original body of C1 is fused to the body of the axis as the **dens,** or **odontoid process;** and (2) the axis has no anterior tubercle on its transverse process.

C7. This vertebra (*Figure 2-3, D*) displays two atypical features: (1) it is the last component of the cervical segment and closely resembles the thoracic vertebrae below, with a long slender spinous process in contrast to the bifid spines of the vertebrae above; and (2) it has no anterior tubercle on its transverse process. Although it resembles a thoracic vertebra, it is distinctly cervical because it does have a transverse foramen.

Thoracic Vertebrae

The 12 thoracic vertebrae (see *Figure 2-2*) exhibit a number of features that distinguish them from other vertebrae: (1) the spinous process is long and slender; (2) the body has an articulating facet for the head of a rib; (3) the transverse process has an articulating facet for the tubercle of a rib; and (4) the body is heart-shaped.

Lumbar Vertebrae

Three features distinguish the five lumbar vertebrae (*Figure 2-4*): (1) they are relatively massive, with bean-shaped bodies; (2) they have no facets for ribs nor do the transverse processes possess transverse foramina, as in the cervical vertebrae; and (3) the spinous processes are not bifid nor slender but square-shaped.

The Sacrum

The five elements of the sacrum (*Figure 2-5*) are fused to form a solid triangular mass. The **spinous processes** are represented posteriorly by a median crest. A **lateral mass** representing fused transverse processes terminates laterally as two ear-shaped articular surfaces for the right and left os coxae. Superiorly, the **sacral promontory** projects anteriorly, and the **sacral canal** continues the vertebral canal inferiorly from the lumbar region. Leaving the sacral canal on either side are four anterior and posterior **pelvic foramina,** which transmit sacral anterior and posterior rami.

The Coccyx

The coccyx is a triangular mass formed by the fusion of four small segments. In humans it represents the *vestigial tail*.

THE ARTICULATED SPINE

The stacked vertebrae and their intervening intervertebral discs make up the total length of the spinal column (*Figure 2-6*). In the neonate the fetal, or **primary, curvature** of the vertebral column is present. A convex cervical secondary curvature appears in the cervical area when the child

39

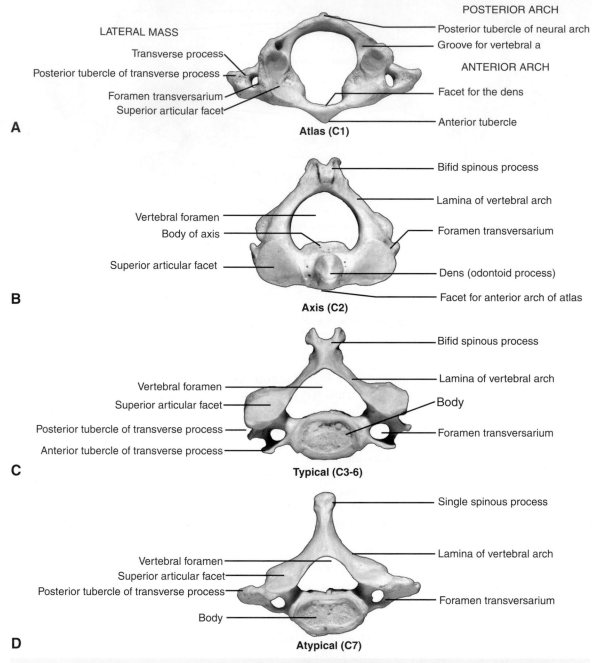

POSTERIOR ARCH

LATERAL MASS

Transverse process —— Posterior tubercle of neural arch

Posterior tubercle of transverse process —— Groove for vertebral a

Foramen transversarium —— ANTERIOR ARCH

Superior articular facet —— Facet for the dens

A —— Anterior tubercle

Atlas (C1)

—— Bifid spinous process

—— Lamina of vertebral arch

Vertebral foramen ——

Body of axis —— Foramen transversarium

Superior articular facet ——

—— Dens (odontoid process)

—— Facet for anterior arch of atlas

B

Axis (C2)

—— Bifid spinous process

—— Lamina of vertebral arch

Vertebral foramen ——

Superior articular facet —— Body

Posterior tubercle of transverse process —— Foramen transversarium

Anterior tubercle of transverse process ——

C

Typical (C3-6)

—— Single spinous process

—— Lamina of vertebral arch

Vertebral foramen ——

Superior articular facet ——

Posterior tubercle of transverse process —— Foramen transversarium

Body ——

D

Atypical (C7)

Figure 2-3 Superior view of cervical vertebrae. **A,** Atlas vertebra (C1). **B,** Axis vertebra (C2). **C,** Typical vertebra (C3 to C6). **D,** Atypical vertebra (C7).

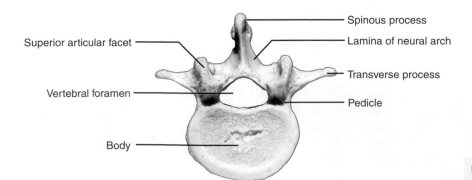

Spinous process

Superior articular facet —— Lamina of neural arch

Transverse process

Vertebral foramen ——

—— Pedicle

Body ——

Figure 2-4 Superior view of lumbar vertebra.

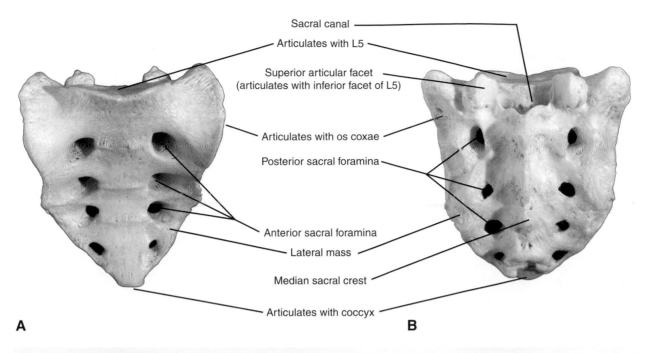

Sacral canal

Articulates with L5

Superior articular facet
(articulates with inferior facet of L5)

Articulates with os coxae

Posterior sacral foramina

Anterior sacral foramina

Lateral mass

Median sacral crest

Articulates with coccyx

A   **B**

Figure 2-5 Sacrum. **A,** Anterior view. **B,** Posterior view.

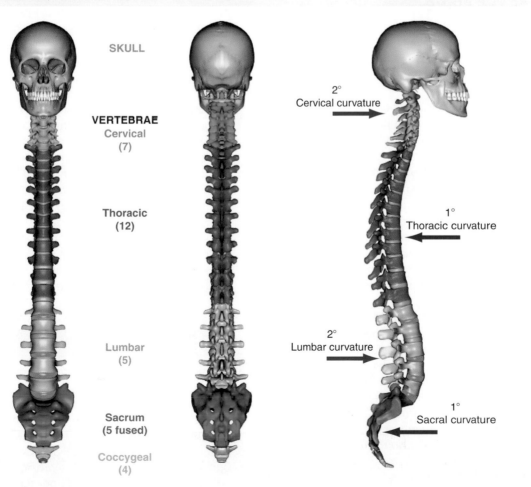

SKULL

VERTEBRAE
Cervical
(7)

Thoracic
(12)

Lumbar
(5)

Sacrum
(5 fused)

Coccygeal
(4)

2°
Cervical curvature

1°
Thoracic curvature

2°
Lumbar curvature

1°
Sacral curvature

Figure 2-6 The articulated spine. **A,** Anterior view. **B,** Posterior view. **C,** Right lateral view.

learns to hold the head erect and to sit up. Similarly, when the child learns to walk, a secondary curvature appears in the lumbosacral region. The curvatures are formed by the intervertebral discs of the curved regions assuming a wedge shape.

> ### CLINICAL NOTES
>
> There are three main types of abnormal curvatures of the spine.
>
> **Kyphosis** is an exaggeration in the primary curvature of the thoracic region. It can be caused by muscle weakness or degenerative changes in the vertebral bodies and intervertebral discs.
>
> **Lordosis** is an exaggeration in the lumbosacral secondary curvature, or small of the back.
>
> **Scoliosis** is an abnormal lateral deviation of the spine. Viewed from behind, the spine should lie in a straight line.

JOINTS OF THE SPINE

Vertebrae articulate with each other between adjacent vertebral bodies; articular facets; and laminae, transverse processes, and spinous processes.

Joints Between Bodies

A symphysis type of joint is found between vertebral bodies (*Figure 2-7*). Hyaline cartilage lines the bony surfaces of the apposing bodies. Interposed is a disc consisting of concentric layers of fibrocartilaginous fibers (**anulus fibrosis**) surrounding a nucleus of fibrogelatinous material (**pulpal nucleus**), which is a remnant of the early notochord. The discs act as shock absorbers and in younger individuals (aged 20 years or younger) are quite strong. **Anterior** and **posterior longitudinal ligaments** run along the anterior and posterior surfaces of the vertebral bodies from the base of the skull to the sacrum, binding the components of the vertebral column together.

Joints Between Articular Facets

Bilateral synovial joints are found between the inferior articulating facets and the superior facets of the vertebra below. The angulations of the articulating facets determine the types of movements in the various segments of the spinal column. The cervical and lumbar vertebrae allow a range of *flexion* (bending forward) and *lateral flexion* (bending to the side). These movements are restricted in the thorax. The lumbar vertebrae can also *rotate* or twist.

Other Intervertebral Joints

Fibrous tissue joins the adjacent laminae, spinous processes, and transverse processes between vertebrae in what is called a *syndesmosis* type of joint.

> ### CLINICAL NOTES
>
> The lower lumbar and upper sacral regions are susceptible to aging and repeated stress that can manifest as **low back pain** possibly radiating down into the buttocks or lower limbs (**sciatica**). There are several causes of low back pain, but two causes can be attributable to degenerative changes in the intervertebral discs, particularly those between L4 and L5 and between L5 and S1.
>
> **Loss of Vertical Dimension**
>
> Compression of the disc and a decrease in the height of the disc can constrict the intervertebral foramen, with resultant entrapment or increased pressure on the spinal nerve as it emerges from the foramen (see *Figure 2-7, B*).
>
> **Herniated Disc**
>
> Flexing the spine anteriorly and laterally causes the disc to bulge posteriorly and to the contralateral side. Time and wear take their toll and can weaken the posterolateral sides of the intervertebral disc and the posterior ligaments. The discs in the lumbosacral region are particularly susceptible to herniation of the **nucleus pulposus**. This herniation involves a rupture through the anulus fibrosis and posterior longitudinal ligament in a posterior or posterolateral direction and impinges on the nerve roots of the cauda equina within the vertebral canal (see *Figure 2-7, C*). The location and extent of the herniation determine the sensory and/or motor symptoms that accompany this condition. The nerve roots usually affected are L5 and S1, two contributors to the sciatic nerve (see Chapter 10). Impingement on roots results in sensory symptoms (pain) along the path of the sciatic nerve (**sciatica**). Impingement on roots can result in variable motor symptoms (e.g., weakness and in extreme cases paralysis of muscles supplied by the sciatic nerve).

> ### CLINICAL NOTES
>
> These synovial joints are also susceptible to acute injury and wear and tear over time and are another source of back pain. Participation in activities to which the individual is unaccustomed and movements that tax the joints can result in inflammation and acute pain, particularly in the cervical and lower back regions. Continued injury can result in chronic pain caused by lax (loose) joint capsules and bony formations around the articular facets that encroach on the intervertebral foramina and the spinal nerves they transmit.

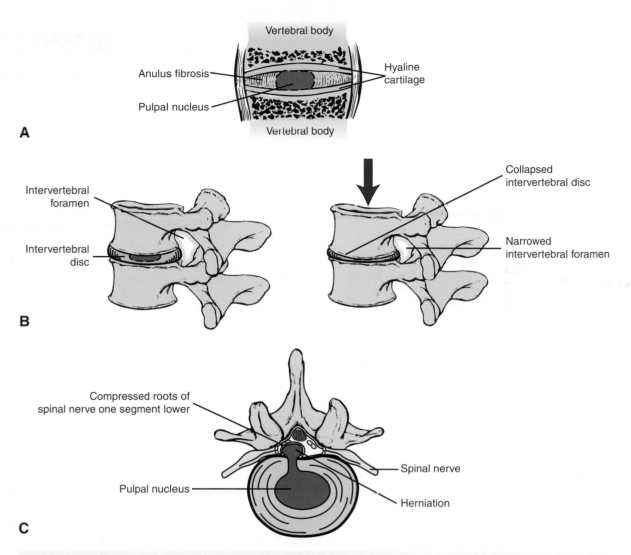

Figure 2-7 A, Coronal section through adjacent vertebral bodies to show intervertebral disc. **B,** Compressed intervertebral disc with resultant narrowing of intervertebral foramen. **C,** Herniated nucleus pulposus of intervertebral disc compressing nerve roots.

2. Surface Features of the Back

The surface features of the back aid in identifying levels of the vertebral column and spinal cord, posterior positions of the thoracic and abdominal viscera for clinical examination. In the erect position the **spine of C7** (vertebra prominens) is normally the only spine visible (*Figure 2-8*). The **median sulcus of the back** lies immediately above the **intergluteal sulcus.** A median sulcus that deviates laterally would indicate scoliosis described previously. To either side of the interior end of the median sulcus are dimples that indicate the positions of the **posterior superior iliac spines** of the os coxae.

3. Spinal Cord

LOCATION AND LENGTH

In the fetus the spinal cord runs from the base of the skull through the entire length of the vertebral canal. As the child grows, the vertebral column grows faster than the spinal cord so that the spinal cord ultimately ends at vertebral level L1 or L2 when the individual is fully grown. The final length is approximately 44 cm.

EXTERNAL FEATURES
Swellings
The spinal cord features two swellings: a **cervical swelling** at spinal cord level C5 to T1, which gives rise

43

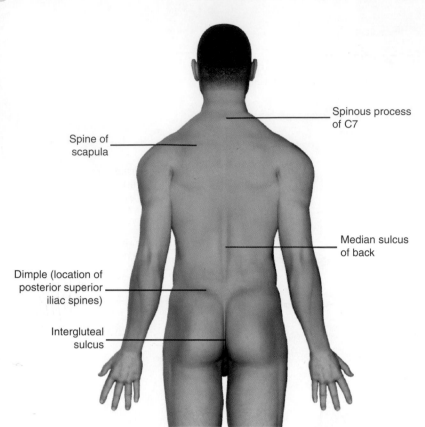

Spinous process of C7

Spine of scapula

Median sulcus of back

Dimple (location of posterior superior iliac spines)

Intergluteal sulcus

Figure 2-8 Surface features of the back.

to the brachial plexus of the upper limb; and a **lumbosacral swelling** at spinal cord level T12 to S4, which gives rise to the *lumbosacral plexus* of the lower limb (*Figure 2-9*).

Spinal Nerves

There are **31 pairs of spinal nerves**, which arise anteriorly and posteriorly as spinal rootlets. The roots join to form spinal nerves proper. Nerves arising from each side of the spinal cord *include* **8 cervical, 12 thoracic, 5 lumbar, 5 sacral,** and **1 coccygeal.**

Because of the discrepancy in length between the spinal cord and the vertebral canal in the adult, the lower lumbar and sacral nerve roots must stream downward to reach and exit through the intervertebral foramina at their respective vertebral levels. The nerve roots descending past the termination of the spinal cord at L2 resemble a horse's tail and are appropriately termed the *cauda equina* (see *Figures 2-9* and *2-10*).

Sulci and Fissures

Longitudinal sulci and fissures groove the surface of the spinal cord. The main ones are the **dorsal median sulcus**, which continues into the substance of the cord as the **dorsal median septum**, and the **ventral median fissure.**

INTERNAL FEATURES

The spinal cord in section consists of a nuclear column of **gray matter,** a surrounding mass of **white matter,** and a **central canal** (*Figure 2-11*).

Gray Matter

This nuclear area can be divided into **posterior (dorsal) horns, anterior (ventral) horns,** an **intermediate area** between the horns, and **intermediolateral horns** (in the thoracic region only). Each of these four areas can be further subdivided into various nuclei based on function, and this information can be found in standard neuroanatomy textbooks.

White Matter

The horns of the gray matter divide the white matter into a **posterior funiculus** between the two posterior horns, an **anterior funiculus** between the anterior horns, and **lateral funiculi** between the anterior and posterior horns. The funiculi can be further subdivided into regions containing specific ascending or descending tracts of fibers.

Central Canal

A narrow canal containing **cerebrospinal fluid (CSF)** runs the length of the spinal cord. It is a remnant of the lumen of the *embryonic neural tube* and is continuous with the ventricular system of the brain.

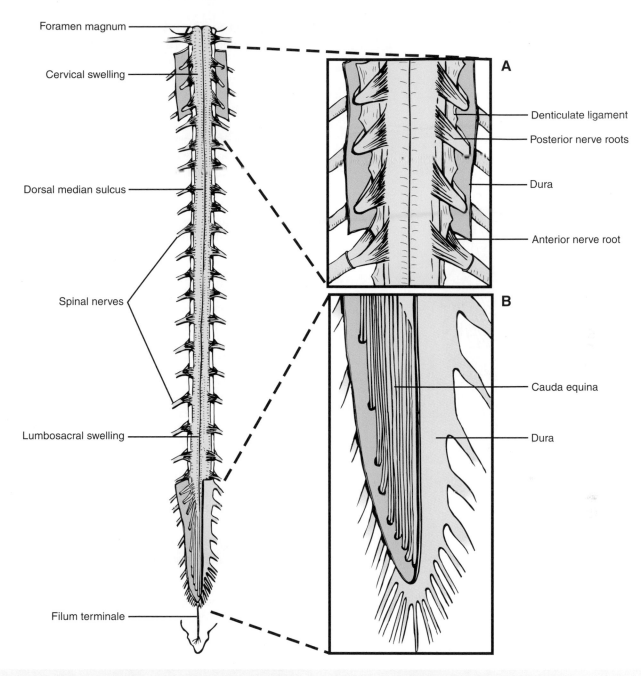

Figure 2-9 Posterior view of exposed spinal cord. **A,** Close-up view of cervical area. **B,** Close-up view of lumbosacral area.

COVERINGS (MENINGES)

The spinal cord and the brain are wrapped in three protective coverings: **pia mater,** the innermost layer; **arachnoid mater,** the intermediate layer; and **dura mater,** the tough membranous outer layer (*Figure 2-12*).

Pia Mater

The pia mater is a fine membrane that covers the spinal cord intimately, following each fissure and groove inward. In addition, it covers the spinal rootlets and extends laterally between the rootlets as a scalloped **denticulate ligament,** which anchors the spinal cord to the walls of the vertebral canal (see *Figures 2-9* and *2-12*). At the end of the spinal cord the pia mater continues inferiorly as the **filum terminale** to anchor the spinal cord to the coccyx below.

Arachnoid Mater

The arachnoid mater is a filmy layer closely applied to the innermost surface of the outer meningeal layer, the dura. Arachnoid means spiderlike, referring to the weblike filaments that extend inward to the pia mater.

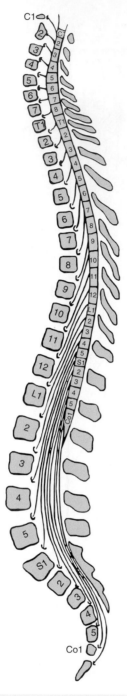

Figure 2-10 Relationship of spinal cord and spinal nerves to vertebral column. Spinal cord ends at vertebral level L2, so remaining lumbar and sacral nerve roots must stream downward to exit at respective intervertebral foramina.

Dura Mater

The dura mater is the outermost layer of the meninges and consists of a tough, heavy, durable membrane.

MENINGEAL SPACES

The meninges are associated with three spaces: the **subarachnoid space, subdural space,** and **extradural (epidural) space.**

Subarachnoid Space

The subarachnoid space lies between the arachnoid layer outwardly and the pia mater inwardly. This space contains CSF, which bathes and protects the spinal cord.

Subdural Space

The subdural space lies just below the dura mater and is a potential space only. Normally this space is obliterated by the underlying pressure of the CSF and opens only under pathological conditions, such as subdural hemorrhage.

Extradural Space

The extradural space lies outside the dura mater but within the bony vertebral canal. It is normally filled with fat.

PROTECTION

The spinal cord is protected by (1) the three layers of meninges, (2) the CSF of the subarachnoid space, and (3) the fat of the extradural space.

BLOOD SUPPLY

The arterial supply to the spinal cord is from a single **anterior spinal artery** and two to four **posterior spinal arteries.** Both sets of arteries are fed by segmental branches of the *vertebral artery* in the cervical region (see Chapter 5), *intercostal arteries* in the thoracic region (see Chapter 3) and *lumbar* and *median sacral branches* in the abdominal region. The venous drainage is to the **vertebral venous plexus,** which drains to the *superior vena cava.*

CLINICAL NOTES

Meningitis

Meningitis is a potentially lethal inflammation of the brain or spinal cord meninges caused by bacterial or viral infections that spread hematogenously (are bloodborne) into the CSF. CSF contains low levels of antibodies and white blood cells, allowing the infection to spread unchecked by the body's defenses. Immediate antibiotic or antiinfective and supportive therapy are necessary.

Spinal Tap

A spinal tap is a method of obtaining CSF for analysis by inserting a needle into the subarachnoid space (*Figure 2-13*). The spinal cord ends at L1 to L2. The dura mater and arachnoid mater, however, continue down to level S2. Thus a needle inserted between the spines at L3-L4 or L4-L5 will pass through the dura mater and arachnoid mater and enter the subarachnoid space without injuring the spinal cord.

Continued

Running through the subarachnoid sac below L2 are the various lumbar and sacral spinal nerve roots collectively called the *cauda equina*. These roots form nerves that ultimately supply the pelvis, perineum, and lower limbs. These nerves are frequently blocked for obstetrical and other surgical procedures. There are two methods for achieving anesthesia in these regions. Both require insertion of a needle between L3 and L4 or L4 and L5.

Epidural anesthesia is accomplished by injecting into the *epidural space*. An epidural drip continues to administer small doses over time. The anesthetic fluid diffuses through the dura mater into the subarachnoid space to contact the nerve roots and cause anesthesia.

Spinal anesthesia requires injection at the same spinal level, but the needle is directed deeper through the dura mater to enter the *subarachnoid space*. The position of the patient, gravity, and the specific gravity of the anesthetic agent are all important factors in this procedure because anesthetic agents can diffuse through the CSF to higher spinal cord levels with unwanted results. If it reaches the thoracic level, the anesthetic can block sympathetic nerves, and if it reaches the cervical level, it can block nerves that supply the diaphragm.

4. Muscles of the Back

The muscles found on the back can be divided into three groups on the basis of position and function. There are **superficial muscles, intermediate muscles, and deep (intrinsic) muscles** of the back. These muscle groups occupy three layers.

SUPERFICIAL GROUP

The superficial group consists of muscles that functionally belong to the upper limb (*Figure 2-14*). They have their origins on the back but insert into the upper limb. These muscles include the **trapezius muscle**, the **latissimus dorsi muscle**, the **levator scapulae muscle**, and the **major** and **minor rhomboid muscles**. These muscles are described with the upper limb muscles in Chapter 9.

INTERMEDIATE GROUP

The intermediate group of muscles is active during *respiration* (*Figure 2-15*) and includes the **serratus posterior superior muscle** and the **serratus posterior inferior muscle**. These muscles are described with the muscles of the thorax in Chapter 3.

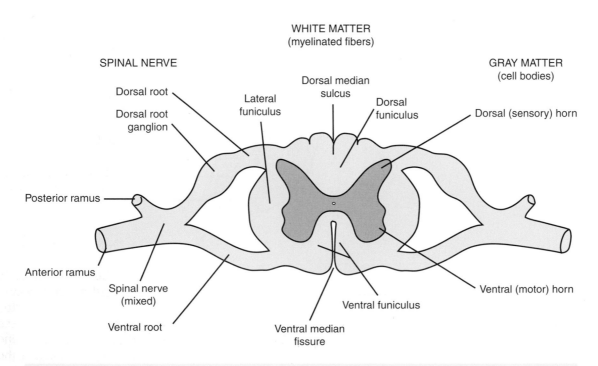

Figure 2-11 Cross section of spinal cord to show internal features.

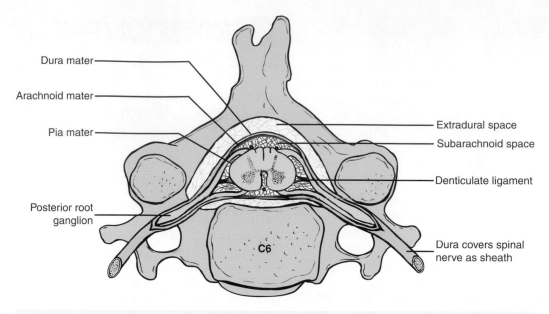

Dura mater

Arachnoid mater

Pia mater

Posterior root
ganglion

Extradural space

Subarachnoid space

Denticulate ligament

Dura covers spinal
nerve as sheath

C6

Figure 2-12 Cervical vertebra with spinal cord, coverings, spinal nerve roots, and spinal nerves in situ.

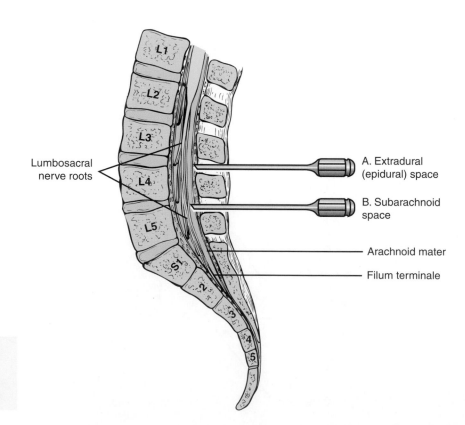

Lumbosacral
nerve roots

A. Extradural
(epidural) space

B. Subarachnoid
space

Arachnoid mater

Filum terminale

Figure 2-13 A, Needle in extradural
(epidural) space for epidural anesthesia
of lumbosacral nerve root. **B,** Needle in
subarachnoid space for cerebrospinal tap
or spinal anesthesia.

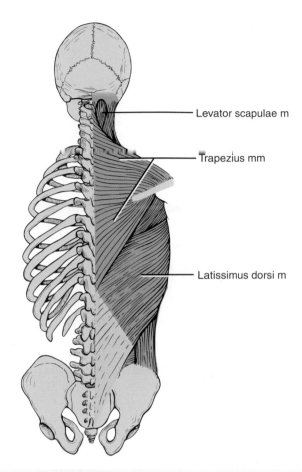

Levator scapulae m

Trapezius mm

Latissimus dorsi m

Figure 2-14 Superficial muscles of back belonging to upper limb.

DEEP GROUP

The deep group of muscles represents the true, or intrinsic, muscles of the back (see *Figures 2-15* and *2-16*). There are many muscles in this group, and memorizing

their individual origins and insertions is pointless. The descriptions that follow* and *Table 2-1* are offered for reference purposes only. There are, however, some basic points that should be learned. In general the muscles originate at lower levels and ascend in staggered fashion to insert into higher levels. Collectively they act to extend the vertebral column and head and to help maintain posture. They receive a segmented blood supply from somatic branches of the aorta and a segmented nerve supply from the posterior rami of spinal nerves.

MOVEMENTS OF THE SPINE

Only the movements of the thoracic and lumbar components of the spine are considered in this chapter, and they are listed in *Table 2-2* along with the muscles that produce the movement (*Figure 2-17*). The ligaments of the vertebral column prevent excessive movement. The movements of the cervical spine and head are considered in Chapter 5.

CLINICAL NOTES

Back Strain

This is a common problem that arises following extreme movements of the back that result in microscopic rupture of intervertebral ligaments or muscle fibers of the intrinsic muscles of the back. This is generally followed by muscles in the surrounding area going into spasm and the sufferer assuming a "lopsided" or "guarded" stance.

---

*Intrinsic Muscles of the Back
The deep group is further divided into three layers.

1. Superficial Layer: The muscle fibers of this layer run from vertebral spines upward and laterally to higher transverse processes. Superiorly the muscle fibers insert into the skull and are termed the *capitis portion* of the muscle.

   Splenius muscle: The fibers of this muscle originate from the spinous processes of the upper six thoracic vertebrae and the lower half of the ligamentum nuchae. They insert into the transverse processes of the upper three cervical vertebrae (cervicis portion) and into the mastoid process and superior nuchal line of the skull (capitis portion).

2. Intermediate Layer: These muscles are collectively called the *erector spinae muscle*. The fibers run from the pelvis to the skull, with several stops along the way, as three parallel bands of muscle.

   Iliocostalis muscle: This is the most lateral column, originating from the iliac crest and lower ribs to ascend six segments at a span into higher ribs. Fibers arising from higher ribs ascend to insert into the posterior tubercles (costal elements) of the cervical vertebrae.

   Longissimus muscle: The longissimus muscle is the intermediate column and runs from transverse process to higher transverse processes. From the sacrum, it ascends to the transverse process of the thoracic vertebrae (thoracis portion), to the transverse process of the cervical

vertebrae (cervicis portion), and to the mastoid process of the skull (capitis portion).

   Spinalis muscle: This is the most medial band of fibers, arising from the sacrum and inserting into ever-higher spinous processes. Inserting at the thoracic level is the thoracis portion and at the cervical level is the cervicis portion.

3. Deep (Innermost) Group: *Transversospinalis muscle* is the collective name given to this layer of muscle because it runs from transverse processes of lower vertebrae upward and medially to vertebral spines at higher levels.

   Semispinalis muscle: This muscle spans at least five vertebrae at a time and inserts into the thoracic spines (thoracis portion), cervical spines and ligamentum nuchae (cervicis portion), and the superior nuchal line of the skull (capitis portion).

   Multifidus muscle: This is a deeper muscle that spans only three vertebrae before ascending higher as another bundle of fibers.

   Rotatores muscle: This muscle is deeper still and spans adjacent vertebrae.

   Minor deep muscles: Interspinales are tiny muscles running from vertebral spines to the next highest spine; intertransversarii are similarly small but run from a transverse process to the next highest transverse process.

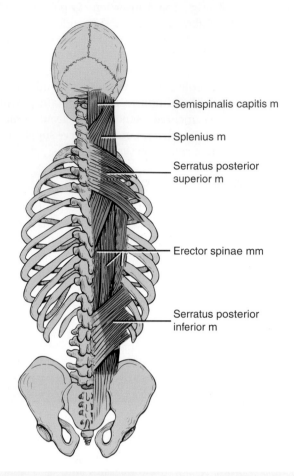

Semispinalis capitis m

Splenius m

Serratus posterior superior m

Erector spinae mm

Serratus posterior inferior m

Figure 2-15 Intermediate and deep (intrinsic) muscles of back.

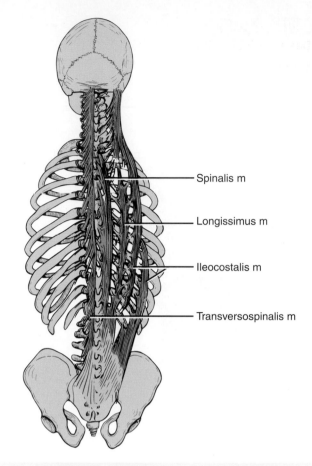

Spinalis m

Longissimus m

Ileocostalis m

Transversospinalis m

Figure 2-16 Deep intrinsic muscles of back. Muscle fibers that insert into thoracic region are termed *thoracis*; into cervical region, *cervicis*; and into skull, *capitis*.

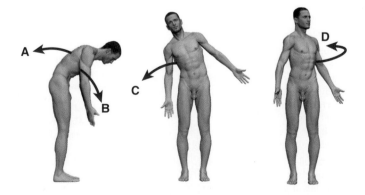

Figure 2-17 Movements of the back. **A, B,** Flexion and extension. **C,** Lateral flexion. **D,** Rotation.

TABLE 2-1

Deep (Intrinsic) Muscles of the Back

Muscle	Origin	Insertion	Action	Nerve
Splenius (capitis and cervicis)	Capitis: lower part of ligamentum nuchae and lower cervical spines	Capitis: mastoid process and superior nuchal line	Together: extend head and neck	Segmented PR of spinal nerves
	Cervicis: spines of T3 to T6	Cervicis: transverse processes of C1 to C4	Individually: flexes head and neck laterally, rotates head to ipsilateral side	
Erector spinae	Inferior origins: iliac crest, spines of sacrum, lumbar and last two thoracic vertebrae Intermediate origins: ribs, transverse processes, and spines	Ribs, transverse processes, and spines of higher vertebrae; skull	Together: extend back Individually: flexes back laterally and rotates back	Segmented PR of spinal nerves
Iliocostalis (lumborum, thoracis, cervicis)	Body of erector spinae, ribs at ever-ascending levels	Lumborum: lower ribs Thoracis: upper ribs Cervicis: transverse processes of C4 to C6 (costal element)		
Longissimus (thoracis, cervicis, capitis)	Body of erector spinae, transverse processes of successively ascending vertebrae	Thoracis: transverse processes of thoracic vertebrae Cervicis: transverse processes of cervical vertebrae Capitis: mastoid process of skull		
Spinalis (thoracis, cervicis, capitis)	Spines of successively ascending vertebrae	Thoracis: spines of thoracic vertebrae Cervicis: spines of cervical vertebrae Capitis: occipital area of skull between superior and inferior nuchal lines		
Transversospinalis	Transverse processes of successively higher vertebrae	Spines of successively higher vertebrae	Together: extend head and spine Individually: flexes laterally and rotates spine	Segmented PR of spinal nerves
Semispinalis (thoracis, cervicis, capitis) spans five to six vertebrae	Transverse processes	Thoracis: spines of thoracic vertebrae Cervicis: spines of cervical vertebrae Capitis: between superior and inferior nuchal lines		

Continued

51

TABLE 2-1

Deep (Intrinsic) Muscles of the Back—cont'd

Muscle	Origin	Insertion	Action	Nerve
Multifidus spans three vertebrae	Transverse processes	Spines of higher vertebrae		
Rotatores spans two vertebrae	Transverse processes	Spines of higher vertebrae		
Interspinales	Spine below	Spine above	Extend and rotate spine	Segmented PR of spinal nerves
Intertransversarii	Transverse process below	Transverse process above	Together: stabilize the spine Individually: flexes the spine laterally	Segmented PR of spinal nerves

PR, Posterior rami.

TABLE 2-2

Muscles Responsible for Movements of Back

	Flexion	**Extension**	**Lateral flexion**	**Rotation**
Abdominal Muscles	Bilateral actions of rectus abdominis, external oblique, internal oblique		Unilateral actions of: external oblique, internal oblique	Unilateral actions of: external oblique, Contralateral actions of: internal oblique
Back Muscles		Bilateral actions of: erector spinae, transversospinalis	Unilateral actions of: erector spinae, transversospinalis	Unilateral actions of: erector spinae, transversospinalis

Review Questions

1. All cervical vertebrae feature _____.
   a. a vertebral body
   b. a bifid spine
   c. anterior and posterior tubercles on the transverse process
   d. an anterior arch
   e. a transverse foramen

2. Which of the following statements concerning typical intervertebral joints is FALSE?
   a. Vertebral bodies are separated by cartilaginous and fibrous elements.
   b. A herniated disc that impinges on anterior roots results in variable sensory symptoms.
   c. Vertebral bodies are bound together by anterior and posterior longitudinal ligaments.
   d. The pulpal nucleus of the intervertebral disc is a remnant of the embryonic notochord.
   e. Articular processes of adjacent vertebrae are separated by synovial joints.

3. The spinal cord, in the adult, extends from the base of the skull to vertebral level _____.
   a. L2
   b. L5
   c. S1
   d. S5
   e. Co1

4. The cauda equina of the spinal cord consists of _____.
   a. anterior and posterior nerve roots
   b. anterior rami
   c. posterior rami
   d. spinal nerves
   e. long extensions of dura mater

5. Pia mater of the spinal cord _____.
   a. is found immediately below the dura
   b. forms lateral supportive structures termed the *denticulate ligaments*
   c. is a tough membrane that protects the spinal cord
   d. is routinely punctured during a spinal tap
   e. is loosely applied to the surface of the spinal cord

6. Scoliosis is _____.
   a. an exaggeration of the primary curvature of the spine
   b. an exaggeration of the lumbosacral secondary curvature of the spine
   c. an exaggeration of the cervical secondary curvature of the spine
   d. a lateral deviation of the spine
   e. a ruptured intervertebral disc

7. Which of the following statements concerning the muscles of the back is FALSE?
   a. The superficial layer of muscles originates on the back and inserts into bones of the upper limb.
   b. The intermediate layer of muscles acts to maintain posture.
   c. The deep intrinsic muscles receive a segmented arterial supply from branches of the aorta.
   d. The deep intrinsic muscles act to extend the spine and head.
   e. The deep intrinsic muscles are innervated by segmented branches of posterior rami of spinal nerves.

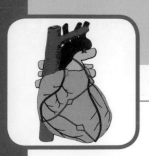

Chapter 3

The Thorax

1. Skeleton and Divisions 54

2. The Thoracic or Chest Wall.................................. 58

3. The Pleural Cavities and Lungs............................ 63

4. The Mediastinum 68

1. Skeleton and Divisions

The thorax, or chest region, is a hollow body cavity enclosed by a thoracic bony and muscular wall. Contained within the thoracic cavity are the major organs of **circulation** and **respiration.**

The thoracic cavity extends superiorly from the dome of the thoracic diaphragm to the cervical region just above the first rib. The diaphragm separates the abdominal cavity below from the thoracic cavity above.

THORACIC SKELETON

The skeleton of the thorax consists of (1) a midline sternum, (2) 12 pairs of ribs and associated costal cartilages, and (3) 12 thoracic vertebrae (*Figure 3-1*). The first ribs, sternum, and first thoracic vertebra comprise the **thoracic inlet.**

Sternum

The sternum, or breast bone, consists of three portions: (1) the **manubrium;** (2) a **body,** which joins the manubrium as a symphysis at the *sternal angle*; and (3) the **xiphoid process,** a small inferior portion (*Figure 3-2*). Superiorly the manubrium of the sternum presents a midline notch and two lateral notches. The midline notch is the **jugular** notch, or **suprasternal notch,** and it can be palpated at the anterior base of the neck. The lateral notches receive the clavicular heads of the upper limb girdle. The extreme lateral borders of the manubrium articulate with the costal cartilages of the first ribs.

The costal cartilages of the second ribs articulate with the sternum at the junction of the manubrium and body. Therefore the **sternal angle** is an important landmark in determining, from the surface, the level of the second rib and the positions of each descending rib. The costal cartilages of the upper seven ribs articulate directly with the sternum.

Ribs

A typical rib consists of (1) a **head,** which articulates with the body of a thoracic vertebra; (2) a neck; (3) a **tubercle,** which articulates with the transverse process of a thoracic vertebra; (4) a **shaft,** or body; (5) an **angle,** at which the rib turns inferiorly and anteriorly; and (6) a shallow **subcostal groove** on the internal inferior surface, which shelters the *intercostal nerve and vessels* (*Figure 3-3*). Anteriorly the typical rib is joined to the sternum by its own **costal cartilage.**

There are three types of ribs:

1. **True ribs** (ribs 1 to 7) attach via their costal cartilages directly to the sternum.
2. **False ribs** (ribs 8 to 10) attach indirectly via their costal cartilages or do not attach at all. The **first rib** (*Figure 3-4*), exhibits all the features of a typical true rib, but it is atypical because it is shorter, flatter, and the highest of the ribs. In addition, a number of important features are found only on the first rib. On the superior aspect from medial to lateral are (1) a **groove for the subclavian vein,** (2) a **scalene tubercle** for attachment of the

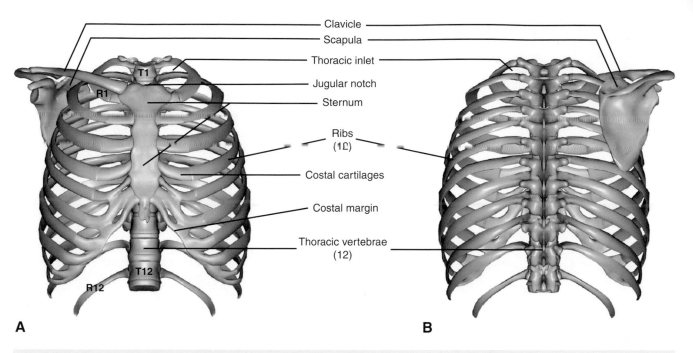

Figure 3-1 Skeleton of thorax. **A**, Anterior view. **B**, Posterior view.

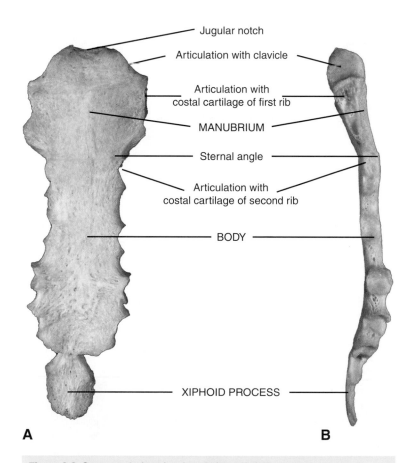

Figure 3-2 Sternum. **A**, Anterior view. **B**, Lateral view.

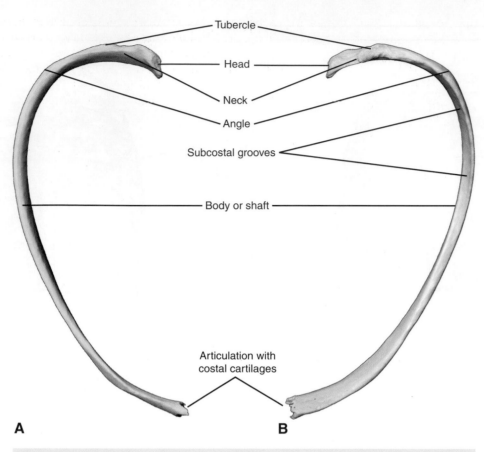

Figure 3-3 Typical right rib. **A,** Superior view. **B,** Inferior view.

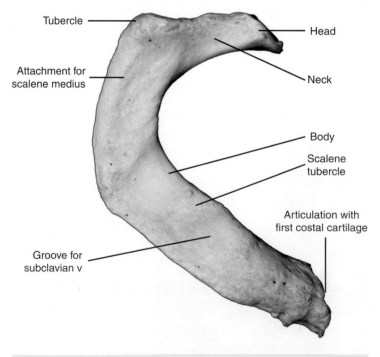

Figure 3-4 Superior view of the first right rib.

scalenus anterior muscle, and (3) a roughened area for the **attachment of the scalenus medius muscle.**

3. **Floating ribs** (ribs 10 to 12) do not attach to the sternum.

Thoracic Vertebrae

In addition to all of the features attributable to a typical vertebra described in Chapter 2, the thoracic vertebrae exhibit the following unique features: (1) the **body** is heart-shaped, (2) the **spinous processes** are long and slender, and (3) the bodies and transverse processes have **facets for articulation with ribs** (*Figures 3-5* and *3-6*).

Figure 3-7 demonstrates the articulation of a rib with a thoracic vertebra. Except for ribs 1, 10, 11, and 12, the head of each rib articulates with the body of its own vertebra and that of the vertebra above. The facets on the vertebral bodies are really *demifacets*, and in the articulated spine the demifacet below and the one above make a complete facet. Ribs 1, 10, 11, and 12 articulate with only their own vertebrae. The tubercles of the ribs articulate with the transverse processes of each thoracic vertebra.

Joints

The joints between the thoracic vertebrae are considered in Chapter 2. The remaining thoracic joints allow movements that result in expansion of the thoracic cavity during inspiration (see *Figure 3-7*). The movements of respiration are discussed later in this chapter, under "Mechanics of Breathing." There are three types of thoracic skeleton joints:

1. **Costovertebral joints** are synovial joints between the heads of the ribs and the vertebral bodies and between the tubercles of the ribs and the transverse processes. They allow the ribs to be elevated or depressed.
2. **Sternocostal joints** are synovial joints between the costal cartilages of the true ribs and the sternum. However, the first rib differs in that its costal cartilage joins the first rib directly to the manubrium as a synchondrosis.

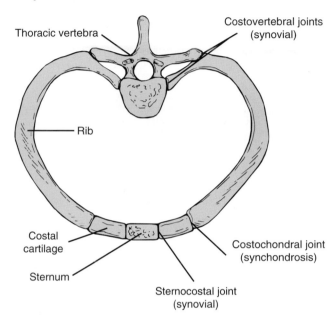

Figure 3-6 Horizontal section through thorax to demonstrate articulation of ribs.

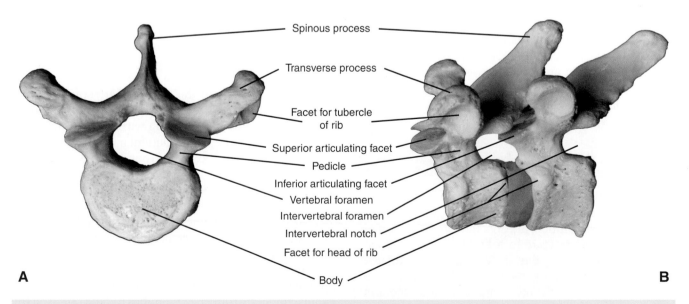

Figure 3-5 A, Superior view of typical thoracic vertebra. **B,** Left lateral view of two articulated vertebrae.

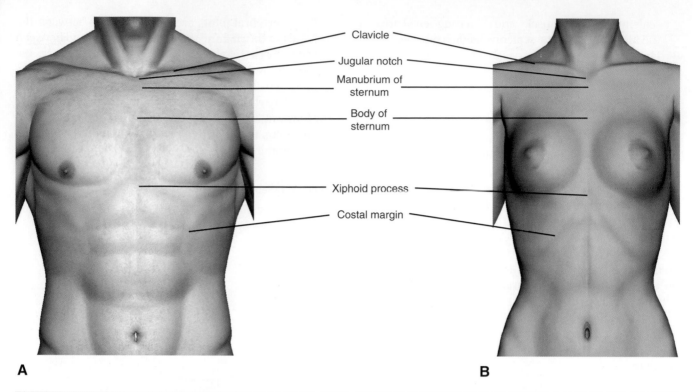

A
B

Figure 3-7 Horizontal section through thorax to demonstrate articulation of ribs. Anterior view of surface features of thorax. **A**, male. **B**, female.

3. **Costochondral joints** are synchondroses between the distal ends of the ribs and their corresponding costal cartilages.

DIVISIONS OF THE THORAX

The thoracic cavity is divided into three main regions: (1) the **right pleural cavity,** (2) the **left pleural cavity** (the pleural cavities contain the lungs), and (3) the **mediastinum,** a midline structure that separates the right and left pleural cavities. The mediastinum is a collection of structures, including the heart and its great vessels, the trachea and esophagus, and other structures. These structures are described later in this chapter.

CLINICAL NOTES

Dislocated, Separated, and Fractured Ribs

A **dislocated rib** is displaced at its sternocostal joint. A **rib separation** is a rib torn from its costal cartilage. A **rib fracture** is a break in the rib itself and often occurs at the angle of the rib. Although painful, rib fractures generally are not reduced and immobilized (as are limb fractures), unless there is evidence of lung or other internal damage.

2. The Thoracic or Chest Wall

SURFACE FEATURES

The Breast

The breast, or mammary gland, arises as modified sweat gland tissue within the superficial fascia of the anterior chest wall and is covered by skin (*Figure 3-8*). In postpubertal women the breast is a large organ capable of lactation. In men and children it is rudimentary.

In women the breast overlies the pectoralis major muscles at the level of ribs 2 to 6. An axillary tail passes laterally and superiorly to the axillary region (armpit). The functional component of the breast consists of 15 to 20 lobules of glandular tissue lying within accumulated fat of the superficial fascia. The glandular ducts empty to the surface through the nipple. Surrounding the nipple is an areola containing areolar glands and ranging from light pink to dark brown. Suspensory ligaments (of Cooper) support the breast by anchoring it to underlying deep fascia. Arterial supply comes from mammary branches of the axillary artery, the internal thoracic artery, and intercostal arteries.

Knowledge of lymphatic drainage is extremely important because malignancies of the breast may spread along lymphatic routes. Lymphatics radiate out from the nipple and communicate with lymph nodes of various

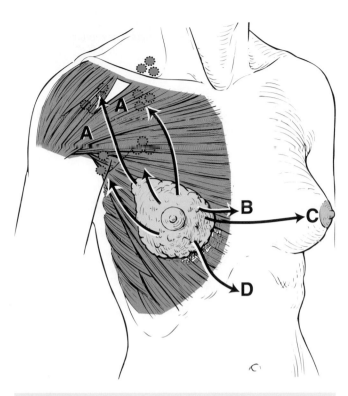

Figure 3-8 Features of female breast and lymph drainage. **A,** Drainage to axillary nodes. **B,** Drainage to internal thoracic nodes of chest wall. **C,** Drainage to opposite breast. **D,** Drainage to nodes of anterior abdominal wall.

regions. The breast is divided into quadrants. The two **lateral quadrants** drain superiorly to nodes of the axilla. The two **medial quadrants** drain to the axillary nodes, the anterior chest wall, and the interior abdominal wall, and they may even drain across the midline to the opposite breast.

Skeletal Landmarks

The following important landmarks in the chest are used to locate underlying structures (*Figure 3-9*):

1. The **suprasternal, or jugular, notch,** located at the anterior base of the neck, is an important landmark for locating the underlying trachea.
2. The **costal margin** is formed by the inferior aspects of costal cartilages 7 through 10. The margins rise on each side to meet in the midline at the xiphoid process. This landmark is used as an aid in locating the correct sternal position for external heart massage during cardiac emergencies.
3. The **sternal angle** is important because the first rib cannot be palpated. The sternal angle marks the position of the second rib. From this position the ribs may be counted externally to locate various areas of the heart below.

The surface anatomy of the heart and lungs is covered in the descriptions of these organs in subsequent sections.

CLINICAL NOTES

Lactation

During pregnancy, glandular tissue hypertrophies. Secretion of colostrum occurs during the third trimester, and production of milk begins soon after giving birth.

Accessory Nipples or Breasts

In lower mammals the multiple mammary glands develop along "milk lines" running from the axilla to the groin. Occasionally in humans of either sex, accessory nipples or breasts may be found along this line.

Gynecomastia

Gynecomastia is the enlargement of the breasts in males. It may occur during puberty but is a transient condition. It may also occur in older men as part of the aging process.

Carcinoma of the Breast

Breast cancer is the most common type of cancer among women and rarely occurs in men. Most cancers initially are detected by the patient as a lump or mass distinctly different from surrounding breast tissue. Others are found during routine mammography. The upper lateral quadrant is the most common site of occurrence. Diagnosis is made after fine-needle biopsy and cytological examination. More advanced lesions interfere with lymphatic drainage, causing local puffiness and an uneven dimpled skin surface termed *peau d'orange* (orange peel). A *mastectomy* is the removal of an entire breast. A radical version is the additional removal of the pectoral muscles and axillary lymph nodes. A *lumpectomy* is the excision of just the lesion and some surrounding tissue.

MUSCLES

Muscular Action

In a sequence not yet completely understood, the thoracic muscles act to stabilize the upper and lower ribs and elevate the remaining ribs to increase thoracic volume during quiet inspiration. During forced inspiration the upper ribs are elevated by the accessory muscles to further increase the thoracic volume.

Extrinsic Thoracic Muscles

The superficial muscles covering the chest wall are actually muscles belonging to other regions and are described in sections that discuss these regions. Muscles of the *upper limb* (see Chapter 9), which originate from the thoracic skeleton, are the pectoralis major and minor, serratus anterior,

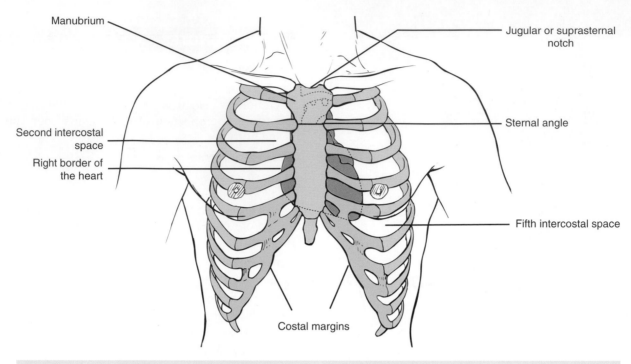

Manubrium

Jugular or suprasternal notch

Sternal angle

Second intercostal space

Right border of the heart

Fifth intercostal space

Costal margins

Figure 3-9 Surface landmarks of anterior chest wall.

latissimus dorsi, rhomboid major and minor, levator scapulae, and trapezius. Muscles of the *anterior abdominal wall* (see Chapter 4), which attach to the thoracic skeleton, are the rectus abdominis, external oblique, internal oblique, and transversus abdominis. Posteriorly, erector spinae and muscles of the *back* (see Chapter 2) attach to the thoracic skeleton.

Accessory Extrinsic Muscles of Respiration

Several muscles of the neck region insert into the skeleton of the upper thorax to elevate the sternum and ribs during forced inspiration. These muscles are the scalenus anterior, scalenus medius, and scalenus posterior and are described fully in Chapter 5, page 151.

Intercostal Muscles

The intercostal muscles of the thorax are involved with the mechanics of breathing. They run from (1) rib to rib, (2) sternum to rib, and (3) vertebra to rib (*Figure 3-10* and *Table 3-1*). The **external intercostal muscles** pass from rib to rib in an anteroinferior direction (in the same direction as the external abdominal oblique muscle) and elevate the ribs during inspiration. The **internal intercostal muscle** passes from rib to rib, perpendicular to the external intercostal muscle, and depresses the ribs during expiration. The **innermost intercostal muscles** run in same direction as the internal intercostal muscles, but the two layers are separated by the intercostal nerves and vessels. The innermost layer is subdivided into the *subcostal* and *transversus thoracis*. They likely aid the internal intercostals in

depressing the ribs. *Figure 3-11* shows that the muscles are not continuous sheets, and in some areas the muscle is replaced by thin membranous tendon. The intercostal muscles are supplied by intercostal nerves.

Back Muscles that Participate in Respiration

The **levator costarum** muscles lie on the posterior aspect of the thorax. They run from transverse processes (C7 to T11) and pass down and laterally to insert into the area between the tubercle and the angle of the rib below. They

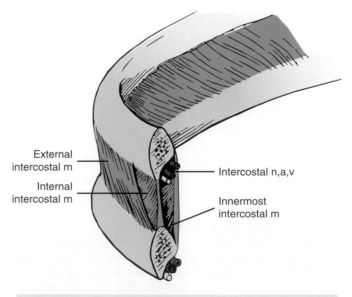

External intercostal m

Internal intercostal m

Intercostal n,a,v

Innermost intercostal m

Figure 3-10 Typical intercostal space.

TABLE 3-1

Muscles of the Thorax

Muscle	Origin	Insertion	Action	Nerve
Intercostals				
External intercostal	Inferior margins of ribs; fibers pass obliquely down and medially	Superior margins of ribs immediately below	Elevate ribs and increase transverse and anteroposterior diameters of thorax for inspiration	AR of thoracic spinal nerves (intercostal nerves)
Internal intercostal	Inferior margins of costal cartilages and ribs; fibers pass obliquely down and laterally at right angles to the externals	Superior margins of costal cartilages and ribs immediately below	Depress ribs and decrease transverse and anteroposterior diameters of thorax for expiration	AR of thoracic spinal nerves (intercostal nerves)
Innermost intercostal. The posterior fibers are termed the *subcostals*; the anterior fibers are termed the *transversus thoracis*	Inferior border of ribs; fibers pass down in same direction as the internal intercostals	Superior margins of ribs immediately below	Depress ribs along with internal intercostals for expiration	AR of thoracic spinal nerves (intercostal nerves)
Back muscles that participate in respiration				
Levator costarum	Transverse processes of C7 and T1-T11 and fibers pass down and laterally	Rib below between tubercle and angle	Elevate ribs and increase thoracic volume for inspiration; help rotate and laterally flex the vertebral column	PR of thoracic spinal nerves
Serratus posterior superior	Ligamentum nuchae and spinous processes of upper two or three thoracic vertebrae; fibers pass down and laterally	Superior borders of the 2nd to 5th ribs just lateral to their angles	Elevate ribs and increase thoracic volume for inspiration	AR of thoracic spinal nerves (intercostal nerves)
Serratus posterior inferior	Spinous processes of lower two lumbar vertebrae; fibers pass upward and laterally	Inferior borders of lower four ribs	Depresses lower ribs and fixes them during expiration	AR of thoracic spinal nerves (intercostal nerves)
Diaphragm (the most important muscle of respiration)	Sternal: inner aspect of xiphoid process Costal: lower six ribs and costal cartilages Lumbar: anterior aspects of bodies of upper two to three lumbar vertebrae as right and left crura	Central tendon of diaphragm	Fleshy fibers pull central tendon of diaphragm inferiorly to increase the superoinferior dimension of the thorax for inspiration	AR of C3, C4, and C5 arise from the cervical and brachial plexuses to form the phrenic nerve

AR, Anterior rami; *PR,* posterior rami.

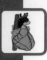

NERVES   ARTERIES

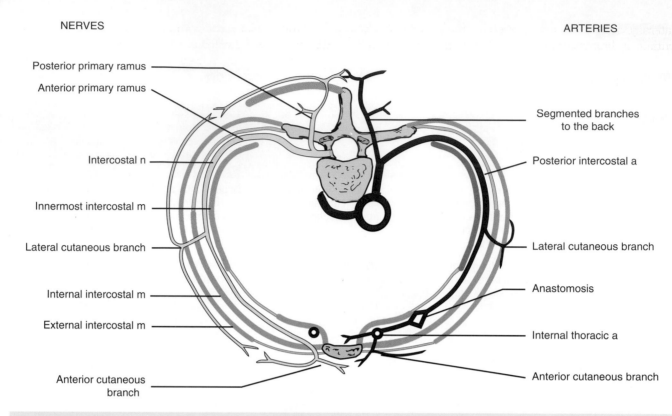

Posterior primary ramus

Anterior primary ramus

Intercostal n

Innermost intercostal m

Lateral cutaneous branch

Internal intercostal m

External intercostal m

Anterior cutaneous branch

Segmented branches to the back

Posterior intercostal a

Lateral cutaneous branch

Anastomosis

Internal thoracic a

Anterior cutaneous branch

Figure 3-11 Origins of intercostal nerves and arteries. Nerves and arteries are shown separately but are bilateral structures and run together with veins as neurovascular bundles.

elevate the ribs during inspiration and are innervated by posterior rami of thoracic spinal nerves.

Diaphragm

The diaphragm is the most important muscle of respiration and its attachments are described in Chapter 4, pages 96 and 97. On contraction, the diaphragm pulls the central tendon inferiorly to increase the vertical dimension of the thorax during inspiration. It is supplied by the right and left phrenic nerves (anterior rami of C3, C4, and C5).

The **serratus posterior superior** and **inferior** are thin, flat muscles on the posterior thoracic wall (see *Figure 2-15*). The superior muscle runs from the lower cervical and upper thoracic vertebral spines downward and laterally to the upper ribs. It elevates the ribs during inspiration. The inferior muscle arises from the upper lumbar and lower thoracic vertebral spines and passes upward and laterally to insert into the lower ribs. It depresses or stabilizes the lower ribs.

INTERCOSTAL BLOOD VESSELS AND NERVES

The intercostal vessels and nerves run between the ribs, under the shelter of the subcostal groove of the more superior rib (see *Figures 3-10* and *3-11*). The vessels and nerves run between the internal and innermost intercostal muscles.

Arteries and Veins

Posterior intercostal arteries arise as paired segmented branches of the thoracic aorta. These arteries run laterally and anteriorly to supply the body wall.

Anterior intercostal arteries arise from the internal thoracic artery. The internal thoracic artery arises from the subclavian artery in the root of the neck, enters the thoracic inlet, and travels down the inner aspect of the chest wall. As it descends, it gives rise to anterior intercostal arteries, which supply the anterior body wall and pass laterally to anastomose with the posterior intercostal arteries.

The internal thoracic artery ends in two terminal branches as it approaches the abdomen by dividing into the *superior epigastric artery* of the anterior abdominal wall and the *musculophrenic artery* of the diaphragm.

Intercostal veins parallel the blood flow of the arteries but in a reverse direction. Anterior intercostal veins empty into the internal thoracic veins. Posterior intercostal veins empty into the azygos and hemiazygos veins. The superior intercostal veins empty into the brachiocephalic veins.

Nerves

Spinal nerves arise from the spinal cord in paired segmented fashion. The anterior rami of these nerves travel laterally and anteriorly with the intercostal vessels as **intercostal nerves**. The *lateral cutaneous branches* are given off laterally, and as the nerves approach the midline, anterior cutaneous branches are given off to the anterior chest wall.

3.   The Pleural Cavities and Lungs

PLEURA

The **right** and **left pleural cavities** are completely enclosed spaces within the thorax that contain the right and left lungs (*Figure 3-12*). Like the peritoneal cavity, the pleural cavity is lined with serous membrane, or **pleura**.

Parietal pleura lines the inner aspect of the pleural cavity. It is subdivided as follows: *Costal pleura* lines the inner aspect of the rib cage, *diaphragmatic pleura* lines the superior aspect of the diaphragm, *mediastinal pleura* covers the mediastinum, and *cervical pleura* bulges up into the neck as the cupola. Where parietal pleura reflects from the mediastinum and diaphragm onto the thoracic wall is important, and the areas of reflection may be plotted based on knowledge of surface anatomy.

Visceral pleura lines the lungs, following all the contours and fissures intimately. Both visceral pleura and

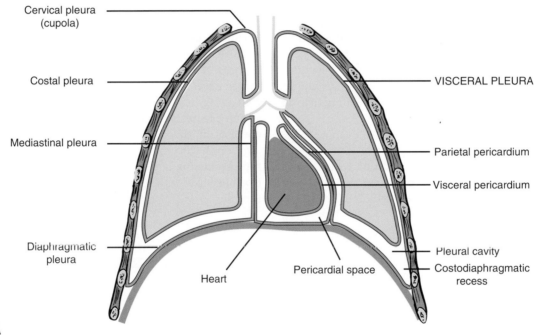

PARIETAL PLEURA

- Cervical pleura (cupola)
- Costal pleura
- Mediastinal pleura
- Diaphragmatic pleura
- Heart

VISCERAL PLEURA

- Parietal pericardium
- Visceral pericardium
- Pericardial space
- Pleural cavity
- Costodiaphragmatic recess

A

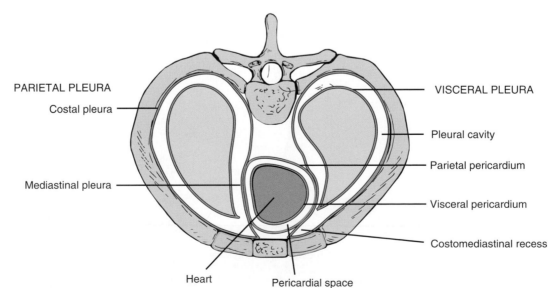

PARIETAL PLEURA

- Costal pleura
- Mediastinal pleura
- Heart
- Pericardial space

VISCERAL PLEURA

- Pleural cavity
- Parietal pericardium
- Visceral pericardium
- Costomediastinal recess

B

Figure 3-12 Sections through thorax to show pleural cavities, mediastinum, and coverings. **A**, Coronal section. **B**, Transverse section.

parietal pleura are continuous at the root of the lung. It is helpful to imagine the lung bud in the developing embryo growing into an empty pleural cavity lined with parietal pleura. As the lung invades the cavity, it carries with it parietal pleura, which eventually covers the lung as visceral pleura.

Pleural recesses are areas where there is a space between reflected layers of pleura. During quiet inspiration the recesses are not filled with lung tissue. There is a *costodiaphragmatic recess* laterally and inferiorly and a *costomediastinal recess* medially and anteriorly.

LUNGS

The lungs are two spongy organs resembling inverted, blunted cones cut in half. They are housed in the right and left pleural cavities. The lungs consist of small, air-filled chambers, or **alveoli**, where exchange of gases (oxygen $[O_2]$ and carbon dioxide $[CO_2]$ takes place with the circulatory system. In turn the alveoli are supported by elastic tissue, which tends to collapse and shrink the lung (**elastic recoil**) during respiratory expiration.

Surfaces and Borders

Each lung exhibits four surfaces, each of which takes the shape of surrounding structures (*Figures 3-13* and *3-14*). The surfaces are (1) the **apex**, which is a rounded superior aspect that bulges up through the thoracic inlet; (2) the **diaphragmatic surface,** or **base,** which rests on the dome of the diaphragm; (3) a **mediastinal surface,** which contacts the midline mediastinum; and (4) the **costal surface,** which is rounded to fit the curved ribs.

Separating the four surfaces are three borders: (1) a sharp **anterior border,** which separates the costal surface from the mediastinal surface; (2) a rounded **posterior** or **vertebral border,** which separates the costal and mediastinal surfaces posteriorly; and (3) the **lower circumferential border,** which separates the diaphragmatic surface from the costal and mediastinal surfaces.

Fissures and Lobes

Both the right and left lungs are divided into lobes by fissures. Both lungs have an **oblique fissure,** which separates each lung into an **upper** and a **lower lobe.** The right lung has a second fissure (the **horizontal fissure**), which creates a third **middle lobe.** Thus the right lung consists of three lobes, and the left lung consists of two lobes. The missing middle lobe of the left lung is represented by a deficiency, the **cardiac notch;** its inferior border is called the *lingula* because it resembles a tongue.

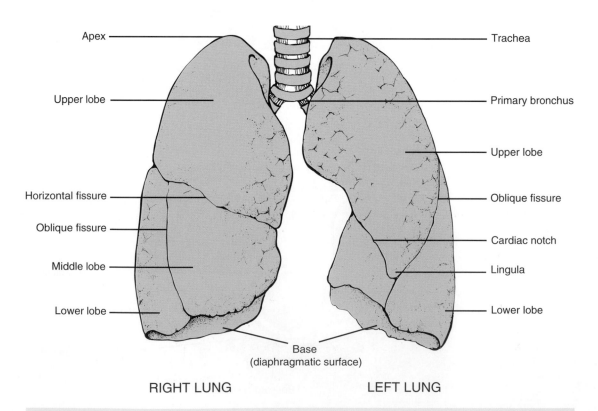

RIGHT LUNG   LEFT LUNG

Figure 3-13 Anterior aspect of lungs.

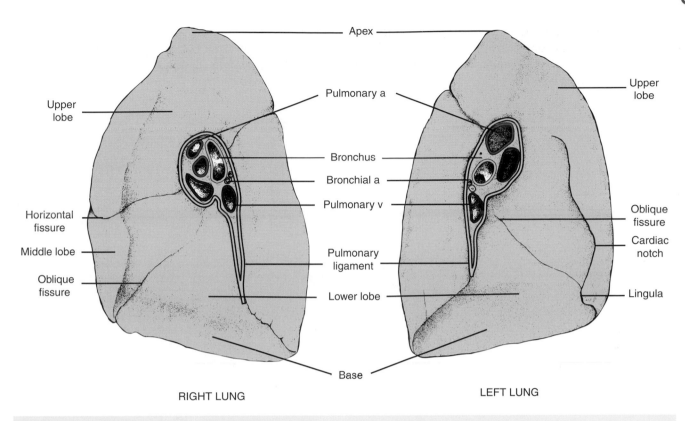

Figure 3-14 Medial or mediastinal surface of lungs.

The Hilum

On the mediastinal aspect of each lung are an exit and entrance (hilum) for blood vessels and air tubes. The **pulmonary artery** from the right ventricle enters the hilum of the lung carrying unoxygenated blood. The **pulmonary vein** leaves the hilum of the lung carrying oxygenated blood.

The **right** and **left bronchi** arise from the midline trachea. They carry air to the hilum of the lung during inspiration and carry air from the hilum during expiration.

The **bronchial artery** arises from the thoracic descending aorta and travels to the hilum to supply lung tissue. In addition, **autonomic nerves** and **lymphatics** enter or leave through the hilum of the lung.

BRONCHI AND BRONCHIAL TREE

The trachea consists of approximately 20 U-shaped, incomplete **cartilaginous rings** strung together with fibroelastic tissue (*Figure 3-15*). The posterior deficient portion is covered with fibrous tissue and involuntary muscle. Approximately half the course of the trachea is within the neck. It continues inferiorly from the larynx in the neck, lying anterior to and paralleling the course of the esophagus. Applied laterally to the trachea are the two lobes of the thyroid gland, connected by an isthmus that crosses the second or third tracheal ring (see Chapter 5).

The trachea descends and enters the inlet of the thorax, passing deep to the sternum, where it is covered by the thymus gland. At vertebral level T5 (sternal angle), the trachea bifurcates into a **right** and **left primary bronchus.** The last tracheal ring features the **carina,** a midline cartilaginous ridge that separates the lumens of the primary bronchi. It is seen during a bronchoscopic examination.

Bronchi and Bronchioles

The **right** and **left primary bronchi** are approximately half the diameter of the trachea. The right bronchus differs from the left, however, in that it is slightly wider, shorter, and in a more direct line with the trachea.

Right Bronchial Tree. The right primary bronchus divides into three **secondary bronchi,** or **lobar** bronchi, one for each of the three lobes. The secondary bronchus to the upper lobe is given off before the primary bronchus plunges through the hilus. Within the right lung the primary bronchus divides to supply secondary bronchi to the middle and lower lobes.

Each lobe of the right lung is further subdivided functionally into **bronchopulmonary** segments. Each secondary bronchus breaks up into **tertiary** or **segmental bronchi** to supply 10 bronchopulmonary segments. Each segment can function independently of the others, and the

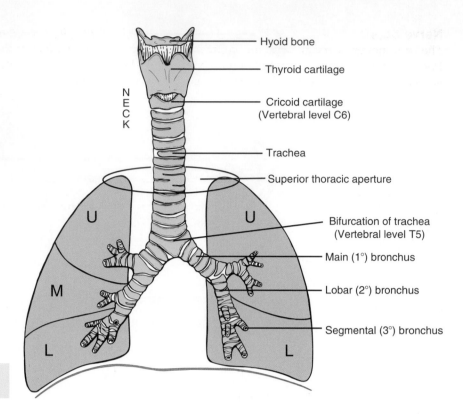

Figure 3-15 Respiratory tract. L, lower lobe; M, middle lobe; U, upper lobe.

Labels in figure:
- Hyoid bone
- Thyroid cartilage
- Cricoid cartilage (Vertebral level C6)
- Trachea
- Superior thoracic aperture
- Bifurcation of trachea (Vertebral level T5)
- Main (1°) bronchus
- Lobar (2°) bronchus
- Segmental (3°) bronchus
- N E C K

thoracic surgeon makes use of this fact when considering the removal of diseased portions of lung tissue without affecting the function of remaining healthy segments.

Within the bronchopulmonary segments the tertiary bronchi continue to divide, decrease in size, and lose their cartilaginous support. When this occurs, the tubes are called **bronchioles** and their walls are supported only by a relative increase in smooth muscle thickness. Spasm of this smooth muscle decreases airflow, a condition known as *asthma*.

CLINICAL NOTES

Aspiration of Foreign Objects

A hazard in a dental office is an aspirated foreign body (e.g., an extracted tooth, a piece of filling material, a root canal instrument) that has fallen past the vocal folds of the larynx into the trachea. Such an object is more likely to enter the right primary bronchus because it is in a more direct line with the trachea. When possible and practicable, a rubber dam should be placed to prevent such an accident.

The bronchioles finally end as **terminal bronchioles,** from which ductules lead off to blind sacs, or *alveoli*, which are one cell thick. Surrounding each alveolus is a capillary network fed by arterioles branching from the pulmonary arteries and drained by venules, which ultimately unite as the pulmonary veins. It is at the capillary level that the gas exchange takes place (CO_2 from capillary to alveolus, O_2 from alveolus to capillary).

Left Bronchial Tree. The scheme of the bronchial tree is precisely the same in the left lung as in the right lung, with the following exceptions: There are only **two lobes** and therefore two secondary bronchi, which divide to form **tertiary bronchi.** Often a pair of bronchopulmonary segments fuse in the superior lobe and a pair of segments fuse in the inferior lobe, resulting in a total of only eight bronchopulmonary segments usually found in the left lung.

BLOOD AND NERVE SUPPLY

Blood Supply

The source and course of the pulmonary vessels, which carry blood for the purpose of gas exchange from the heart to the lungs and back, are considered in the discussion of the heart. The lung tissue receives its own supply of blood from the **bronchial arteries** (see *Figure 3-31*), which branch from the descending aorta and follow the bronchi and bronchioles to the parenchyma of the lung. Paralleling the arterial supply but running in the opposite direction are lymph vessels, which ultimately drain to the bronchomediastinal trunk (see *Figure 3-32*).

Nerve Supply

The autonomic nervous system controls the lungs. **Parasympathetic efferents** are pulmonary branches of the vagus nerve (cranial nerve X). **Sympathetic efferents** are derived mainly from the second, third, and fourth ganglia of the sympathetic trunk. Both autonomic components form a pulmonary nerve plexus around the pulmonary vessels at the hilus of the lung and surround and follow the vessels as they pass into the lung.

Vagal efferent parasympathetic fibers are *bronchoconstrictors* and *secretomotor*. Efferent sympathetic fibers function as bronchodilators. Therefore adrenaline, or epinephrine, which mimics sympathetic effects, dilates constricted bronchioles brought about by asthmalike attacks (see Clinical Notes box on page 68).

The nerve supply to each component of parietal pleura is exactly the same supply as that of the adjacent structures; that is, the phrenic nerve, which supplies the diaphragm and mediastinum, supplies adjacent pleura. Intercostal nerves supply costal pleura.

MECHANICS OF BREATHING

Respiration consists of two phases: air is inhaled during inspiration and exhaled during expiration (*Figure 3-16*).

Inspiration

A number of muscles function during inspiration. The muscles involved perform one basic function: They act to decrease the pressure within the sealed pleural cavities by *enlarging the volumes* of the pleural cavities. Increasing the volume *lowers the pressure* and *causes higher atmospheric pressure from outside to fill the lungs with air* via the bronchial tree.

Inspiration is achieved by enlarging the pleural cavity in three planes: (1) The *transverse diameter* is increased by the action of the intercostal muscles, raising the ribs at the costovertebral and costosternal joints and swinging them laterally (like a pail with two raised handles); (2) the *anteroposterior diameter* is increased when the right and left rib pairs raise as a unit (like the handle of a pail) around the right and left costovertebral joints, causing the sternum to move anteriorly; and (3) the *vertical plane* is enlarged by the action of the diaphragm contracting downward (much like a plumber's helper).

During **forced inspiration**, accessory muscles are brought into action. The scalene muscles of the neck raise the first two ribs, and the muscle raises the manubrium. Extremely labored breathing may involve the pectoral muscles and the serratus anterior muscle.

Expiration

Normal expiration, or **quiet expiration,** is *passive*. On relaxation of the muscles of respiration, the elastic recoil of the lung tissue forces air out.

During **forced expiration** the abdominal muscles contract to raise the intraabdominal pressure while the diaphragm relaxes. The result is a relative rise in intrathoracic pressure to forcefully expel air from the lungs.

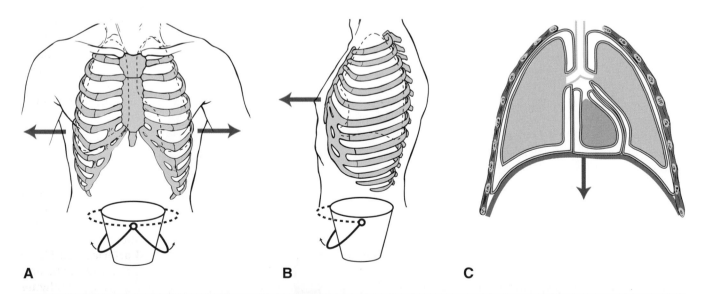

A **B** **C**

Figure 3-16 Thoracic volume is increased in three planes during inspiration. **A,** Transverse increase is illustrated using pail with two handles. Lifting handles is like raising right and left ribs at the costovertebral and costosternal joints. **B,** Anteroposterior increase is illustrated using pail with one handle. Lifting handle is like raising right and left ribs as a unit at costovertebral joints. **C,** Vertical dimension is increased by downward pull of diaphragm.

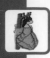

CLINICAL NOTES

Lung Emphysema

Emphysema results in a decreased number of air spaces distal to the terminal bronchioles and destruction of elastic tissue necessary for elastic recoil during quiet normal expiration. The result is breathlessness on exertion and labored chest movements to provide sufficient oxygen. In advanced cases the ribs are horizontal and in a constant state of inspiration (the individual is "barrel-chested"). The accessory muscles of the neck and chest are very active in this distressing condition and are made more effective by the patient holding on to a table surface to stabilize the shoulder girdle. Emphysema is a possible consequence of long-term smoking.

Pneumothorax

Pneumothorax is the presence of air in the pleural cavity caused by a puncture through the thoracic wall or a spontaneous rupture through the lung surface. In either case the lung is exposed to atmospheric pressure, collapses as a result of elastic recoil of the lung tissue, and ceases to function. Internal ruptures of lung are diagnostic on physical examination and chest radiographs because the mediastinum shifts to the opposite side.

Resections

A diseased lung that is no longer treatable may be totally (pneumonectomy) or partially resected. Lobes and pulmonary segments function individually, and a lobe or a bronchopulmonary segment may be removed without affecting the function of the remaining opposite lung or segments of the remaining lung.

Bronchial Asthma

Asthma causes spasm of smooth muscle in the bronchial tree, inflammation of the respiratory mucosa, and production of mucus. One method of drug therapy uses β-adrenergic drugs (e.g., epinephrine) to dilate the bronchial smooth muscle and open the airway.

Pigmented Lungs

Upon their initial view of a lung, students are always amazed that it is spotted with black pigment. The black spots are produced by carbon particles from city air and/or tobacco smoke. Carbon particles at the gas exchange interface are carried by phagocytes to the periphery and surfaces of the lung, where they are visible as black specks. Healthy lungs of young people not exposed to atmospheric pollutants and tobacco smoke are a healthy pink.

4. The Mediastinum

The mediastinum is a group of midline structures that separates the right and left pleural cavities. It is covered on its right and left surfaces with mediastinal pleura (see *Figure 3-12*).

The **mediastinum** contains (1) the heart and its great vessels, (2) the thoracic trachea and bronchi, (3) the thoracic esophagus, (4) the vagus nerves, (5) the phrenic nerves, and (6) the thoracic duct. The mediastinum is divided into four areas as follows (*Figure 3-17*):

1. The **middle mediastinum** contains the heart and its fibrous sac of pericardium. It sits behind the body of the sternum.
2. The **anterior mediastinum** is a small, fat-filled space between the middle mediastinum and the body of the sternum. Here the right and left pleural reflections just fail to meet as they approach the midline.
3. The **superior mediastinum** occupies the space between the thoracic inlet and the middle mediastinum below. It contains the great vessels of the heart and the upper portions of the thoracic trachea and esophagus.

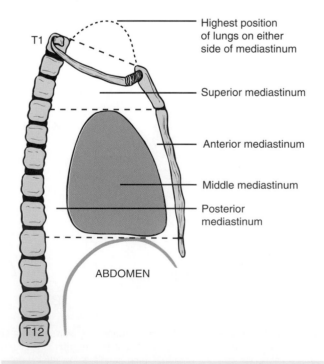

Figure 3-17 Divisions of mediastinum.

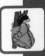

4. The **posterior mediastinum** occupies the area posterior to the middle mediastinum and the diaphragm, which curves down to vertebral level T12.

THE MIDDLE MEDIASTINUM

The middle mediastinum is occupied by the heart contained within the pericardial sac, in the same way that the lungs occupy the pleural cavity.

Pericardial Sac

Pericardium is composed of two layers: (1) an outer layer of tough *fibrous tissue*, which is adherent to the diaphragm below, and (2) an inner layer of *serous membrane* (see *Figure 3-12*). It is helpful to imagine the developing heart invading the serous-lined pericardial sac. As the heart bulges into the sac, it pushes the serous layer ahead of it, which remains adherent to the surface of the heart as **visceral pericardium** or **epicardium**.

Parietal serous pericardium lines the inner aspect of the fibrous sac. The small space between the parietal and visceral pleura, termed the pericardial cavity, is filled with serous fluid.

The Heart

A basic description of the heart and its relationship to the rest of the circulatory system is presented in Chapter 1.

Shape and Position. The heart is classically described as approximating the size and shape of a clenched fist.

However, the hearts found in laboratory specimens tend to be larger, a reflection of an older population and chronic cardiovascular and pulmonary disease. In addition, the size of the heart depends on whether the heart was fixed in diastole or systole. The heart sits within the thorax above the diaphragm, immediately behind the body of the sternum (*Figure 3-18*). It lies closer to the anterior than to the posterior chest wall.

The superior border of the heart is at the level of the sternal angle (second costal cartilage). The right border follows a roughly parallel course immediately to the right of the body of the sternum inferiorly to the level of the fifth intercostal space. The inferior border passes to the left above the xiphoid process to a point 10 cm (the width of a hand) to the left of the midline. The inferior border ends to the left at the fifth intercostal space or the sixth rib, as the apex of the heart. The left border then runs obliquely upward toward the sternal angle.

Disposition of the Chambers. The adult heart does not quite resemble the simplified four-chambered box described in Chapter 1, page 15. During heart development, it rotates counterclockwise, causing the right side to be carried over onto the anterior surface and the left side to extend onto the posterior surface. The resulting disposition of the chambers is shown in *Figures 3-19* and *3-20*.

The **right atrium** forms the entire right surface and border of the heart and about one fourth of the anterior surface. The **right ventricle** occupies most of the anterior surface and forms two thirds of the inferior border. The **left ventricle**

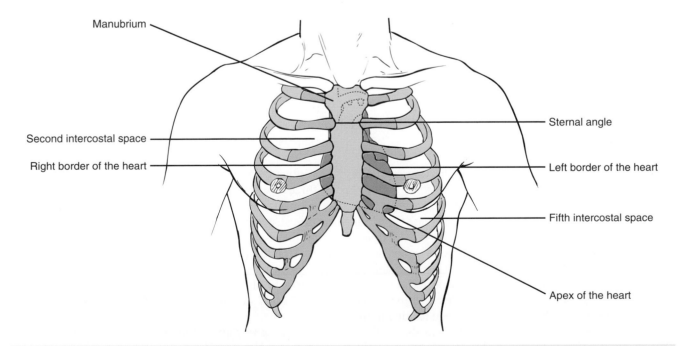

Figure 3-18 Position of heart in relation to skeleton of anterior chest wall.

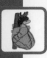

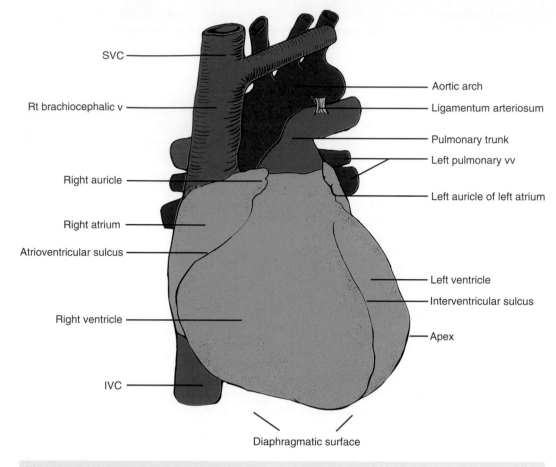

SVC

Rt brachiocephalic v

Right auricle

Right atrium

Atrioventricular sulcus

Right ventricle

IVC

Aortic arch

Ligamentum arteriosum

Pulmonary trunk

Left pulmonary vv

Left auricle of left atrium

Left ventricle

Interventricular sulcus

Apex

Diaphragmatic surface

Figure 3-19 Anterior surface of heart. *IVC*, Inferior vena cava; *SVC*, superior vena cava.

forms nearly all of the left border and a small piece of the left inferior border, which is termed the *apex*. The left ventricle makes up a large portion of the posterior surface. The **left atrium** is entirely on the posterior aspect of the heart.

The auricles are earlike appendages of the atria. The right auricle embraces the base of the aorta; the left auricle embraces the base of the pulmonary trunk. Both are visible from the anterior aspect.

Surfaces and Features. The heart presents three surfaces and an apex. The **sternocostal surface** (see *Figures 3-18* and *3-19*) is the anterior aspect of the heart, which should be visualized on the anterior chest surface following the previous description and using a knowledge of surface anatomy. The anterior surface is almost completely overlapped by the lungs. The **diaphragmatic surface** rests on but is not adherent to the diaphragm below. The **base** or **posterior surface** (see *Figure 3-20*) consists mainly of the left atrium and left ventricle. The **apex** of the heart may be seen beating in the left fifth intercostal space about 10 cm from the midline. Two grooves on the surface of the heart mark the underlying septa, which separate the four chambers of the heart.

The **atrioventricular sulcus** indicates the septum separating the two atria from the two ventricles. It runs in almost a vertical plane. Because it encircles the heart like a crown, it is also called the *coronary sulcus*.

The **interventricular sulcus** indicates the septum separating the right and left ventricles. It is usually divided into an anterior interventricular and posterior interventricular sulcus.

The Heart Wall. The heart, like all hollow viscera, consists of three layers: (1) an outer serous layer, (2) a middle muscular layer, and (3) an inner lining. Specifically the names for the structures forming the heart wall are the **epicardium** (or visceral pericardium), a serous layer that covers the external aspect of the heart; the **myocardium,** a layer of cardiac involuntary muscle that originates from and inserts into fibrous rings surrounding the valve orifices; and the **endocardium,** an inner lining of endothelium.

Entrances and Exits. Entering the right atrium are the superior and inferior venae cavae carrying deoxygenated blood from the system (*Figure 3-21*). The superior vena

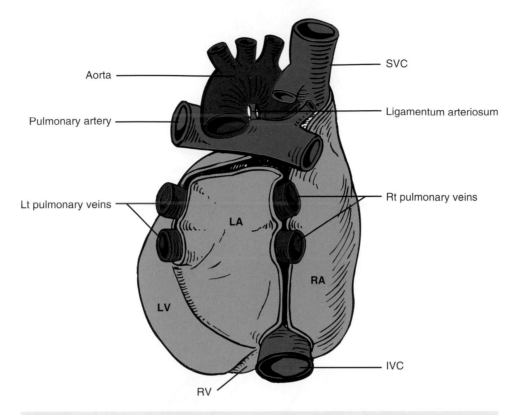

Figure 3-20 Posterior (basal) surface of heart. *IVC*, Inferior vena cava; *SVC*, superior vena cava; *RA*, right atrium; *LA*, left atrium; *RV*, right ventricle; *LV*, left ventricle.

cava returns blood from the head and upper limb and thorax; the inferior vena cava returns blood from the lower limbs and abdomen.

Upon contraction of the atrium, blood passes through the right atrioventricular valve to the right ventricle. Upon contraction of the ventricle, blood leaves the heart to pass to the right and left lungs via the pulmonary arteries. Blood gases are exchanged in the lung, and oxygenated blood returns via pulmonary veins to the left atrium. Upon contraction of the atrium, blood passes through the left atrioventricular valve to the left ventricle. Upon contraction of the left ventricle, oxygenated blood passes to the system via the aorta and its branches.

Internal Features of the Heart Chambers

Right Atrium. The right atrium is a relatively thin-walled receiving chamber for the incoming contents of the superior and inferior venae cavae (*Figure 3-22*). In addition, blood returning from the heart muscle via the coronary sinus empties into the right atrium. Internally the right atrium presents a number of significant features:

1. The **orifice of the superior vena cava** lies superiorly. It is not guarded by valves.
2. The **orifice of the inferior vena cava** lies inferiorly and is guarded by a small, rudimentary, crescent-shaped valve.

3. The **crista terminalis** is a vertical ridge running between the orifices of the two venae cavae. It divides the atrium into a relatively smooth posterior wall and a roughened anterior wall. It represents the junction between the sinus venosus and the heart in the developing heart of the embryo.
4. The **pectinate muscles** radiate out at right angles from the crista terminalis and travel in a roughly parallel but interconnected transverse course.
5. The **fossa ovalis** is an oval depression on the smooth posterior border immediately above the valve of the inferior vena cava. It represents the obliterated **foramen ovale**, a prenatal shunt from right to left atrium (see Chapter 1, page 18). The *anulus ovalis* is a slightly raised ridge surrounding the fossa ovalis.
6. The **right auricle** is an appendage of the right atrium, and its lumen is continuous with the atrial lumen. Externally the right auricle embraces the base of the aorta.
7. The **right atrioventricular valve** lies inferiorly and to the left of the inferior vena cava orifice. It is commonly called the *tricuspid valve*, which describes the three leaf-like (cusp) components of the valve. The orifice of the valve leads to the right ventricle.
8. The **coronary sinus** returns blood from the heart walls and opens into the right atrium just above the atrioventricular orifice.

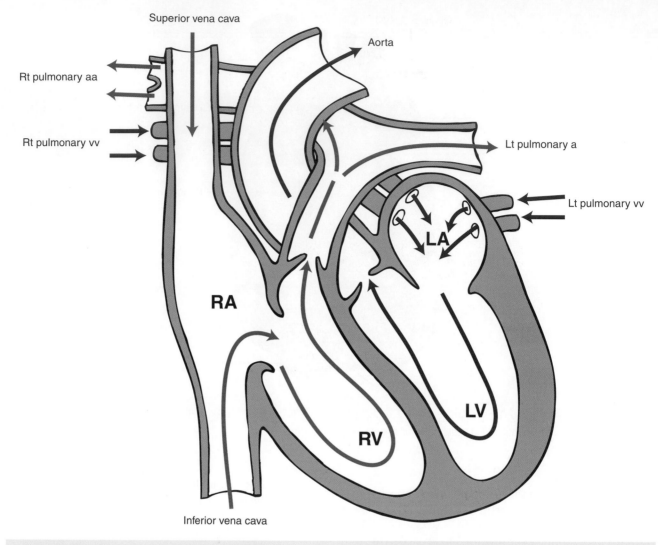

Figure 3-21 Flow of blood through chambers of heart.

9. The **sinoatrial** and **atrioventricular nodes** are localized areas of specialized myocardial tissue in the right atrium. They are not visible on gross inspection of the cadaver heart, but their locations are described. The sinoatrial node, the pacemaker of the heart, is located at the junction of the superior vena cava and the right atrium. The atrioventricular node, the relay station, is located in the septum above the opening of the coronary sinus. The roles of the sinoatrial and atrioventricular nodes are described on page 77.

Right Ventricle. The right ventricle is a thicker-walled chamber than the atrium and represents a pumping chamber (*Figure 3-23*). It receives blood from the right atrium via the right atrioventricular valve. The internal features are as follows:

1. **Trabeculae carneae** are ridges of cardiac muscles that give the internal aspect a roughened appearance.

2. The **right atrioventricular valve**, or **tricuspid valve**, consists of three cusps, and the bases of these are anchored to a tendinous ring around the valve orifice. The free edges of the cusps project into the lumen of the right ventricle. They prevent backflow of blood into the right atrium during ventricular systole.

3. **Chordae tendineae** are thin, tendinous cords or strings that pass from the free edges of the cusps to papillary muscles.

4. **Papillary muscles** anchor the chordae tendineae and the cusps to the heart wall. The papillary muscles contract concurrently with the contraction of the ventricles and ensure that the tips of the cusps seal the orifice without being blown back into the right atrium.

5. The **pulmonary valve** guards the exit of blood from the right ventricle to the pulmonary artery. It is a pocket valve and consists of three pockets, which lie flattened against the lumen of the orifice when empty. After contraction of the right ventricle and the escape of

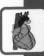

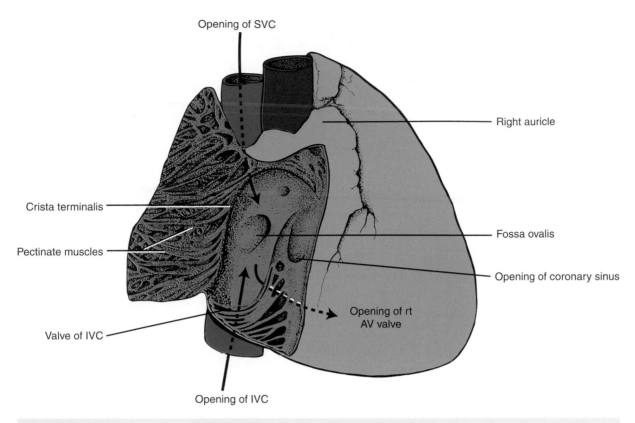

Opening of SVC

Right auricle

Crista terminalis

Fossa ovalis

Pectinate muscles

Opening of coronary sinus

Opening of rt
AV valve

Valve of IVC

Opening of IVC

Figure 3-22 Internal features of opened right atrium. *AV,* Atrioventricular; *IVC,* inferior vena cava; *SVC,* superior vena cava.

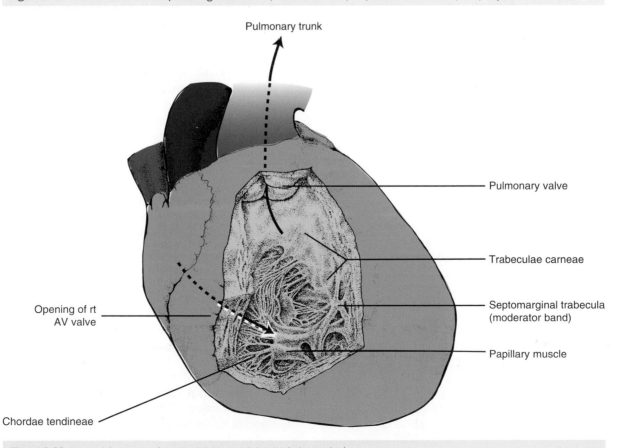

Pulmonary trunk

Pulmonary valve

Trabeculae carneae

Septomarginal trabecula
(moderator band)

Opening of rt
AV valve

Papillary muscle

Chordae tendineae

Figure 3-23 Internal features of opened right ventricle. *AV,* Atrioventricular.

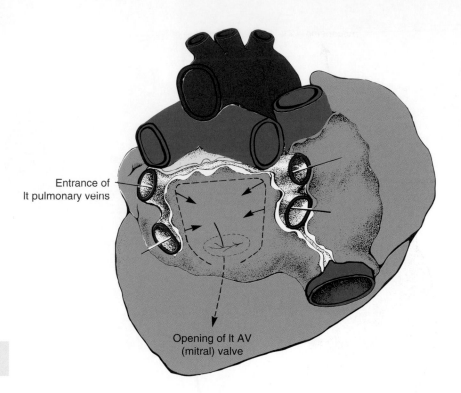

Entrance of
lt pulmonary veins

Opening of lt AV
(mitral) valve

Figure 3-24 Internal features of left atrium.
AV, Atrioventricular.

blood to the pulmonary trunk, backflow of blood fills the pockets and closes the valve, preventing further backflow into the right ventricle.

6. The **septomarginal trabecula** (moderate band) contains impulse-conducting cardiac fibers from the interventricular septum to the anterior papillary muscle.

Left Atrium. The left atrium is a thin-walled receiving chamber for incoming contents of the pulmonary veins from the lungs (*Figure 3-24*). Two **right** and two **left pulmonary veins** enter through four separate orifices. Draining the left atrium is the **left atrioventricular valve,** or bicuspid or **mitral valve,** described next.

Left Ventricle. The left ventricle is a pumping chamber that pumps blood to the entire body (*Figure 3-25*). As a result, the ventricular walls are even thicker than the right ventricular walls. Within the left ventricle are structures that are similar to those found in the right ventricle:

1. **Trabeculae carneae** are ridges of cardiac muscle that roughen the internal aspect of the ventricle.

2. The **left atrioventricular valve,** or **mitral valve,** is similar to its right counterpart except that it consists of only two cusps (bicuspid). To the early anatomists the two cusps resembled a bishop's mitre (i.e., tall hat with pointed front and rear panels) and hence the term *mitral valve.*

3. **Chordae tendineae** and **papillary muscles** function in the same manner as on the right side and prevent the blowing out of the valves into the left atrium during ventricular contraction.

4. The **aortic valve** is a three-pocket valve identical in design and function to the pulmonary valve. It prevents regurgitation of blood from the aorta back into the left ventricle.

Auscultation of Heart Valves. The heart valves may be auscultated (listened to) with a stethoscope to distinguish between normal and abnormal heart sounds and to detect heart murmurs as the chambers undergo successive contractions (*Figure 3-26*). Normally one hears two distinct sounds: *lub-dup.* The first sound (*lub*) is produced by the contraction of the ventricles and the closure of the atrioventricular (systole). The second sound (*dup*) is produced by the audible closure of the aortic and pulmonary valves during relaxation (diastole). It is important to know where to place the stethoscope to listen to each of the heart valves.

The areas of auscultation are remote from the actual heart valve sites because the valve sites are closely packed together in diagonal fashion from the left second sternocostal articulation to the right sixth sternocostal articulation. In addition, they are obscured by the sternum. However, valve sounds are carried along with blood flow and detected where blood flow deflects off the heart wall.

Thus the **mitral valve** is best heard at the heart apex, the **tricuspid valve** at the left lower aspect of the sternal border, and the **pulmonary valve** at the left sternal border second interspace. The **aortic valve** is the only one heard on the right sternal border at the second interspace.

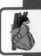

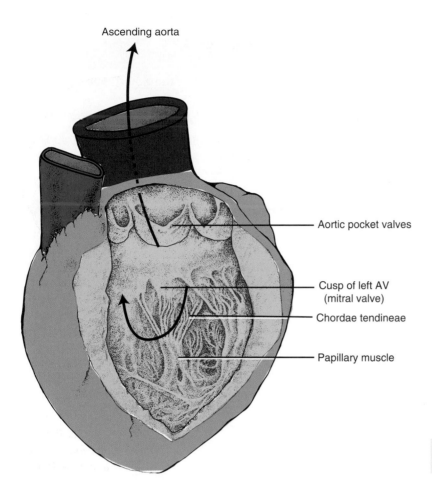

Ascending aorta

Aortic pocket valves

Cusp of left AV
(mitral valve)

Chordae tendineae

Papillary muscle

Figure 3-25 Internal features of opened left
ventricle of heart. *AV,* Atrioventricular.

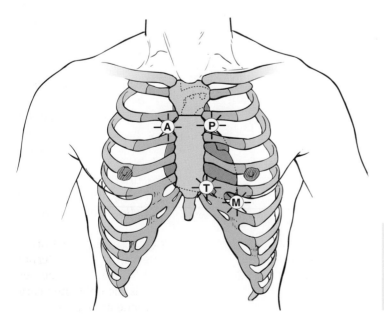

Figure 3-26 Sites of auscultation of heart sounds. **A** (aortic)
is detected at the second interspace, right sternal border. **P**
(pulmonary) is heard at the left sternal border second interspace. **M** (mitral) is best heard at heart apex in fifth interspace. **T** (tricuspid) is heard at lower left aspect of sternal
border.

CLINICAL NOTES

Damaged Heart Valves

Some patients have a history of damaged heart valves. The damage may be congenital or acquired following a disease such as rheumatic fever, which may result in an inflamed heart, or carditis. Carditis may damage heart valves, resulting in two types of conditions. *Valvular insufficiency* is incomplete closure of a heart valve or a leaky valve permitting the backflow of blood. A mitral valve insufficiency, for example, allows blood to leak back into the left atrium during ventricular systole. *Valvular stenosis* is the narrowing of a heart valve orifice, which interferes with the volume of blood flowing into or out of a chamber. A mitral valve stenosis, for example, prevents the complete emptying of blood to the left ventricle. This condition can be corrected with a mitral valve replacement.

In either case insufficiency or stenosis over time will put stress on the affected chambers, increase their work load, and depending on which valve is diseased, cause hypertrophy of the right (pulmonary) or the left (systemic) side of the heart. The heart can enlarge or hypertrophy to a certain extent, and then it will go into failure.

Heart Murmur

The turbulence generated by blood flowing through damaged valves produces a characteristic sound that can be heard with a stethoscope.

Prophylactic Antibiotics for Oral Surgical and Dental Procedures

Patients with damaged heart valves run the risk of acquiring *subacute bacterial endocarditis*, a blood-borne bacterial infection of the endocardial lining of the heart. Any dental or oral procedure that results in bleeding can send a shower of streptococcal bacteria into the bloodstream (bacteremia). These bacteria settle and produce vegetative growths on damaged heart valves. Untreated conditions can be fatal. Preventing this condition in patients with known heart valve damage requires that a large prophylactic dose of antibiotic be given 1 hour before any dental or oral procedure that can result in bleeding. This dose should be followed by a smaller dose 6 hours after the procedure.

Blood Vessels

Coronary Arteries. The **right** and **left coronary arteries** are the first pair of arteries to arise from the aorta (see *Figure 3-31*). They arise just above the aortic valve, where the aortic valves dilate somewhat as the aortic sinus. The **aortic sinus** is divided into right, left, and posterior parts by the pocket valves. The right and left coronary arteries arise from the right and left aortic sinuses, respectively, to supply the heart wall (*Figure 3-27*).

The **right coronary artery** passes inferiorly in the anterior atrioventricular sulcus, supplying blood to cardiac tissue. At the inferior margin of the heart it gives off

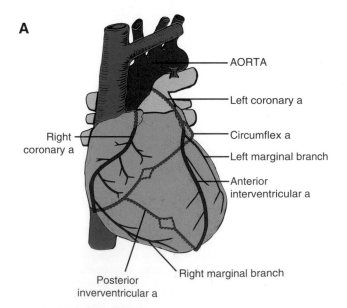

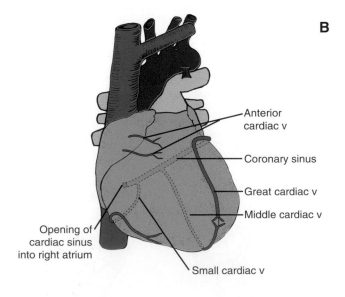

Figure 3-27 Blood vessels of heart. **A**, Arterial supply. **B**, Venous drainage.

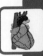

the *right marginal branch* and then turns posteriorly and ascends in the posterior atrioventricular sulcus until it reaches the posterior interventricular groove. There it divides into two branches. One branch continues posteriorly in the atrioventricular sulcus to anastomose with the circumflex artery. The other branch turns obliquely downward toward the apex of the heart to anastomose with the anterior interventricular branch of the left coronary artery.

The **left coronary artery** travels between the left atrium and pulmonary trunk to reach the atrioventricular or coronary sulcus, where it gives off two terminal branches. The **anterior interventricular** branch descends in the sulcus toward the apex of the heart. It curves around posteriorly to anastomose with the posterior interventricular branch of the right coronary artery. The **circumflex branch** travels around to the posterior aspect of the heart in the atrioventricular sulcus. It descends obliquely to anastomose with the terminal part of the right coronary artery.

Coronary Veins. A single large vein, termed the *coronary sinus*, travels in the posterior atrioventricular sulcus toward the right atrium of the heart, which it enters. The various cardiac veins of the heart drain into this coronary sinus.

The **great cardiac vein** receives venous blood as it travels up the anterior interventricular sulcus. As it approaches the atrioventricular sulcus, it turns sharply posteriorly and to the right as the coronary sinus. Here it receives a tributary from the left atrium, the **oblique vein**, and a second tributary, the **posterior vein of the left ventricle**. As the coronary sinus approaches the right atrium, it receives the **middle cardiac vein**, traveling in the posterior interventricular sulcus, and small cardiac veins.

Small **anterior cardiac veins** of the right ventricle drain directly to the right atrium. An undetermined small amount of blood passes to and from the heart wall via small veins called *venae cordis minimae*. They take blood directly from the chambers to the heart wall and back again.

Innervation

Intrinsic Control of Heartbeat. A specialized conduction system exists in the heart (*Figure 3-28*). This system initiates the heartbeat and conducts this impulse to cardiac muscle to effect the heartbeat, or contraction.

The **sinoatrial node** is a small aggregation of specialized cardiac muscle tissue on the superior aspect of the crista terminalis at the junction of the superior vena cava and the right atrium. It acts as a pacemaker and initiates the heartbeat. The initiated impulse (about 70 beats/min) spreads out over the atrial walls and causes them to contract and fill the ventricle.

The **atrioventricular node** contains similar specialized cardiac tissue. It is located in the atrioventricular septum

---

CLINICAL NOTES

Coronary Atherosclerosis

Coronary atherosclerosis is a progressive narrowing (stenosis) of the coronary arteries caused by the deposition of lipid plaque (atheromas) below the intima of the vessels.

Cardiac Ischemia

Ischemia refers to oxygen-deprived tissue. In this case, occluded or stenosed cardiac arteries deliver less oxygen to the myocardium.

Angina Pectoris

Angina means pain, and *pectoris* refers to the chest region. Angina pectoris occurs when cardiac ischemia places sufficient stress on the myocardium to result in a characteristic pain that may range from a severe, constricting, substernal pain to a vague discomfort in the chest. The pain may radiate to the left shoulder, medial aspect of the left arm, back, throat, and jaws. Angina is elicited by increased demands on the myocardium that occur during an increase in physical activity. Pain subsides upon rest. If prescribed, a tablet of nitroglycerine may be placed under the tongue; the tablet is rapidly absorbed into the blood to dilate the occluded vessels and relieve the angina.

Myocardial Infarction

A myocardial infarction occurs when a coronary vessel is completely occluded and the block of myocardium supplied becomes necrotic and dies. Myocardium does not regenerate; the necrotic or dead tissue is replaced by scar tissue.

Coronary Angioplasty

Angioplasty involves the passage of a catheter to an occluded coronary vessel. A tiny balloon is inflated at the end of the catheter to dilate the vessel lumen and increase the blood flow.

Coronary Bypass

Coronary bypass is a surgically created shunt to bypass a diseased portion of the coronary arteries. For the graft an expendable segment of the great saphenous vein is removed from the patient's lower limb. The vein is reversed in direction before it is grafted in place so that the arterial flow is not impeded by the valves in the vein.

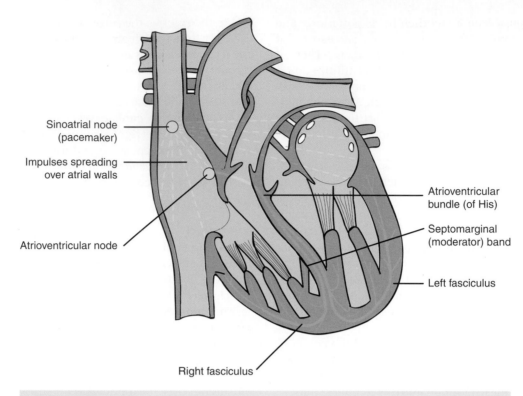

Sinoatrial node
(pacemaker)

Impulses spreading
over atrial walls

Atrioventricular node

Atrioventricular
bundle (of His)

Septomarginal
(moderator) band

Left fasciculus

Right fasciculus

Figure 3-28 Scheme of conducting system of heart.

just above the opening of the coronary sinus. It picks up the impulses from the atrial walls and relays the impulses down the interventricular septum via a bundle of specialized cardiac muscle cells (**bundle of His**), which are capable of conduction.

The bundle of His divides into right and left portions, which descend in the interventricular septum to distribute the impulses to the right and left ventricular walls, causing them to contract. Conduction fibers also travel to the papillary muscles in both ventricles to effect a simultaneous contraction with the ventricles and thereby prevent damage and leakage at the atrioventricular valves.

Extrinsic Modification of the Heartbeat. The autonomic nervous system can modify the rate at which the pacemaker sinoatrial node initiates the heartbeats. **Parasympathetic fibers** from the vagus nerve *slow* the heartbeat, whereas **sympathetic fibers** from the sympathetic trunk *speed up* the heartbeat.

The **cardiac plexus** is a collection of both parasympathetic and sympathetic fibers found on the inferior aortic arch border anterior to the bifurcation of the trachea. It receives preganglionic vagal fibers, which synapse in the plexus. It also receives postganglionic sympathetic fibers, which had previously synapsed in the cervical ganglia of the sympathetic trunk. Parasympathetic and sympathetic efferents leave the cardiac plexus and pass to the heart to modify the heartbeat.

Afferent, or Sensory, Cardiac Nerves. Afferent nerve fibers accompany sympathetic nerves to carry visceral

feedback to the central nervous system (CNS). These impulses normally are not perceived at a conscious level. However, when cardiac muscle is rendered ischemic because of impaired blood flow, impulses rise to a conscious level through this pathway and are perceived as pain or **angina pectoris.**

CLINICAL NOTES

Electrocardiogram

The impulses generated by the sinoatrial node that eventually spread over the atria and through the conducting system can be detected, amplified, and recorded on a chart or electrocardiogram.

Heart Block

The anterior interventricular artery supplies the interventricular septum. Should this artery be occluded and an infarct occur in this area, it could damage the atrioventricular bundle, cutting one or both ventricles from their conducting system. The ventricles will continue to beat on their own but at a reduced rate. This condition, termed a *heart block*, is treatable with the surgical subcutaneous placement of a **pacemaker** attached to a wire threaded through the venous system to the wall of the right ventricle.

Continued

The cardiac component of the cardiopulmonary resuscitation involves restarting circulation by applying manual pressure to the sternum (external heart massage).

Cardiac Dysrhythmias

Dysrhythmias are irregular beats that occur when there is interference with the conducting system. This can result in a variety of conditions, such as accelerated heart rate (tachycardia), decelerated heart rate (bradycardia), and premature atrial or ventricular beats. In addition, chaotic signals can cause twitching (fibrillation) of the atria or the ventricles. Ventricular fibrillation is a more serious condition because of impaired systemic circulation.

ANTERIOR MEDIASTINUM

The anterior mediastinum contains connective tissue and fat, a bit of thymus gland, and some lymph nodes.

SUPERIOR AND POSTERIOR MEDIASTINUM

It is more efficient to consider the structures of the superior and posterior mediastinum as single units because they pass from one to the other (*Figures 3-29* and *3-30*).

Trachea and Bronchi

The trachea and bronchi are described on page 65 with the lung.

Esophagus

The esophagus is a tubelike portion of the gastrointestinal tract; extends from the pharynx at vertebral level C6 to the abdomen at vertebral level T11. It has three components: (1) a cervical, (2) a thoracic, and (3) a short abdominal portion.

The esophagus has four constrictions: (1) at its origin or pharyngeal end, (2) where it passes the aortic arch in the superior mediastinum, (3) at the bifurcation of the trachea, and (4) where it passes through the diaphragm.

Both ends of the esophagus exhibit a sphincter: (1) The pharyngeal end is guarded by the cricopharyngeus muscle to prevent the swallowing of air, and (2) the abdominal end is controlled by the cardiac sphincter to prevent regurgitation of stomach contents.

Thoracic Esophagus. The esophagus enters the thorax and superior mediastinum through the thoracic inlet, anterior to vertebral bodies and posterior to the trachea. It continues into the posterior mediastinum and at vertebral levels T8, T9, and T10; the aortic arch and descending aorta intervene between the vertebral bodies and the esophagus below the level of the heart. Here the esophagus is suspended by a mesoesophagus from the aorta

behind, which frees the esophagus somewhat to pass anteriorly and slightly to the left as it passes through the diaphragm.

Blood Supply. The esophagus picks up blood vessels as it descends. In the cervical region it receives branches from the laryngeal arteries. In the thorax it receives a variable number of visceral branches from the aorta. In the abdomen it receives branches from the short and left gastric arteries.

Nerve Supply. The esophagus picks up autonomic nerves as it descends. In the cervical region it receives sympathetic fibers from the cervical sympathetic ganglia and parasympathetic fibers from recurrent laryngeal branches of the vagus nerve. In the thorax and abdomen sympathetic supply is from the sympathetic trunk, and parasympathetic supply is from the vagus nerves.

In the superior mediastinum the right and left vagus nerves form a plexus around the esophagus (esophageal plexus) and follow the esophagus as it continues into the posterior mediastinum and through the diaphragm into the abdomen. Within the abdomen the vagus nerves are reconstituted as the **anterior** and **posterior vagal trunks.**

Aorta

Within the thorax the aorta is divided for descriptive purposes, into the ascending aorta, aortic arch, and descending or thoracic aorta (*Figure 3-31*).

CLINICAL NOTES

Lodging of Foreign Objects

The areas of constriction slow the passage of food at these levels and represent sites where accidentally swallowed objects or an overly large bolus of food can lodge. The first constriction, or cricopharyngeus constriction, is the most common site where obstructions in children can occur.

Esophageal Dysphasia

Dysphasia is difficulty in swallowing that can be caused by several conditions. Partial obstructions produced by tumors in adjacent structures or carcinoma of the esophagus itself can cause dysphasia. In addition, motor disorders can interfere with esophageal peristalsis.

Heartburn

Despite the name, heartburn is an irritated esophagus caused by a reflux of acidic gastric contents past the cardiac sphincter. This reflux results in a burning sensation in the chest deep to the sternum.

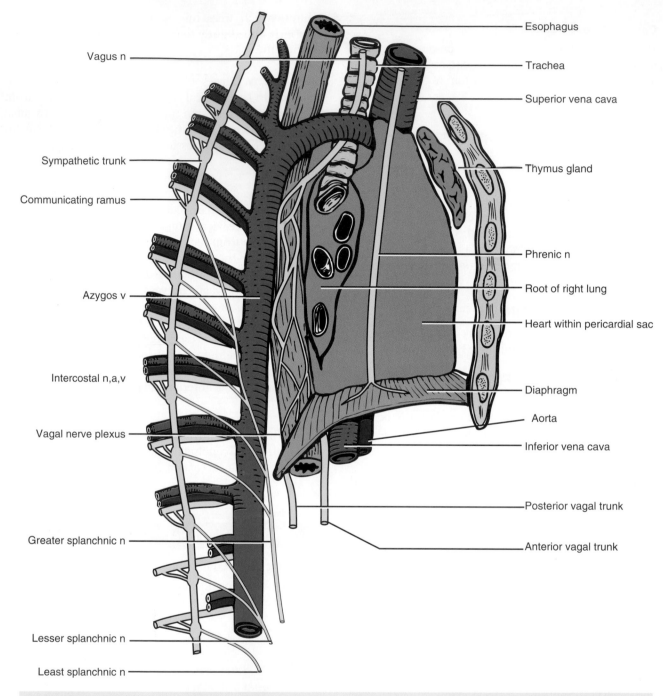

Vagus n

Sympathetic trunk

Communicating ramus

Azygos v

Intercostal n,a,v

Vagal nerve plexus

Greater splanchnic n

Lesser splanchnic n

Least splanchnic n

Esophagus

Trachea

Superior vena cava

Thymus gland

Phrenic n

Root of right lung

Heart within pericardial sac

Diaphragm

Aorta

Inferior vena cava

Posterior vagal trunk

Anterior vagal trunk

Figure 3-29 Lateral view of right mediastinum. Right lung has been removed.

Ascending Aorta and Its Branches. The ascending aorta originates at the aortic orifice and, arching slightly to the left, passes superiorly to the level of the second costal cartilage. Above the aortic valves, the ascending aorta bulges slightly as the **aortic sinus.** The three valves divide the sinus into a right, left, and posterior portion. Arising from the right and left coronary sinuses are the **right** and **left coronary arteries,** respectively.

Aortic Arch and Its Branches. The aortic arch begins at the level of the second costal cartilage and arches to the left so that its superior border lies at about the midpoint of the manubrium. In addition to arching to the left, it arches posteriorly and descends to vertebral level T4, where it continues inferiorly as the **descending aorta.**

Brachiocephalic Artery. The branchiocephalic artery is the first branch to arise from the aortic arch. It passes upward posteriorly to the right sternoclavicular joint and at this

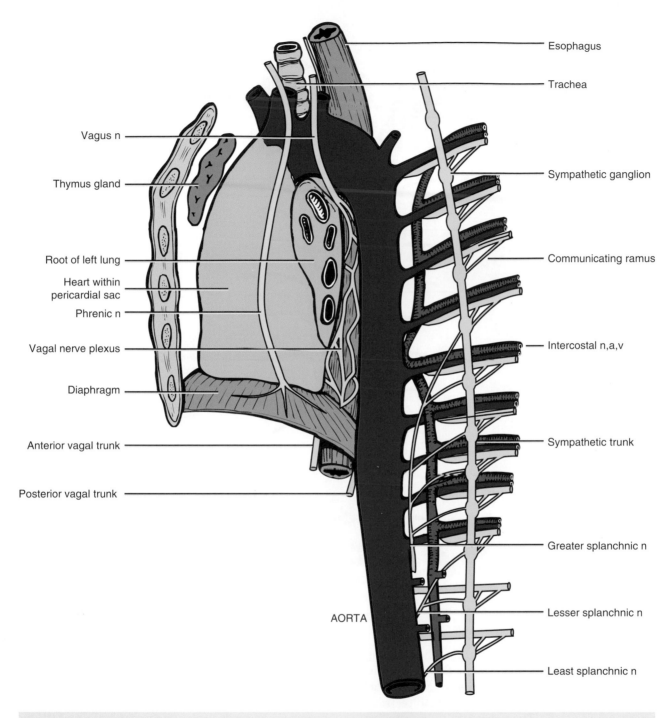

Vagus n

Thymus gland

Root of left lung

Heart within
pericardial sac

Phrenic n

Vagal nerve plexus

Diaphragm

Anterior vagal trunk

Posterior vagal trunk

AORTA

Esophagus

Trachea

Sympathetic ganglion

Communicating ramus

Intercostal n,a,v

Sympathetic trunk

Greater splanchnic n

Lesser splanchnic n

Least splanchnic n

Figure 3-30 Lateral view of left side of mediastinum. Left lung has been removed.

level divides into the **right common carotid artery,** which ascends to the neck, and the **right subclavian artery,** which enters the upper limb.

Left Common Carotid Artery. The left common carotid artery arises from the apex of the aortic arch posterior to the left sternoclavicular joint. It ascends through the left side of the neck.

Left Subclavian Artery. The left subclavian artery arises immediately distal to the left common carotid artery and passes to the left upper limb.

Descending (Thoracic) Aorta. The descending aorta continues inferiorly from the aortic arch from vertebral level T4. It turns slightly to the right and comes to lie anterior to the vertebral bodies within the posterior mediastinum. It descends through the posterior mediastinum, providing unpaired visceral branches to thoracic viscera and paired somatic branches to the thoracic wall. The thoracic aorta ends by passing through the diaphragm to become the **abdominal aorta** at vertebral level T12.

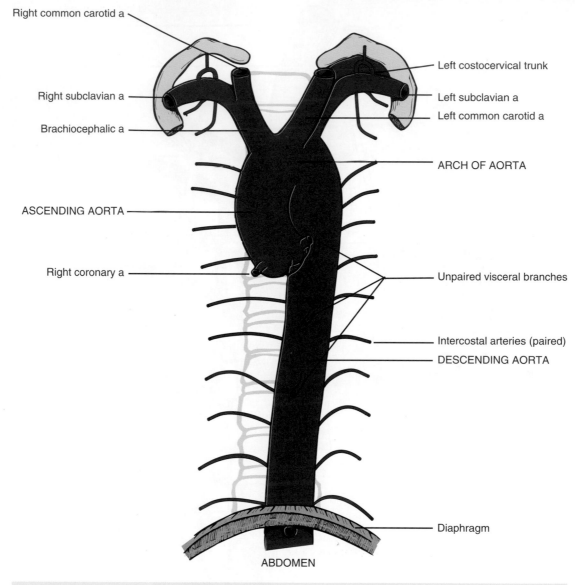

Right common carotid a

Left costocervical trunk

Right subclavian a

Left subclavian a

Brachiocephalic a

Left common carotid a

ARCH OF AORTA

ASCENDING AORTA

Right coronary a

Unpaired visceral branches

Intercostal arteries (paired)

DESCENDING AORTA

Diaphragm

ABDOMEN

Figure 3-31 Thoracic aorta and its branches.

Visceral branches supply the lungs, the esophagus, and the pericardium and diaphragm. **Somatic branches** consist of the lower nine posterior intercostal arteries and the subcostal artery, which arise directly from the descending aorta. (The upper two intercostal arteries arise from the costocervical trunk, a branch of the subclavian artery.)

Veins of the Thorax. There are three main veins or groups of veins to consider in the thorax: (1) the inferior vena cava, (2) the superior vena cava and its tributaries, and (3) the azygos and hemiazygos systems of veins (*Figure 3-32*).

Inferior Vena Cava. The inferior vena cava drains the lower limbs and the abdomen, pierces the diaphragm through the central tendon, rises in the thorax for 1 to 2 cm, and ends abruptly in the inferior aspect of the right atrium of the heart.

Superior Vena Cava and Its Tributaries. The superior vena cava basically drains the upper limbs and the head and neck. It is formed by a union of the **right** and **left brachiocephalic veins** at the level of the first costal cartilage behind the manubrium. The superior vena cava then descends behind the body of the sternum to the level of the third costal cartilage, where it enters the right atrium of the heart.

The **brachiocephalic veins** are formed by a union of the **internal jugular veins** and the **subclavian veins** at the root of the neck behind the sternoclavicular joints. The left vein passes to the right to join the descending right brachiocephalic vein at the level of the first costal cartilage.

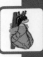

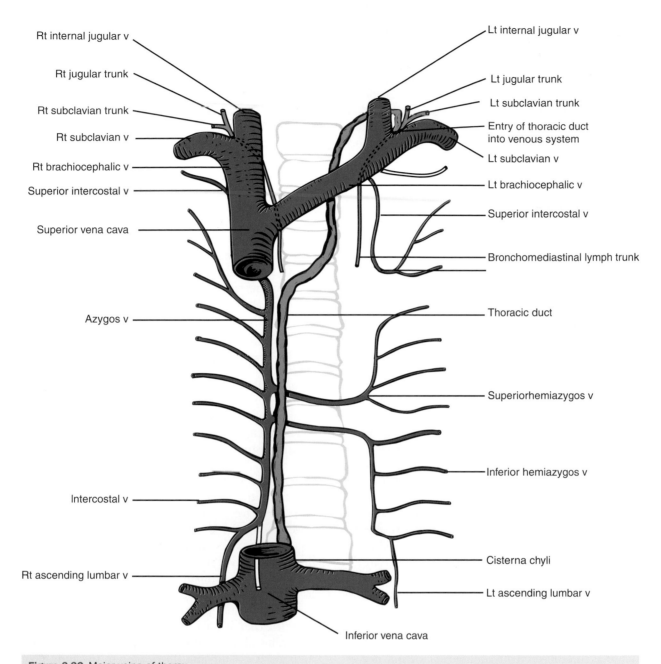

Rt internal jugular v

Rt jugular trunk

Rt subclavian trunk

Rt subclavian v

Rt brachiocephalic v

Superior intercostal v

Superior vena cava

Azygos v

Intercostal v

Rt ascending lumbar v

Lt internal jugular v

Lt jugular trunk

Lt subclavian trunk

Entry of thoracic duct into venous system

Lt subclavian v

Lt brachiocephalic v

Superior intercostal v

Bronchomediastinal lymph trunk

Thoracic duct

Superiorhemiazygos v

Inferior hemiazygos v

Cisterna chyli

Lt ascending lumbar v

Inferior vena cava

Figure 3-32 Major veins of thorax.

The Azygos and Hemiazygos System of Veins. The azygos and hemiazygos system of veins drains the thoracic wall (see *Figure 3-32*). Ascending from the abdomen to the thorax are the **right** and **left ascending lumbar veins**. The right ascending lumbar vein passes through the diaphragm and continues to rise as the **azygos vein**. It picks up all the *intercostal veins* except the *highest intercostal*, which drains to the *right brachiocephalic vein*. At the level of the third to fourth thoracic vertebrae, the azygos vein arches anteriorly over the root of the right lung to empty into the **superior vena cava**.

The left ascending lumbar vein continues up into the thorax as the **inferior hemiazygos vein** and drains the lower intercostal veins. It ascends to approximately vertebral level T8 and then crosses the midline to join the azygos vein on the right side. An **accessory**, or **superior**, **hemiazygos vein** drains the fourth, fifth, sixth, and seventh intercostal veins as it descends to the level of T8, where it crosses to the right to enter the azygos vein. The upper three intercostal veins join to form the *superior intercostal vein*, which ascends to drain to the *left brachiocephalic vein*.

The Thoracic Duct

The thoracic duct begins in the abdomen as a small sac called the *cisterna chyli*. Draining to the cisterna chyli are the lymphatics of the *lower extremities*, the *pelvis*, and the *abdomen.* Arising from the cisterna chyli is the **thoracic duct,** which enters the thorax through the aortic opening in the diaphragm. It then ascends within the thorax between the azygos vein and the aorta. Within the thorax, it picks up visceral lymphatic drainage via the **bronchomediastinal trunk.** As the duct approaches the root of the neck, it swings to the left, arches around the left internal jugular vein, and ends by emptying its contents into the confluence of the left internal jugular and left subclavian veins.

Nerves of the Thorax

Four types of nerves are found within the thorax: intercostal nerves, the sympathetic trunk and its branches, the phrenic nerve and its branches, and the vagus nerve (see *Figures 3-29* and *3-30*).

Intercostal Nerves. The intercostal nerves arise from the spinal cord as **anterior rami** of spinal nerves T1 to T12. Spinal nerve T12 is not intercostal but lies below the twelfth rib. For this reason it is called the *subcostal nerve.* The intercostal and subcostal nerves sweep laterally and then anteriorly and medially to supply the musculature of the thoracic walls and return cutaneous sensation from skin of the chest wall and the upper anterior abdominal wall.

Sympathetic Trunk and Its Branches. The scheme of the sympathetic division of the autonomic nervous system is outlined in Chapter 1 on pages 28 to 30. Within the thorax the right and left sympathetic trunks run laterally to the thoracic vertebral bodies. The trunks continue upward to the cervical region and downward to the abdominopelvic region. The thoracic component is covered by parietal pleura.

Incoming **white rami communicantes** run from the intercostal nerves to the ganglia of the sympathetic trunk. Outgoing postganglionic **gray rami communicantes** pass back to the intercostal nerves to be distributed along with the intercostal nerves. Some preganglionic fibers do not synapse in the sympathetic chain of ganglia. Rather, they leave as three discrete myelinated **splanchnic nerves:** greater, lesser, and least splanchnic nerves. The splanchnic nerves pierce the crura of the diaphragm, enter the abdomen, and synapse in the various preaortic ganglia of the abdomen. Postganglionic fibers supply abdominal viscera (see *Figure 4-15*).

Phrenic Nerve. The phrenic nerve arises from the neck from **anterior rami of spinal nerves C3, C4, and C5** (see *Figures 5-18* and *5-20*). It descends along the anterior surface of the scalenus anterior muscle and enters the thoracic inlet anterior to the subclavian artery. It then descends along the lateral aspect of the mediastinum, covered by mediastinal pleura, to the diaphragm below (see *Figures 3-29* and *3-30*). The phrenic nerve carries both efferent and afferent fibers to and from the diaphragm.

The Vagus Nerve (Cranial Nerve X). The vagus nerves exit from the skull through the jugular foramina, descend through the neck in the carotid sheaths, and enter the thoracic inlet anterior to the subclavian arteries (see *Figures 5-14* and *5-20*). As the right vagus nerve passes the right subclavian artery, it gives rise to the **right recurrent laryngeal nerve,** which then loops under the right subclavian artery and ascends in the neck lateral to the trachea to enter the larynx from below. Its distribution is followed in the section dealing with the larynx.

The **left recurrent laryngeal nerve** arises from the left vagus nerve after the vagus nerve passes anterior to the aortic arch. The left recurrent laryngeal nerve loops around the aortic arch and ascends in the neck alongside the trachea to enter the larynx on the left side.

Both vagus nerves descend posteriorly to the root of the lung and provide branches to the **pulmonary plexus** and branches to the **cardiac plexus.** The vagus nerves then converge on the esophagus and descend through the thorax as a nerve plexus surrounding the esophagus. Within the abdomen the vagus nerves form up again as the **anterior** and **posterior vagal trunks.**

Cardiac and Pulmonary Plexuses. The cardiac plexus is found below the aortic arch and anterior to the tracheal bifurcation. It receives sympathetic postganglionic fibers from the cervical sympathetic ganglia via cardiac nerves. It receives preganglionic parasympathetic fibers from the vagus nerves, which synapse within the cardiac plexus. Outgoing fibers pass to the heart (sympathetic fibers speed up the heartbeat; parasympathetic fibers slow the heartbeat).

The pulmonary plexus surrounds the pulmonary vessels at the root of the lung. Sympathetic fibers come from the cardiac plexus; parasympathetic fibers arise from the vagus nerves. Outgoing fibers pass to the lung (sympathetic fibers dilate the bronchioles; parasympathetic fibers constrict the bronchioles).

Thymus Gland

The thymus gland consists of lymphoid tissue (see *Figures 3-29* and *3-30*). It is relatively large in the child, reaches a maximum absolute weight during puberty, and thereafter begins to atrophy and to be replaced by adipose tissue. In the adult cadaver it is hardly noticeable in the superior and anterior mediastina. The thymus gland produces T lymphocytes.

Review Questions

1. The anterior intercostal arteries arise from the
   _____.
   a. ascending aorta
   b. internal thoracic artery
   c. subclavian artery
   d. posterior intercostal arteries
   e. descending aorta

2. The right primary bronchus _____.
   a. divides into two primary bronchi within the right lung
   b. is slightly longer than the left primary bronchus
   c. arises from the trachea at vertebral level C6
   d. is slightly narrower that the right primary bronchus
   e. is most likely to transmit aspirated foreign objects

3. Quiet, passive expiration is accomplished by
   _____.
   a. recoil of the elastic tissue of the lungs
   b. contraction of the diaphragm
   c. increased abdominal pressure
   d. contraction of the external intercostal muscles
   e. contraction of the serratus anterior muscles

4. A stethoscope placed at the right sternal border, second Interspace would pick up the sounds of the _____.
   a. pulmonary valve
   b. valve of the inferior vena cava
   c. left atrioventricular (mitral) valve
   d. right atrioventricular (tricuspid) valve
   e. aortic valve

5. Which of the following structures does NOT pass through the diaphragm?
   a. The azygos vein
   b. The superior vena cava
   c. The esophagus
   d. The greater splanchnic nerves
   e. The inferior vena cava

6. The visceral blood supply to lung tissue is mainly from _____.
   a. pulmonary arteries
   b. pericardiophrenic arteries
   c. intercostal arteries
   d. bronchial arteries
   e. internal thoracic arteries

7. Which of the following statements concerning the azygos vein is FALSE?
   a. It arises from the right ascending lumbar vein.
   b. It empties into the right brachiocephalic vein.
   c. It receives blood from the right posterior intercostal veins.
   d. It receives blood from the left posterior intercostal veins via the hemiazygos veins.
   e. It is situated in the posterior mediastinum.

8. Which of the following structures is NOT a feature of the right ventricle of the heart?
   a. pectinate muscles
   b. moderator (septomarginal) band
   c. pulmonary valve
   d. trabeculae carneae
   e. tricuspid atrioventricular valve

9. The left coronary artery bifurcates to form the circumflex artery and the _____.
   a. posterior interventricular artery
   b. anterior interventricular artery
   c. transverse artery
   d. middle cardiac artery
   e. marginal artery

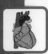

Questions 10 through 12

Match each of the following descriptions with appropriate lettered nerves found in the illustration of the right mediastinum.

10. _____ increases peristalsis of the gut.

11. _____ decreases peristalsis of the gut.

12. _____ is derived from branches of the cervical and brachial plexuses.

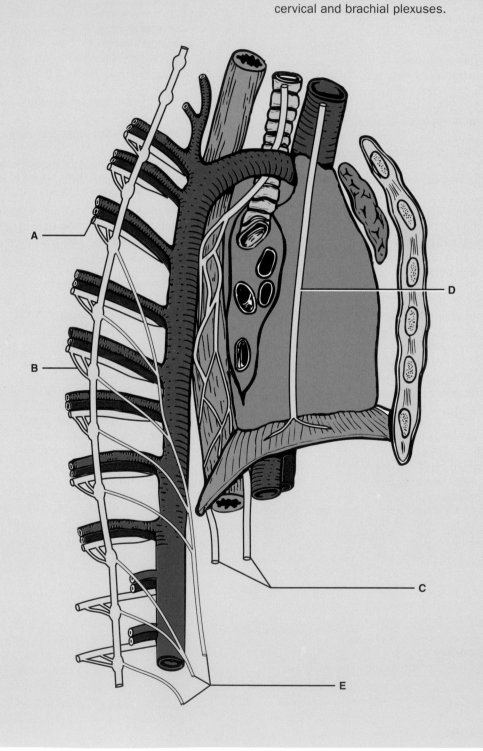

Chapter 4

The Abdomen, Pelvis, and Perineum

1. Skeleton and Subdivisions 87
2. The Abdominal Walls 89
3. Peritoneum and the Peritoneal Cavity 99
4. Blood and Nerve Supply to the Abdomen........... 101
5. The Abdominal Viscera 104

1. Skeleton and Subdivisions

The abdomen (including the pelvis) is a large body cavity containing the major portion of the digestive tract and the viscera of the genitourinary system. Enclosing the abdominal cavity are a muscular anterolateral abdominal wall, a muscular thoracic diaphragm superiorly, a muscular and bony posterior wall, and a muscular and membranous pelvic diaphragm below.

The abdominopelvic cavity extends from the floor of the pelvis inferiorly and rises in a dome superiorly to the level of the fifth intercostal space within the thoracic cage.

SKELETON OF THE ABDOMEN

The skeleton of the abdomen consists of a thoracic component, a vertebral component, and a pelvic component (*Figure 4-1*).

Thoracic Component

Because the abdominal cavity extends up into the thoracic cage, the thorax between the fifth intercostal space above to the costal margin below should be considered, along with the abdominal skeleton. The thoracic cage is discussed on pages 54 to 57.

Vertebral Component

The lower thoracic vertebrae, the lumbar vertebrae, the sacrum, and the coccyx form the vertebral component of the abdominal skeleton. These structures are described on pages 40 to 43.

Pelvic Component

Os Coxae (Hip Bone). The right and left **os coxae** comprise the lower limb girdle and take part in the hip joint (see Chapter 10). In addition, they join with the sacrum and the coccyx to form the **pelvic cavity**, which houses and protects several pelvic viscera. The os coxae is originally formed from three separate bones that fuse as one complete bone by about the sixteenth year. The bones are the ilium, ischium, and pubis, and they lend their names to the three regions of the single adult os coxae (*Figure 4-2*).

The **ilium** superiorly consists of a flared, flattened plate with a concave medial surface and ends superiorly as the iliac crest. The iliac tubercle is a small bony elevation on the superior lateral aspect of the iliac crest. The right and left iliac tubercles mark the widest points on an articulated pelvis. These points can be palpated and represent anthropological landmarks used to measure the width of the pelvis (bicristal diameter). The anterior aspect of the iliac crest exhibits two small elevations called the anterior inferior and the anterior superior iliac spines.

The **ischium** is represented mainly by the ischial tuberosity, which bears the weight of the body when a person is in an upright, seated position.

The **pubis** meets its fellow of the opposite side anteriorly at the pubic symphysis, a semimovable joint that loosens in women to expand the birth canal before childbirth. Lateral to the symphysis is the pubic tubercle. The inguinal ligament connects the pubic tubercle to the anterior superior iliac spine.

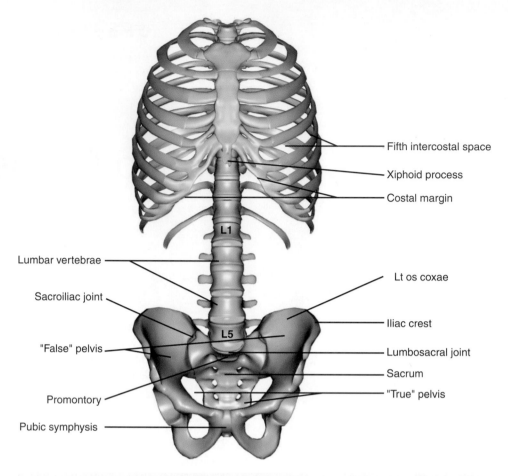

Figure 4-1 Skeleton of abdomen.

The pubis and ischium unite to form the obturator foramen, which is largely obliterated in life by a membrane. All three bony elements meet and contribute to the cup-shaped acetabulum on the lateral aspect, which receives the head of the femur. Projecting posteriorly from the ischium is the ischial spine, which divides the posterior aspect into the greater sciatic notch above (which transmits the sciatic nerve) and the lesser sciatic notch below.

Pelvic Cavity. The pelvic cavity is divided into an **upper (false) pelvis,** limited entirely by the iliac crests, and a **lower (true) pelvis,** surrounded by the right and left pubis, the ischium, and the sacrum, which extends into the lower pelvis as the promontory. The basic difference between typical male and female pelvises is that the diameter of the lower pelvis of a woman generally is larger to allow passage of a baby's head during childbirth.

DIVISIONS OF THE ABDOMEN

To facilitate descriptions of abdominal visceral locations, the abdomen is divided into regions (*Figure 4-3*). There are two systems in common use. One divides the abdomen into

CLINICAL NOTES

Bone Grafts

The iliac crest is a convenient site for harvesting bone to aid surgical procedures that require transplants for bone reconstruction. A relatively noninvasive technique uses a power-driven trephine (a cylindrical saw) to remove a core of bone from the anterior iliac crest for use in maxillofacial (oral) surgery. The grafts are used to fill in bony defects (cleft palates) and to augment alveolar bone for eventual dental implants.

four quadrants based on the median sagittal plane in the abdomen intersecting with a transverse plane. This effectively divides the abdomen into upper left, upper right, lower left, and lower right quadrants.

The other system divides the abdomen into nine regions based on two sagittal and two transverse planes through the abdomen.

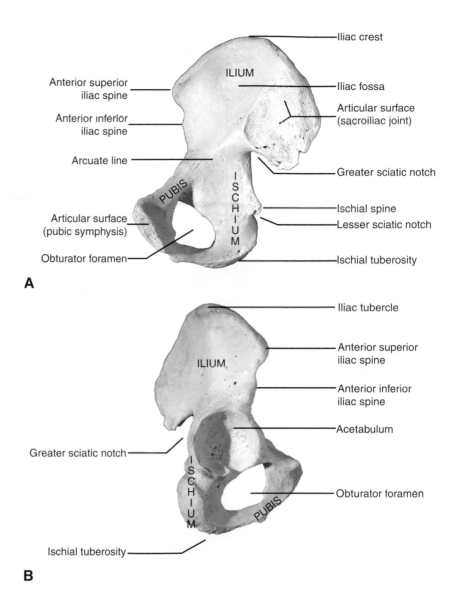

Figure 4-2 Right os coxae (hip bone). **A,** Medial view. **B,** Lateral view.

1. The **sagittal planes** are located by a line joining the midclavicular point to the midpoint of the inguinal ligament. These are located on the right and left sides.
2. The **transverse planes** are located by a line joining the most inferior points of the costal margins (approximately vertebral level L3) and a line joining the right and left iliac tubercles on the superior aspects of the iliac crests (approximately vertebral level L5).

   The four planes divide the abdomen into nine regions.

2. The Abdominal Walls

The abdominal cavity is enclosed by four walls: (1) an anterolateral wall, (2) a posterior wall, (3) a superior wall (thoracic diaphragm), and (4) an inferior wall (pelvic diaphragm).

ANTEROLATERAL ABDOMINAL WALL
Surface Features

Palpable abdominal landmarks are the costal margins and the xiphoid process, the iliac crests, the superior and inferior anterior iliac spines, and the pubic tubercles (*Figure 4-4*). In thin, muscular individuals a linear depression runs in the midline of the abdomen from the xiphoid process to the symphysis pubis. It represents the underlying linea alba, which is the union of right and left muscular aponeuroses. The linea semilunaris is a curved line lateral to the midline. It represents the lateral limits of the rectus abdominis muscle. Transverse bands running from the linea semilunaris and the midline represent underlying tendinous insertions of the rectus abdominis muscle. The umbilicus (belly button) is the scarred result of the postnatal closure of the umbilical cord. A slight crease runs from

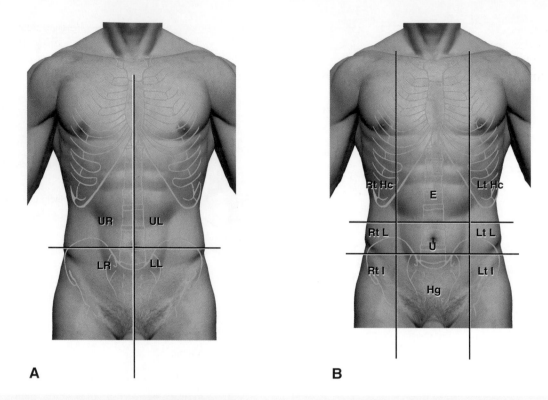

A

B

Figure 4-3 Divisions of abdomen. **A,** Four quadrants based on two planes. *UR,* Upper right; *UL,* upper left; *LR,* lower right; *LL,* lower left. **B,** Nine regions based on four planes. *Rt Hc,* Right hypochondriac; *Lt Hc,* left hypochondriac; *E,* epigastric; *Rt L,* right lumbar; *Lt L,* left lumbar; *U,* umbilical; *Rt I,* right iliac; *Lt I,* left iliac; *Hg,* hypogastric.

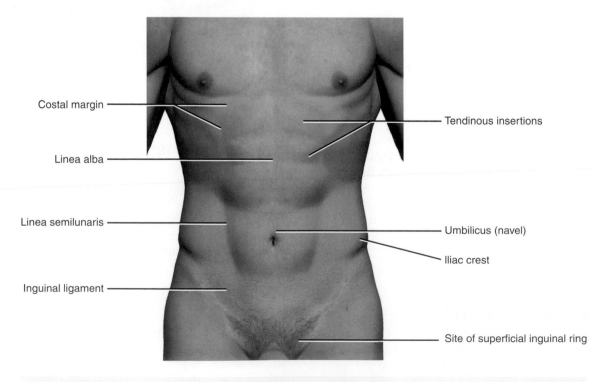

Costal margin — Tendinous insertions

Linea alba

Linea semilunaris — Umbilicus (navel)

Iliac crest

Inguinal ligament

Site of superficial inguinal ring

Figure 4-4 Surface features of anterior abdominal wall.

the anterior superior iliac spine toward the pubic tubercle. It represents the position of the inguinal ligament. Just above and medial to the pubic tubercle is the site of the superficial inguinal ring, the site of indirect inguinal hernias.

Layers

From outward within, the layers that compose the anterolateral abdominal wall below the skin are the (1) superficial fascia, (2) deep fascia, (3) muscles and aponeurosis, (4) transversalis fascia, (5) extraperitoneal layer, and (6) peritoneum (*Figure 4-5*).

Superficial Fascia. The superficial fascia, or subcutaneous fatty layer (**tela subcutanea**), of the abdominal wall is usually divisible into two layers.

1. **Camper's fascia**, the more superficial layer that contains a variable amount of fat
2. **Scarpa's fascia**, a deeper layer that contains relatively less fat and is more membranous in structure; considered a separate layer when placing sutures during closing after abdominal surgery

Deep Fascia. The deep fascia of the abdomen is even more membranous and covers the underlying muscle layer.

Muscles and Aponeuroses. Four pairs of bilateral muscles and their flattened tendons, or **aponeuroses**, contribute to the anterolateral abdominal wall (*Table 4-1* and *Figure 4-6*). There are three pairs of flat muscles (external oblique muscle, internal oblique muscle, and transverse abdominis muscle) and one pair of straplike muscles (rectus abdominis muscle). The three flat muscles are layered in sheets, but the fiber directions of each muscle run in different directions, resulting in a strong laminated muscular unit. Each muscle is fleshy laterally and forms membranous aponeuroses medially. As the aponeuroses of the three flat muscles approach the midline, they form a **membranous sheath** that wraps around the rectus abdominis muscle.

The **external oblique muscle** is the outermost of the group and runs from the lower ribs downward and medially. As the muscle fibers approach the midline, they give way to a membranous aponeurosis, which forms a portion of the anterior sheath of the rectus abdominis muscle. It then meets its counterpart of the opposite side in the midline linea alba. The inferior fibers attach on the iliac crest and form a tendinous free border running from the anterior superior iliac spine to the pubic tubercle. This tendinous free border folds inward on itself and is called the *inguinal ligament*.

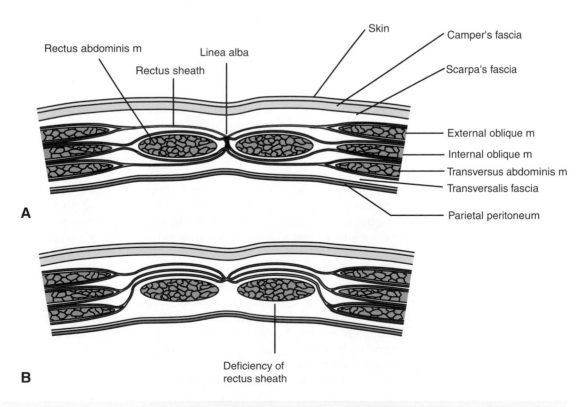

Figure 4-5 Transverse sections through anterior abdominal wall to demonstrate its layers. **A,** Above level of the umbilicus. **B,** Above pubic symphysis.

TABLE 4-1

Muscles of the Anterior Abdominal Wall

Muscle	Origin	Insertion	Action	Nerve
External oblique	External aspects of lower 8 ribs	Iliac crest, aponeurosis of anterior abdominal wall at linea alba	Increase abdominal pressure	Segmented AR of thoracic spinal nerves
Internal oblique	Lumbodorsal fascia, iliac crest, inguinal ligament	Costal cartilages of last 3 ribs, linea alba of abdominal aponeurosis	Increase abdominal pressure	Segmented AR of thoracic spinal nerves
Transversus abdominis	Internal aspects of lower 6 costal cartilages, lumbodorsal fascia, iliac crest, inguinal ligament	Linea alba of abdominal aponeurosis	Increase abdominal pressure	Segmented AR of thoracic spinal nerves
Rectus abdominis	Pubic symphysis, pubic crest	Anterior aspect of xiphoid process, anterior aspects of costal cartilages 5, 6, and 7	Increase abdominal pressure, flex vertebral column	Segmented AR of thoracic spinal nerves

AR, Anterior rami.

The **internal oblique muscle** originates from the iliac crest and runs upward and medially to insert into the costal margin, the linea alba, and the pubis, along with the underlying transverse abdominis muscle, as the conjoint tendon. The internal oblique muscle becomes aponeurotic as it approaches the midline and takes part in the formation of the rectus sheath.

The **transversus abdominis muscle** is the innermost of the three flat muscles and originates from the lumbodorsal fascia, iliac crest, inguinal ligament, and lower costal cartilages. It runs in a transverse direction medially to insert as an aponeurosis, along with its opposite fellow, into the midline linea alba. It also forms a part of the membranous sheath for the rectus abdominis muscle. The lower fibers, along with the lower fibers of the internal oblique muscle, insert into the pubis as the conjoint tendon.

The **rectus abdominis muscle** runs inferiorly from the costal margin and lower thoracic cage to the pubis. The muscle is enclosed in a membranous sheath formed by the aponeuroses of the three flat muscles. The muscle inserts via three tendinous insertions into the anterior wall of the membranous sheath, in addition to its inferior attachment to the pubis.

The formation of the **rectus sheath** is rather complicated, as shown in *Figure 4-5.* Two representative cuts through the muscle layer are shown. At level A the internal oblique apilioneurosis splits to encircle the rectus abdominis muscle. At level B all of the aponeuroses are anterior to the muscle, leaving a deficiency in the sheath posteriorly. The **arcuate line** marks the limit of the aponeurotic contribution to the posterior wall of the bed of the rectus sheath. Below this arcuate line, only the transversalis fascia separates the rectus abdominis muscle from the underlying peritoneum.

The muscles of the anterior wall function in two ways: (1) flexion and rotation of the trunk, and (2) compression of the anterior wall. First, the right and left oblique muscles, acting together with the rectus abdominis muscle, flex the trunk. Unilateral contractions of the oblique fibers, however, result in a rotation or twisting of the trunk.

Second, the abdominal muscles, acting in concert when the back is stabilized, tense the anterolateral abdominal wall to protect underlying viscera. They contract to aid in raising intra-abdominal pressure during forced expiration, coughing, sneezing, defecation, micturition, and childbirth.

Transversalis Fascia. Transversalis fascia is a layer of deep fascia in which the fibers run in a transverse direction. It lies immediately deep to the anterolateral abdominal muscles and the rectus sheath.

Extraperitoneal Layer. The extraperitoneal layer, a fatty, connective tissue layer, is interposed between the transversalis fascia and the deeper peritoneum. Abdominal organs form in this layer during embryological development.

Peritoneum. The deep, fatty, extraperitoneal layer becomes membranous and continuous with the more organized connective tissue of the peritoneal layer below. Deeper still is a smooth, glistening layer of mesothelial cells, which line the peritoneal cavity. Peritoneum and the contents of the abdomen are discussed on page 99.

Inguinal Region

The inguinal region is superior to the medial portion of the inguinal ligament. Here the lower fibers of the internal oblique and transversus abdominis muscles do not

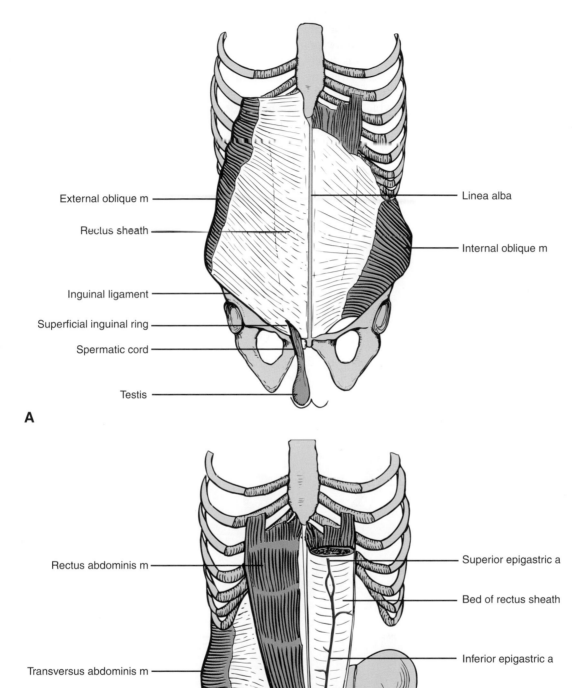

Figure 4-6 Muscles of anterior abdominal wall. **A,** External oblique muscle is shown on left and deeper internal oblique muscle on right. **B,** Transversus abdominis muscle and rectus abdominis muscle are shown on left. Rectus abdominis muscle has been cut superiorly and inferiorly to show bed of rectus sheath and epigastric arteries on right.

insert into the inguinal ligament but rather insert as the conjoint tendon into the pubis, leaving a free inferior gap (see *Figure 4-6*). The external oblique aponeurosis covers this gap incompletely, its inferior medial fibers diverging as a triangular opening as it approaches the pubis. The opening is the **superficial inguinal ring**, which serves as the external opening of the **inguinal canal**. The canal is formed by the deficiency of the transversus abdominis and internal oblique muscles and their conjoint tendon posteriorly and the external oblique aponeurosis anteriorly.

Issuing from this canal in males is the **spermatic cord**, from which the testis is suspended within the scrotum. In females the **round ligament** of the uterus passes through the canal to attach to the labium majus.

Spermatic Cord. The gonads develop within the extraperitoneal layer of the abdomen (*Figure 4-7*). The **gubernaculum** extends from this site down to the developing scrotum in males and to the labia majora in females. It marks the path for the descent of the testes in males.

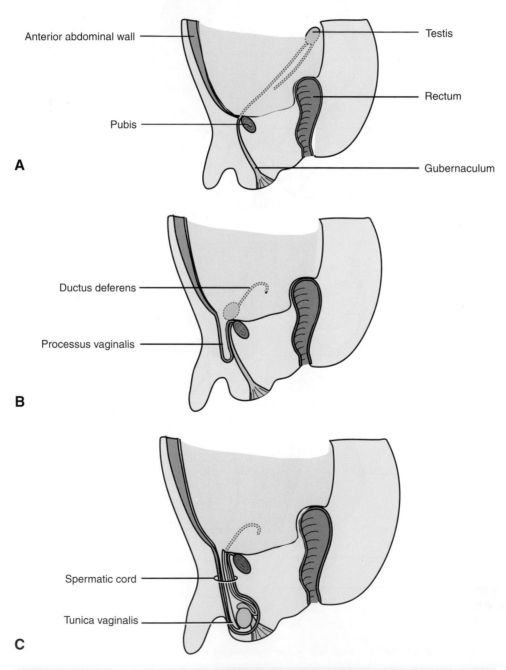

Figure 4-7 Development and descent of testes and formation of spermatic cord. **A,** Two months in utero. **B,** Three months in utero. **C,** At birth.

During the third prenatal month in the male fetus, a portion of peritoneum (processus vaginalis) begins to pouch outward through the transversalis fascia, through the inguinal canal, and down into the scrotum. It is guided by the previous descent of the **gubernaculum.** As the processus vaginalis passes through each layer from deep to superficial, it drags with it portions of each layer. These layers eventually form the coverings of the spermatic cord.

The stage is now set for the descent of the testes. These glands develop within the extraperitoneal layer and in the seventh intrauterine month follow the processus vaginalis down to the scrotum. They drag with them the ductus deferens and the testicular blood supply from the abdominal aorta. The resulting deficiency in the transversalis fascia is the **deep inguinal ring.**

In the female fetus the ovaries descend slightly but remain with the pelvis. The gubernaculum becomes fibrous and persists as the **round ligament of the uterus** running from the lateral aspects of the uterus through the inguinal canal to the skin of the labia majora.

Layers.   The spermatic cord consists of five layers:

1. **External spermatic fascia,** derived from the external oblique aponeurosis
2. **Cremaster muscle,** derived from internal oblique and transversus abdominis muscles; is under involuntary control and lifts the testes up toward the warm abdomen when the area is exposed to cold temperatures (A cremaster reflex can be elicited by stroking the superior aspect of the inner thigh.)
3. **Internal spermatic fascia,** derived from the transversalis fascia
4. **Loose areolar tissue,** derived from the extraperitoneal layer
5. **Remnants of the processus vaginalis**

For the last layer, the superior portion of the processus obliterates. If it remains patent, an inguinal hernia can result. The inferior portion wraps around the testes to form a fluid-filled space termed the *tunica vaginalis.* The space affords the testes some movement in the scrotum.

Contents.   The spermatic cord contains four structures that are associated with the testes: (1) the **ductus (vas) deferens**, which carries sperm back into the abdomen to the seminal vesicle; (2) the **testicular artery**, which is a branch of the abdominal aorta; (3) the **pampiniform plexus** of veins that form up as the **testicular vein**, which is emptying into the inferior vena cava of the abdomen; and (4) the **vessels** and **nerves** of **the ductus deferens**, which supply the ductus.

Scrotum.   The skin of the anterolateral abdominal wall continues inferiorly to form the scrotum that contains the testes. The superficial fascia contains the **dartos muscle**, a thin layer of nonstriated muscle that contracts and puckers the skin of the scrotum in response to cold.

Blood and Nerve Supply

The anterolateral abdominal wall is supplied by the lower six intercostal nerves of the thorax, which stream downward and medially to the abdomen. Inferiorly, the abdominal wall is supplied by two branches of the first lumbar anterior ramus. These are named specifically as the **iliohypogastric** and **ilioinguinal nerves,** and they supply the skin and musculature of the lower aspect of the anterolateral abdominal wall.

The arterial supply is from two sources. Posteriorly segmented branches of the aorta follow the spinal nerves. Anteriorly segmented branches arise from the **superior** and **inferior epigastric arteries** running in the bed of the rectus sheath (see *Figure 4-6*). The superior epigastric artery arises superiorly as a continuation of the internal thoracic artery; the inferior epigastric artery arises inferiorly from the external iliac artery. The two epigastric arteries anastomose above the umbilicus and supply the contents of the rectus sheath and the sheath itself. Collateral branches from the epigastric arteries anastomose with the aortic collateral vessels posteriorly.

CLINICAL NOTES

Vasectomy

Vasectomy is an elective surgical procedure in men for the purpose of birth control. The ductus (vas) deferens is exposed bilaterally through relatively small openings in the anterosuperior wall of the scrotum. The ducts are sectioned and ligated, resulting in sterility but not impotency. The prostate gland and seminal vesicles still contribute secretions to the ejaculate.

Undescended Testis (Cryptorchidism)

The testes normally descend into the scrotum during the eighth or ninth month in utero. Occasionally one or both testes fail to descend and remain in the abdomen. The empty scrotum after birth is a clue. Without surgical intervention the testes fail to produce sperm in the higher temperatures of the abdominal cavity, resulting in infertility.

Continued

Inguinal Hernia—cont'd

Intra-abdominal pressures are relatively high and become higher still with expulsive contractions of the abdominal muscles. Consequently, weak spots in the abdominal wall may collapse and allow passage of a section of bowel. The most common site of an abdominal hernia is the inguinal region. Inguinal hernias are either indirect or direct.

An **indirect hernia** is more common in young boys and results when the processus vaginalis persists and allows a loop of bowel to penetrate the deep inguinal ring and enter the inguinal canal along with the spermatic cord and pass through the external inguinal ring down into the scrotum. In girls the herniated bowel and abdominal wall coverings pass into the labium majus.

Direct hernias occur in older men and do not pass through the internal inguinal ring. Instead, they push through a weakened abdominal wall just medial to the

inguinal canal and do not assume the coverings of the spermatic cord. However, the gut ultimately bulges through the external ring, making the determination of whether it is direct or indirect difficult.

Hydrocele

An overproduction of fluid within the tunica vaginalis results in swelling of the scrotum—hydrocele.

Varicocele

Varicocele results when the pampiniform plexus of veins draining the testis becomes tortuous and dilated, assuming the feeling of a "bag of worms." It usually occurs on the left side and may be a reflection of the drainage of the left testicular vein into the left renal vein. The condition is not serious but is thought to lead to a diminished sperm output on the affected side because of the increase in temperature.

SUPERIOR ABDOMINAL WALL

The diaphragm is a fibromuscular partition that separates the abdominal cavity below from the thoracic cavity above. It does not lie in a flat plane but rather domes upward; therefore abdominal contents just below the diaphragm are found to be within the lower confines of the thoracic rib cage, yet still technically within the abdominal cavity.

Origins of the Thoracic Diaphragm

The muscular slips of the diaphragm originate from three sites of attachment (*Figure 4-8*). **Sternal slips** arise from the posterior aspect of the xiphoid process. **Costal slips** originate from the internal surfaces of the lower six costal cartilages and the twelfth rib. **Lumbar attachments** arise as a right crus from the vertebral bodies and discs of L1, L2, and L3, and a left crus arising from the vertebral bodies and discs of L1 and L2. The two crura cross each other to form the median arcuate ligament through which enters the abdominal aorta. Tendons arching from the crura to the transverse processes of L1 form medial arcuate ligaments. Tendons arching from the transverse processes of L1 to the midpoints of the twelfth ribs form lateral arcuate ligaments.

Insertion of the Diaphragm

The fleshy fibers of the diaphragm converge and insert into the **central tendon,** which is roughly clover-shaped.

Structures Passing Through the Diaphragm

Several structures pass either through the diaphragm or between the diaphragm and the body wall on their way to or from the abdomen.

1. The **aorta** enters the abdomen through the median arch between the two crura.
2. The **inferior** vena cava passes out of the abdomen to the thorax through its own opening in the central tendon about 2 to 3 cm from the midline.
3. The **esophagus** passes through its own opening formed by the fibers of the right crus. The muscle fibers around the opening are arranged in sphincterlike fashion, so as the diaphragm contracts, the sphincteric action of the diaphragm prevents gastric contents from being squeezed back up into the esophagus.
4. The **thoracic duct** passes through the median arch along with the aorta.
5. The **azygos vein** passes through the right crus; the **hemiazygos vein** passes through the left crus.
6. The **posterior** and **anterior vagal trunks** pass into the abdomen, along with the esophagus, through the esophageal opening.
7. The **splanchnic nerves** (preganglionic sympathetic branches from the sympathetic trunk of the thorax) pass through the crura of the diaphragm.
8. The **sympathetic trunks** pass behind the medial arcuate ligament to enter the abdomen.
9. The **superior epigastric arteries** are continuations of the internal thoracic arteries that pass anteriorly between the sternal and costal origins of the diaphragm.

Functions of the Diaphragm

The main function of the diaphragm is **respiration**. The contracting muscle fibers pull down on the central tendon during thoracic inspiration. The mechanisms involved with inspiration and expiration are discussed in Chapter 3, page 67.

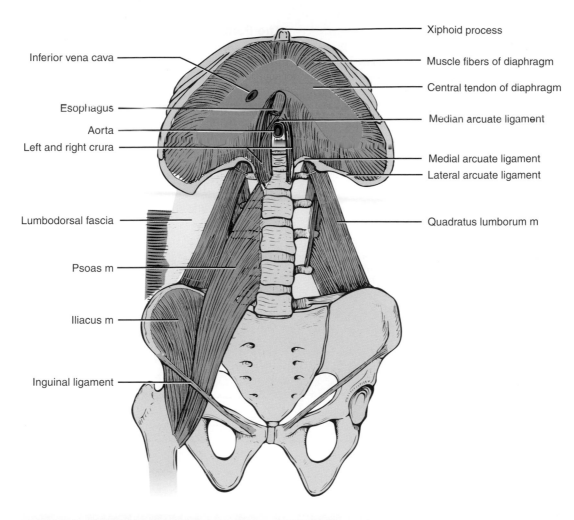

Xiphoid process

Inferior vena cava

Muscle fibers of diaphragm

Central tendon of diaphragm

Esophagus

Median arcuate ligament

Aorta

Left and right crura

Medial arcuate ligament

Lateral arcuate ligament

Lumbodorsal fascia

Quadratus lumborum m

Psoas m

Iliacus m

Inguinal ligament

Figure 4-8 Superior wall (diaphragm) and posterior wall of abdomen.

Other functions of the diaphragm include **esophageal constriction** during inspiration to prevent gastric regurgitation and aiding in inferior vena caval blood flow to the heart within the thorax.

Nerve Supply of the Diaphragm

The diaphragm originates early in development from the cervical region, and as it descends during development it drags its cervical nerve and blood supply along with it. The **phrenic nerve** is the motor and sensory supply to the diaphragm. It arises in the neck from *anterior rami* of *spinal nerves* C3, C4, and C5. The phrenic nerve descends through the thoracic inlet and travels inferiorly on either side of the middle mediastinum to reach the diaphragm (see Chapter 3, page 84).

Blood Supply of the Diaphragm

Arterial supply to the diaphragm is from the internal thoracic artery via the **pericardiophrenic** and **musculophrenic arteries** and from aortic branches via **intercostal** and **phrenic arteries**.

POSTERIOR ABDOMINAL WALL

The posterior abdominal wall consists of skin and fascia, bone (including the lumbar and thoracic vertebrae, the lower ribs, and the os coxae), and a fleshy component consisting of three muscles (see *Figure 4-8*).

The quadratus lumborum muscle is flat and runs from the twelfth rib and all the lumbar transverse processes down to the iliac crest. Unilaterally the muscle helps bend the vertebral column to the same side. Its nerve supply is from anterior rami of upper lumbar nerves.

The psoas major and iliacus muscles are generally considered as a unit (iliopsoas muscle), and it is actually a muscle of the lower limb described in Chapter 10.

INFERIOR ABDOMINAL WALL

The inferior abdominal wall is funnel-shaped. The cup portion of the funnel is represented by the levator ani muscles; the stem of the funnel is represented by the rectum passing inferiorly through the pelvic outlet.

Muscles

The levator ani muscles originate along the internal aspects of the os coxae (*Figure 4-9* and *Table 4-2*). The fibers run medially and inferiorly toward the rectum to blend with the longitudinal smooth muscle of the rectum. A portion of each levator ani muscle runs from the ischial tuberosity to the coccyx and is given a special name, the *coccygeus muscle.*

The levator ani muscles help draw the rectum superiorly during defecation. The muscle is deficient anteriorly to allow passage of the urethra in men and the urethra and the vagina in women (see also *Figure 4-37*).

The Perineum

The levator ani muscles form not only the floor of the abdominopelvic cavity but also the roof of the most inferior aspect of the trunk, the perineum. Superficially the perineum is that area bounded by the thighs and the buttocks. On a deeper plane, the perineum is bounded by the ischiopubic rami converging on the pubic symphysis anteriorly and the sacrotuberous ligaments converging on the coccyx posteriorly.

These boundaries roughly define a diamond-shaped area. If a line is drawn joining the right and left ischial tuberosities, the perineum is further divided into a **posterior anal triangle** and an **anterior urogenital triangle.**

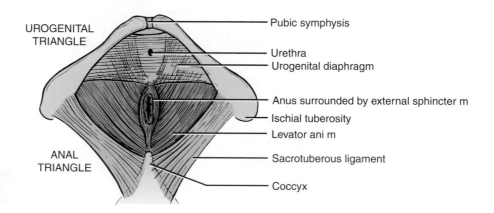

UROGENITAL TRIANGLE

ANAL TRIANGLE

Pubic symphysis
Urethra
Urogenital diaphragm
Anus surrounded by external sphincter m
Ischial tuberosity
Levator ani m
Sacrotuberous ligament
Coccyx

Figure 4-9 Inferior wall (pelvic diaphragm) of abdomen.

TABLE 4-2

Muscles of Superior, Posterior, and Inferior Abdominal Walls

Muscle	Origin	Insertion	Action	Nerve
Superior				
Thoracic diaphragm	Internal aspect of xiphoid process, inner aspects of costal cartilages, crura on lumbar vertebrae L1-L3, and superior aspect of rib 12	Central tendon of diaphragm	Inspiration; increases volume of thoracic cavity	Phrenic nerve
Inferior				
Levator ani	Internal aspect of os coxae and obturator internus fascia	Anterior and lateral aspects of coccyx, anococcygeal ligament, anal canal wall, perineal body, side of the prostate gland (male), side of vaginal wall (female)	Raises anal canal for defecation; supports prostate gland (male), sphincter for vagina (female); forms floor of pelvic cavity	AR of spinal nerves S3 and S4
Posterior				
Quadratus lumborum	Lumbodorsal fascia, iliac crest	Transverse processes of L1-L4, inferior aspect of rib 12	Flexes spine laterally, depresses rib 12	AR of spinal nerves T12, L1-L3
Iliopsoas	Iliac: iliac fossa of os coxae Psoas: all lumbar vertebrae	Both portions insert into lesser trochanter of femur	Flex and rotate thigh medially	Femoral nerve and AR of spinal nerves L2-L4

AR, Anterior rami.

Anal Triangle. The anal triangle is the posterior half of the perineum. A fat-filled space between the inferior surface of the levator ani muscles and the medial aspect of the pelvic walls is termed the ***ischiorectal fossa.*** This space allows the rectum to expand during defecation.

Urogenital Triangle. The urogenital triangle is the anterior half of the perineum. Stretched across, between the pubic rami, is the **urogenital diaphragm,** which presents a free border posteriorly. Contained within this diaphragm is a thick fibrous **perineal membrane** inferiorly; the **sphincter urethrae muscle** above; and another, more delicate, fibrous membrane superiorly. The superior membrane and the inferior perineal membrane sandwich the muscle fiber of the sphincter urethrae.

In men the muscle fibers surround the urethra. In women these fibers surround the vagina, with a few fibers surrounding the more anteriorly placed urethra. Further descriptions of the male and female perineum are presented later in this chapter.

3. Peritoneum and the Peritoneal Cavity

Peritoneum is a lining tissue consisting of a single inner layer of squamous cell mesothelium and a thin, supporting, and nutritive outer layer of connective tissue. Peritoneum lines the primitive gut cavity rather simply, but as abdominal structures develop in the extraperitoneal layer and push the overlying peritoneum into the abdominal cavity, complex folds of peritoneum result.

NOMENCLATURE

To understand the distribution of peritoneum within the hollow abdominal cavity, consider the schematic representation of a transverse section through the abdomen in *Figure 4-10.*

1. **Parietal peritoneum** lines the inner abdominal body walls.
2. **Visceral peritoneum** covers the viscera, or organs.
3. The **peritoneal cavity** is the space between the visceral and parietal layers. Serous fluid occupies this limited space and lubricates the mobile viscera.
4. **Mesentery** is a double-layered fold of peritoneum that suspends some abdominal organs in the peritoneal cavity. Mesenteries are attached to and continuous with the peritoneum of the posterior body wall. It is through these mesenteries that vessels and nerves pass to and from the suspended viscera. The mesenteries act somewhat like a leash, allowing a certain degree of movement in those portions of gut that possess a mesentery.
5. **Retroperitoneal viscera** are those that do not possess a mesentery. These organs lie within the extraperitoneal layer of the abdominal wall.
6. An **omentum** is a double-layered fold of peritoneum that is somewhat like a mesentery but joins two viscera.
7. **Ligaments** (of peritoneum) are specifically named folds of peritoneum that are part of mesenteries or omenta.

DEVELOPMENT OF THE GUT AND PERITONEUM

To better understand the complexities of the peritoneal linings, it is advantageous to consider the development of the gut during embryonic life. *Figure 4-11* shows the primitive gut, which is essentially a tube suspended from the posterior body wall by a dorsal mesentery. Running to the suspended gut through the dorsal mesentery are three branches of the abdominal aorta: (1) the **celiac trunk,** which supplies the foregut; (2) the **superior mesenteric artery,** which supplies the midgut; and (3) the **inferior mesenteric artery,** which supplies the hindgut.

Two glands develop as outgrowths of the gut. The **liver** develops anteriorly in the primitive ventral mesentery, which extends superiorly from the umbilicus. The **pancreas** develops posteriorly in the dorsal mesentery. Both glands drag along their respective blood supplies from the

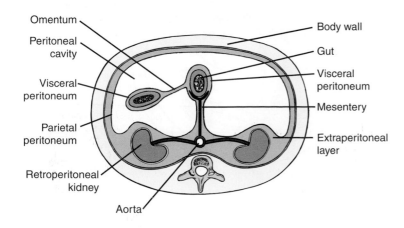

Figure 4-10 Scheme of disposition of the peritoneum within abdominal cavity.

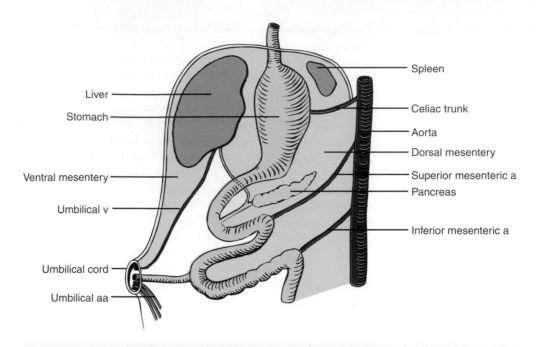

Figure 4-11 Developing abdominal viscera, peritoneum, and blood supply (sixth week prenatal).

gut as they develop. The spleen also develops in the dorsal mesentery.

As the individual develops and the gut elongates and differentiates, some sections of the gut rotate and their mesenteries become adherent to the body wall, rendering them no longer mobile.

Figure 4-12, A, shows a transverse section through the developing abdomen. As indicated, the stomach and spleen move to the left, and the liver moves to the right. *Figure 4-12, B,* represents a later stage in development, with the liver now occupying most of the upper right quadrant and the stomach and spleen occupying the upper left quadrant. In addition, the mesentery of the stomach becomes

adherent to the posterior body wall and is lost. In like manner, the mesenteries of the duodenum, ascending colon, descending colon, and rectum are fused to the posterior body wall, and these sections of gut become "retroperitoneal." With blunt dissection, these obliterated mesenteries can be restored in the laboratory and occasionally in actual abdominal surgery (as needed).

As a result, only the following structures retain a mesentery; that is, they are suspended from the posterior body wall by a double-layered fold of peritoneum: the jejunum, ileum, transverse colon, and sigmoid, or pelvic, colon. Although the mesentery of the stomach is lost during development, the stomach remains suspended by the

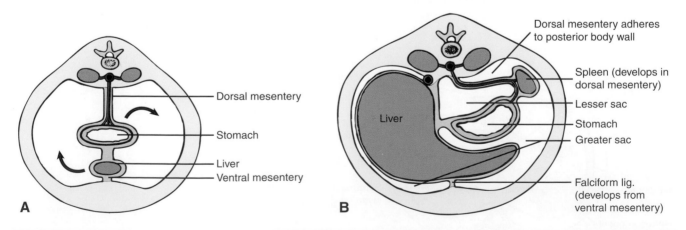

Figure 4-12 Horizontal sections through abdomen. **A,** Before gut rotation (sixth week prenatal). **B,** After gut rotation (eleventh week prenatal).

greater and lesser omenta. The remaining structures do not possess a mesentery in the adult and are said to be **retroperitoneal.**

The liver does not have a mesentery, nor is it considered retroperitoneal. Rather, it is suspended from the diaphragm and posterior body wall by a broad-based peritoneal attachment, called the *coronary ligament*, which is described along with the liver (on page 115).

4. Blood and Nerve Supply to the Abdomen

The arterial supply and nerve supply to the abdominal structures arise from the thorax and pass through the diaphragm. The thoracic components of these structures are described in Chapter 4.

ARTERIAL SUPPLY: THE ABDOMINAL AORTA

The **descending aorta** of the thorax passes through the diaphragm to become the abdominal aorta (*Figure 4-13*). It descends on the posterior body wall to the pelvis, and at vertebral level L4 it divides into two terminal branches:

the **right** and **left common iliac arteries.** These, in turn, divide into the **right** and **left external iliac arteries,** which descend to supply the lower limb, and the **right** and **left internal iliac arteries,** which supply pelvic structures. The abdominal aorta gives off a number of branches within the abdomen before terminating as the common iliac arteries at vertebral level L4.

Somatic Branches

Inferior Phrenic Arteries. The inferior phrenic arteries arise from the aorta as it passes through the diaphragm. The right and left branches then ascend to supply the inferior aspect of the diaphragm.

Lumbar Arteries. Although there are five lumbar arteries, only the first four pairs arise from the aorta. The fifth pair arises from the internal iliac arteries, which then turn laterally to supply the lower abdominal wall. Anteriorly the segmented lumbar arteries anastomose with collateral branches of the superior and inferior epigastric arteries.

Median Sacral Artery. The small branch of the median sacral artery continues inferiorly from the bifurcation of the aorta to supply the anterior aspect of the sacral area. It may supplement the supply of the fifth lumbar arteries.

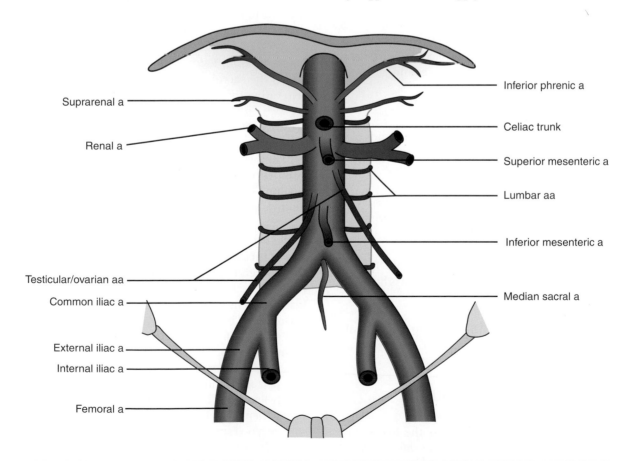

Suprarenal a
Renal a
Testicular/ovarian aa
Common iliac a
External iliac a
Internal iliac a
Femoral a

Inferior phrenic a
Celiac trunk
Superior mesenteric a
Lumbar aa
Inferior mesenteric a
Median sacral a

Figure 4-13 Branches of abdominal aorta.

Unpaired Branches to the Gut and Associated Glands

Three unpaired branches arise from the abdominal aorta to supply the gut and its associated glands, the liver, the pancreas, and the spleen. Each of the three branches supplies the derivatives of the embryonic foregut, midgut, and hindgut. These branches are described in detail later in this chapter along with the descriptions of the abdominal viscera they supply.

Celiac Trunk. The celiac trunk arises as a short stem at vertebral level T12, L1, just below the diaphragm, and immediately breaks up into three main branches. These three branches of the celiac trunk supply foregut derivatives within the abdomen (i.e., abdominal esophagus, stomach, the duodenum [proximal to the entrance of the bile duct], the liver and gallbladder, part of the pancreas, and the spleen).

Superior Mesenteric Artery. The superior mesenteric artery arises immediately below the celiac trunk and supplies derivatives of the midgut (i.e., the distal half of the duodenum, jejunum, ileum, cecum and appendix, ascending colon, and transverse colon). Its territory ends at the left colic flexure. It also supplies the distal half of the duodenum and the inferior portion of the pancreas.

Inferior Mesenteric Artery. The inferior mesenteric artery arises at vertebral level L3 and supplies derivatives of the hindgut distal to the left colic flexure (i.e., descending colon, pelvic or sigmoid colon, and rectum).

Paired Branches to the Glands of the Genitourinary System

Three paired collateral branches supply the glands of the genitourinary system, and they originate in proximity to each other from the aorta.

Suprarenal Arteries. Suprarenal arteries arise either directly from the aorta or from the renal arteries. They supply the suprarenal glands.

Renal Arteries. The renal arteries originate from the aorta at vertebral level L1-L2. They simply pass laterally to supply the right and left kidneys.

Testicular/Ovarian Arteries. Of the group, the testicular/ovarian arteries are the most inferior pair. They travel inferiorly to supply the gonads.

VENOUS RETURN: THE INFERIOR VENA CAVA

The external iliac veins, which drain the lower limbs, and the **internal iliac veins**, which drain the pelvis, unite within the pelvis to form the **right and left common iliac veins** (*Figure 4-14*).

The right and left common iliac veins unite at vertebral level L5 to form the **inferior vena cava**. As the inferior vena cava passes upward through the abdomen, it picks up several tributaries. Superiorly the inferior vena cava passes through the diaphragm to enter the thorax and pour its venous flow into the right atrium.

Somatic Branches

The somatic branches correspond to the somatic arterial branches.

Inferior Phrenic Veins (Paired). The inferior phrenic veins drain the inferior aspect of the diaphragm. They either drain directly to the superior aspect of the inferior vena cava or to the paired ascending lumbar veins.

Lumbar Veins (Paired). Five pairs of lumbar veins drain the body walls. Only the upper four lumbar veins drain to the inferior vena cava. The fifth drains directly or indirectly to the common iliac vein. Paralleling the inferior vena cava on either side are **ascending lumbar veins,** which arise from the common iliac veins and ascend on the posterior abdominal wall through the diaphragm to the thorax, where they become the azygos and hemiazygos veins. As they ascend in the abdomen, they communicate with the lumbar veins and therefore provide an alternative route for venous flow from the body wall.

Median Sacral Vein (Unpaired). The median sacral vein drains the sacral region and joins the left common iliac vein rather than the inferior vena cava.

Tributaries of Genitourinary Glands (Paired)

The renal veins receive venous blood from the right and left kidneys. The suprarenal veins receive venous blood from the right and left suprarenal glands. The testicular/ovarian veins receive venous blood from the male testicles or the female ovaries.

Tributaries of the Gastrointestinal Tract and Associated Glands

Venous return from the gastrointestinal tract does not return directly to the inferior vena cava (see *Figure 4-27*). Instead, veins returning from the gut join to form the **portal vein.** The portal vein enters the liver, carrying nutrients absorbed from the gut. Within the liver the portal vein ultimately ends as a capillary bed; at this level, nutrients are exchanged for processing and storage within the liver. The portal capillary beds are drained by **hepatic veins,** which leave the liver to enter the inferior vena cava as several **hepatic veins.**

The blood supply and return of the gut therefore passes through two sets of capillaries: the first in the gut itself and the second in the liver. This is referred to as a *portal system.*

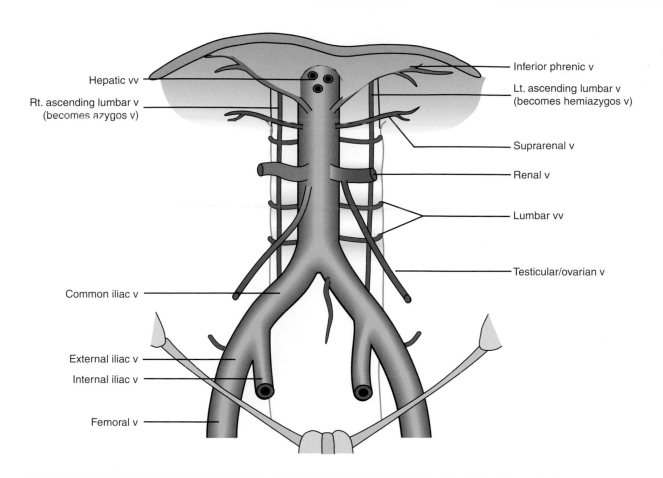

Hepatic vv

Rt. ascending lumbar v
(becomes azygos v)

Inferior phrenic v

Lt. ascending lumbar v
(becomes hemiazygos v)

Suprarenal v

Renal v

Lumbar vv

Testicular/ovarian v

Common iliac v

External iliac v

Internal iliac v

Femoral v

Figure 4-14 Tributaries of inferior vena cava.

NERVES OF THE ABDOMEN

Somatic Nerves

The anterior rami of the lower six thoracic spinal nerves and the first lumbar nerve supply the various layers of the anterolateral abdominal walls. Two branches of the anterior rami of L1, the **iliohypogastric** and **ilioinguinal nerves,** supply the lower portion of the abdominal wall (see *Figure 10-20*).

The anterior rami of lumbar nerves L1 to L4 unite and divide within the substance of the psoas muscle to form the lumbar plexus. Branches of the **lumbar plexus** supply a portion of the lower limb and consequently are considered in Chapter 10 with the lower limb.

Similarly, the anterior rami of L4 and L5 and S1 to S4 unite to form the **sacral plexus,** the branches of which provide motor and sensory nerves to the perineum and the remainder of the lower limb.

Autonomic Nerves

Sympathetic Nerves. The scheme of the sympathetic nervous system is outlined in Chapter 1 (pages 27 to 30) and is illustrated in *Figure 1-26*.

Greater, lesser, and **least splanchnic nerves** arise bilaterally from the thoracic sympathetic trunks and, with-

out synapsing in the sympathetic trunk, pass inferiorly through the diaphragm to the abdomen (*Figure 4-15*). In addition, **lumbar splanchnic nerves** arise from the lumbar portion of the sympathetic trunk.

Within the abdomen are collections of secondary neurons, which are associated with the abdominal aorta and its branches (**preaortic ganglia**). The largest collection is the **celiac ganglion** and its associated plexus, found around the celiac trunk. Smaller ganglia and plexuses surround the superior mesenteric, inferior mesenteric, renal, and testicular/ovarian arteries. Within these ganglia the splanchnic (thoracic and lumbar) nerves synapse. The postganglionic fibers are distributed to the various abdominal viscera as hitchhiking nerve fibers along the abdominal arteries.

Parasympathetic Nerves. Parasympathetic innervation of the abdominal viscera is shared by the *vagus nerves* (supplying the gut up to the left colic flexure) and the *pelvic splanchnic nerves* (supplying the gut distal to the left colic flexure and pelvic organs).

Vagus Nerves. Within the thorax the right and left vagus nerves form a plexus around the esophagus. As the esophagus passes through the diaphragm into the

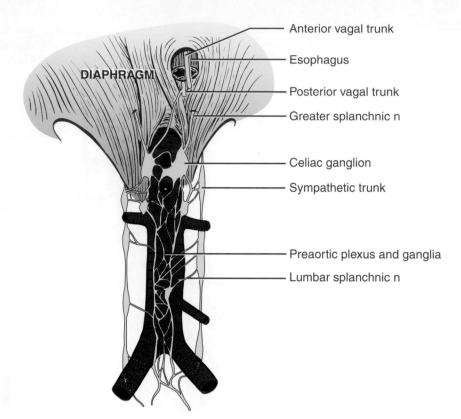

Anterior vagal trunk

Esophagus

Posterior vagal trunk

Greater splanchnic n

Celiac ganglion

Sympathetic trunk

Preaortic plexus and ganglia

Lumbar splanchnic n

DIAPHRAGM

Figure 4-15 Autonomic nerves of abdomen.

abdomen, the vagal plexus regroups as the **anterior** and **posterior vagal trunks.** The anterior vagal trunk supplies the liver and biliary apparatus, gastric pylorus, duodenum, and pancreas. The posterior vagal trunk supplies the remainder of the stomach, then passes to and joins the celiac plexus. Vagal fibers are then distributed, along with the branches of the celiac plexus, to the gut and its derivatives proximal to the left colic flexure.

Pelvic Splanchnic Nerves. Within the pelvis, parasympathetic outflows from spinal nerve levels S2 to S4 join the inferior mesenteric plexus as **pelvic splanchnic nerves** and are then distributed along with the branches of the plexus. They supply the gut distal to the left colic flexure and the pelvic viscera.

Parasympathetic fibers of the abdomen travel to their sites of innervation as preganglionic fibers and synapse with secondary neurons within the substance of the organ they supply.

5. The Abdominal Viscera

THE GUT (ALIMENTARY CANAL)

The embryonic gut develops simply as a food tube (see Figure 1-31), beginning at the oral cavity and ending at the anus. In the adult the scheme is the same except for a few developmental changes resulting in a more complex

disposition (*Figure 4-16*). The gut is transformed from a straight tube to one that is dilated in parts and tightly coiled in other parts to accommodate 6 to 7 m of gut in a relatively small abdominal cavity. The gut wall generally consists of four layers: (1) an outer layer of **visceral peritoneum**, (2) a layer of **smooth muscle** (*outer longitudinal fibers* and *inner circular fibers*), (3) a **submucosal layer**, and (4) an inner lining of **mucous membrane.**

Components

A short description of the oral cavity, pharynx, and esophagus is presented to outline the continuity of the gut proximal to the abdomen.

The **oral cavity** is where the ingestion of food takes place and where food is prepared for subsequent digestion. Food is chewed into a manageable bolus with the teeth, and saliva is added to the food to facilitate the formation of the bolus. The swallowing reflex is voluntarily initiated in the oral cavity, pushing the bolus into the pharynx.

The **pharynx** is a common chamber for food and air and it is encircled posteriorly and laterally by three involuntary constrictor muscles, which push the bolus down through the funnel-shaped pharynx. Within the pharynx the air channel divides anteriorly from the food tube behind, and food is prevented from entering the airway by the epiglottis, which functions like a trap door. At the level of C6 the pharynx becomes the esophagus.

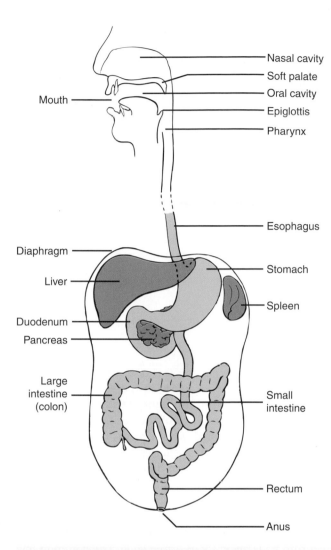

Nasal cavity
Soft palate
Oral cavity
Epiglottis
Pharynx

Mouth

Esophagus

Diaphragm
Liver

Stomach

Spleen

Duodenum
Pancreas

Large
intestine
(colon)

Small
intestine

Rectum

Anus

Figure 4-16 Scheme of gastrointestinal system.

The **esophagus** is a muscular tube that serves only to propel food through the neck and thorax to the abdomen. In the thorax the esophagus passes through the diaphragm and for about 2 to 3 cm descends into the abdomen. It then abruptly dilates to become the stomach at the cardiac orifice. The thoracic portion of the esophagus is described further in Chapters 3 (pages 79 to 81) and 5 (page 158).

The **stomach** is a dilated, J-shaped structure situated in the upper left quadrant. The stomach ends as the pylorus distally, and gastric contents travel through the pyloric sphincter to the tubelike duodenum.

The **duodenum** is a relatively short section of the gut (about 25 cm long) that is disposed on the posterior wall of the abdomen in the shape of a C. Distally it turns abruptly inferiorly as the jejunum and ileum of the small intestine.

The **jejunum** and **ileum** consist of approximately 6 to 7 m of coiled muscular tubing that occupies a large area within the abdominal cavity. They are attached to the posterior body wall by a mesentery.

The **large intestine** ascends on the right side of the posterior abdominal wall, crosses over to the left side, descends, and then turns toward the midline in the pelvic area to become the rectum.

The **rectum** carries food residue inferiorly, where it is evacuated through the anus.

Associated Glands and Viscera

The **liver** and **pancreas** develop as outgrowths of the gut and thus receive the same blood supply as the gut. The liver occupies the upper right quadrant of the abdomen under the shelter of the diaphragm. The pancreas lies nestled within the arms of the C-shaped duodenum. The tail of the pancreas extends to the left, behind the stomach, to touch the hilus of the spleen. The **spleen** is an organ containing lymphoid tissue that is tucked up under the diaphragm on the left side.

Stomach

The esophagus, after passing inferiorly through the diaphragm, follows an abdominal course for 2.5 cm and then dilates to form the stomach. Although generally described as being shaped like a J, the actual size, shape, and position of the stomach depend on its physiological state and on body build among individuals. The proximal and distal ends of the stomach are fixed, leaving the midportion relatively mobile. The average capacity of a stomach is approximately 1 L.

Position. The stomach lies within the upper left quadrant, with its proximal end immediately below the left dome of the diaphragm. Other relationships include the liver to the right; the spleen, pancreas, and left kidney posteriorly; and the anterolateral abdominal wall anteriorly.

Features

Cardiac Portion. The esophagus is subjected to sphincteric action by the diaphragm (*Figure 4-17*). In addition, as the esophagus enters the stomach, modified circular muscle at the **cardiac orifice** provides additional control of the entrance to the stomach. The area adjacent to the cardiac orifice is the cardiac portion of the stomach. To the left of the cardiac orifice, the stomach bulges upward as the **fundus,** and this area is usually seen on radiograms as containing a bubble of gas.

Pylorus. The stomach followed to the right begins to narrow down at the **pyloric antrum,** which subsequently leads to the relatively narrower pyloric canal. The stomach ends at the **pyloric sphincter,** which contains a concentration of circular smooth muscle and controls the release of gastric contents to the duodenum.

Body. Between the pylorus and the cardiac portion of the stomach is the body of the stomach.

Curvatures. The curved right superior border of the stomach is called the *lesser curvature,* and similarly the curved left inferior border is called the *greater curvature.*

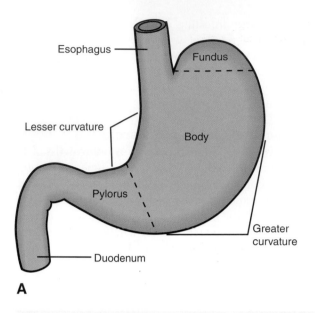

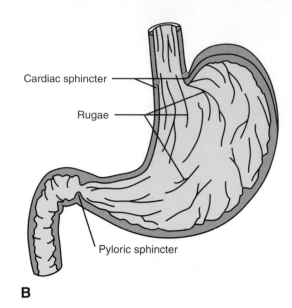

Figure 4-17 Features of stomach. **A,** External. **B,** Internal.

Rugae. The mucosa within the stomach is thrown into longitudinal folds, or rugae. They allow for distension as the stomach fills up with ingested food. They also increase considerably the surface area of the stomach for purposes of gastric secretion. Gastric rugae can be seen in post–barium meal radiographs.

Stomach Wall and Function. An important function of the stomach is to break up and mix ingested food. The muscular coat is correspondingly modified to perform this mixing function, and in addition to the normal longitudinal and circular muscle layers, a third inner oblique layer is present in the stomach.

The stomach adds gastric juices to the food in the form of enzymes such as pepsin (secreted by the chief cells) and hydrochloric acid (secreted from parietal cells). Chief and parietal cells are not found in the pylorus. However, mucous glands are found throughout the stomach as well as throughout the remainder of the gut.

Peritoneal Coverings and Attachments. The stomach is covered with *visceral peritoneum* (*Figure 4-18*). It is connected to other viscera by two omenta: the *lesser* and the *greater omenta* (see also *Figure 4-29*).

Lesser Omentum. The lesser omentum connects the lesser curvature of the stomach and the proximal 3 cm of duodenum to the liver above. The margin of the lesser omentum ends abruptly as a free edge. The **common bile duct, portal vein,** and **hepatic artery** pass through the lesser omentum in this area. Immediately posterior to the free edge is the **epiploic foramen,** which connects the **greater** and **lesser sacs.**

CLINICAL NOTES

Gastroesophageal Reflux Disease

Incompetence of the lower esophageal sphincters allows regurgitation (reflux) of highly acidic stomach contents back into the esophagus and occasionally into the oral cavity. The lining of the esophagus is not designed for the acid medium and becomes inflamed (esophagitis), producing pain in the form of "heartburn." Chronic cases can result in ulcers, strictures, and occasionally considerable hemorrhage. Gravity plays a role, and in addition to antacids and other medications, patients are advised to refrain from eating too close to their bedtimes and to raise the head of the bed by 6 inches.

Hiatus Hernia

A hiatus hernia is a protrusion of a portion of the stomach through the thoracic diaphragm. There are two types. A sliding hiatus hernia is one in which the abdominal esophagus and some of the cardiac portion slide up through the diaphragm into the thorax. In a paraesophageal hiatus hernia the abdominal esophagus and cardiac portion of the stomach remain below the diaphragm, but a portion of the fundus pops up on the left through the diaphragm to lie adjacent to the thoracic esophagus.

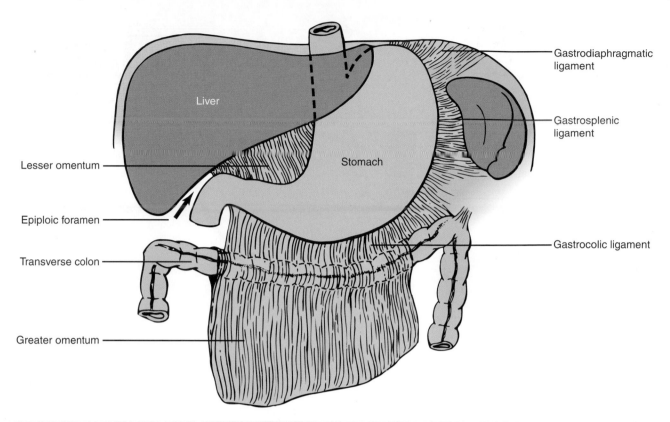

Figure 4-18 Peritoneal coverings and attachments of stomach.

Greater Omentum. The greater omentum connects the greater curvature of the stomach to three separate structures. Therefore it is divided into three separate components or ligaments: (1) the **gastrocolic ligament**, which runs from the greater curvature of the stomach down into the abdomen like an apron, recurves upward, and attaches to the transverse colon; (2) the **gastrosplenic ligament,** which runs from the curvature to the spleen; and (3) the **ligament,** which runs from the greater curvature, becoming continuous with the parietal peritoneum of the diaphragm.

The gastrocolic portion of greater omentum drapes down into the abdomen as a fatty apron before recurring superiorly to contact and cover the transverse colon. The greater omentum can migrate toward areas of infection (e.g., a burst appendix) and attempts to wall off the infection.

Arterial Supply. The blood supply to the stomach is derived from all three branches of the celiac trunk (*Figure 4-19*). The **celiac trunk** arises from the anterior aspect of the aorta just below the diaphragm and travels approximately 1 or 2 cm before dividing into three terminal branches.

Left Gastric Artery. The **left gastric artery** passes to the left, runs superiorly to the level of the esophagus, and then turns inferiorly along the lesser curvature. It supplies the stomach.

Splenic Artery. The **splenic artery** passes to the left behind the stomach and the lesser sac, along the superior border of the pancreas. On reaching the hilus of the spleen it divides into two branches: the **short gastric artery** and the gastro-omental artery. The short gastric artery runs superiorly along the greater curvature to the stomach. The **left gastro-omental artery** descends along the greater curvature to supply the stomach and the greater omentum.

Common Hepatic Artery. The **common hepatic artery** passes to the right and divides near the duodenum into two branches: the hepatic artery and the gastroduodenal artery. The **hepatic artery** ascends to supply the liver, and on the way it gives off the **right gastric artery,** which supplies the lesser curvature of the stomach and anastomoses with the left gastric artery. The hepatic artery continues superiorly and gives off a **cystic artery** to the gallbladder. It then divides into the right and left branches that supply the liver.

The **gastroduodenal artery** passes inferiorly posterior to the duodenum and divides into two branches. The **superior pancreaticoduodenal artery** supplies part of the pancreas and the duodenum. The **right gastro-omental artery** swings to the left along the greater curvature of the stomach to anastomose with the left gastro-omental artery. It supplies portions of the stomach and the greater omentum.

Summary of Arterial Supply. In summary, the stomach is supplied by (1) the **left gastric artery,** a direct branch of the celiac trunk; (2) the **right gastric artery,** a branch of the *common hepatic artery* by way of the *hepatic artery;*

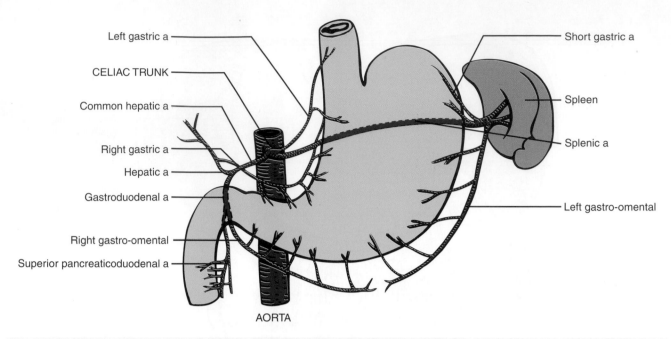

Left gastric a

CELIAC TRUNK

Common hepatic a

Right gastric a

Hepatic a

Gastroduodenal a

Right gastro-omental

Superior pancreaticoduodenal a

Short gastric a

Spleen

Splenic a

Left gastro-omental

AORTA

Figure 4-19 Arterial supply to stomach.

(3) the **short gastric**, branching off from the *splenic artery;* (4) the **left gastro-omental artery,** another branch of the *splenic artery;* and (5) the **right gastro-omental artery,** a branch of the *common hepatic artery* by way of the *gastroduodenal* and *common hepatic arteries.*

Venous Return. The veins of the stomach parallel the names and courses of the arteries that supply the stomach. The **right** and **left gastric veins** drain directly to the portal vein. The **short gastric vein** and the **left gastro-omental vein** join the splenic vein, which drains to the portal vein. The **right gastro-omental** vein drains to the superior mesenteric vein, which joins the splenic vein to form the portal vein (see *Figure 4-28*).

CLINICAL NOTES

Peptic Ulcers

A peptic ulcer is a circumscribed erosion of the protective mucosa that occurs in regions of the gut exposed to acid and pepsin. Ulcers most commonly occur in the first few centimeters of the duodenum as **duodenal ulcers** or along the lesser curvature of the stomach as **gastric ulcers.** Initial, conservative treatment consists of a regimen of neutralizing acids and other medications that promote healing; surgery is required only for cases that involve complications, are suggestive of malignancy, or do not respond to initial treatment.

Duodenum

The gut distal to the pylorus marks the beginning of the small intestine, and the first section of small intestine is the duodenum (*Figure 4-20*). The duodenum lies in the form of a C on the posterior body wall, encircling the head and neck of the pancreas within its arms. It is about 25 cm long.

Position. The duodenum is somewhat centrally located on the posterior body wall. Its proximal end begins 2 or 3 cm to the right of the midline. Its distal portion ends 2 or 3 cm to the left of the midline. Only 5 cm separates the proximal and distal ends. The abdominal aorta and the inferior vena cava lie posteriorly. Within the arms of the C lie the head and neck of the pancreas.

Parts. The duodenum is classically divided into four parts, each part corresponding to a portion of the C.

The **first part** (superior) is about 5 cm long and runs posteriorly and to the right, where it contacts the liver above and the neck of the gallbladder.

The **second part** (descending) descends for about 10 cm, paralleling the inferior vena cava and the medial border of the right kidney behind. Both the common bile duct and the pancreatic duct empty their secretions into the second portion of the duodenum through a common opening on the concave aspect of the C (*Figure 4-21*).

The **third part** (horizontal) turns to the left at the level of the third lumbar vertebra and passes in a horizontal plane to the left for about 10 cm.

The **fourth part** (ascending) turns abruptly upward for 2 cm or so and then becomes the proximal end of the jejunum.

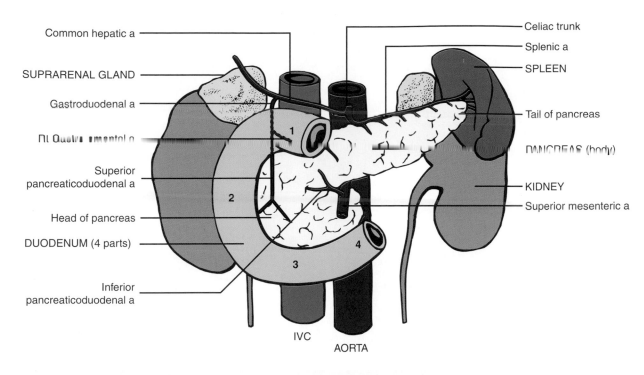

Common hepatic a

SUPRARENAL GLAND

Gastroduodenal a

Dt Gastro omental a

Superior
pancreaticoduodenal a

Head of pancreas

DUODENUM (4 parts)

Inferior
pancreaticoduodenal a

Celiac trunk

Splenic a

SPLEEN

Tail of pancreas

PANCREAS (body)

KIDNEY

Superior mesenteric a

IVC

AORTA

Figure 4-20 Duodenum, pancreas, spleen, and kidneys in situ. *IVC,* Inferior vena cava.

Wall of the Duodenum and Its Function. The duodenal wall is relatively thick and consists of the four coats found throughout the gut. The internal mucous membrane lining is thrown into many circular folds (plicae circulares) and contains numerous duodenal glands. It is in the second part of the duodenum that enzymes from the pancreas and bile from the liver are added to the ingested food (see *Figure 4-21*). The opening is into the concave midportion of the second part and is seen internally opening through an elevation termed the *major duodenal papilla.* Immediately above the papilla is the **minor duodenal papilla,** which marks the entrance of the accessory pancreatic duct into the duodenum.

Smooth muscle sphincters guard the openings of the common bile duct, pancreatic duct, and the ampulla that control the flow of bile and pancreatic enzymes to the duodenum as needed.

Peritoneal Attachments. The duodenum for most of its length is retroperitoneal. Only a variable proximal few centimeters retain a short mesentery. As the fourth part of the duodenum ascends and curves abruptly anteriorly to become the jejunum, the mesentery that supports the remainder of the small intestine begins.

Arterial Supply. The blood supply to the duodenum is derived from the **celiac trunk** and the **superior mesenteric artery.** The division between their territories of supply is approximately the level of the entrance of the bile duct

in the second part. It also marks the division between the foregut and the midgut.

The **superior pancreaticoduodenal artery** arises indirectly from the celiac trunk in the following manner: celiac trunk, common hepatic artery, gastroduodenal artery, and finally the superior pancreaticoduodenal artery. It follows the inner curve of the duodenum and supplies the superior aspects of the pancreas and duodenum.

The **inferior pancreaticoduodenal artery** is the first branch of the superior mesenteric artery. It supplies the inferior portion of the pancreas and duodenum.

Venous Return. The superior and **inferior pancreaticoduodenal veins** transport the venous return from the duodenum to the portal vein via the superior mesenteric vein.

Jejunum and Ileum

The fourth, ascending, portion of the duodenum becomes the jejunum. At this point the small intestine assumes a mesentery, allowing it a degree of mobility. Although there is no clear demarcation, the jejunum is described as being the proximal two fifths of the mobile small intestine (excluding the duodenum), and the ileum is the remaining distal three fifths. The mobile section of the small intestine is roughly 6 to 7 m long.

Position. The jejunum and ileum occupy a central position framed superiorly and laterally by the large intestine.

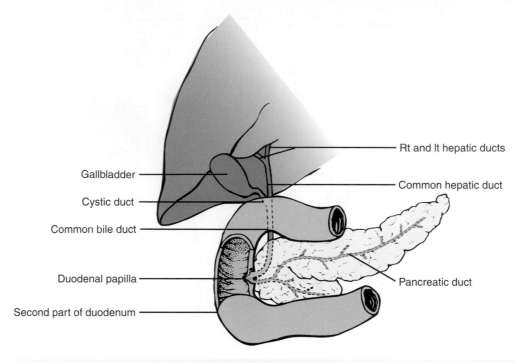

Figure 4-21 Biliary apparatus and pancreatic duct.

Labels (top to bottom, left side): Gallbladder — Cystic duct — Common bile duct — Duodenal papilla — Second part of duodenum

Labels (right side): Rt and lt hepatic ducts — Common hepatic duct — Pancreatic duct

Draped anteriorly over the coils of small intestine is the greater omentum.

Peritoneal Attachments. The jejunum and ileum are slung from the posterior body wall by a mesentery. The root of the **mesentery** (where the double-layered peritoneum of the mesentery reflects onto the body wall as parietal peritoneum) is only 15 to 20 cm long and runs diagonally from the duodenal junction to the ileocolic junction (*Figure 4-22*).

From this rather short base the mesentery must support 6 to 7 m of small gut on its periphery. The arrangement can be compared with a collapsed fan and accounts for the convoluted arrangements within the abdomen. On initial inspection it is virtually impossible to determine which end is which. By placing the hands on either side of the mesentery, the dissector or surgeon can immediately determine the direction from proximal to distal. It is through the mesentery that the nerve and blood supplies travel to the small intestine.

Small Intestine Wall and Function. The mucous membrane of the small intestine is suited for absorption (*Figure 4-23*). The surface area of the mucosa is greatly increased for absorption in the following manner: The mucous membrane is thrown into many circular folds (**plicae circulares**), and the folds are further covered by microscopic fingerlike projections called *villi*. Each villus contains an arteriole, a capillary bed into which digested food is absorbed, and a venule, which transports the venous blood containing the absorbed nutrients to mesenteric veins. In addition, each villus contains a central lymphatic capillary or lacteal,

which absorbs fats. Among the villi are crypt openings leading to the **intestinal glands (of Lieberkühn)**, which secrete digestive enzymes.

Jejunum and Ileum Contrasted and Compared. In general, the diameter of the small intestine decreases from proximal to distal, and digestive activity and absorption of digested foods diminish from proximal to distal (see *Figure 4-23*). This gradual functional change is reflected in slight morphological differences as the jejunum gradually becomes the ileum.

For comparison, the **jejunum** has a thicker muscular wall for more active peristalsis, has a mucosal inner lining of greater diameter for absorption, and has more plicae circulares and more villi for greater absorption. The **ileum**, on the other hand, has more mesenteric fat, more lymphoid tissue (Peyer's patches) to handle waste materials, and a more complex arterial configuration.

Arterial Supply. The blood supply to the small intestine is derived from the **superior mesenteric artery** (see *Figure 4-22*). A dozen or more **intestinal branches** are given off, which travel through the mesentery to the small gut. Distally the arteries join as loops, or **arcades**. Arising from the arcades are straight branches, or **vasa recti**, which supply the gut itself.

Venous Drainage. Venous return drains to **small intestinal tributaries** of the **superior mesenteric vein**. The superior mesenteric vein joins the splenic vein to form the

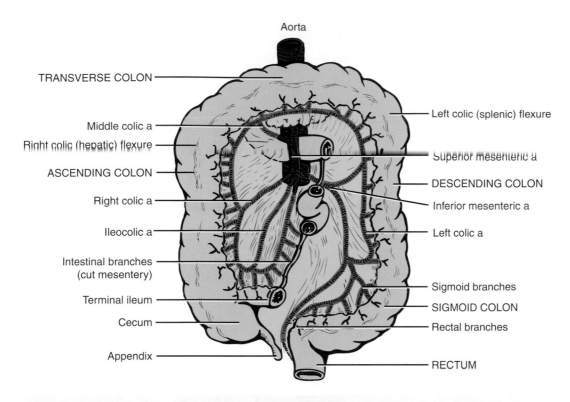

Aorta

TRANSVERSE COLON

Middle colic a

Right colic (hepatic) flexure

ASCENDING COLON

Right colic a

Ileocolic a

Intestinal branches
(cut mesentery)

Terminal ileum

Cecum

Appendix

Left colic (splenic) flexure

Superior mesenteric a

DESCENDING COLON

Inferior mesenteric a

Left colic a

Sigmoid branches

SIGMOID COLON

Rectal branches

RECTUM

Figure 4-22 Arterial supply to small and large intestines. The transverse colon has been raised for clarity.

portal vein, which transports absorbed elements from the gut to the liver for processing (see *Figure 4-28*).

Large Intestine, or Colon

The colon extends from the ileocolic junction to the anus (see *Figure 4-22*). It is about 1.5 m long and diminishes in diameter from proximal to distal.

Position. The colon sits within the abdomen like a large question mark, with its lateral and superior borders flanking the loops of small intestine.

Features and Parts. The colon differs from the small intestine in a number of ways. The lumen is of a greater diameter. The longitudinal smooth muscle coat consists of only three longitudinal bands, called *teniae coli* (*Figure 4-24, A*). The teniae originate at the base of the appendix and can be traced continuously throughout the length of the large intestine (excluding the rectum). The large intestine exhibits sacculations, or **haustra,** caused by the contracted teniae coli. Small bags of fat-filled peritoneum, called **appendices epiploicae,** hang from the outer peritoneal coat of the colon (see *Figure 4-24, B*).

The large intestine consists of the cecum and appendix, ascending colon, transverse colon, descending colon, sigmoid colon, rectum, and anal canal.

Cecum and Appendix. The ileum ends at the **ileocecal orifice,** which pouts into a rather large baglike struc-

ture within the right iliac fossa called the *cecum* (see *Figure 4-24, B*). Guarding the orifice is a slitlike **ileocecal valve,** which prevents regurgitation of colonic contents back into the ileum. Opening into the cecum about 2 cm below the orifice is a blind-ended diverticulum, the **vermiform appendix** (*vermiform,* "like a worm"). The appendix varies greatly in length (from 5 to 18 cm) and contains a considerable amount of lymphoid tissue within its submucosa.

Ascending Colon. The colon ascends from the cecal area on the right side to the inferior aspect of the liver, where it deflects and turns sharply as the **right colic flexure,** or **hepatic flexure.** The ascending colon is the shortest portion of the large intestine. It is fixed to the posterior body wall and is retroperitoneal.

CLINICAL NOTES

Appendicitis

Because of the concentration of lymphoid tissue, the appendix can become infected (appendicitis) just as the tonsillar lymphoid area of the oropharynx (tonsillitis) can. An infected appendix, however, is a hollow structure; if not removed in time, it could burst, releasing its contents into the peritoneal cavity, causing inflammation of the peritoneum (**peritonitis**).

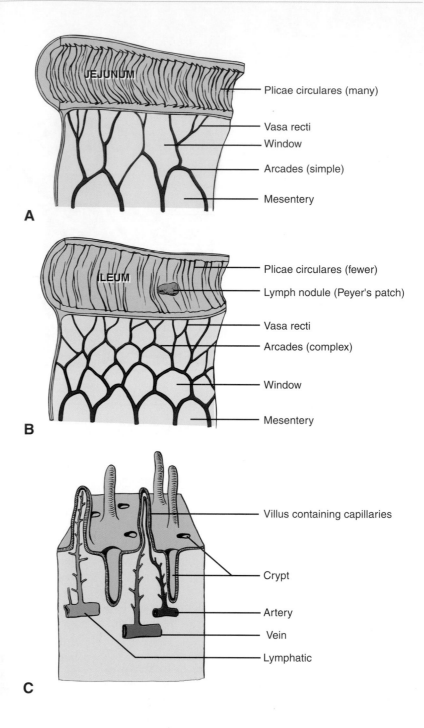

Plicae circulares (many)

Vasa recti

Window

Arcades (simple)

Mesentery

A

Plicae circulares (fewer)

Lymph nodule (Peyer's patch)

Vasa recti

Arcades (complex)

Window

Mesentery

B

Villus containing capillaries

Crypt

Artery

Vein

Lymphatic

C

Figure 4-23 Small intestine. **A,** Features of jejunum. **B,** Features of ileum. **C,** Close-up of intestinal villi and crypts.

Transverse Colon. The transverse colon has a mesentery (*transverse mesocolon*), is movable, and hangs down into the abdomen for a variable distance. At its lowest point it extends to the umbilical level or lower. As the colon approaches the left side, it ascends to the level of the spleen and deflects sharply downward on the left as the descending colon. The flexure is the **left colic flexure,** or the **splenic flexure.**

Descending Colon. The descending colon is nonmobile, and its descent parallels the lateral border of the left kidney.

At the level of the left iliac crest, the colon turns medially as the sigmoid, or pelvic, colon.

Sigmoid Colon. At this point the colon once more becomes mobile by acquiring a mesentery. It follows an S-shaped course within the pelvic cavity, and at the middle of the sacrum the large intestine takes a straight course downward as the rectum.

Rectum and Anal Canal. Although the term *rectum* means straight, it follows the curvature of the sacrum to the level of the pelvic diaphragm, where it makes an almost

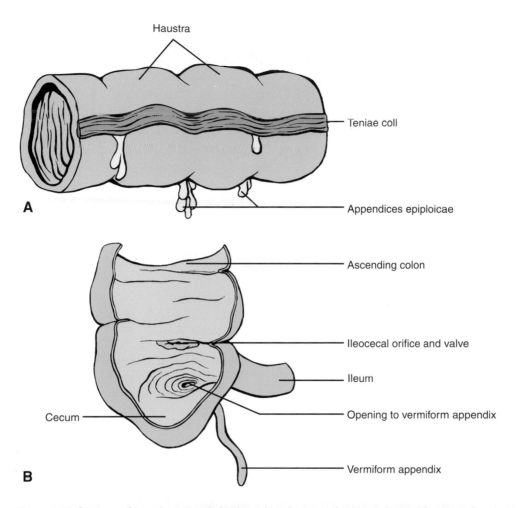

Figure 4-24 Sections of large intestine. **A,** Distinguishing features of colon. **B,** Internal features of cecum.

90-degree turn as the **anal canal** (approximately 4 cm long) (*Figure 4-25*). The rectum exhibits no sacculations, and the longitudinal layer of smooth muscle is intact; that is, the teniae are not found on the rectum.

Two sphincter muscles, which control expulsion of contents, surround the anal canal. The **internal sphincter ani** is a thickened portion of the circular muscular coat and is therefore involuntary (under parasympathetic control). The **external sphincter ani** is formed from the levator ani muscles and is under voluntary control. The levator ani muscles draw the anal canal upward over the feces during defecation.

Wall of the Colon and Its Function. The mucous membrane lining of the large gut contains no villi. However, cryptic mucous glands are present. The surface of the mucosal lining is designed for *water absorption.* The contents of the colon are feces, and the consistency of the feces ranges from fluid in the ascending colon to semifluid in the transverse colon, to varying degrees of hardness as it passes from the descending to the sigmoid colon.

The lining of the rectum differs from that of the rest of the large gut. Transverse folds of mucous membrane protrude into the lumen in three areas, probably to prevent inadvertent passage of fecal materials. A series of vertical ridges of mucous membrane, called *anal columns,* are found within the anal canal. Small transverse folds join the lower ends of the columns as *anal valves.* Small veins within these folds can become tortuous or varicose, resulting in *hemorrhoids.* Distally the anal canal exits from the body at the anus. A white line separates the mucous membrane of the anal canal from the skin of the anus externally.

Peritoneal Attachments. Certain sections of the large intestine have retained their dorsal mesenteries. Other sections had mesenteries, but they were subsequently obliterated during embryonic development of the gut.

The cecum generally hangs free in the right iliac fossa, supported by one or two short mesenteries. The appendix is supported by its own mesentery, the *mesoappendix,* and because the appendix is mobile, its position may be quite

113

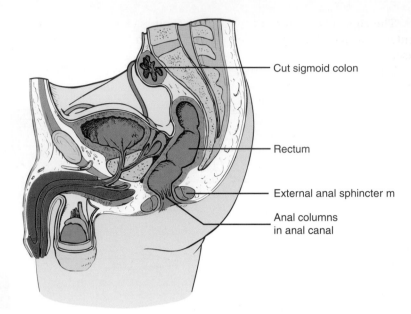

Figure 4-25 Median section through pelvis to show rectum and anal canal.

Cut sigmoid colon

Rectum

External anal sphincter m

Anal columns in anal canal

variable. The ascending colon is retroperitoneal and therefore fixed. However, the transverse colon is supported by a mesentery, the *transverse mesocolon;* consequently the transverse colon may occupy a variable position within the abdominal cavity. The descending colon is retroperitoneal, but the sigmoid colon is suspended by a V-shaped mesentery. The rectum is retroperitoneal.

Arterial Supply. The colon is supplied by branches of the superior and inferior mesenteric arteries (see *Figure 4-22*).

Superior Mesenteric Artery. The **ileocolic artery** arises from the superior mesenteric artery, travels through the mesentery toward the ileocecal junction, and gives off a number of branches. An *ileal* branch travels back to the ileum in a recurrent path to supply the distal end of the ileum. An *appendicular* branch travels through the mesoappendix to supply the appendix. (This branch is tied off during the course of an appendectomy.) *Cecal* branches supply the cecum, and *colic* branches ascend to supply the ascending colon.

CLINICAL NOTES

Colonoscopy

The colon can be inspected using a flexible fiber-optic *colonoscope* that is inserted into the anal canal and negotiated through the rectum, sigmoid colon, and ascending colon. There may be some difficulty negotiating the left colic (splenic) flexure on attempting to enter the transverse colon and further difficulty in navigating around the right colic (hepatic) flexure to the descending colon. The examination ends at the cecum because the colonoscope cannot pass the ileocecal valve. As suspicious areas and polyps are encountered, they can be excised and removed for further inspection in the pathology laboratory.

Rectal Examination

Digital examination of the rectal canal and lower rectum is a common procedure in adults because approximately 75% of colonic cancer occurs in the rectum. In addition, the prostate gland can be palpated in men to detect overgrowth and possible prostate cancer. In late pregnancy the cervix can be palpated to detect imminent delivery.

Hemorrhoids

The rectal veins drain to the inferior mesenteric vein, which in turn drains to the hepatic portal system of veins. Rectal veins also anastomose with veins that drain via the internal and common iliac vein to the inferior vena cava. This communication between the hepatic portal and inferior vena cava systems is termed a *portosystemic anastomosis.* Portal hypertension can result in engorged and tortuous rectal veins, termed *hemorrhoids* or commonly called *piles.* Another cause of hemorrhoids is excessive straining during defecation, as in chronic constipation.

The **right colic artery** arises from the superior mesenteric artery. It supplies the superior portion of the ascending colon.

The **middle colic artery** travels through the transverse mesocolon to supply the transverse colon.

Inferior Mesenteric Artery. The **inferior mesenteric artery** arises from the abdominal aorta approximately 5 cm below the superior mesenteric artery. It passes to the left and breaks up into three terminal branches: (1) the left colic artery; (2) sigmoid arteries; and (3) rectal branches to supply the descending colon, sigmoid colon, and rectum, respectively.

Venous Return. The cecum, ascending, and transverse colon are drained by tributaries of the **superior mesenteric vein.** The descending colon, sigmoid colon, and rectum are drained by tributaries of the **inferior mesenteric vein,** which drains to the splenic vein. The superior and inferior mesenteric veins unite to form the portal vein, which transports venous return from the colon to the liver (see *Figure 4-28*).

The Liver

The liver is a large organ that weighs approximately 2 kg and occupies the upper right quadrant of the abdominal cavity. It is dark red and soft, adapting its shape to its neighboring structures. It is extremely friable and easily lacerated, totally unlike the consolidated, relatively hard structure found in the dissecting laboratory. The liver sits under the diaphragm in the upper right quadrant and is sheltered anteriorly by the lower right rib.

Surfaces and Features. The liver presents two surfaces: a smooth **diaphragmatic surface,** which includes the anterior, superior, and posterior aspects of the liver, and a **visceral surface,** which takes the shape of the abdominal contents inferior to the liver (*Figure 4-26*). These are, from right to left, the right colic flexure, the right kidney, the duodenum, and the stomach.

Hooking the liver upward to expose the posterior and inferior surfaces allows the four lobes of the liver to be delineated quite readily (see *Figure 4-26, B*). A grouping of

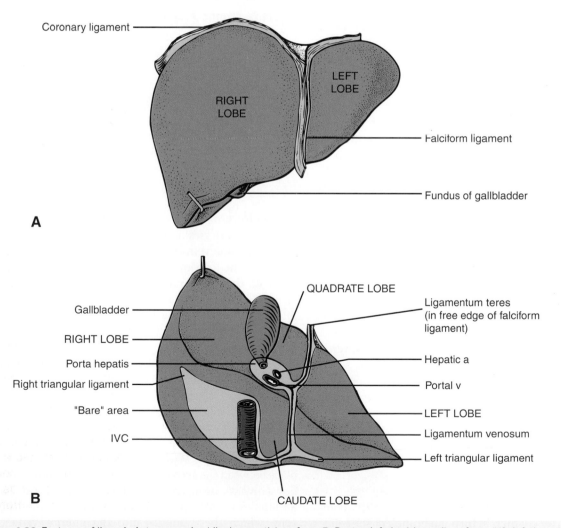

Figure 4-26 Features of liver. **A,** Anterosuperior (diaphragmatic) surface. **B,** Posteroinferior (visceral) surface. *IVC,* Inferior vena cava.

115

fissures and fossae on this view takes the form of an H. The left vertical bar contains the ligamentum venosum posteriorly and the ligamentum teres anteriorly. The right vertical bar contains the inferior vena cava posteriorly and the gallbladder anteriorly. The horizontal crosspiece, called the *porta hepatis* ("gateway of the liver"), is the site of entrance of the hepatic arteries and the portal vein. It is also the site of exit of the right and left hepatic ducts. Dispersed around the various lines of the H are the four lobes of the liver. The right lobe lies to the right of the inferior vena cava and the gallbladder. The left lobe lies to the left of the ligamentum teres and the ligamentum venosum. The quadrate lobe lies between the gallbladder, the ligamentum teres, and the porta hepatis. The caudate lobe lies between the inferior vena cava, the ligamentum venosum, and the porta hepatis. The caudate lobe projects into the lesser sac.

Peritoneal Attachments
Coronary Ligament. The liver is covered with visceral peritoneum (see *Figure 4-26, B*). Posteriorly the visceral peritoneum reflects back onto the diaphragm as the diaphragmatic peritoneum (see *Figure 4-29*). The somewhat circular area of reflection is fairly extensive and is called the *coronary ligament* (*corona,* meaning "crown"). Cutting through this ligament to remove the liver from the abdomen reveals the so-called **bare area** of the liver, an area devoid of visceral peritoneum.

Falciform Ligament. The falciform ligament is all that remains of the primitive ventral mesentery (see *Figure 4-11*). It is a double-layered, sickle-shaped membrane that extends upward from the umbilicus on the inner aspect of the anterior wall to the anterior aspect of the liver. At the liver the falciform ligament splits to the right and left to become continuous with the coronary ligament. The free edge of the sickle-shaped membrane contains a thick, round ligament, or **ligamentum teres.** This is a remnant of the umbilical vein (see Chapter 1, pages 18 and 19).

Ligamentum Venosum. The ligamentum venosum is the **obliterated ductus venosus,** which once connected the umbilical vein, as it approached the porta hepatis, to the inferior vena cava. It represents a former *fetal bypass of the liver* (see Chapter 1, pages 18 and 19).

Lesser Omentum. The lesser omentum is a double-layered sheet of mesentery that joins the liver above to the stomach below (*Figure 4-27*). Running through the omentum toward the porta hepatis of the liver are the **common bile duct,** the **hepatic artery,** and the **portal vein**.

The right side of the lesser omentum is a free edge. Posterior to the free edge is the opening to the lesser sac (epiploic foramen).

Blood Flow to the Liver
Hepatic Artery. The hepatic artery arises from the common hepatic artery, which in turn is a branch of the celiac trunk (see *Figure 4-19*). The hepatic artery passes upward in the free edge of the lesser omentum. As it approaches the porta hepatis it divides into a right and a left branch, each supplying right and left halves of the liver, respectively. The hepatic artery supplies the tissue of the liver with oxygenated blood.

Portal Vein. The portal vein ultimately drains the blood returning from the digestive tract and the spleen and transports the products of digestion to the liver for processing (*Figure 4-28*). The portal vein forms in the following manner. The **inferior mesenteric vein,** which drains *hindgut derivatives,* unites with the **splenic vein,** which drains the *foregut derivatives.* The **superior mesenteric vein,** which drains *midgut derivatives,* joins the splenic vein to form the **portal vein.** The portal vein travels upward within the lesser omentum and divides into right and left branches as it approaches the porta hepatis. It supplies both halves of the liver.

CLINICAL NOTES

Portosystemic Anastomoses
The portal system anastomoses with the inferior vena cava at the distal portion of the rectum and the distal end of the esophagus. Venous varicosities (enlarged and tortuous veins) could result from increased portal pressure (portal hypertension). Danger lies in the possible bursting of these vessels in the esophageal area. Varicosities in the rectal area are more a nuisance than a danger and are termed *hemorrhoids*.

Venous Return. All of the blood supplied to the liver from the **hepatic arteries** and the **portal vein** eventually drains via the **hepatic veins** to the **inferior vena cava** (see *Figure 4-28*). As the inferior vena cava comes into intimate contact with the liver on the posterior aspect of the liver, two or more hepatic veins arise from the liver to pass directly into the inferior vena cava.

Structure and Function. Fibrous septa separate liver tissue into small functional units, or *lobules*. Each lobule consists of several sheets of epithelial cells, which radiate out from a central vein. At the periphery of each lobule (between adjoining lobules) are small branches of the hepatic artery, portal vein, and hepatic duct. The vessels empty their blood into the spaces between the epithelial sheets (sinusoids). Within the sinusoids, exchanges take place between the epithelial cells and the blood as the blood flows inward toward the central vein. The central veins of all lobules ultimately come together to form the hepatic vein, which then empties into the inferior vena cava. Within the liver sheets are small ducts, termed *canaliculi*.

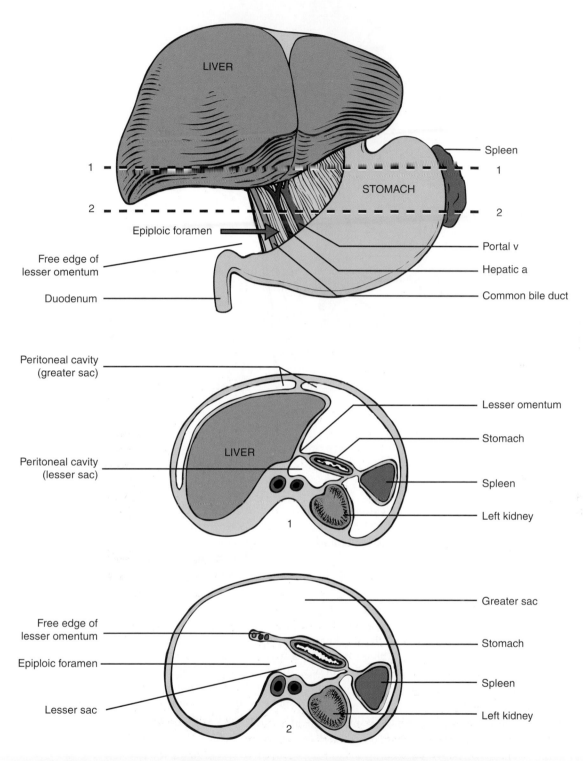

Figure 4-27 Transverse sections through abdomen at two levels to demonstrate structures passing to and from liver through lesser omentum. Section 1 passes through the lower aspect of the liver. Section 2 passes through the epiploic foramen.

The canaliculi carry bile manufactured by the liver cells in the opposite direction to that of the blood flow. The bile canaliculi flow toward the periphery of the lobule, emptying into bile ducts that ultimately empty into the right and left hepatic ducts. The functions of the liver can be divided into four main categories.

Metabolic Functions. The liver metabolizes the products of digestion brought by the portal vein from the intestines.

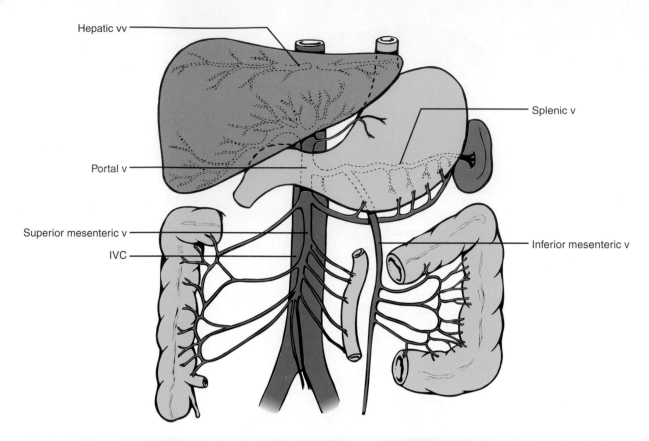

Hepatic vv

Splenic v

Portal v

Superior mesenteric v

IVC

Inferior mesenteric v

Figure 4-28 Hepatic portal system of veins. *IVC,* Inferior vena cava.

In the liver, blood glucose is transformed to *glycogen* and stored. When the concentration of blood glucose is low, the glycogen in the liver is converted back to glucose and released to the body through the bloodstream.

The liver stores vitamin A, which is essential for the maintenance of the mucous membrane. In addition, *vitamins D* and B_{12} and iron in the form of *ferritin* are stored in the liver.

Storage and Filtration of Blood. The liver acts as a blood *reservoir* and can store 500 to 1000 mL of blood within the sinusoids. The liver contains phagocytic cells, which protrude into the blood sinusoids to filter bacteria from the blood.

During fetal development the liver functions as *hemopoietic tissue* and produces both leukocytes and erythrocytes.

Bile Production and Secretion. *Bile* is produced by the liver cells from diet or stored cholesterol and from bilirubin, a breakdown product of phagocytosed erythrocytes. Bile is collected by the biliary system of ducts, which transport it to the duodenum, where it acts to emulsify fats.

Production of Blood Coagulating Factors. *Fibrinogen, prothrombin, accelerator globulins,* and so on, are produced in the liver. Heparin, an anticoagulant, is not manufactured by the liver but rather by its connective tissue septa

containing mast cells. Heparin is manufactured in connective tissue throughout the body.

Biliary Apparatus. The liver continuously produces bile. The **bile canaliculi** within the liver lobules drain the bile to intralobular ducts. In turn, these ducts drain to **interlobular ducts.** The interlobular ducts ultimately form the **right** and **left hepatic ducts** (see *Figure 4-21*).

Below the porta of the liver the right and left hepatic ducts join to form the **common hepatic duct.** Arising from the common hepatic duct is a diverticulum, or sac, called the *gallbladder,* which stores and concentrates bile. A short **cystic duct** joins the common hepatic duct to form the **common bile duct,** which transports the bile inferiorly to the duodenum.

The **gallbladder** is found on the visceral surface of the liver, hanging inferiorly so that its rounded fundus peeks out below the sharp anterior inferior border of the liver at about the level of the ninth costal cartilage in the right midclavicular plane. It holds about 25 mL, and it is here that the bile is concentrated.

Between meals the entrance of the bile duct into the duodenum is closed by a sphincter. Bile is manufactured continuously, and the excess tracks back into the gallbladder.

During a meal the bile passages open and the stored bile travels back through the cystic duct to the common bile duct. The common bile duct passes downward through the free edge of the lesser omentum, runs posteriorly to the first part of the duodenum, and then curves to enter the midpoint of the second part of the duodenum.

The common bile duct joins with the pancreatic duct distally to form a common chamber, called the *ampulla.* The ampulla then discharges bile and pancreatic enzymes into the duodenum. The distal end of the common bile duct is controlled by a sphincter, which opens to release bile during a meal.

Pancreas

The pancreas is a soft, glandular organ about 20 cm long (see *Figures 4-20* and *4-21*). Its long axis lies transversely in the abdomen against the posterior body wall.

Features and Parts. The pancreas can be divided into three main areas: the head, body, and tail. The *head* sits within the arms of the C-shaped duodenum at lumbar vertebral level L1-L2. The head lies directly in front of the inferior vena cava, the aorta, and the right renal vessels. The superior mesenteric artery issuing from the aorta separates the uncinate process from the rest of the head. The *body* extends to the left for 12 to 15 cm and ends as the *tail*, which touches the hilus of the spleen. The stomach lies anterior to the pancreas, separated from it by the lesser sac.

Peritoneum. The pancreas is entirely covered by peritoneum anteriorly and is therefore retroperitoneal. This peritoneum provides a base for the attachment of the transverse mesocolon (*Figure 4-29*).

CLINICAL NOTES

Jaundice

Obstruction of the flow of bile through the biliary tree results in a backup of bile and release of excess bilirubin into the bloodstream. This results in yellowing of the skin (French, *jaune*), mucous membranes, and whites of the eyes.

Gallstones

In the process of concentration of the bile within the gallbladder, bile salts may precipitate as sludge or solid stones. Blockage results in considerable pain (biliary colic) referred to the epigastric region and may necessitate the removal of the gallbladder (**cholecystectomy**). Removal poses no problem with digestion because bile is stored within the remainder of the biliary tree and the sphincter of the common bile duct continues to control the passage of bile into the duodenum.

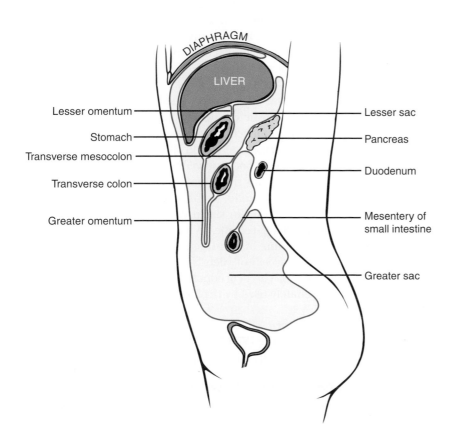

Figure 4-29 Median section through abdomen to show disposition of peritoneum.

Structure and Function. The pancreas consists of two glands in one: the exocrine and endocrine portions.

Exocrine Portion. The various lobules of the pancreas are drained by ductules, which eventually drain into a **main pancreatic duct.** The pancreatic duct traverses the length of the pancreas left to right from within, picking up tributaries as it goes. Along with the common bile duct, it empties its secretions into the ampulla of the duodenum. The distal end of the pancreatic duct is guarded by a sphincter. The ampulla empties into the duodenum through an opening in the **major duodenal papilla.** A second, or **accessory, pancreatic duct** occasionally enters the duodenum independently of the main duct through an opening in the **minor duodenal papilla.** The exocrine secretions of the pancreas consist of digestive enzymes concerned with protein, carbohydrate, and fat breakdown.

Endocrine Portion. The pancreas contains special clusters of cells, or **islets of Langerhans,** scattered throughout its substance. These cells produce **insulin,** an agent necessary for sugar metabolism.

Arterial Supply. Like the duodenum, the pancreas is supplied by branches of both the celiac trunk and the superior mesenteric artery. The **splenic artery** arises from the *celiac trunk* and passes to the left on its way to the spleen by grooving the superior border of the pancreas. As it contacts the pancreas, it supplies it with small branches.

CLINICAL NOTES

Pancreatitis

The close relationship of the common bile duct and the pancreatic duct and their common entry into the ampulla of the duodenum occasionally pose problems. Obstruction within the ampulla by a gallstone can cause a backup of bile into the pancreas, resulting in **acute pancreatitis** (inflammation of the pancreas).

The **superior pancreaticoduodenal artery** is an ultimate branch of the *celiac trunk.* It arises from the gastroduodenal branch and passes inferiorly between the head of the pancreas and the duodenum to supply both structures.

The **inferior pancreaticoduodenal artery** arises from the *superior mesenteric artery,* travels superiorly between the pancreatic head and the duodenum, and supplies both structures.

Venous Drainage. Corresponding veins drain venous blood from the pancreas to the portal system. The **splenic vein** receives tributaries from the superior surface of the pancreas and passes to the left to help form the portal vein. The **superior** and **inferior pancreaticoduodenal veins** drain directly to the portal vein.

Spleen (Lien)

The spleen is about 13 cm by 7 cm (see *Figures 4-18, 4-19,* and *4-20*). It lies in the upper left quadrant of the abdomen, and its superior surface assumes the rounded shape of the diaphragm above. It is protected under ribs 9, 10, and 11 laterally. It lies no farther medially than the midaxillary line.

Features and Parts. The spleen presents two surfaces: a smooth diaphragmatic surface superiorly and laterally and a visceral surface medially and inferiorly. The visceral surface assumes its shape from the greater curvature of the stomach, the left kidney, and the left colic flexure, with which it makes contact. The anterior border is notched.

The business end of the spleen is the hilus, which is centrally located on the visceral surface. Contacting the hilus is the tail of the pancreas, and running to and from the hilus are the splenic vessels.

Peritoneum. The spleen develops in the primitive dorsal mesogastrium (mesentery of the developing stomach). The mesogastrium fuses with the peritoneum of the posterior body wall during development, but the spleen remains attached to the stomach by the **gastrosplenic ligament,** a portion of the greater omentum (see *Figure 4-12*). The **splenorenal ligament** attaches the spleen to the left kidney. The two peritoneal ligaments allow the spleen a degree of mobility. The spleen itself is covered with visceral peritoneum except at the hilus.

Structure and Function. The spleen is like a sponge surrounded by elastic connective tissue and smooth muscle cells. Elastic connective tissue septa divide the spleen into many compartments, within which are networks of cells surrounded by blood sinusoids.

The spleen has three main functions. First, the spleen produces *lymphocytes.* Second, it is a *storehouse for blood,* and by increasing in size it can store up to one sixth of the total blood volume. When needed, it adds blood to the circulation by contracting. Third, the spleen *filters circulating blood* of debris and *breaks down worn-out erythrocytes.* The byproducts of red blood cell breakdown are ultimately used by the liver to produce bile.

Blood Supply. The spleen is supplied by the **splenic artery,** a branch of the celiac trunk. It is drained by the **splenic vein,** which helps form the portal vein.

A Review of Peritoneal Reflections

Figure 4-29 offers a review of the relationship of various abdominal organs and the continuity of parietal and visceral peritoneum. The peritoneal cavity is divided into two regions: the greater and lesser sacs. The **lesser sac** is the enclosed area behind the stomach; the **greater sac** is the remainder of the peritoneal cavity. The two sacs communicate only via the epiploic foramen.

CLINICAL NOTES

Splenectomy (Surgical Removal of the Spleen)

Although the spleen is protected by the ribs, it can be damaged following trauma to the upper left quadrant. If ruptured, the spleen bleeds profusely and is difficult to repair because the tissue is extremely friable (tears easily). The spleen is not essential to life in humans and may be surgically removed if it is injured and not reparable following trauma to the spleen.

CLINICAL NOTES

Acute Peritonitis

Peritonitis, a serious condition, is an inflammation of the visceral and parietal peritoneum and is most often caused by infections that result from perforations of the gut and leakage of gut contents into the peritoneal cavity. Common causes are a burst appendix releasing its contents into the greater sac, or a peptic ulcer that has perforated into the lesser sac. Spread from one area to the other can take place through the epiploic foramen.

URINARY SYSTEM

The urinary system consists of the right and left kidneys, the right and left ureters, the bladder, and the urethra (*Figure 4-30*).

Kidneys

The shape of the kidney is self-descriptive. Each kidney is approximately 10 cm long, 5 cm wide, and 2.5 cm thick. The kidneys lie on the posterior body wall, with the long axes parallel to the vertebral column. The kidneys are angled against the vertebral column so that the medial border is more anterior to the lateral border (see *Figure 4-10*).

Position. Posteriorly the upper portion of each kidney is sheltered by the eleventh and twelfth ribs. The lower halves are protected only by muscles of the posterior abdominal wall. Therefore the lower halves are more susceptible to trauma. The left kidney is slightly higher than the right.

Medially the bodies of the last thoracic vertebra and vertebrae L1 to L3 separate the right and left kidneys.

Anterior to the vertebral bodies are the inferior vena cava and the aorta.

Anteriorly the right kidney contacts the suprarenal gland above, the liver, and the hepatic flexure of the colon below. The left kidney contacts the suprarenal gland, the stomach, the spleen, the jejunum, and the splenic flexure of the colon.

Features and Parts. The lateral border of the kidney is rounded; the medial border is concave and contains a vertical slit through which the ureter and the renal vessels pass to and from the kidney. The concave area is the **hilus of the kidney;** the vertical slit is the **renal sinus.**

Peritoneum. The kidneys occupy a retroperitoneal position. Under the peritoneum the kidneys are enveloped in a cushioning layer of perirenal fat. Anchoring the kidney to the posterior body wall is a layer of fibrous renal fascia, which is deficient below. A kidney could slip through this deficiency and become a "floating kidney." The left kidney is joined to the spleen by the splenorenal ligament.

Structure and Function. The **nephron** is the basic functional unit of the kidney. It consists of a number of parts (*Figure 4-31*).

The **glomerulus** is a twisted ball of capillary-like tubes. The arterioles of the kidney approximate the glomerulus to form a *renal corpuscle.* The fine tubes of the glomerulus filter the arterial blood. An efferent arteriole leaves the glomerulus and ends in an adjacent capillary bed, which is drained by renal venules.

The filtrate from the glomerulus passes to the **proximal convoluted tubule,** the **loop of Henle,** and then the **distal convoluted tubule.** Water, glucose, and sodium are reabsorbed into the bloodstream within this system. Waste products are retained, and adjacent nephrons empty the final filtrate into a **collecting tubule,** which is eventually discharged to the ureters.

Figure 4-31, A, represents a coronal section through a kidney to display the gross internal features of the kidney.

The **cortex** is the pale, granular outer layer, or bark, of the kidney. Contributing to the granular appearance are glomeruli, distal and proximal convoluted tubules, and the proximal portions of the collecting tubules.

The **medulla** is the inner, darker area that appears striped and consists of approximately six *renal pyramids,* of which the apices point toward the hilus of the kidney. The pyramids of the medulla contain loops of Henle and collecting tubules (distal portions).

Renal columns are found between the pyramids and represent cortical tissue. **Medullary rays** are streaks of medullary tissue that extend into the cortex from the base of the pyramids. The **renal papilla** is the apex of the medullary pyramid, and it is here that the collecting tubules pour their contents into receiving cuplike structures.

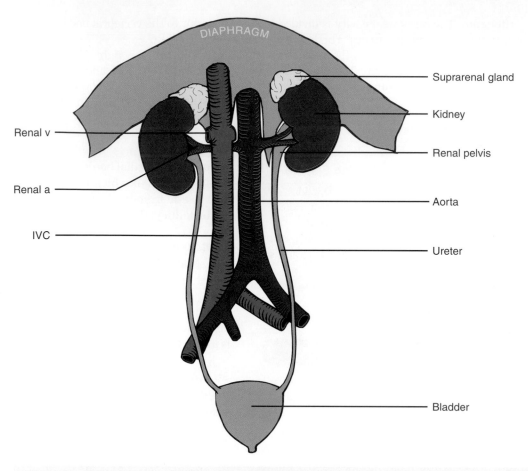

Figure 4-30 Components of the urinary system and the blood supply to the kidneys.

The **minor calyces** are those cuplike structures that receive secretions from the renal papillae. Several minor calyces unite to form a major calyx. About three **major calyces** are found in the kidney, and these unite to form the **renal pelvis.** The ureters drain the renal pelvis to the bladder in the pelvis below.

Blood Supply. The **renal artery** arises from the abdominal aorta, passes laterally, and enters the hilus of the kidney (see *Figure 4-30*). The right renal artery passes behind the inferior vena cava. As the artery enters the hilus, it gives off a branch that passes superiorly to the suprarenal gland. Within the sinus of the kidney the renal arteries end as several *interlobar arteries*, which course peripherally through the renal columns to reach the cortex. Here they bifurcate at right angles as *arcuate arteries*, which run parallel below the cortex and then anastomose with each other to form *arcades*. From the arcades, interlobular arteries pass peripherally into the cortex to give off the afferent arterioles to the glomeruli. The capillary beds are adjacent to the glomeruli. Efferent arterioles leave the glomeruli and then drain to the capillary beds.

Venules leave the capillary beds and eventually coalesce as the **renal veins.** The renal veins leave the hilus of each kidney anterior to the artery. The left renal vein usually receives tributaries from the left testicular/ovarian vein, the left phrenic vein, and the suprarenal vein. The right and left renal veins drain to the inferior vena cava.

Ureters

The **ureter** is a muscular tube that carries urine from the kidneys down to the bladder within the pelvis. It is approximately 25 cm long, with its proximal half within the abdomen and the distal half within the pelvis. The **renal pelvis** is funnel-shaped and collects urine from the **calyces** within the kidney. The pelvis then narrows down to the thick-walled muscular ureter, which then milks the urine down to the bladder by peristaltic action.

The ureters travel inferiorly just below the parietal peritoneum of the posterior body wall. As they enter the pelvis, they pass anterior to the common iliac arteries.

The blood supply to the ureters is by region. Proximally they receive branches from the *renal arteries*; the midportions receive contributions from the *testicular/ovarian arteries*; and the distal portions receive branches from *vesicle arteries* (arteries that supply the bladder).

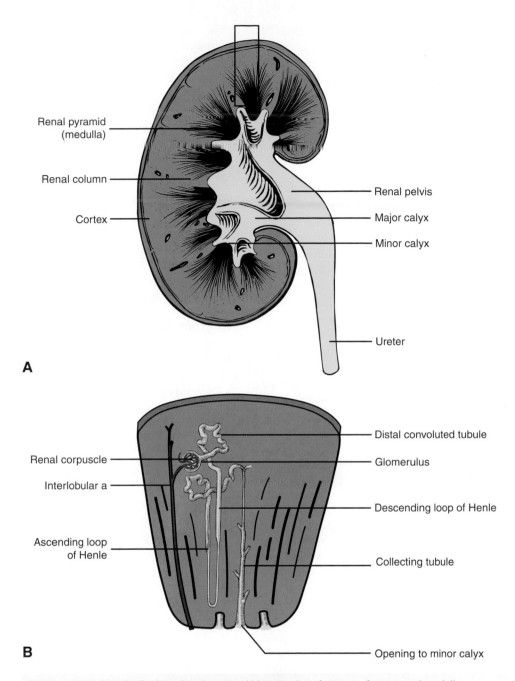

Figure 4-31 **A,** Longitudinal section through a kidney to show features of cortex and medulla.
B, Magnified section of kidney showing components of a nephron.

The Bladder

The **urinary bladder** is a hollow, thick-walled receiving and holding chamber for urine. It has a maximum capacity of approximately 500 mL, and because it constantly fills and is periodically emptied, its shape changes. It generally is described as being pyramidal in shape, but this description is based on an empty bladder in an embalmed cadaver. The pyramid presents a triangular superior surface and two triangular lateral surfaces that slope toward each other inferiorly. The base of the pyramid is directed posteriorly.

Position. The anterior border of the bladder rests against the inner aspect of the pubic bones (see *Figures 4-40* and *4-42*). The superior aspect is covered with peritoneum and as the bladder fills, it bulges superiorly, lifting the overlying peritoneum with it.

In males, intestinal loops lie superiorly; in females the uterus flops over the superior aspect of the bladder. The prostate gland is applied to the posterior aspect of the male bladder, and the gland is anterior to the rectum. In women the vagina and the cervix of the uterus intervene between the rectum and the posterior aspect of the bladder.

123

Entrances and Exit. The right and left ureters pass to the posterior aspect of the bladder, converge inferiorly, and then pass through the wall of the bladder obliquely to open into the lumen of the bladder about 2.5 cm apart (see *Figure 4-37*). The openings are only 2.5 cm above the funnel-shaped exit of the bladder, which is the beginning of the urethra. The two openings of the ureters above and the exit of the urethra below form an equilateral triangle known as the *trigone of the bladder.*

Structure and Function (Micturition). The lumen of the bladder is lined with transitional epithelial mucosa adapted for stretching. The walls contain smooth muscle fibers running in various directions, and these collectively are called the *detrusor muscle.* Smooth muscle forms an internal urethral sphincter as the urethra exits from the bladder. Pelvic splanchnic parasympathetic nerves are motor to the detrusor muscle and inhibitory to the sphincter muscles. As the bladder fills and stretch receptors in the mucosa are stimulated, an involuntary parasympathetic reflex is set up, which stimulates the detrusor muscle to contract. In the infant the internal sphincter relaxes and allows the bladder to void. In early childhood (in the second or third year) we learn to control the relaxation of the internal sphincter through toilet training and suppress reflex voiding.

CLINICAL NOTES

Urinary Calculi (Stones)

Calculi, or stones, can occur anywhere in the urinary tract and can result in obstruction of urine, pain, and infection. A stone in the ureter causes the peristaltic contractions to increase, resulting in considerable pain (**ureteral** or **renal colic**). Visceral afferents transmit the impulses via spinal nerves, and the pain is perceived as coming from referred sites: flank, lumbar, inguinal, and genital areas. Dependent on size and composition, stones may be passed spontaneously. If not, intervention may be called for, ranging from noninvasive **shock wave lithotripsy** using ultrasound that pulverizes the stone to open surgery.

Blood Supply. The urinary bladder is supplied by the **superior** and **inferior vesical arteries**, which arise from the internal iliac artery and are drained by veins of the same name that empty to the internal iliac vein.

Urethra

The male and female urethras are considered with the genital tracts.

SUPRARENAL GLANDS

Right and left suprarenal glands are perched like caps on the superior poles of the right and left kidneys (see *Figure 4-30*). The right gland is pyramidal in shape and wedged into the interval between the inferior vena cava and the upper pole of the right kidney. The left suprarenal gland is shaped like a half-moon and spills farther down the medial border of the left kidney.

Structure and Function

Structurally and functionally the suprarenal gland consists of two distinct parts: the cortex and medulla (*Figure 4-32*).

The **cortex** forms a thick outer layer and is involved with the production of a group of *steroid hormones*, such as cortisone. These hormones regulate salt and water balance, carbohydrate metabolism, production of collagen, and production of sex hormones responsible for secondary sex characteristics.

The **medulla** is really modified nervous tissue and functions as a sympathetic ganglion. Adrenaline and noradrenaline are secreted by the medulla. Adrenaline, or epinephrine, amplifies the effects of the sympathetic system and is poured into the circulation during periods of stress.

Blood Supply

The arteries to the suprarenal glands enter the glands through the hilus of the gland located on the anterior surface. Three arteries generally supply the suprarenal glands: (1) suprarenal branches arising directly from the aorta, (2) suprarenal branches arising from the renal arteries, and (3) suprarenal branches arising from the phrenic arteries. Corresponding veins drain the venous

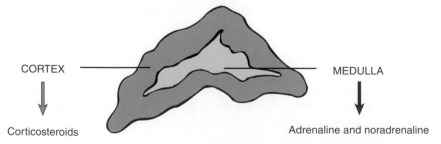

CORTEX — Corticosteroids

MEDULLA — Adrenaline and noradrenaline

Figure 4-32 Section through a suprarenal gland to show cortex and medulla.

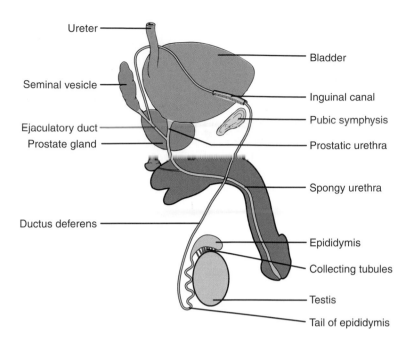

Figure 4-33 Scheme of male genital system.

return from the suprarenal glands directly or indirectly to the inferior vena cava.

THE MALE GENITAL SYSTEM

The genital system is composed of organs that represent our primary sex characteristics. They are the recognizable features that distinguish the male sex from the female sex at birth. During adolescence, secondary sex characteristics appear, further distinguishing the sexes and the adult from the child.

The male sex organs consist of the testes, the epididymis, the ductus deferens, the seminal vesicles, prostate gland, and the penis and urethra (*Figure 4-33*).

Testes

The development and prenatal descent of the testes are discussed in the section on the anterolateral abdominal wall and the inguinal region. The testes lie within the scrotal sac outside the abdominal cavity. Each testis is ovoid in shape and about 4 cm long.

A white, thick fibrous coat, the **tunica albuginea,** surrounds the testis (*Figure 4-34*). The posterior portion of the tunic is the **mediastinum,** from which fibrous septa containing blood vessels and nerves pass to the interior of the testis and thus divide the testes into roughly 250 compartments, or lobules. Each lobule contains one or more convoluted **seminiferous tubules,** which are about 50 cm long when unraveled. Cells line the seminiferous tubules, and some cells produce the male hormone **testosterone;** other cells ultimately develop as **spermatozoa,** which are shed into the lumen of the tubules.

The various seminiferous tubules converge on the mediastinum toward a network of tubules termed the

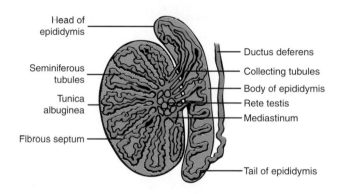

Figure 4-34 Longitudinal section through a testis to show internal features.

rete testis. From the superior aspect of the rete testis, a dozen or more **collecting tubules** leave the testis as efferent ductules, which transport the spermatozoa to the overlying **epididymis.**

Epididymis

The epididymis is a caplike structure that sits on the superior and posterior aspects of the testes. It is tapered from distal to proximal and has a *head*, a *body*, and a *tail*. Although the epididymis is only 6 cm long, its contents consist of a tightly coiled tube that can reach a length of several meters if uncoiled. At the inferior pole of the testis, the epididymis finally unravels as a single large duct, which then loops superiorly as the **ductus deferens.** The spermatozoa are stored within the epididymis, pending ejaculation.

Ductus Deferens

The ductus deferens ascends along the medial aspect of the epididymis to become a constituent of the **spermatic cord,**

125

which traverses the **inguinal canal** of the anterolateral abdominal wall to enter the abdomen. The ductus crosses the pelvic brim and passes medially to cross over the ureter. It then descends on the posterior wall of the bladder, dilates as the **ampulla**, and then joins with the duct of the **seminal vesicle** to form the **ejaculatory duct.**

Seminal Vesicles

Seminal vesicles are paired glands stuck to the posterior wall of the bladder (see *Figures 4-33* and *4-35*). The seminal vesicles do not store sperm as the name suggests; rather, they produce a *sticky secretion* for semen formation. The duct of the seminal vesicle joins with the distal end of the ampulla of the ductus deferens to form an **ejaculatory duct.** The right and left ejaculatory ducts empty their contents, sperm and secretions, into the **prostatic portion** of the **urethra** (see *Figure 4-32*).

CLINICAL NOTES

Prostate Enlargement

Benign overgrowth of the middle lobe may partially obstruct the drainage of urine into the urethra and slow the urinary stream during micturition. Overgrowth of the entire gland may be checked with rectal palpation.

Prostate Gland

The prostate gland lies below the neck of the bladder and surrounds the proximal 3 cm of the urethra (**prostatic urethra**) (see *Figures 4-33, 4-35,* and *4-37*). The gland is classically described as being the size of a walnut. It has a **middle lobe**, which bulges anteriorly into the base of the bladder in the middle of the trigone.

The prostate gland contains smooth muscle and glandular material. The gland produces a *watery secretion* that is expelled by the smooth muscle during ejaculation. This secretion passes to the prostatic urethra through tiny openings in the prostatic urethra to join the sperm and seminal vesicle secretions and finally form the ejaculate, or semen.

Bulbourethral Glands

Bulbourethral glands are tiny glands about 1 cm wide found within the urogenital diaphragm. They empty a *mucous type of secretion* into the urethra as a further contribution to the ejaculate (see *Figure 4-33*).

Penis

The penis consists of a root affixed to the perineum and a shaft suspended from the root (*Figures 4-36* and *4-37*). Within, the penis is made up of *three cylinders* composed of erectile tissue, or tissue rich in blood supply.

Right and Left Corpora Cavernosa. Each corpus cavernosum originates as a root, or **crus**, of the penis from the

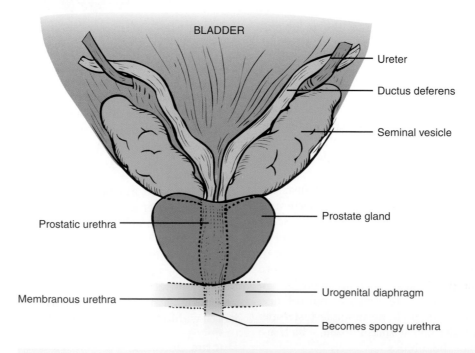

Figure 4-35 Posterior aspect of base of bladder to show relationships of ductus deferens, seminal vesicles, and prostate gland to urethra.

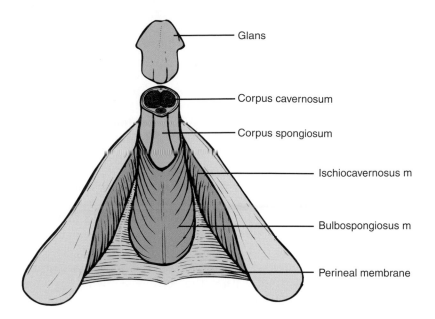

Figure 4-36 Interior view of perineum to show components of penis.

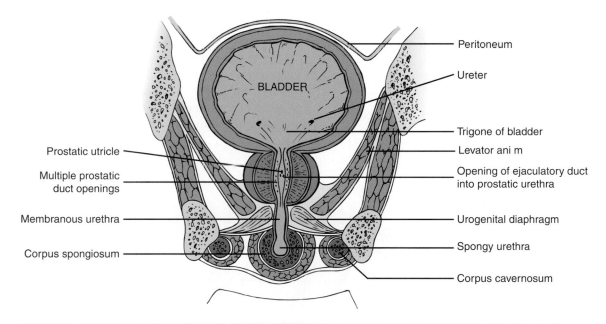

Figure 4-37 Coronal section through male pelvis to show bladder, urethra, and prostate gland.

pubic rami. The crura converge as two cylinders as they pass anteriorly and help form the shaft of the penis.

Corpus Spongiosum. The corpus spongiosum is a third midline cylinder that originates from the perineal membrane as the **bulb of the penis.** The corpus spongiosum passes forward below and between the two corpora cavernosa. Passing into the bulb from above is the **membranous urethra,** which now becomes the **spongy urethra.** The urethra passes longitudinally through the corpus spongiosum to the tip of the penis. The corpus spongiosum itself ends distally as a dilation, or the **glans,** of the penis. The glans is

covered by a fold of skin called the ***prepuce.*** This fold may be removed surgically at birth for ritualistic or hygienic reasons (circumcision).

Muscles. Striated muscle surrounds the erectile tissue of the two crura (**ischiocavernosus muscle**) and the bulb (***bulbospongiosus muscle***). The muscles act to *maintain an erection.* The bulbospongiosus muscle also aids in expelling urine during micturition and semen during ejaculation.

Blood and Nerve Supply. The arterial blood supply is ultimately from the internal iliac artery via the **internal**

pudendal artery. Arising from the internal pudendal artery is the **dorsal artery of the penis** and the **deep artery of the penis.** Both arteries supply the cavernous erectile tissue with blood via tortuous *helicine arteries*.

The erectile tissue of the penis is under autonomic control. In general, parasympathetic fibers from spinal nerves S2 and S3 via the hypogastric plexus cause the helicine arteries to dilate, thus filling the cavernous tissue. Venous outflow is blocked by the action of the dilated arteries pressing on the accompanying veins. Thus the erectile tissue becomes engorged with blood, and erection results.

Ejaculation. When the erect penis is stimulated physically, sympathetic stimulation of the epididymis sets up peristaltic waves to empty sperm into the ductus deferens. The sperm are further propelled up the ductus deferens by peristaltic waves to the prostatic urethra, where secretions are added by the seminal vesicles and the prostate gland to produce semen. The bulbourethral glands add a small amount of fluid to the ejaculate. The seminal fluid is then expelled along the urethra, aided by contractions of the bulbospongiosus muscle.

THE FEMALE GENITAL SYSTEM

The female genital system consists of the ovaries, the uterine tubes, the uterus, the vagina, and external genitalia (*Figure 4-38*).

Ovaries

The ovaries are paired structures that correspond to the testes of the male. They too develop in the fatty extraperitoneal layer adjacent to the developing kidneys and migrate down to the lateral wall of the pelvis. Here each ovary is suspended by a mesentery or mesovarium.

The ovary is not covered by peritoneum as are the other abdominopelvic contents. The outer layer consists of specialized germinal cells overlying an inner core of fibrous stroma. During embryonic development, germinal cells invade the underlying connective tissue. Some of these germinal cells eventually develop into **oögonia**; others form the follicles. After menarche (the first menstrual period), ova are found within the stroma at various levels of maturation. Once a lunar month, every 28 days on average, one ovum ruptures the surface lining and finds itself within the peritoneal cavity. By some unknown mechanism it is drawn to the opening of the uterine tube.

Uterine Tubes

The uterine tubes are bilateral, hollow, muscular tubes about 10 cm long. They extend from the area approximating the ovary laterally to the lumen of the uterus medially. The tubes run along the superior free edge of the broad ligaments of the uterus. The mouth of each tube is the funnel-shaped **infundibulum**, which opens like a trumpet

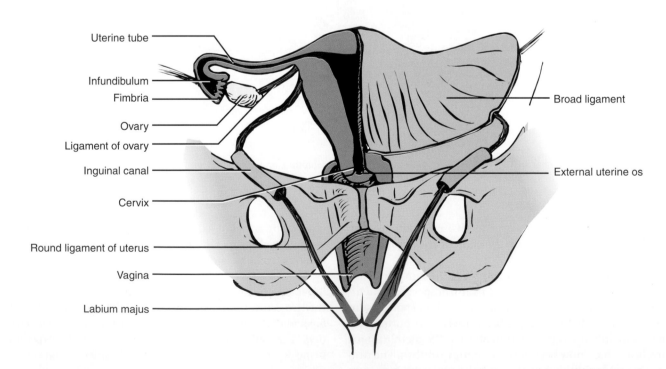

Uterine tube
Infundibulum
Fimbria
Ovary
Ligament of ovary
Inguinal canal
Cervix
Round ligament of uterus
Vagina
Labium majus

Broad ligament
External uterine os

Figure 4-38 Scheme of female genital system. On left side, peritoneum has been stripped away and uterus and vagina sectioned longitudinally to reveal lumina of right uterine tube, uterus, and vagina.

into the peritoneal cavity adjacent to the ovary. Around the opening, or ostium, of each tube are fingerlike projections called *fimbria*. These fimbria help attract and direct the shed ovum into the uterine tube. The uterine tube narrows somewhat proximally as it approaches the uterus. This portion is termed the *isthmus*. The isthmus passes through the wall of the uterus to enter the lumen of the uterus. The tubes are lined with ciliated columnar epithelium, which guides the ovum toward the uterus. If intercourse takes place around the time of ovulation, fertilization may occur. The ovum generally is fertilized within the uterine tube. The fertilized ovum then continues, propelled through the tube by peristaltic action and the waving cilia, toward the cavity of the uterus, where implantation takes place.

Uterus

The uterus is a thick-walled, pear-shaped, muscular, hollow organ within the pelvis. It is about 7 to 8 cm long, 5 cm wide, and 3 cm thick. It is made up of four portions, which are, from superior to inferior, (1) a rounded *fundus*, which protrudes up into the pelvis; (2) a *body*; (3) an *isthmus*; and (4) a narrow *cervix*, or neck.

The uterus lies between the urinary bladder anteriorly and the rectum posteriorly (see *Figure 4-42*). The entire uterus is tilted forward (anteverted). The uterus is also flexed anteriorly at the cervical-isthmus junction (anteflexed).

The cavity of the uterus in nonpregnant women is capillary-thin in an anteroposterior direction, with the anterior and posterior walls almost touching. In the coronal plane the cavity roughly approximates the external configuration. At the upper lateral extremities of the cavity the lumens of the right and left uterine tubes become continuous with the uterine cavity. Inferiorly the cavity narrows at the isthmus and cervix. The internal uterine os connects the isthmus cavity with that of the cervix. The external uterine os connects the cavity of the cervix with that of the vagina below.

Peritoneal Coverings and Supporting Ligaments. The uterus is covered superiorly, anteriorly, and posteriorly by peritoneum. To understand the uterus and its coverings, picture the uterus as a headless person with the arms held out at the sides and the wrists bent backward. The arms represent the uterine tubes, which curve posteriorly to approximate the ovaries. The fingers represent the fimbria. A sheet thrown over our pictured person is the uterine peritoneum. The same sheet drapes over the outstretched arms as a double-layered fold. This fold represents the *broad ligament*, which anchors the uterus to the lateral wall of the pelvic cavity and inferiorly to the pelvic floor. Attached to the posterior aspect of the broad ligament is the round ligament, or *mesovarium*, which supports the

ovary. Attached to the uterus just below the entrance of the uterine tubes is the *round ligament* (a remnant of the prenatal gubernaculum), which runs from the outer body of the uterus down through the broad ligament to the internal inguinal ring. Here it passes through the inguinal canal and ultimately attaches to the inner aspect of the labium majus. The round ligament follows the same course as the spermatic cord in men but lends support to the uterus.

Structure and Function. The walls of the uterus are made up of the same components that basically line hollow viscera: serous coat, smooth muscle, submucosa, and mucosa.

Serous Coat. The serous coat is the peritoneum and its supporting connective tissue base.

Myometrium. The myometrium is the muscular coat; it contains an oblique layer of smooth muscle as well as the longitudinal and circular layers. The smooth muscle contracts and relaxes rhythmically at all times. It contracts more forcibly during menstruation, causing cramps, and during the last stage of pregnancy for eventual expulsion of the baby during the birth process.

Endometrium. The endometrium is a specialized layer of mucous membrane that proliferates to form a thick lining to coincide with ovulation. Once each lunar month, an ovum is shed from the ovary, caught by the fimbria, and propelled through the uterine tube to the cavity of the uterus. If the ovum is fertilized within the uterine tube, the fertilized ovum implants in the prepared endometrium and proceeds to develop a placenta. If fertilization does not take place, all but the basal layer of endometrium is sloughed off and passes out through the vagina, along with the resulting hemorrhage, as menstrual discharge. This event is commonly called a *period*.

After several days, repair to the endometrium is initiated and the endometrium is built up once again in anticipation of the eventuality of receiving a fertilized ovum. On average, the entire cycle takes 28 days, and in the mature woman (after puberty) it takes place more or less on a regular cyclic basis until the onset of menopause.

Vagina

The vagina is a muscular tube about 10 cm long. It leads from the external uterine os of the uterus to the vestibule of the external genitalia. The cervix of the uterus extends downward into the anterior superior aspect of the vagina, creating four reflections, or fornices (anterior, posterior, and bilateral).

Anterior to the vagina is the bladder; the rectum is located posteriorly. Surrounding the vagina are portions of the levator ani muscles. The external vaginal opening is partially obstructed in the virgin woman by a fold of membrane called the *hymen*.

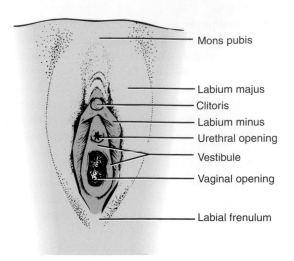

Figure 4-39 Features of external female genitalia.

- Mons pubis
- Labium majus
- Clitoris
- Labium minus
- Urethral opening
- Vestibule
- Vaginal opening
- Labial frenulum

External Genitalia

The vagina and the urethral orifice both open into a common area termed the *vestibule* (*Figure 4-39*). The vestibule is bound on either side by two sets of lips, or labia. Opening into the vestibule are several mucous glands. The greater vestibular (Bartholin's) glands are relatively large mucous glands that open via short ducts into the vestibule.

Labia Minora. Immediately lateral to the vestibule is a pair of thin folds of skin containing no fat. Anteriorly they meet in the midline, and posteriorly they blend with the labia majora to form the *labial frenulum*, or *fourchette.*

Labia Majora. Lateral to the labia minora are two outer lips, each consisting of a layer of skin overlying a ridge of fat. Hair covers the lateral aspects of the labia. Anteriorly the labia majora are continuous with a midline fatty mound covered by skin, the *mons pubis.*

CLINICAL NOTES

Episiotomy
During delivery of an infant, the attending physician often will enlarge the vestibular opening by cutting the fourchette to accommodate the large head of the infant and to prevent tearing of the tissues. The procedure is termed an *episiotomy.*

Clitoris. The clitoris is the homologue of the male penis. However, it is much smaller in size than the penis, and it is not traversed by the urethra as the penis is in men. Instead, the female urethra empties into the vestibule between the clitoris anteriorly and the vagina posteriorly. Anteriorly the labia minora meet at the clitoris and help form a fold of skin, or *prepuce*, over the clitoris. Like the penis, the clitoris contains two corpora cavernosa and a glans (*Figure 4-40*).

Relationships of Pelvic Viscera

Male Pelvis. The relationships of the pelvic viscera are apparent in a median section through the pelvis (*Figure 4-41*). Anteriorly the section is through the pubic symphysis, and immediately posterior is the urinary bladder. In the cadaver the urinary bladder is empty, in a collapsed state, and hardly noticeable. In life, however, as the bladder fills, it bulges upward into the abdominal cavity, lifting its covering of periosteum as it expands.

At the base of the bladder is the prostate gland, wrapped around the prostatic portion of the urethra. Closely applied to the back of the bladder are the seminal vesicles, converging like a V toward the neck of the bladder, where the ductus deferens of each side joins the seminal

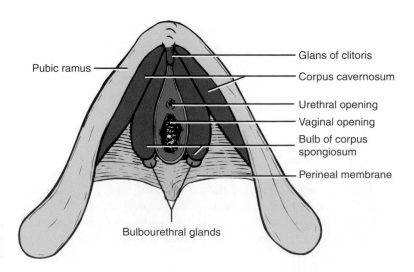

- Glans of clitoris
- Corpus cavernosum
- Urethral opening
- Vaginal opening
- Bulb of corpus spongiosum
- Perineal membrane

Pubic ramus

Bulbourethral glands

Figure 4-40 Components of female external genitalia.

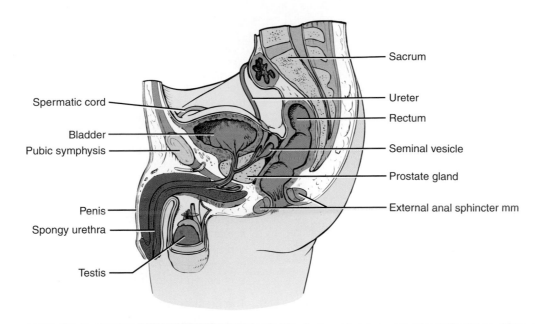

Sacrum

Ureter

Rectum

Seminal vesicle

Prostate gland

External anal sphincter mm

Spermatic cord

Bladder

Pubic symphysis

Penis

Spongy urethra

Testis

Figure 4-41 Median section through a male pelvis to show relationships of pelvic structures.

vesicular ducts to form a right and a left ejaculatory duct, which pierce and enter the prostatic urethra.

Posterior to the bladder and the glands are the rectum and anal canal, through which the prostate gland may be palpated during a physical examination. Posterior to the rectum is the bony sacrum.

Female Pelvis. As in men the urinary bladder in the female pelvis is located immediately behind the pubis (*Figure 4-42*). There is no prostate gland surrounding the exiting urethra. The urethra runs inferiorly, paralleling the anterior wall of the vagina. Both the vagina and urethra open into the common vestibule below.

Extending downward into the vagina superiorly is the uterus, which leans forward over the superior aspect of the urinary bladder. Immediately posterior is the rectum, following the curvature of the bony sacrum behind.

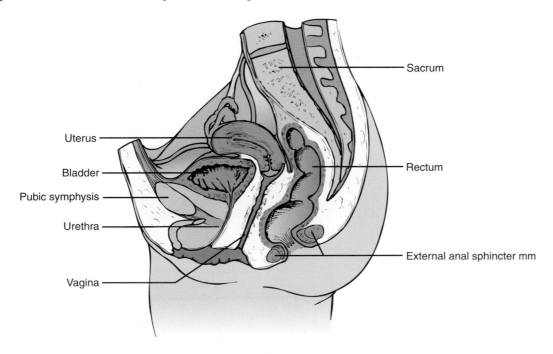

Sacrum

Rectum

External anal sphincter mm

Uterus

Bladder

Pubic symphysis

Urethra

Vagina

Figure 4-42 Median section through a female pelvis to show relationships of pelvic structures.

Review Questions

1. Which of the following statements concerning the anterior abdominal wall is FALSE?
   a. In women the inguinal canal transmits the round ligament of the uterus.
   b. Indirect inguinal hernias pass through the internal inguinal ring and assume spermatic cord coverings.
   c. The linea alba represents the midline union of the right and left abdominal aponeuroses.
   d. The posterior wall (bed) of the rectus sheath ends inferiorly at the arcuate line.
   e. The anterior abdominal muscles contract during forceful inspiration.

2. The superior epigastric artery arises from the _____.
   a. internal thoracic artery
   b. abdominal aorta
   c. external iliac artery
   d. iliohypogastric artery
   e. internal iliac artery

3. Branches of the celiac trunk directly or indirectly supply all the following EXCEPT the _____.
   a. distal end of the esophagus
   b. distal end of the duodenum
   c. spleen
   d. superior aspect of the pancreas
   e. gallbladder

4. Which statement concerning the lesser omentum is TRUE?
   a. The epiploic foramen lies immediately posterior to its free edge.
   b. It joins the porta hepatis of the liver to the greater curvature of the stomach.
   c. It contains the hepatic veins.
   d. It contains the superior mesenteric artery.
   e. It contains the inferior vena cava.

5. The inferior vena cava receives direct tributaries from all of the following EXCEPT the _____.
   a. liver
   b. suprarenal gland
   c. testes
   d. posterior abdominal wall
   e. spleen

6. The sigmoid colon _____.
   a. has a mesentery
   b. is supplied by the superior mesenteric artery
   c. receives its parasympathetic supply from the vagus nerve
   d. begins at the left colic flexure
   e. is a derivative of the midgut

7. The jejunum, in contrast to the ileum, shows all the following features EXCEPT _____.
   a. a thicker muscular layer
   b. more lymphoid tissue
   c. a greater diameter
   d. more plicae circulares
   e. more villi

8. The spleen _____.
   a. is normally palpable below the left costal margin
   b. manufactures erythrocytes during the fetal period
   c. drains its venous return to the inferior vena cava
   d. contacts the head of the pancreas
   e. is essential to life

9. The prostate gland _____.
   a. is approximately the size of a pea
   b. adds a thick yellow secretion to the ejaculate
   c. stores its secretions in the seminal vesicles
   d. may be palpated below the skin just posterior to the scrotum
   e. may obstruct the passage of urine following overgrowth of the middle lobe

Questions 10 through 13

Match each of the following features or descriptions with the appropriate lettered structures found on the illustration of the posterior inferior aspect of the liver.

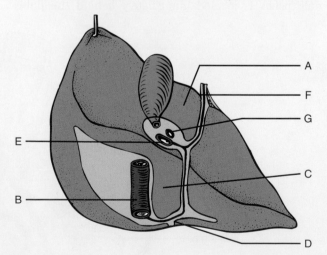

10. _____ caudate lobe

11. _____ a vestige of the umbilical vein

12. _____ a vestige of the ductus venosus

13. _____ the vessel that receives the venous return from the liver

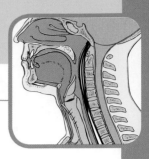

Chapter 5

The Neck

1. Skeleton and Surface Anatomy 133

2. Coverings and Regions 136

3. The Anterior Triangle 140

4. The Posterior Triangle 150

5. The Root 155

6. The Suboccipital Region 159

7. The Prevertebral Region 163

8. Movements of the Neck 164

1. Skeleton and Surface Anatomy

The neck (cervix) is the relatively narrow and flexible portion between the head above and the chest below. It transports a food tube, an air tube, and a neurovascular bundle between these two areas. In addition, the upper limbs originate from the cervical region during their embryological development. Their blood and nerves course through the base of the neck as they pass to and from the upper limb.

THE CERVICAL SKELETON

The skeleton of the neck consists of a vertebral unit and a visceral unit (*Figure 5-1*). In addition, bones of the upper limb girdle, inferior aspect of the skull, and the superior aspect of the thoracic skeleton help provide attachment for muscles of the neck.

Skeleton of the Vertebral Unit

Seven cervical vertebrae compose the vertebral unit of the neck. Descriptions of typical vertebrae C3 to C6 and atypical vertebrae (C1-atlas, C2-axis, and C7) are presented in Chapter 2. The cervical vertebrae should be reviewed at this point.

Skeleton of the Visceral Unit

The skeleton of the visceral unit consists of the hyoid bone, the larynx, and trachea (*Figure 5-2*). These structures are briefly described here; more detailed descriptions are presented subsequently in Chapter 7 in the section dealing with the pharynx and larynx.

Hyoid Bone. The hyoid bone is a floating bone just below the mandible (see *Figure 5-2*). It is a ∪-shaped bone with the prongs, or horns, of the ∪ facing posteriorly. The hyoid bone consists of three parts: (1) a *rectangular body* to which is appended; (2) a pair of *lesser horns*, which project upward and backward; and (3) a pair of *greater horns*, which project posteriorly.

Thyroid Cartilage. Immediately below the hyoid bone is the thyroid cartilage. It consists of two flat plates, or laminae, joined anteriorly. From above, the thyroid cartilage appears ∨-shaped, with the point of the ∨ facing anteriorly and the deficiency posteriorly.

Attached to the posterolateral aspects of the cartilage are two pairs of horns. *Superior horns* project upward; *inferior horns* project downward. The external aspect of the laminae exhibits a ridge called the *oblique line*. The anterior union of the two laminae project forward as the *thyroid prominence*, or the Adam's apple.

Other Bones. Additional bones that belong to other regions are noted here because they provide attachments for various cervical structures. These are the base of the skull and the mandible (see Chapter 6), the scapula and the clavicle of the upper limb girdle (see Chapter 9), and the manubrium of the sternum and the first rib (see Chapter 3).

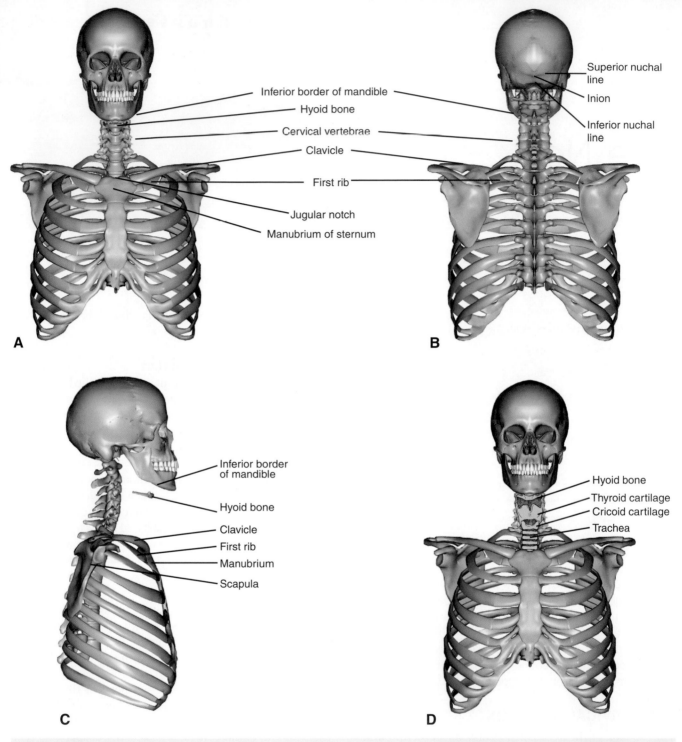

Figure 5-1 Skeleton of cervical region. **A,** anterior view. **B,** posterior view. **C,** right lateral view. **D,** anterior view of larynx and trachea in relation to cervical skeleton.

SURFACE ANATOMY

Posteriorly, the neck is an upward extension of the back, that is, a group of back extensor muscles overlying the cervical vertebrae (see Chapter 2) (*Figure 5-3*).

Anteriorly is a series of important landmarks. Below the chin (*submental*) and below the inferior border of the mandible (*submandibular*) is the soft-tissue, muscular diaphragm that forms the floor of the mouth. This area funnels downward toward a succession of palpable midline landmarks. The lower border of the mandible and chin can be palpated easily. Immediately below the chin is the body of the U-shaped **hyoid bone**. Below the hyoid

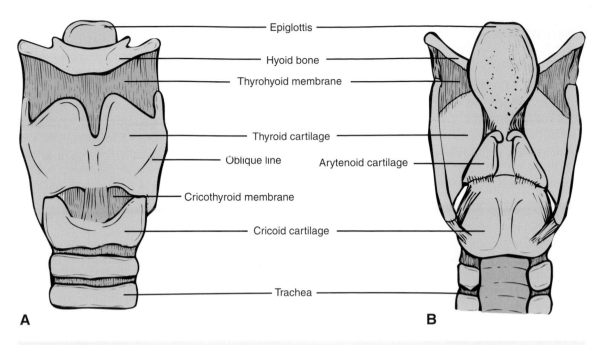

Epiglottis

Hyoid bone

Thyrohyoid membrane

Thyroid cartilage

Oblique line

Arytenoid cartilage

Cricothyroid membrane

Cricoid cartilage

Trachea

A

B

Figure 5-2 Skeleton of larynx. **A,** Frontal view. **B,** Posterior view.

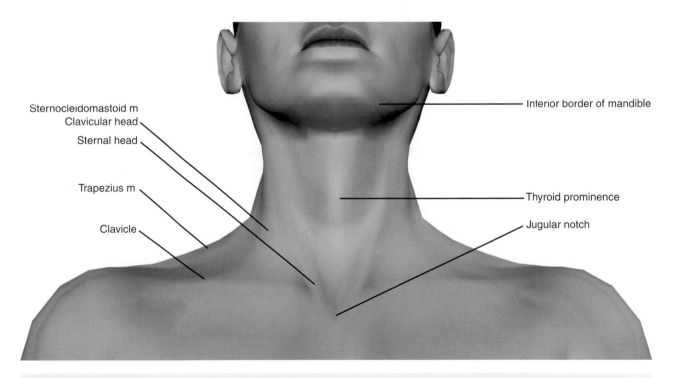

Sternocleidomastoid m
Clavicular head
Sternal head

Trapezius m

Clavicle

Interior border of mandible

Thyroid prominence

Jugular notch

Figure 5-3 Surface features of anterior aspect of the neck.

bone, in descending order, are the **thyrohyoid space,** a dip immediately below the hyoid bone; the **thyroid prominence** (Adam's apple) of the thyroid cartilage; the **cricothyroid space,** an important landmark for performing an emergency cricothyrotomy; the arch of the **cricoid** cartilage; and the trachea, descending from the cricoid cartilage down to where it disappears behind the **jugular notch** of the manubrium. The clavicles extend laterally on either side of the manubrium of the sternum to form the anterior aspect of the base of the neck.

2. Coverings and Regions

FASCIAL COVERINGS

Immediately deep to the skin of the neck is a layer of **superficial fascia**. Deeper still is an intricate covering of **deep cervical fascia**. These fasciae compartmentalize the structures of the neck (*Figure 5-4*). Between the various compartments are spaces occupied by loose areolar tissue. These fascial compartments are potential routes through which infection can spread from one site to another.

Superficial Fascia and Platysma Muscle

The superficial fascia is a subcutaneous layer that contains a variable amount of *fat, superficial lymph nodes, cutaneous nerves* and *vessels* that supply the overlying skin, and a thin muscle (the *platysma*).

Platysma muscle is a thin, wide sheet of muscle that covers the anterior and lateral aspects of the neck (*Figure 5-5*). It is a superficial muscle related to the superficial muscles of facial expression, and therefore it lies within the superficial fascia of the neck. It originates from *pectoral fascia* below the clavicle and sweeps upward to the *inferior border of the mandible*. The more lateral fibers continue superiorly and medially to blend into the *risorius muscle*, which inserts into the angle of the mouth. The medial fibers decussate as they approach and insert into the inferior border of the mandible.

The platysma acts to *tense the skin* of the neck if the mandible is stabilized by the muscles of mastication. The platysma also purportedly helps *depress the mandible*. Its motor supply is from cervical branches of the facial nerve (cranial nerve VII), the cranial nerve that also supplies the muscles of facial expression.

Deep Cervical Fascia

Deep Investing Fascia. Below the superficial fascial layer is a thin sheet of deep cervical fascia that wraps around the entire circumference of the neck—like a collar. This fibrous collar has superior attachments to the skull and inferior attachments to the sternum and pectoral girdle. As it encircles the neck, it splits to pass around and form the sheath of two large muscles, the *sternocleidomastoid* and the *trapezius*. The detailed attachments are rather complicated and are presented for reference purposes.*

Visceral (Pretracheal) Fascia

Contents. The visceral fascia lies deep to the deep investing fascia and forms a sheath around the **visceral unit of the neck.** Contained within the visceral unit are the **pharynx,** which continues below vertebral level C6 as the **esophagus;** the **larynx,** which continues below vertebral level C6 as the **trachea;** and the **thyroid gland,** which is found lateral to the trachea and larynx as two lateral lobes joined by an *isthmus* across the midline. Visceral fascia that surrounds the pharynx is called *buccopharyngeal fascia;* the visceral fascia surrounding the trachea and esophagus is referred to as the *pretracheal fascia,* despite the fact that it surrounds the visceral unit.

Attachments. The visceral fascia arises superiorly from the hyoid bone and from a shared attachment with the pharynx to the base of the skull. Inferiorly the visceral fascia extends into the superior mediastinum of the thorax to blend in with the pericardium of the heart.

Prevertebral Fascia

Contents. The prevertebral fascia surrounds the **cervical vertebral unit.** The vertebral unit includes the following components: the **seven cervical vertebrae**, the **cervical portion of the spinal cord** and **eight pairs of spinal nerves (C1 to C8)**, **anterior vertebral muscles** that *flex* the neck, and posterior vertebral muscles that extend the neck. The prevertebral fascia extends laterally on either side to surround the brachial plexus and subclavian vessels as they pass from the neck to the axilla. This covering is called the *axillary sheath.*

Attachments. Superiorly the prevertebral fascia extends from the base of the skull, forming a sheath around the vertebral column and its musculature as they descend through the neck. Inferiorly the posterior portion of the sheath blends with the investing fascia of the musculature of the back, and the anterior portion blends with the anterior longitudinal ligament of the thoracic vertebrae.

Alar Fascia. The alar fascia is formed by a division of the anterior component of the prevertebral fascia to form two potential spaces between the posterior vertebral unit and the anterior visceral unit. The alar fascia binds to the transverse processes on either side to limit the space laterally.

---

* **Superiorly** the fascia attaches to the inferior border of the mandible, inferior border of the body of the hyoid bone, angle of the mandible, the inferior border of the zygomatic arch, and the mastoid and styloid processes. Because the fascia splits to enclose the sternocleidomastoid and trapezius muscles, it shares their attachment to the mastoid process, superior nuchal line, and external occipital protuberance of the skull. At the inferior aspect of the skull, the deep investing fascia also splits to pass around and help form the fibrous capsules of the parotid and submandibular glands.

Inferiorly the deep investing fascia attaches to the manubrium of the sternum, clavicles, and spines of the scapula along with the

sternocleidomastoid and trapezius muscles, which it ensheathes. As it descends to the manubrium, it divides into two sheets: an anterior one attaching to the anterosuperior aspect of the manubrium and a posterior one attaching to the posterosuperior aspect of the manubrium. This creates a space, the **suprasternal space (of Burns)**, that contains some areolar tissue, fat, and lymph nodes. It also contains some portions of the inferior thyroid veins and the anterior jugular venous arch.

Posteriorly the deep investing fascia gains attachment to the ligamentum nuchae, a membranous extension of the cervical spines.

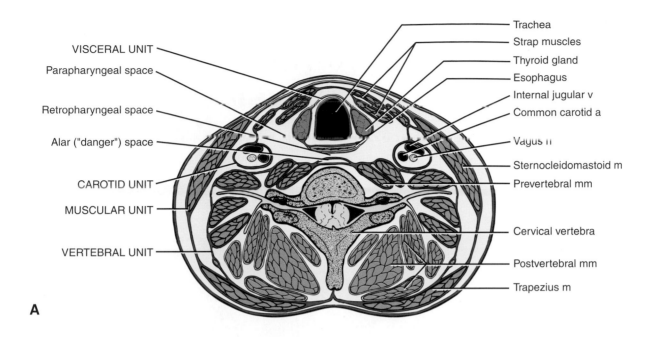

VISCERAL UNIT

Parapharyngeal space

Retropharyngeal space

Alar ("danger") space

CAROTID UNIT

MUSCULAR UNIT

VERTEBRAL UNIT

Trachea
Strap muscles
Thyroid gland
Esophagus
Internal jugular v
Common carotid a
Vagus n
Sternocleidomastoid m
Prevertebral mm

Cervical vertebra

Postvertebral mm

Trapezius m

A

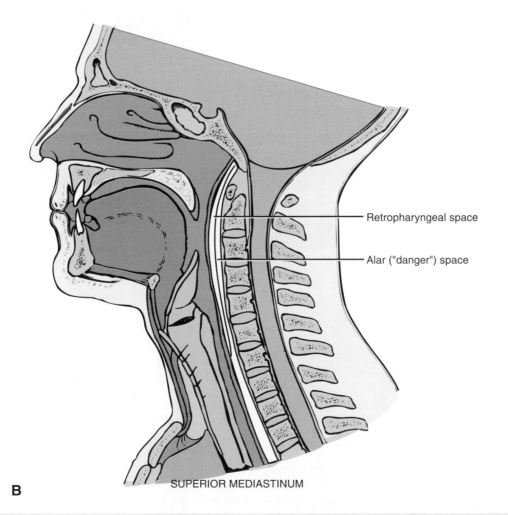

Retropharyngeal space

Alar ("danger") space

B   SUPERIOR MEDIASTINUM

Figure 5-4 Fascia of neck. **A,** Cross section to demonstrate fascial compartments of neck. **B,** Sagittal section to show continuity of cervical fascia and fascial spaces with mediastinum.

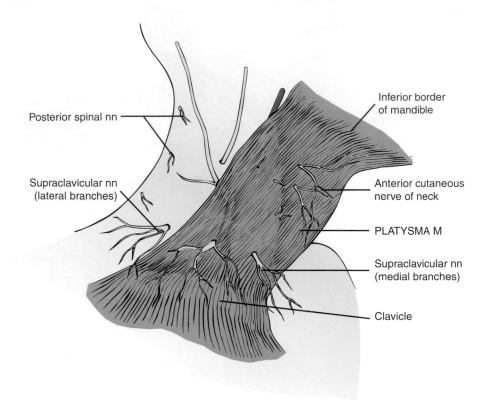

Posterior spinal nn

Supraclavicular nn
(lateral branches)

Inferior border
of mandible

Anterior cutaneous
nerve of neck

PLATYSMA M

Supraclavicular nn
(medial branches)

Clavicle

Figure 5-5 Platysma muscle.

Carotid Sheaths
Contents. Lateral to the visceral unit are bilateral tubes of fascia extending from the base of the skull to the thoracic inlet. Contained within the carotid sheaths are the **common carotid artery,** the **internal jugular vein,** and the vagus nerve (**cranial nerve X**).

Attachments. Superiorly the carotid sheath attaches to the base of the skull around the carotid canal, which transmits the internal carotid artery, and the jugular foramen, which transmits the internal jugular vein and the vagus nerve. The carotid sheath blends anteriorly with the visceral fascia and posteriorly with the prevertebral fascia as it descends in the neck; its inferior limits are the visceral and prevertebral fascia.

Potential Fascial Spaces

Loose areolar connective tissue fills the spaces between the various layers of deep cervical fascia. They are potential spaces and become actual spaces only when invaded and displaced by infective material (pus) or occasionally by air (surgical emphysema). There are two important fascial spaces to consider.

Retropharyngeal Space. The retropharyngeal space is a potential space between the visceral unit anteriorly and the vertebral unit posteriorly. It extends from the base of the skull down to the superior mediastinum. It is packed with loose connective tissue that allows a degree of up-and-down movement between the visceral and vertebral units during swallowing.

Alar Space. The alar space is a subdivision of the retropharyngeal space created by the alar fascia previously

---

CLINICAL NOTES

Mediastinitis

Massive infections of dental origin can break through into the retropharyngeal and alar spaces and track down to the mediastinum below, resulting in infection and inflammation of the mediastinum (mediastinitis). A more detailed description of the spread of dental infection is presented in Figure 11-32.

Surgical Emphysema

Emphysema is a pathological condition in which air or gas is abnormally present within or between tissues. Inappropriate oral surgery procedures can introduce air under pressure into the fascial issue planes. If it occurs near the surface, a characteristic "crackling" is produced on palpation. If the air is forced into the retropharyngeal or alar fascial space, it can rapidly track to the mediastinum. This condition is described in Figure 11-32.

described. It also extends from the base of the skull above to the superior mediastinum below, and it has been dubbed by some as the *danger space*.

REGIONS

To facilitate the study of a seemingly complicated area, the neck is divided into two major areas, or triangles, by the **sternocleidomastoid muscle** (*Figure 5-6*). The area anterior to this muscle and below the inferior border of the mandible is the *anterior triangle of the neck*. The area posterior to the sternocleidomastoid muscle is the *posterior triangle of the neck*, which is limited posteriorly by a second large muscle, the **trapezius.**

The sternocleidomastoid and trapezius muscles developed from a single muscular sheet during prenatal development and therefore share the same nerve supply. During

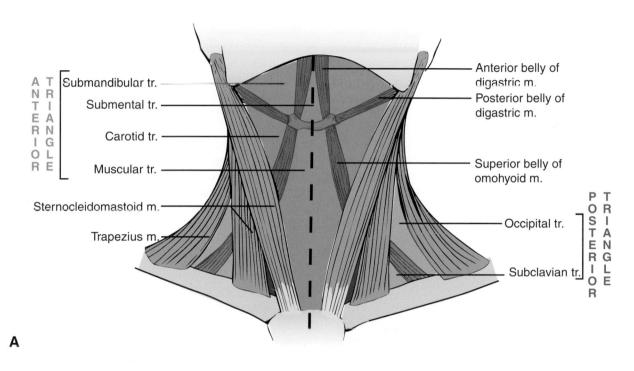

A

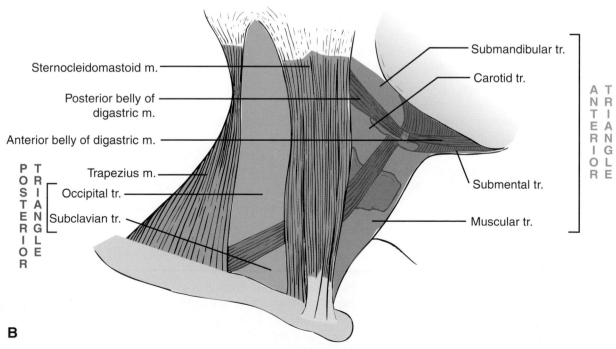

B

Figure 5-6 Key muscles of neck that delineate anterior and posterior triangles. **A,** Anterior view. **B,** Right lateral view.

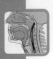

development a cleft develops between them, and they separate to form the borders of the posterior triangle of the neck.

Sternocleidomastoid Muscle

Origins. The sternocleidomastoid muscle arises as two heads from the manubrium of the sternum (sterno portion) and the superior aspect of the medial third of the clavicle (cleido portion).

Insertions. The two heads blend as they pass obliquely upward and backward to insert into the mastoid process of the skull and the lateral half of the superior nuchal line of the skull.

Actions. The sternocleidomastoid muscles, acting bilaterally, flex the neck. Singly they act to flex the head laterally and rotate the head to the opposite side. During forced inspiration the sternocleidomastoid muscles pull upward on the sternum to further increase the intrathoracic volume.

Nerve Supply. The nerve supply to the sternocleidomastoid muscle is primarily from the **spinal accessory nerve** (**cranial nerve XI**). In addition, motor and proprioceptive fibers arise from anterior rami (AR) of spinal nerves C2 and C3.

CLINICAL NOTES

Torticollis (Wry Neck)

The term *torticollis* literally means a twisted neck. **Spasmodic torticollis** occurs in adults and is characterized by unilateral spasms of the sternocleidomastoid and trapezius muscles and possibly the deeper muscles of the neck.

Congenital torticollis results from damage to the sternocleidomastoid muscle following a difficult delivery. Damaged muscle fibers and a hematoma (localized hemorrhage producing a swelling) develop into scar tissue that causes spasm. The neck is pulled to the ipsilateral side, and the face is turned to the contralateral side.

Trapezius Muscle

The trapezius muscle is expansive and covers a number of regions. It is a superficial muscle of the back, a muscle of the upper limb girdle, and a cervical muscle (see *Figure 2-14*).

Origins. The trapezius muscle arises from the external occipital protuberance, the medial half of the supe-

rior nuchal line, the ligamentum nuchae, and the lower cervical and all the thoracic spines.

Insertions. The fibers originating from the head insert into the lateral third of the clavicle, and the remaining fibers insert into the acromion and spine of the scapula.

Actions. The trapezius muscle contracts to elevate and rotate the scapula. Its cervical portion, acting bilaterally, can extend the head. Singly it can rotate the head and face to the opposite side.

Nerve Supply. The motor nerve supply is primarily from branches of the **spinal accessory nerve** (**cranial nerve XI**). In addition, it receives motor and proprioceptive branches from AR of spinal nerves C3 and C4.

Triangles

The sternocleidomastoid and trapezius muscles divide the neck into two major areas, or triangles. Other key muscles further subdivide these triangles into smaller component triangles: (1) the **anterior triangle** of the neck and its component muscular, carotid, submandibular, and submental triangles and (2) the **posterior triangle** of the neck and its component occipital and subclavian triangles.

3. The Anterior Triangle

The anterior triangle occupies the anterior portion of the neck as an inverted triangle, its base consisting of the inferior border of the mandible and its apex directed downward toward the manubrium of the sternum (*Figure 5-7*). Like the posterior triangle the anterior triangle has depth and should be considered a region. Therefore, in addition to three boundaries, it has a roof, a floor, and several contents.

BOUNDARIES

The **anterior boundary** is the midline of the neck (i.e., straight line running from the base of the chin above to the jugular notch of the sternum below). The **posterior boundary** is formed by the anterior border of the sternocleidomastoid muscle. The **superior border** is the bony inferior border of the mandible. For ease of description the anterior triangle of the neck is further divided into smaller component triangles (see *Figure 5-6*).

Muscular Triangle

The muscular triangle occupies the anterior aspect of the neck below the hyoid bone. It is bounded by the superior belly of the omohyoid muscle, the sternocleidomastoid muscle, and the midline of the neck. It contains the infrahyoid strap muscles of the neck.

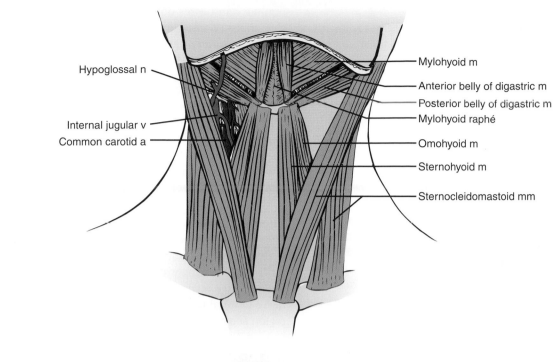

Hypoglossal n

Internal jugular v

Common carotid a

Mylohyoid m

Anterior belly of digastric m

Posterior belly of digastric m

Mylohyoid raphé

Omohyoid m

Sternohyoid m

Sternocleidomastoid mm

A

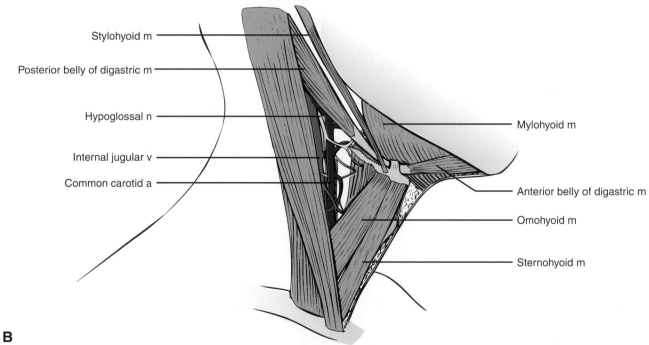

Stylohyoid m

Posterior belly of digastric m

Hypoglossal n

Internal jugular v

Common carotid a

Mylohyoid m

Anterior belly of digastric m

Omohyoid m

Sternohyoid m

B

Figure 5-7 Anterior triangle of neck and its contents. **A,** Anterior view. **B,** Right lateral view.

Carotid Triangle

The carotid triangle is bounded by the superior belly of the omohyoid muscle, the posterior belly of the digastric muscle, and the sternocleidomastoid muscle. It contains the common carotid artery and its branches; the internal jugular vein and its tributaries; cranial nerves X, XI, and XII; and several branches of the cervical plexus.

Submandibular Triangle

The boundaries of the submandibular triangle are the inferior border of the mandible and the upper borders of the posterior and anterior bellies of the digastric muscle. This region contains the submandibular gland, submandibular lymph nodes, the lingual and facial arteries, cranial nerve XII, and the nerve to the mylohyoid muscle.

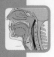

Submental Triangle

As the name implies, the submental triangle is below the chin (mens) and is bounded by the right and left anterior bellies of the digastric muscle and the body of the hyoid bone. The submental triangle is a midline structure. The other triangles are bilateral.

ROOF

The posterior triangle and anterior triangle are covered by skin, superficial fascia containing platysma muscle, and deep investing fascia of the neck.

Superficial Veins

The detailed venous drainage of the face is described with the study of the face in Chapter 7. To summarize, the anterior portion of the face is drained by the **facial vein,** and the posterior portion of the face is drained by the **retromandibular vein.** Both veins leave the face and drain inferiorly to the neck. The retromandibular vein at the angle of the jaw divides into anterior and posterior divisions (Figure 5-8).

The **anterior division of the retromandibular vein** unites with the facial vein to form the **common facial vein,** which drains to the internal jugular vein below the sternocleidomastoid muscle.

The **posterior division of the retromandibular vein** unites with the **posterior auricular vein** to form the **external jugular vein** just below the lobe of the ear. The external

jugular vein passes obliquely downward over the sternocleidomastoid muscle to enter the posterior triangle.

The **anterior jugular vein** originates in the submental region, drains the anterior aspect of the neck, and descends on either side of the midline to a point just above the jugular notch of the manubrium. Here it dives deep to the origin of the sternocleidomastoid muscle, emerging in the posterior triangle, where it empties to the external jugular vein. A **communicating vein** joins the common facial vein above to the anterior jugular vein below. The right and left anterior jugular veins occasionally may be joined across the midline by the **anterior jugular arch.**

Superficial Nerves

The **transverse cervical nerve** of the neck originates in the posterior triangle and passes across the sternocleidomastoid muscle to supply skin overlying the anterior triangle of the neck (see *Figure 5-5*). The **cervical branch of the facial nerve (cranial nerve VII)** passes inferiorly from the parotid region above to supply the platysma muscle.

FLOOR

The floor of the anterior triangle of the neck is formed by the pharynx, the larynx, and the thyroid gland. These structures are posteroinferior extensions and relations of the oral and nasal cavities and are therefore described in Chapter 7.

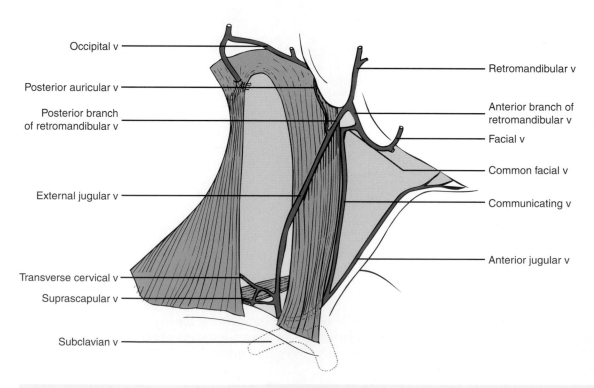

Occipital v

Posterior auricular v

Posterior branch of retromandibular v

External jugular v

Transverse cervical v

Suprascapular v

Subclavian v

Retromandibular v

Anterior branch of retromandibular v

Facial v

Common facial v

Communicating v

Anterior jugular v

Figure 5-8 Superficial venous drainage of neck.

CONTENTS

The anterior triangle of the neck contains a number of muscles, arteries, veins, and nerves.

Muscles

The muscles of the anterior triangle are grouped according to position and function (see *Figures 5-7, 5-9,* and *Table 5-1*). **Suprahyoid muscles** originate above the hyoid bone: **infrahyoid muscles** originate below the hyoid bone. Both sets of muscles insert directly or indirectly into the hyoid bone.

Infrahyoid Muscles. Four infrahyoid straplike muscles are present on either side of the neck: two superficial muscles (omohyoid and sternohyoid muscles) and two deeper muscles (sternothyroid and thyrohyoid muscles).

Omohyoid Muscle. The omohyoid muscle consists of a superior and an inferior belly. The **inferior belly of the omohyoid muscle** is actually an upper limb girdle muscle and originates from the superior border of the scapula. It runs anteriorly and medially across the posterior triangle of the neck and narrows down to an intermediate tendon. The tendon passes through a sling of fascia attached to the clavicle that deflects the muscle upward and medially as the **superior belly of the omohyoid muscle**. The superior belly passes deep to the sternocleidomastoid muscle, emerges into the anterior triangle, and inserts into the body of the hyoid bone.

Sternohyoid Muscle. The sternohyoid muscle arises from the posterior aspect of the manubrium of the sternum and the head of the clavicle. The fibers pass upward, over the anterior aspect of the trachea and larynx, and insert into the body of the hyoid bone above.

Sternothyroid Muscle. The sternothyroid muscle runs deep to the sternohyoid muscle, originating from the posterior aspect of the manubrium of the sternum and inserting above into the oblique line of the thyroid cartilage.

Thyrohyoid Muscle. The thyrohyoid muscle originates from the oblique line of the thyroid cartilage and passes upward to insert into the body of the hyoid bone.

Functions. The infrahyoid and suprahyoid muscles always contract bilaterally, never singly, unless a motor nerve lesion renders a muscle of one side paralyzed. The infrahyoid muscles act to depress the hyoid bone and the larynx, as occurs during swallowing. They also aid indirectly in depressing the mandible.

Nerve Supply. All of the infrahyoid muscles are supplied by AR of spinal nerves C1, C2, and C3 via the **cervical plexus** and **ansa cervicalis** (see *Figure 5-12*). The cervical plexus is described as one of the nerve contents of the anterior triangle.

Suprahyoid Muscles. Five pairs of muscles originate above the hyoid bone and insert into the hyoid bone below (see *Figure 5-7*).

Posterior Belly of the Digastric Muscle. The posterior belly of the digastric muscle originates from the base of the skull, specifically from the *digastric notch* deep to the mastoid process. Its fleshy belly converges as an intermediate tendon as it travels down toward the greater horn of the hyoid bone. It is not a fixed insertion but rather passes through a tunnel of fascia and then shares this tendon with another muscle, the anterior belly of the digastric muscle.

Anterior Belly of the Digastric Muscle. The anterior belly originates as the same intermediate tendon. It passes

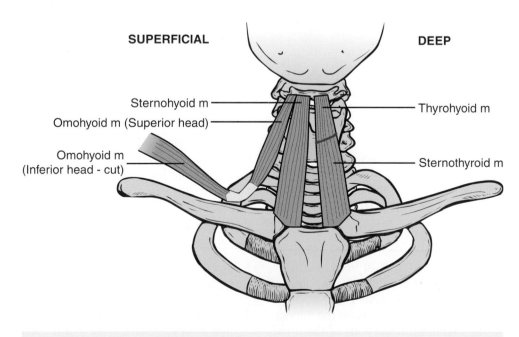

Figure 5-9 Infrahyoid (strap) muscles of neck.

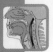

TABLE 5-1

Muscles of the Anterior Triangle*

Muscle	Origin	Insertion	Action	Nerve
Infrahyoid				
Omohyoid	Inferior belly: superior border of scapula	Inferior belly: intermediate tendon	Depresses hyoid bone and larynx	Ansa cervicalis (AR of C1, C2, C3)
	Superior belly: intermediate tendon	Superior belly: body of hyoid bone, lower border		
Sternohyoid	Manubrium of sternum, posterior aspect	Body of hyoid bone, lower border	Depresses hyoid bone and larynx	Ansa cervicalis (AR of C1, C2, C3)
Sternothyroid	Manubrium of sternum, posterior aspect	Oblique line of thyroid cartilage	Depresses larynx	Ansa cervicalis (AR of C1, C2, C3)
Thyrohyoid	Oblique line of thyroid cartilage	Body and greater horn of hyoid bone, lower border	Depresses hyoid bone	Thyrohyoid branch of hypoglossal nerve (hitchhiking branches of AR of C1)
Suprahyoid				
Digastric (posterior belly)	Digastric notch of temporal bone at base of skull	Intermediate tendon, which passes through sling of fascia on greater horn of hyoid bone	Raises hyoid bone	Facial nerve (cranial nerve VII)
Digastric (anterior belly)	Intermediate tendon	Digastric fossa of mandible	Elevates hyoid bone	Nerve to mylohyoid (cranial nerve V3)
Mylohyoid	Mylohyoid line on medial aspect of mandibular body	Median raphé and body of hyoid bone	Elevates hyoid bone, base of tongue, and floor of mouth	Nerve to mylohyoid (cranial nerve V3)
Geniohyoid	Inferior genial tubercle of mandible	Body of hyoid bone	Elevates hyoid bone, protracts hyoid bone	AR of C1
Stylohyoid	Styloid process	Greater horn of hyoid bone	Elevates hyoid bone	Facial nerve (cranial nerve VII)

AR, Anterior rami of spinal nerves.

*See Table 5-2 for discussion of the platysma and sternocleidomastoid muscles.

upward and forward as a second fleshy belly, inserting into the digastric fossa of the mandible (a small depression on the inner aspect of the inferior border just off the midline).

Mylohyoid Muscle. The mylohyoid muscle is a broad, flat muscle that originates from the mylohyoid ridge on the medial aspect of the mandible. The fibers pass downward and medially to insert into a midline raphé anteriorly and the body of the hyoid bone posteriorly. The midline raphé is formed by the common attachment, or interdigitation, of fibers of the right and left mylohyoid muscles.

Geniohyoid Muscle. Although a true suprahyoid muscle, the geniohyoid is not fully described here. Rather, it is included as a structure considered with the floor of the mouth described in Chapter 7. The geniohyoid is found deep to the mylohyoid muscle, running from the inferior genial tubercles of the mandible to the body of the hyoid bone.

Stylohyoid Muscle. The stylohyoid muscle originates from the styloid process of the temporal bone and passes downward and forward to insert on the greater horn of the hyoid bone. Its tendinous insertion splits to pass around the intermediate tendon of the digastric muscles.

Functions. Upon contraction the suprahyoid muscles raise the hyoid bone and larynx when the mandible is stabilized. They can also act, along with the infrahyoid muscles, to help depress the mandible.

Nerve Supply. Unfortunately the nerve supply to the suprahyoid muscles is not uniform.

1. The *posterior belly of the digastric muscle* is supplied by **cervical branches of the facial nerve (cranial nerve VII).**
2. The *anterior belly of the digastric muscle* receives its motor supply from a branch of the **third division of the trigeminal nerve** (i.e., the **nerve to mylohyoid**).

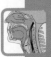

3. The *mylohyoid muscle* receives motor fibers from the **nerve to mylohyoid**, a branch of the **third division of the trigeminal nerve**.
4. The *geniohyoid muscle* receives its motor supply from the **cervical plexus** (i.e., a branch of the **AR of spinal nerve C1**), which travels along with the hypoglossal nerve.
5. The *stylohyoid muscle*, like the posterior belly of digastric muscle, is supplied by **cervical branches of the facial nerve** (cranial nerve VII).

Arteries

The arteries of the anterior triangle are all derived from the common carotid artery (*Figure 5-10*).

Common Carotid Artery. The common carotid artery originates in the superior mediastinum of the thorax. The right common carotid artery arises from the brachiocephalic artery; the left common carotid artery arises directly from the arch of the aorta.

The common carotid artery passes upward through the thoracic inlet to enter and ascend through the neck within the carotid sheath. It gives off no branches as it ascends above the omohyoid muscle to the anterior triangle of the neck. As the artery approaches the level of the hyoid bone, it dilates slightly as the **carotid sinus**. Within the walls of the sinus are *baroreceptors* (*baro*, meaning "pressure", as in *barometer*), proprioceptive nerve endings of the glossopharyngeal and vagus nerves that measure changes in blood pressure. This feedback information helps regulate blood pressure. Posterior to the carotid sinus is the **carotid body**, a small structure containing *chemoreceptors*, proprioceptive endings of the glossopharyngeal and vagus nerves that measure blood gases, carbon dioxide excess, and reduced oxygen tension in the arterial blood. This feedback information helps regulate heart rate and respiration.

At the level of the hyoid bone the common carotid artery divides into terminal branches: the **internal carotid** and the **external carotid arteries**.

Internal Carotid Artery. The internal carotid artery leaves the anterior triangle superiorly and continues upward to the *carotid canal* at the base of the skull. It gives off no branches as it ascends to enter the skull.

CLINICAL NOTES

Carotid Pulse

The **carotid pulse** is readily felt on the side of the neck in the interval between the superior border of the thyroid cartilage and the anterior border of the sternocleidomastoid muscle. It is the preferred site for detecting a pulse in cardiopulmonary resuscitation (CPR).

External Carotid Artery. The external carotid artery remains external and travels upward to the face via the parotid region. At its origin it immediately gives off the

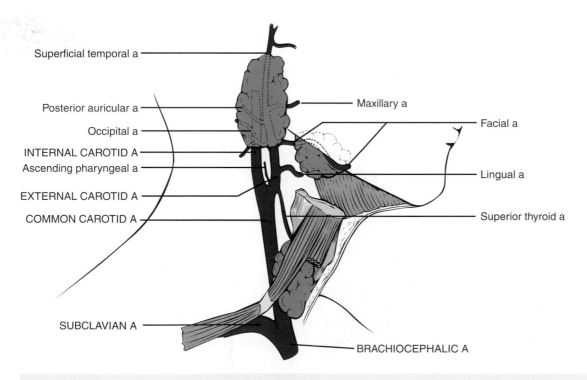

Figure 5-10 Common carotid artery and branches.

Superficial temporal a
Posterior auricular a
Occipital a
INTERNAL CAROTID A
Ascending pharyngeal a
EXTERNAL CAROTID A
COMMON CAROTID A
SUBCLAVIAN A
Maxillary a
Facial a
Lingual a
Superior thyroid a
BRACHIOCEPHALIC A

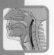

first of six collateral branches, which at least originate within the confines of the anterior triangle.

Superior Thyroid Artery. The superior thyroid artery loops downward and medially deep to the infrahyoid muscles to enter and supply the superior portion of the thyroid gland. On the way it gives off two branches: a *superior laryngeal branch*, which passes between the hyoid and thyroid cartilage to supply the larynx within, and a *sternocleidomastoid branch*, which supplies a portion of that muscle.

Lingual Artery. The lingual artery passes deep to the posterior belly of the digastric muscle, runs anteriorly through the submandibular region deep to the hyoglossus muscle, and then supplies the tongue.

Facial Artery. The facial artery runs anteriorly under the posterior belly of the digastric muscle to enter the submandibular region. It is pushed up into the interval between the medial aspect of the body of the mandible and the external surface of the mylohyoid muscle by the submandibular gland. The facial artery then takes a lateral course, curls over the inferior border of the mandible, and ascends to supply the anterior portion of the face.

Ascending Pharyngeal Artery. The ascending pharyngeal artery arises from the medial aspect of the external carotid artery; travels upward to the base of the skull; and along the way supplies the pharynx, soft palate, and auditory tube.

Occipital Artery. The occipital artery passes posteriorly deep to the posterior belly of the digastric muscle and then deep to the mastoid process of the skull. It sends a muscular branch to the sternocleidomastoid muscle and then ascends in the occipital area to supply the occipital portion of the scalp.

Posterior Auricular Artery. The posterior auricular artery arises to supply the skin overlying the mastoid process and scalp behind the ear.

Terminal Branches. The external carotid artery ends within the parotid region as *two terminal branches*: (1) the **superficial temporal artery,** which ascends to the scalp anterior to the ear, and (2) the **maxillary artery,** which passes deep to the neck of the condyle to enter the infratemporal region of the face. These two terminal branches are discussed with the parotid and infratemporal regions in Chapter 7.

Veins

All the veins of the anterior triangle, except the anterior jugular vein, drain to the internal jugular vein (*Figures 5-8* and *5-11*).

The **internal jugular vein** emerges from the jugular foramen at the base of the skull. It descends through the neck along with the vagus nerve and the internal carotid artery, within the carotid sheath. As the internal jugular vein descends, it picks up the following tributaries:

1. **Veins of the pharyngeal plexus** return venous blood from the pharynx and drain into the internal jugular vein near the angle of the jaw.
2. The **facial vein,** draining the anterior aspect of the face, unites with the anterior branch of the retromandibular vein to form the **common facial vein.** The common

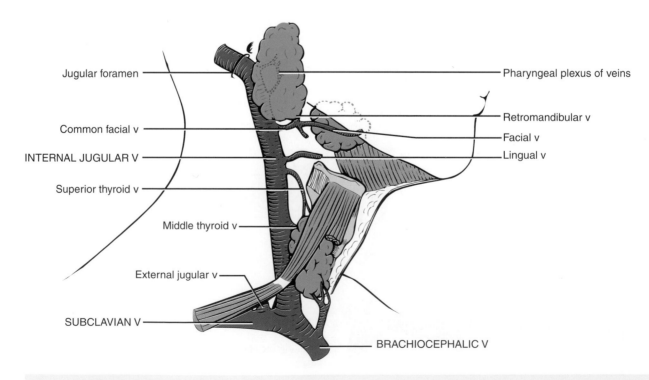

Figure 5-11 Internal jugular vein and tributaries.

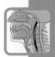

facial vein drains to the internal jugular vein above the hyoid bone.

3. The **lingual vein** drains the tongue and floor of the mouth and enters the internal jugular vein just below the common facial vein.

4. The **superior thyroid vein** drains the thyroid gland and part of the larynx and drains to the internal jugular vein at the level of the hyoid bone.

5. The **middle thyroid vein** drains the thyroid gland and drains to the internal jugular vein at the level of the cricoid cartilage. There is no equivalent middle thyroid artery.

The internal jugular vein then passes deep to the sterno-cleidomastoid muscle and leaves the anterior triangle to enter the root of the neck. Here it joins the **subclavian vein**, forming the **brachiocephalic vein**. The right and left brachiocephalic veins join in the superior mediastinum to form the **superior vena cava** (see Chapter 3, pages 82 and 83).

Nerves

Three cranial nerves and one nerve plexus are found within the anterior triangle of the neck (see *Figures 5-12* and *5-13*).

Accessory Nerve. The accessory nerve (cranial nerve XI) emerges from the **jugular foramen** at the base of the skull, crosses the internal jugular vein within the anterior triangle, and then leaves the area by piercing the upper portion of the sternocleidomastoid muscle and supplying it. The

accessory nerve then travels across the posterior triangle toward the trapezius muscle, which it enters and supplies (see "Posterior Triangle" in the following section).

Hypoglossal Nerve. The hypoglossal nerve (cranial nerve XII) emerges from the **hypoglossal (anterior condylar) canal** at the base of the skull and descends externally to the carotid sheath. It passes deep to the posterior belly of the digastric muscle to enter the anterior triangle. It loops anteriorly under the digastric tendon to enter the submandibular portion of the anterior triangle. Here it disappears between the mylohyoid muscle and the hyoglossus muscle to supply the muscles of the tongue (see Chapter 7).

Cervical Plexus. The AR of spinal nerves C1 to C4 combine to form the cervical plexus. In general, posterior branches of the plexus pass to the posterior triangle and emerge as the **lesser occipital nerve**, the **great auricular nerve**, the **anterior cutaneous nerve of the neck**, and the **supraclavicular nerves**. Several **small motor branches** (not illustrated) arise to supply the levator scapulae, and the scalene muscles of the posterior triangle. In addition, branches of C3 and C4 of the cervical plexus unite with C5 of the brachial plexus to form the **phrenic nerve**. *Anterior branches* of the cervical plexus pass forward to form a superior and inferior root that unite as a loop in the neck or **ansa cervicalis**.

Superior Root. The AR of spinal nerve C1 passes forward to hitchhike with the hypoglossal nerve (cranial nerve XII). As the hypoglossal nerve curves anteriorly toward the

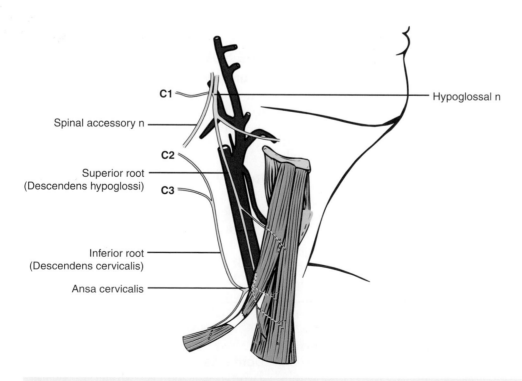

C1

Spinal accessory n

C2

Superior root
(Descendens hypoglossi)
C3

Inferior root
(Descendens cervicalis)

Ansa cervicalis

Hypoglossal n

Figure 5-12 Nerves of anterior triangle (accessory and hypoglossal nerves and cervical plexus).

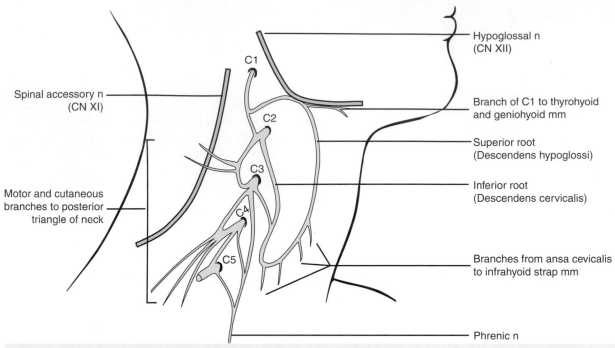

Figure 5-13 Cervical plexus and branches. (NOTE: C5 belongs to brachial plexus.)

submandibular region, this hitchhiking branch leaves the hypoglossal nerve and descends along the surface of the carotid sheath. Some of the hitchhiking fibers of C1 continue anteriorly with the hypoglossal nerve and leave further distally to supply the *thyrohyoid and geniohyoid muscles.*

Inferior Root. Cervical plexus branches originating from AR of C2 and C3 descend in the neck posterior to, but paralleling, the superior root. At the level of the larynx the two roots come together as a loop, or ansa (the ansa cervicalis). From the **ansa cervicalis**, branches arise to *supply motor fibers to the infrahyoid muscles.*

Vagus Nerve. The vagus nerve (cranial nerve X) emerges from the jugular foramen and passes inferiorly within the carotid sheath between the internal jugular vein and internal carotid artery (*Figure 5-14*). As it descends in the neck, it gives rise to the following branches.

Meningeal branches arise and immediately reenter the skull through the jugular foramen to supply sensory branches to the dura of the posterior cranial fossa.

Pharyngeal branches pass to the pharynx. They join sympathetic fibers and the pharyngeal portion of the glossopharyngeal nerve (cranial nerve IX) to form the *pharyngeal plexus* of nerves (motor from cranial nerve X, sensory from cranial nerve IX, and sympathetic from the superior cervical ganglion).

Cardiac branches arise and descend in the neck to the superior mediastinum, where they end as the vagal contribution to the *deep cardiac plexus,* which acts to slow the heartbeat.

The **superior laryngeal** nerve divides into (1) an *internal laryngeal nerve,* a large sensory nerve that pierces the thyrohyoid membrane and is sensory from laryngeal mucosa above the vocal folds and (2) an external laryngeal nerve, which descends to supply the cricothyroid muscle of the larynx.

THE SUBMANDIBULAR TRIANGLE (REGION)

Boundaries
The boundaries of this component region of the anterior triangle are the inferior border of the mandible above and the anterior and posterior bellies of the digastric muscle below (*Figure 5-15*).

Roof
The same structures that form the roof of the anterior triangle form the roof of the component submandibular region.

Floor
The floor of the triangle is formed by two flat muscles: the mylohyoid muscle, described previously as a suprahyoid muscle, and the hyoglossus muscle, which is considered with the tongue in Chapter 7.

Contents
Two types of glands, two nerves, two arteries, and two veins are found within the submandibular region.

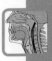

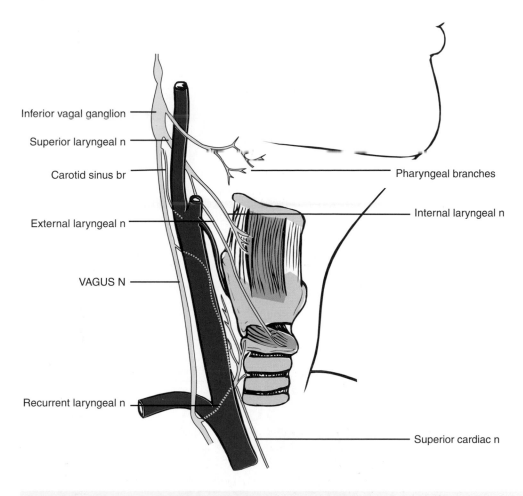

Figure 5-14 Vagus nerve within neck.

Labels: Inferior vagal ganglion, Superior laryngeal n, Carotid sinus br, External laryngeal n, VAGUS N, Recurrent laryngeal n, Pharyngeal branches, Internal laryngeal n, Superior cardiac n

Submandibular Gland. The submandibular gland is a large salivary gland that produces and secretes mixed mucus and serous saliva. It possesses two continuous portions. A **superficial portion** fills the interval between the mylohyoid muscle and the submandibular fossa of the mandible. The gland then wraps around the free posterior border of the mylohyoid muscle as a **deep portion,** which is above the mylohyoid muscle within the floor of the mouth. The submandibular duct continues anteriorly from the deep portion of the gland for approximately 3 cm and empties into the oral cavity just below the tongue (see "Floor of Mouth" in Chapter 7).

Submandibular Lymph Glands. A cluster of submandibular lymph glands, or nodes, is found in this region. They are one of several groups of lymph nodes that form a ring around the base of the skull. Draining to the submandibular lymph nodes are lymphatics of the oral cavity; therefore oral infections could manifest as enlarged palpable lymph nodes (see "Lymphatics of the Head and Neck" in Chapter 8).

Hypoglossal Nerve. The hypoglossal nerve was noted in the anterior triangle. It passes anteriorly deep to the digastric tendon to enter the submandibular region; it then leaves the region by traveling between the mylohyoid and hyoglossus muscles on its way to supply the muscles of the tongue.

Mylohyoid Nerve. The mylohyoid nerve arises as a small branch from the **inferior alveolar nerve** within the infratemporal region. It descends on the medial aspect of the mandibular ramus through a small *mylohyoid groove* to appear under the inferior border of the mandible in the submandibular region. It runs forward to supply motor fibers to the *mylohyoid muscle* and the *anterior belly of digastric muscle.*

Facial Artery. After leaving the external carotid artery, the facial artery enters the submandibular region, where it is pushed upward by the submandibular gland into the interval between the mylohyoid muscle and the medial aspect of the mandible. The artery loops down-

149

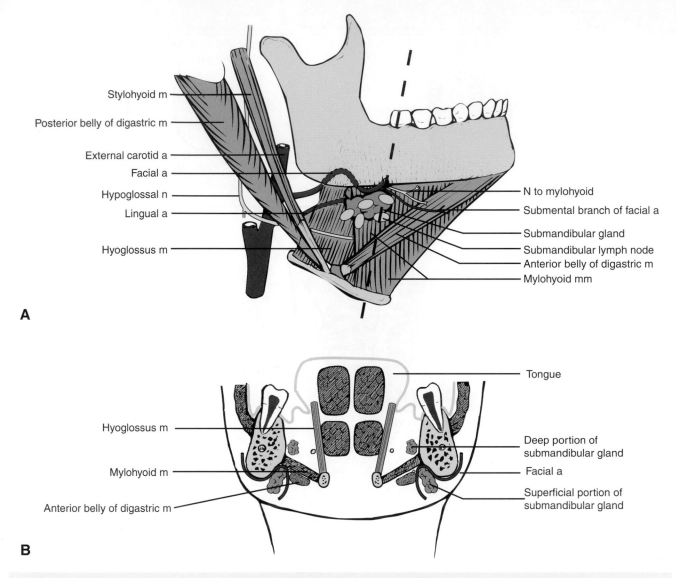

Figure 5-15 Submandibular region and its contents. **A,** Right lateral view. **B,** Coronal section through submandibular region.

ward and externally to reappear at the antegonial notch of the mandible. At this point the pulse of the facial artery may be palpated as it passes through the shallow notch. From here the facial artery ascends to the face (see Figure 7-4).

Within the submandibular region it gives off the following branches: **ascending palatine** and **tonsillar branches** to the soft palate and palatine tonsils, respectively; **glandular branches** to the submandibular gland; and the **submental artery** to the chin, which travels with the mylohyoid nerve.

Lingual Artery. The lingual artery travels forward from the external carotid artery and passes deep to the posterior belly of the digastric muscle to enter the submandibular region. It leaves again by passing deep to the hyoglossus muscle to enter the floor of the mouth, where it supplies the tongue and the structures of the floor of the mouth.

Lingual and Facial Veins. Lingual and facial veins are the companion veins to the facial and lingual arteries and were described as tributaries of the internal jugular vein (see Figure 5-11).

4. The Posterior Triangle

The posterior triangle of the neck occupies the lateral aspect of the neck; its apex is directed toward the skull and its base toward the clavicle. The posterior triangle has depth and properly should be considered a region. Therefore, in addition to three boundaries, it has a roof, a floor, and several contents.

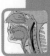

BOUNDARIES

The **anterior boundary** is formed by the posterior border of the sternocleidomastoid muscle. The **posterior boundary** is formed by the anterior border of the trapezius muscle, and the **inferior border** is formed by the middle third of the clavicle (see *Figure 5-6* and *Table 5-2*).

ROOF

From superficial to deep, the structures forming the roof of the posterior triangle are **skin, superficial fascia and platysma muscle,** and **deep investing fascia of the neck.** The platysma muscle was described with the anterior triangle of the neck.

FLOOR

The floor of the posterior triangle is formed by a series of five muscles and their overlying prevertebral deep fascia (*Figure 5-16*). Each muscle originates from cervical vertebrae and therefore is a muscular component of the vertebral unit. From the top of the triangle downward, the floor muscles are the splenius capitis, levator scapulae, scalenus posterior, scalenus medius, and scalenus anterior muscles.

Splenius Capitis Muscle

The splenius capitis muscle is a postvertebral muscle of the back and is described in Chapter 2, page 49. It originates from the ligamentum nuchae (a membranous posterior

---

TABLE 5-2

Muscles of the Posterior Triangle

Muscle	Origin	Insertion	Action	Nerve
Platysma	Superficial fascia of deltoid and pectoral regions	Inferior border of mandible, some fibers sweep upward and blend with risorius	Tightens the skin of the neck, depresses mandible	Facial nerve (cranial nerve VII)—cervical branch
Sternocleidomastoid	Manubrium and medial third of clavicle	Mastoid process and lateral half of superior nuchal line	Bilateral: flexes neck Individually: draws head to shoulder, turns face to opposite side	Spinal accessory nerve, AR of C2 and C3
Trapezius	Spines of all thoracic and cervical vertebrae, ligamentum nuchae, inion, and superior nuchal line	Spine and acromion of scapula, lateral third of clavicle	*Head* Bilateral: extends head Individually: tilts chin to opposite side *Limb girdle* Rotates and adducts scapula, elevates scapula and clavicle	Spinal AR of C3 and C4
Splenius capitis	Lower part of ligamentum nuchae, lower cervical spines	Mastoid process and superior nuchal line	Bilateral: extends head Individually: flexes head laterally, rotates head to ipsilateral side	Segmented PR of cervical spinal nerves
Levator scapulae	Transverse processes of 4 upper cervical vertebrae	Superior portion of vertebral border of scapula	Elevates scapula, rotates scapula	Dorsal scapular nerve
Scalenus posterior	Transverse processes of vertebrae C5 and C6	Superior aspect of second rib	Bilateral: flexes neck Individually: flexes neck laterally	AR of C5 to C8
Scalenus medius	Transverse processes of C2 to C7	Superior aspect of first rib	Bilateral: flexes neck Individually: flexes neck laterally	AR of C3 and C4
Scalenus anterior	Transverse processes of vertebrae C3 to C6	Scalene tubercle of first rib	As above NOTE: The scalene muscle and sternocleidomastoid aid in forced inspiration by elevating the ribs and sternum	AR of C5 to C8

AR, Anterior rami of spinal nerves; *PR,* posterior rami of spinal nerves.

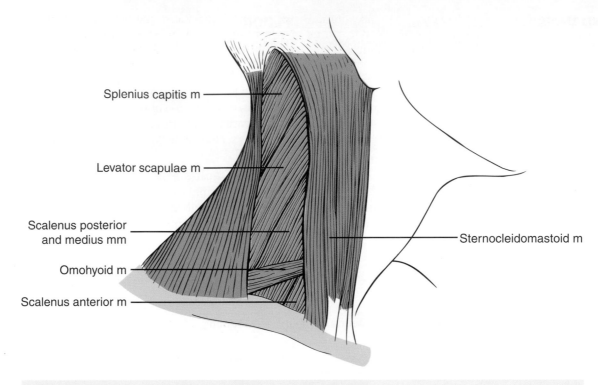

Figure 5-16 Muscles of floor of posterior triangle.

extension of the cervical spines) and the lower cervical and upper thoracic spines. The fibers run upward and laterally, inserting into the mastoid process and the lateral aspect of the superior nuchal line.

Bilaterally the splenius capitis muscles act to extend the head. Singly the muscle rotates the head to the same side. It receives its motor supply from posterior rami of spinal nerves C4 to C8.

Levator Scapulae Muscle
The levator scapulae muscle originates from the transverse processes of vertebrae C1 to C4. Its fibers sweep downward and laterally to insert into the upper vertebral border of the scapula.

Bilaterally both muscles can extend the neck and elevate the scapula. The levator scapulae receives its motor supply from AR of spinal nerves C3 and C4.

Scalenus Posterior and Medius Muscles
The scalenus posterior and medius muscles originate from the posterior tubercles of all the cervical vertebrae. The scalenus medius inserts into the superior surface of the first rib. The scalenus posterior continues further inferiorly to insert into the second rib. Bilaterally the muscles act to flex the neck. Singly each muscle flexes the neck to the same side. During forced inspiration the muscles raise the first and second ribs. The motor nerve supply is from AR of spinal nerves C3 to C8.

Scalenus Anterior Muscle
The scalenus anterior muscle originates from anterior tubercles of transverse processes C3 to C6. It inserts below into the scalene tubercle of the first rib. The actions of the scalenus anterior are identical to those of the scalenus medius and posterior muscles. Its nerve supply is from AR C5 to C8.

CONTENTS
The following structures are found at least in part within the confines of the posterior triangle and are to be considered as contents: the external jugular vein, some cutaneous nerves of the neck, some motor nerves of the neck, and some upper limb structures passing through the posterior triangle.

External Jugular Vein
The **external jugular vein** is formed by the union of the **posterior auricular vein** and the *posterior branch* of the **retromandibular vein** just below the lobe of the ear (see *Figure 5-8*). The external jugular vein passes obliquely downward over the sternocleidomastoid muscle to enter the posterior triangle, where it receives three tributaries:

1. The **transverse cervical vein,** which drains the posterolateral aspect of the neck
2. The **suprascapular vein,** which drains the suprascapular region of the back

3. The **anterior jugular vein,** which drains the anterior aspect of the neck and descends on either side of the midline to a point just above the jugular notch of the manubrium

The anterior jugular vein dives deep to the origin of the sternocleidomastoid muscle, emerging in the posterior triangle, where it empties to the external jugular vein. A *communicating vein* joins the common facial vein above to the anterior jugular vein below. The right and left anterior jugular veins occasionally may be joined across the midline by the *anterior jugular arch*. The external jugular vein ends by running deep to the clavicle to enter the **subclavian vein.**

Cutaneous Nerves

The cervical plexus was described with the anterior triangle of the neck. Four branches of the cervical plexus arise from the posterior triangle deep to the posterior border of the sternocleidomastoid muscle. Cutaneous branches radiate from a single area at the midpoint of the posterior border of the sternocleidomastoid muscle (*Figure 5-17*).

The **lesser occipital nerve** (AR of spinal nerves C2 and C3) ascends along the posterior border of the sternocleidomastoid muscle to carry sensation from the skin of the occipital region behind the ear.

The **great auricular nerve** (AR of spinal nerves C2 and C3) ascends on the sternocleiomastoid muscle to the ear. It supplies skin overlying the mastoid region, a portion of

the auricle, and somewhat overlaps the trigeminal territory of the parotid and masseteric cutaneous areas.

The **transverse cervical nerve** (AR of spinal nerves C2 and C3) crosses the sternocleidomastoid muscle to supply overlying skin of the anterior aspect of the neck.

Supraclavicular nerves (AR of C3 and C4) stream downward over the clavicle as lateral, intermediate, and medial groups of branches to skin overlying the acromial, deltoid, and pectoral regions.

CLINICAL NOTES

Local Anesthesia

Knowledge of the disposition of these nerves is important when a block anesthetic of the skin of the neck is to be administered. A single injection of local anesthetic agent at the midpoint of the posterior border of the sternocleidomastoid muscle blocks all four sets of cutaneous nerves of the neck.

Motor Nerves

Accessory Nerve. The spinal accessory nerve (cranial nerve XI) passes through the jugular foramen to enter the neck below. It travels inferiorly and posteriorly through the anterior triangle and plunges into the sternocleidomastoid muscle and supplies it. It then crosses the posterior triangle to enter the trapezius muscle and supplies it.

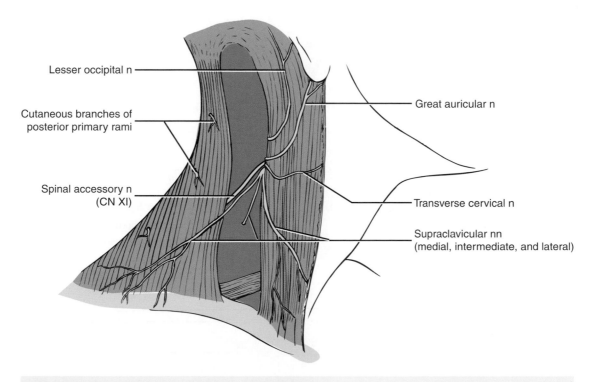

Lesser occipital n
Cutaneous branches of posterior primary rami
Spinal accessory n (CN XI)
Great auricular n
Transverse cervical n
Supraclavicular nn (medial, intermediate, and lateral)

Figure 5-17 Nerves of posterior triangle. *CN,* Cranial nerve.

The accessory nerve (cranial nerve XI) appears in the posterior triangle as it emerges from under the midpoint of the posterior border of the sternocleidomastoid muscle (see *Figure 5-17*). It runs obliquely downward along the surface of the levator scapulae muscle, disappears under the anterior border of the trapezius muscle, and supplies it.

Motor Nerves to Upper Limb Muscles and Muscles of the Floor. AR of spinal nerves C3 to C8 arise as various branches within the triangle floor to supply muscles of the floor and the rhomboids and serratus anterior muscles of the upper limb.

Phrenic Nerve. Although the phrenic nerve is not technically part of the posterior triangle, it is near enough and important enough to consider at this point. The phrenic nerve arises from converging AR of spinal nerves C3, C4, and C5 (see *Figure 5-13*). The phrenic nerve then descends along the surface of the scalenus anterior muscle and enters the thoracic cavity below (*Figure 5-18*).

Within the thorax the right and left phrenic nerves descend on either side of the mediastinum and end by supplying motor and proprioceptive fibers to the diaphragm (see Figures 3-29 and 3-30).

Upper Limb Structures Passing Through the Posterior Triangle. The major vein, artery, and nerve of the upper limb pass through the base of the posterior triangle on their way to or from the upper limb (see *Figure 5-18*).

Subclavian Vein. Within the upper limb the **basilic** and **brachial veins** unite within the axilla to form the **axillary vein** (see Figure 9-31). As the axillary vein crosses the first rib, it becomes the **subclavian vein.** Within the posterior triangle it picks up the **external jugular vein** and then joins the **internal jugular vein** of the neck to form the **brachiocephalic vein** medial to the insertion of the scalenus anterior muscle. Within the superior mediastinum below, the right and left brachiocephalic veins unite to form the **superior vena cava.**

Subclavian Artery. The right subclavian artery arises from the **brachiocephalic artery;** the left subclavian artery arises from the **arch of the aorta** within the superior mediastinum of the chest. The arteries arch upward and over the first rib and at this point are separated from the subclavian vein by the insertion of the scalenus anterior muscle. On crossing the first rib the subclavian artery becomes the **axillary artery.**

Several branches are given off within the root of the neck before its brief appearance within the posterior triangle. One of these branches, the **thyrocervical trunk,** gives off two cervical branches of its own that pass through the posterior triangle:

1. The **transverse cervical artery,** the companion artery to the vein of the same name, which drains to the external jugular vein
2. The **suprascapular artery,** which passes to the suprascapular region of the back and is the companion artery

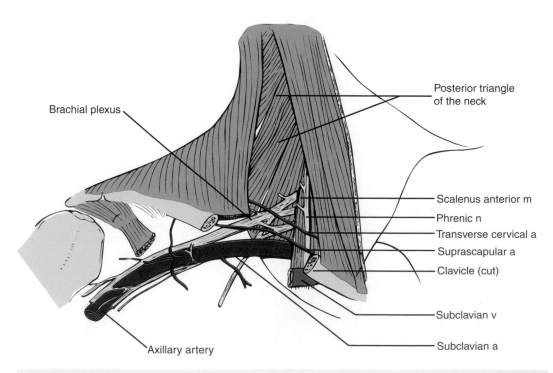

Figure 5-18 Upper limb structures within posterior triangle.

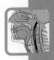

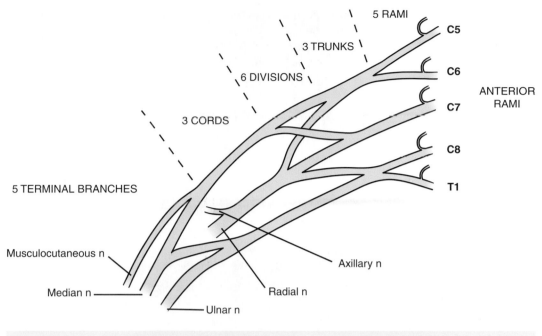

Figure 5-19 Brachial plexus.

to the vein of the same name, which drains to the external jugular vein

Both of these cervical arteries pass anteriorly to the scalenus anterior muscle, clamping the phrenic nerve to that muscle.

The Brachial Plexus. Deep within the neck, AR of spinal nerves C5 to C8 and T1 unite to form the brachial plexus in the following manner (see *Figures 5-18* and *5-19*).

Five Roots. AR of spinal nerves C5 to C8 and T1 are the five roots of the brachial plexus.

Three Trunks. The roots of C5 and C6 unite to form the *upper trunk*, C7 continues on as the *middle trunk*, and C8 and T1 unite to form the *lower trunk*. The trunks pass over the first rib between the insertions of the scalenus anterior and scalenus medius muscles.

Six Divisions. After passing over the first rib to the axilla below, the trunks divide to form two divisions each (an anterior and a posterior division from each of the trunks), making a total of six divisions.

Three Cords. The three posterior divisions unite to form the *posterior cord*. The superior two anterior divisions unite to form the *lateral cord*. The inferior anterior division forms the *medial cord*.

Five Upper Limb Nerves. The lateral cord gives rise to the *musculocutaneous nerve* and a portion of the *median nerve*. The medial cord gives rise to part of the *median nerve* and the entire *ulnar nerve*. The posterior cord gives rise to the *radial nerve* and the *axillary nerve*. The distribution of the upper limb nerves is presented in Chapter 9 (see Figure 9-28).

5. The Root

The root of the neck is the junction between the neck above and the thorax below. It is immediately above the thoracic inlet, through which pass a number of important cervical structures to or from the thorax below.

BOUNDARIES

The thoracic inlet is bounded (1) **anteriorly** by the manubrium of the sternum; (2) **laterally** by the first ribs, which slope upward as they pass posteriorly to articulate with vertebra T1; and (3) **posteriorly** by vertebra T1 (*Figure 5-20*).

CONTENTS

The root of the neck contains major blood vessels, nerves, and cervical viscera (see *Figure 5-20*).

Blood Vessels and Lymphatic Trunks

The subclavian artery, subclavian vein, thoracic duct, and right lymphatic duct pass through the root of the neck.

Subclavian Artery. The right subclavian artery arises from the **brachiocephalic artery;** the left subclavian artery arises directly from the **arch of the aorta** within the superior mediastinum. The subclavian artery arches upward over the first rib and then descends over the first rib to become the axillary artery en route to the upper limb. The subclavian artery crosses the first rib posterior

155

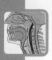

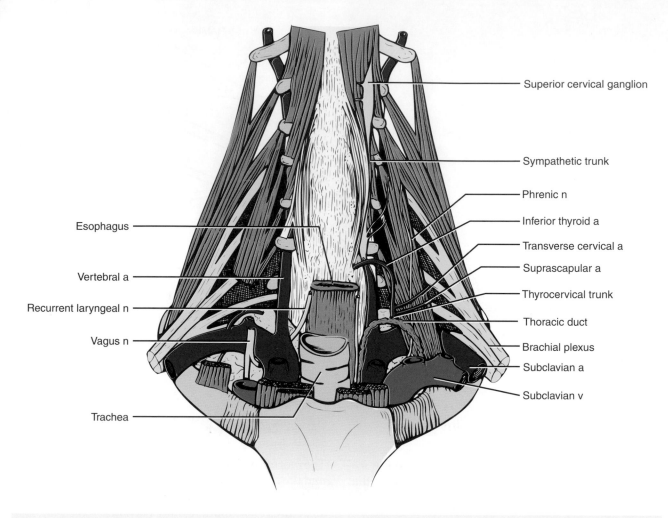

Esophagus

Vertebral a

Recurrent laryngeal n

Vagus n

Trachea

Superior cervical ganglion

Sympathetic trunk

Phrenic n

Inferior thyroid a

Transverse cervical a

Suprascapular a

Thyrocervical trunk

Thoracic duct

Brachial plexus

Subclavian a

Subclavian v

Figure 5-20 Root of neck.

to the insertion of the scalenus anterior muscle. Several branches arise from the subclavian artery.

The **vertebral artery** is the first branch to arise from the subclavian artery. It ascends in the root of the neck to enter the transverse foramen of vertebra C6. Beyond the root of the neck it ascends through successively higher transverse foramina to reach the foramen magnum. It enters the skull, joins the opposite vertebral artery, and supplies the brain as the *basilar artery.*

The **internal thoracic artery** runs inferiorly through the thoracic inlet and parallel to the body of the sternum. It descends on the internal aspect of the anterior chest wall, giving off segmented anterior intercostal branches. It supplies branches to the diaphragm and then passes inferiorly to supply the upper anterior abdominal wall as the **superior epigastric artery.**

The **thyrocervical trunk** arises as a short stem and abruptly divides into two cervical branches and one thyroid branch. The **suprascapular artery** crosses the scalenus anterior muscle, enters the posterior triangle, and passes posteriorly to the suprascapular region of the back. The **transverse**

cervical artery crosses the scalenus anterior muscle to enter the posterior triangle to supply lateral structures of the neck. The **inferior thyroid artery** ascends in the neck and arches medially and downward to enter and supply the inferior portion of the thyroid gland. A large muscular branch travels straight upward from the arch of the inferior thyroid artery as the **ascending cervical artery.**

The **costocervical trunk** is a short branch that supplies muscles of the root of the neck and sends branches to the upper two intercostal spaces (see *Figure 3-31*).

Subclavian Vein. The **axillary vein** ascends from the axilla to the level of the lateral border of the first rib and becomes the subclavian vein. It crosses the first rib anterior to the insertion of the scalenus anterior muscle. The subclavian receives three venous tributaries in the root of the neck: the **internal thoracic vein,** the **external jugular vein,** and the **vertebral vein.**

Thoracic Duct. The thoracic duct arises from the thorax behind the esophagus. It arches laterally behind the carotid

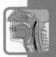

sheath and joins the confluence of the left internal jugular and left subclavian veins. The **subclavian, internal jugular,** and **bronchomediastinal lymph trunks** may join the thoracic duct proximal to its termination, or they may enter the venous system separately in the same area.

Right Lymphatic Duct. On the right side the **bronchomediastinal, jugular,** and **subclavian lymphatic trunks** may join as a short **right lymphatic** duct before entering the confluence of the right subclavian and right internal jugular veins.

Nerves

Vagus Nerve. The vagus nerve (cranial nerve X) leaves the skull through the jugular foramen and descends in the neck within the carotid sheath. The vagus nerves pass through the thoracic inlet to enter the superior mediastinum. The right vagus nerve passes anterior to the right subclavian artery. The left vagus nerve passes anterior to the arch of the aorta. As the vagus nerves cross these vessels, they give rise to the recurrent laryngeal nerves.

Recurrent Laryngeal Nerve. On the right side the recurrent laryngeal nerve arises below the subclavian artery and then loops up behind the artery to ascend in the neck.

On the left side the left recurrent laryngeal nerve loops upward around the arch of the aorta.

Both recurrent laryngeal nerves ascend in the neck along the posterolateral border of the trachea to the level of the cricoid cartilage (vertebral level C6). Here they enter and help supply the larynx.

Sympathetic Trunk. The sympathetic trunk passes upward from the superior mediastinum through the thoracic inlet (*Figure 5-21*). It continues up the neck outside and posterior to the carotid sheath. In the cervical region the sympathetic trunk receives no white communicating rami, but it does give rise to gray rami, which join and travel with cervical spinal nerves.

In the cervical region, the eight sympathetic ganglia coalesce as three major swellings:

1. The **inferior cervical ganglion** is found just above the subclavian artery. Its postganglionic branches are *gray communicating rami* to spinal nerves C7 and C8 and *cardiac branches* to the heart. The inferior cervical ganglion occasionally is found fused with the ganglion of T1 as the **stellate ganglion.**
2. The **middle cervical ganglion** is found at vertebral level C6 opposite the cricoid cartilage. Its postganglionic

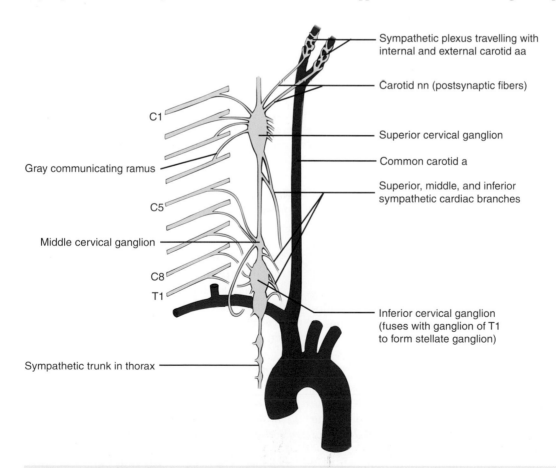

Figure 5-21 Sympathetic trunk within neck and branches.

branches are gray communicating rami to spinal nerves C5 and C6, cardiac branches to the heart, and glandular branches to the thyroid gland.

3. The **superior cervical ganglion** is a long, fusiform ganglion about 2 to 3 cm long, stretching from vertebral level C1 to level C2 or C3. Its postganglionic branches are *gray communicating rami* to spinal nerves C1 to C4, *cardiac branches* to the heart, *glandular branches* to the thyroid gland, and *carotid branches* that follow the external and internal carotid arteries as a perivascular nerve plexus.

Sympathetic Supply to the Head. The entire sympathetic nerve supply to the head region is via the sympathetic nerve plexus surrounding the carotid arteries. Thus, in considering the sympathetic supply to a structure in the head, merely look for the closest branch of the internal or external carotid artery.

CLINICAL NOTES

Horner's Syndrome

If the sympathetic trunk below the superior cervical ganglion is cut, compressed, or damaged, the following facial symptoms appear on the affected side: flushing of the skin, dry skin (anhidrosis), constricted pupil, drooping of the eyelid (ptosis), and sunken eyeball (enophthalmos). Tumors of the apical portion of the lung extend up into the root of the neck and can compress cervical sympathetic fibers and produce these symptoms.

Cervical Viscera

Thyroid Gland. The thyroid gland is somewhat H-shaped, with a right and a left lobe on either side of the cervical portion of the trachea (*Figure 5-22*). An isthmus of glandular material joins the lobes across the anterior aspect of the trachea at the level of the second or third tracheal rings. The upper poles of the gland are limited superiorly by the origins of the overlying sternothyroid muscles at the oblique line of the thyroid cartilage.

The gland is encapsulated and ductless. It is an endocrine gland that manufactures and secretes **thyroxine**, a hormone that controls the basal metabolic rate.

Development and Adult Vestiges. The gland develops as a down growth of oropharyngeal epithelium, which migrates toward the anterior aspect of the neck as a cord of epithelial cells (*Figure 5-23*). It then develops on the anterior aspect of the trachea as the thyroid gland. The cord of epithelial cells is called the *thyroglossal duct* and disappears soon after development of the gland.

In the adult the proximal end of the thyroglossal duct persists as the **foramen cecum** of the tongue. The distal portion of the duct may persist as an extra **pyramidal lobe**, which peaks upward in the midline from the isthmus to the hyoid bone above.

Blood Supply. The blood supply to the gland is from two sources: (1) the **superior thyroid artery**, a branch of the external carotid artery, and (2) the **inferior thyroid artery**, a branch of the thyrocervical trunk.

The venous drainage is via the **superior thyroid vein** to the internal jugular vein, the **middle thyroid vein** to the internal jugular vein, and the **inferior thyroid veins** to the brachiocephalic vein.

CLINICAL NOTES

Thyroglossal Cysts

Clumps of epithelial cells occasionally may persist along the primitive route of the thyroglossal duct and give rise to **thyroglossal cysts** within the neck in the same way that persistent odontogenic epithelial cells can give rise to dental cysts in the jaws.

CLINICAL NOTES

Thyroid Ima Artery

In approximately 10% of the population, a third artery, the **thyroid ima artery**, arises from the brachiocephalic trunk and ascends in the midline to the isthmus of the thyroid gland. It is of no consequence, but its possible presence must be taken into consideration before performing a tracheostomy to preclude arterial hemorrhage.

Nerve Supply. The nerve supply is from sympathetic glandular branches of the three cervical ganglia of the sympathetic trunk.

Parathyroid Glands. There are four parathyroid glands—two on the right and two on the left. They are small (about 5 mm wide) and are embedded in the posterior capsule of the thyroid gland. They are endocrine glands that secrete parathyroid hormone (PTH), which controls the metabolism of calcium in the body.

Esophagus. The esophagus descends in the neck from the pharynx at vertebral level C6 (see *Figure 5-20*). It passes through the thoracic inlet between the vertebral column behind and the trachea in front. It is described in Chapters 3 (page 79) and 4 (page 105).

Trachea. The trachea descends anterior to the esophagus from the cricoid cartilage of the larynx (see *Figure 5-20*).

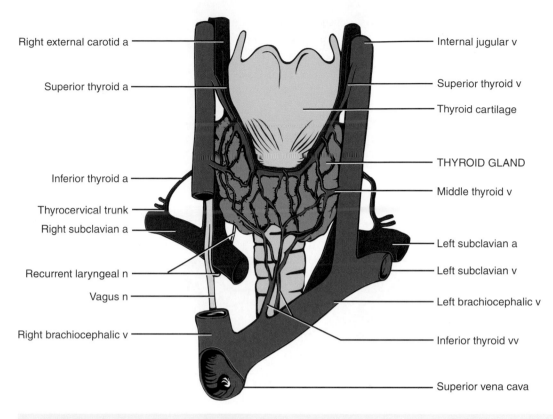

Figure 5-22 Thyroid gland and its blood supply.

Right external carotid a

Superior thyroid a

Inferior thyroid a

Thyrocervical trunk

Right subclavian a

Recurrent laryngeal n

Vagus n

Right brachiocephalic v

Internal jugular v

Superior thyroid v

Thyroid cartilage

THYROID GLAND

Middle thyroid v

Left subclavian a

Left subclavian v

Left brachiocephalic v

Inferior thyroid vv

Superior vena cava

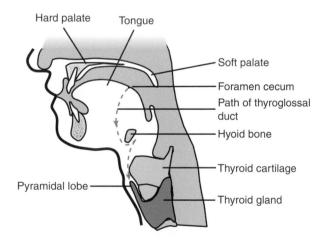

Figure 5-23 Median section of adult head showing path taken by developing thyroid gland.

Hard palate

Tongue

Soft palate

Foramen cecum

Path of thyroglossal duct

Hyoid bone

Thyroid cartilage

Thyroid gland

Pyramidal lobe

It passes through the thoracic inlet to the thorax below (see Chapter 3, page 66).

6.   The Suboccipital Region

The suboccipital region is the area between the occipital portion of the skull above and the posterior aspects of the atlas and axis below.

LOCATION

The suboccipital region is located deep to the trapezius and semispinalis capitis muscles (see Chapter 2, pages 49 and 50). It is a triangular region spanning the area between the spine of the axis and the superior nuchal line of the skull.

CONTENTS

The suboccipital region contains two articulations between the head and neck, four small back muscles, one artery, and two nerves (*Figure 5-24*).

Joints of the Suboccipital Region

The features of the **base** and **occipital region of the skull** are described in Chapter 6, Figure 6-8, and the features of the axis and atlas are described in Chapter 2, Figure 2-4.

Atlanto-occipital Joint. The atlanto-occipital joint is the articulation between the superior articulating facets of the atlas and the occipital condyles of the skull (*Figures 5-25* and *5-26*). It is a bilateral synovial joint that permits a rocking or nodding movement of the head on the atlas ("yes" movements). The ligaments that span the joint are the anterior and posterior atlanto-occipital membranes.

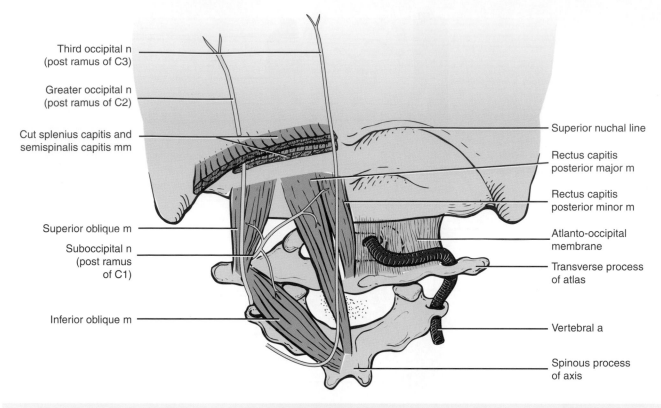

Third occipital n
(post ramus of C3)

Greater occipital n
(post ramus of C2)

Cut splenius capitis and
semispinalis capitis mm

Superior oblique m

Suboccipital n
(post ramus
of C1)

Inferior oblique m

Superior nuchal line

Rectus capitis
posterior major m

Rectus capitis
posterior minor m

Atlanto-occipital
membrane

Transverse process
of atlas

Vertebral a

Spinous process
of axis

Figure 5-24 Suboccipital region and its contents. Trapezius and semispinalis capitis muscles have been cut on left side to show suboccipital muscles and nerves of region. On right, suboccipital muscles have been removed to show course of vertebral artery through region.

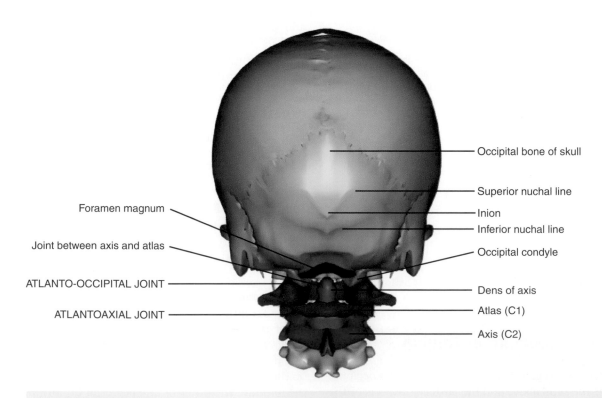

Foramen magnum

Joint between axis and atlas

ATLANTO-OCCIPITAL JOINT

ATLANTOAXIAL JOINT

Occipital bone of skull

Superior nuchal line

Inion

Inferior nuchal line

Occipital condyle

Dens of axis

Atlas (C1)

Axis (C2)

Figure 5-25 Articulated atlas and axis.

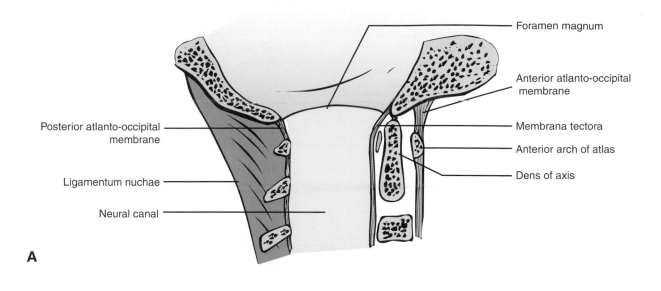

Foramen magnum

Anterior atlanto-occipital membrane

Membrana tectora

Anterior arch of atlas

Dens of axis

Posterior atlanto-occipital membrane

Ligamentum nuchae

Neural canal

A

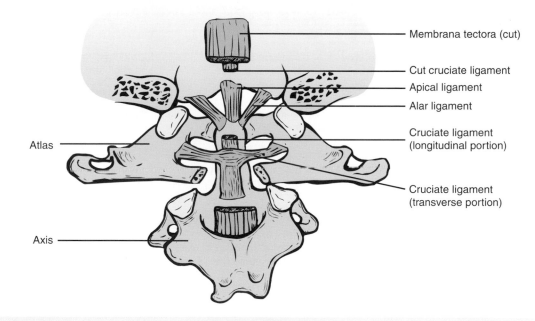

Membrana tectora (cut)

Cut cruciate ligament

Apical ligament

Alar ligament

Cruciate ligament (longitudinal portion)

Cruciate ligament (transverse portion)

Atlas

Axis

B

Figure 5-26 Atlanto-occipital and atlantoaxial joints. **A,** Median view. **B,** Posterior view.

Atlantoaxial Joint. The atlantoaxial joint is the synovial articulation between the superior articulating facets of the axis and the inferior articulating facets of the atlas. In addition, a third articulation takes place between the dens of the axis and the anterior arch of the atlas.

Movement of this joint is around a vertical axis and allows the face to turn from side to side ("no" movements). The supporting ligament is the **transverse ligament,** a *horizontal component* of the **cruciate ligament** to be described. The transverse ligament runs from the inner aspect of the lateral mass of the atlas to the opposite side, binding the bulbous tip of the dens to the anterior arch of the atlas as a cuff, or ligamentous ring. This permits the vertical rotation between the axis and the atlas.

Ligaments That Span Both Joints. Several ligaments run from the axis to the occipital bone and thus span and stabilize both atlanto-occipital and atlantoaxial joints. Bilateral **alar ligaments** run from the tip of the dens up to the inner lip of the foramen magnum at its anterior border. The **apical ligament** passes upward in the midline to the same area.

The **longitudinal portion** of the **cruciate ligament** runs from the body of the axis up to the inner anterior lip of the foramen magnum.

161

The **posterior longitudinal ligament** of the spine continues superiorly as the membrana tectoria, joining the body of the axis to the internal aspect of the basiocciput. It covers the underlying alar, apical, and cruciate ligaments.

Muscles

Four muscles are contained within the area and, acting bilaterally, serve as *extensors of the head* (see *Figure 5-24* and *Table 5-3*). Unilateral contractions rotate the head to the same side.

1. The **obliquus capitis superior** runs from the tip of the transverse process of the atlas upward to the occiput between the superior and inferior nuchal lines.
2. The **obliquus capitis inferior** arises from the spine of the axis and passes obliquely upward and laterally to insert into the tip of the transverse process of the atlas.
3. The **rectus capitis posterior minor** runs from the posterior tubercle of the atlas upward to the occiput below the inferior nuchal line.

TABLE 5-3

Vertebral Muscles of the Neck

Muscles	Origin	Insertion	Action	Nerve
Postvertebral Muscles*				
Obliquus capitis superior	Transverse process of atlas	Above inferior nuchal line of occipital bone	Individually: rotates head laterally Bilateral: extends head	Suboccipital nerve (PR of C1)
Obliquus capitis inferior	Spine of axis	Transverse process of atlas	Individually: rotates atlas and skull about dens Bilateral: extends head	Suboccipital nerve
Rectus capitis posterior major	Spine of axis	Inferior nuchal line of occipital bone	Individually: rotates head laterally Bilateral: extends head	Suboccipital nerve
Rectus capitis posterior minor	Posterior tubercle of atlas	Below inferior nuchal line of occipital bone	Individually: flexes head laterally Bilateral: extends head	Suboccipital nerve
Prevertebral Muscles†				
Longus colli	Transverse processes and bodies of vertebrae C3 to T3	Anterior tubercles of atlas and vertebrae C3, C4, and C5 Bodies of vertebrae T1, T2, and T3	Individually: flexes neck laterally Bilateral: flexes head	AR of C2 to C8
Longus capitis	Anterior tubercles of vertebrae C3 to C6	Basiocciput at base of skull	Individually: flexes and rotates head laterally Bilateral: flexes head	AR of C1 to C4
Rectus capitis anterior	Lateral mass of atlas	Basiocciput anterior to foramen magnum	Individually: rotates head Bilateral: flexes head	AR of C1 and C2
Rectus capitis lateralis	Transverse process of atlas	Jugular process of occipital bone	Individually: flexes head laterally Bilateral: flexes head	AR of C1 and C2

AR, anterior rami of the spinal nerves; *PR*, Posterior rami of the spinal nerves.
* See Table 2-3 for discussion of splenis capitis and semispinalis capitis.
† See Table 5-2 for discussion of scalene muscles and levator scapulae.

4. The **rectus capitis posterior major** arises from the spine of the axis and attaches to the occiput below the inferior nuchal line.

Vertebral Artery

The vertebral artery arises from the subclavian artery in the root of the neck and ascends to the transverse foramen of C6. It enters the foramen and ascends through successively higher transverse foramina to the level of the axis. At this point the artery turns slightly laterally to loop through the transverse foramen of the atlas. It then loops medially, occupying a groove just above the superior articulating facet of the atlas. The vertebral artery then turns abruptly upward, pierces the posterior atlanto-occipital membrane, and enters the skull through the foramen magnum. The vertebral arteries ascend on the ventral lateral aspect of the brainstem and then unite in the midline at the level of the pons as the **basilar artery**. The basilar artery is a major source of blood supply to the brain.

Nerves

Three nerves arise in the suboccipital region. These nerves are branches of posterior primary rami of spinal nerves C1, C2, and C3. The **suboccipital nerve** (C1), a motor nerve, arises above the posterior arch of the atlas. It supplies the muscles of the region. There are no cutaneous branches of C1. The **greater occipital nerve** (C2), a sensory branch, arises above the transverse process of the axis. It ascends up the back of the neck, pierces the overlying muscles of the region, and continues up to innervate the back of the head and posterior scalp. A small **third occipital** nerve arises above the transverse process of vertebra C3 and ascends to the scalp. It supplies a narrow strip of occipital skin on either side of the midline.

7. The Prevertebral Region

The prevertebral region is the area anterior to the bodies of the cervical vertebrae. This area is padded with prevertebral muscles (*Figure 5-27*), which are covered with prevertebral fascia. In general, prevertebral muscles act to flex the head and neck (*Figure 5-28*; *Table 5-4*).

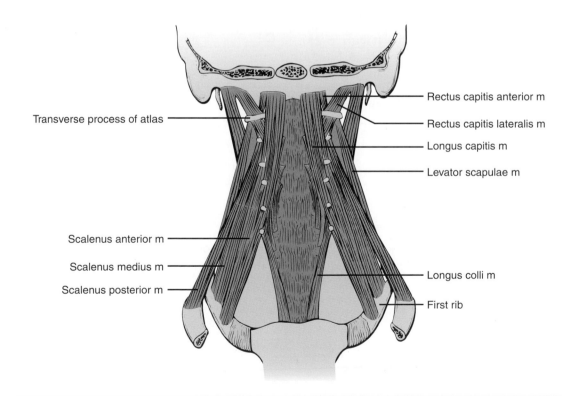

Transverse process of atlas

Scalenus anterior m
Scalenus medius m
Scalenus posterior m

Rectus capitis anterior m
Rectus capitis lateralis m
Longus capitis m
Levator scapulae m

Longus colli m
First rib

Figure 5-27 Prevertebral muscles of neck.

MUSCLES

1. The **scalene muscles**—anterior, medius, and posterior— were considered with the muscles of the floor of the posterior triangle.
2. The **levator scapulae muscle** was described with the posterior triangle of the neck.
3. The **longus colli muscle** extends from the bodies of the vertebrae from T3 upward and ends at the anterior tubercle of the atlas.
4. The **longus capitis muscle** arises from anterior tubercles of C3 to C6 and inserts in the basiocciput above.
5. The **rectus capitis anterior muscle** runs from the lateral mass of the atlas up to the basiocciput.
6. The **rectus capitis lateralis muscle** extends from the transverse process of the atlas upward to the jugular process of the occipital bone (see *Figure 5-27* and *Table 5-3*).

NERVE SUPPLY

The flexor muscles of the prevertebral area are supplied by branches of AR of cervical spinal nerves.

8. Movements of the Neck

The muscles of the neck are capable of producing 3 pairs of movements: flexion and extension, right and left lateral flexion, and right and left rotation (Figure 5-28). The muscles responsible for these movements are listed in Table 5-4. Movements within the neck take place at the cervical intervertebral joints. Movement at the head takes place at the atlanto-occipital joint for flexion and extension (yes movement); and at the pivitol atlantoaxial joint for rotation (no movement).

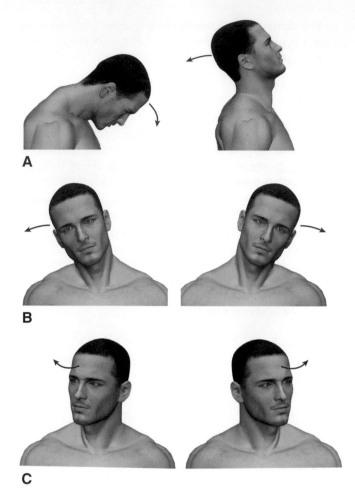

Figure 5-28 Movements of head and neck. **A,** flexion (chindown) extension (head back). **B,** right and left lateral flexion. **C,** Right and left rotation.

TABLE 5-4

Muscles Responsible for Movements of Head and Neck

Flexion	Extension	Lateral flexion	Rotation
Bilateral actions of: scalene, sternocleidomastoid, longus colli	Bilateral actions of: semispinalis capitis, semispinalis cervicis	Ipsilateral actions of: iliocostalis cervicis, longissimus capitis, longissimus cervicis	Ipsilateral actions of: rotatores, semispinalis capitis, semispinalis thoracis
		Contralateral actions of: sternocleidomastoid, trapezius	Contralateral actions of: sternocleidomastoid, trapezius

Review Questions

1. The retropharyngeal space lies between the visceral unit of the neck and the
_____.
   a. vertebral unit
   b. axillary sheath
   c. carotid sheath
   d. deep investing fascia of the neck
   e. superficial fascia of the neck

2. A local anesthetic injected into the midpoint of the posterior border of the sternocleidomastoid muscle would anesthetize all of the following cutaneous areas EXCEPT the
_____.
   a. posterior aspect of the neck
   b. lower part of the ear
   c. anterior aspect of the neck
   d. upper pectoral region
   e. deltoid regions

3. Which of the following statements concerning muscles of the neck is FALSE?
   a. Bilateral contractions of the sternocleidomastoid and scalene muscles aid in forced inspiration.
   b. Bilateral contractions of the platysma muscle can aid in depression of the mandible.
   c. Bilateral contractions of suprahyoid and infrahyoid muscles can aid in depression of the mandible.

   d. Unilateral contractions of the sternocleidomastoid muscle draw the face to the ipsilateral (same) side.
   e. Bilateral contractions of the splenius capitis muscles extend the head.

4. The inferior thyroid artery arises from the
_____.
   a. common carotid artery
   b. external carotid artery
   c. costocervical trunk
   d. thyrocervical trunk
   e. suprascapular artery

5. The posterior ramus of C2 gives rise to the
_____.
   a. transverse cervical nerve
   b. greater occipital nerve
   c. suprascapular nerve
   d. great auricular nerve
   e. lesser occipital nerve

6. All of the following nerves originate completely or in part from the cervical plexus EXCEPT the
_____.
   a. nerve to thyrohyoid
   b. phrenic nerve
   c. nerve to mylohyoid
   d. transverse cervical nerve
   e. ansa cervicalis

Questions 7 through 10
Match each of the numbered labeled cervical muscles with the appropriate lettered nerve supply in the illustration. Lettered nerves may be chosen once, more than once, or not at all.

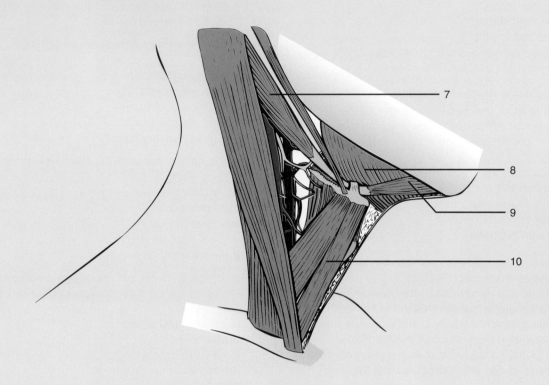

A. _____ trigeminal nerve
B. _____ facial nerve
C. _____ accessory nerve
D. _____ cervical plexus
E. _____ hypoglossal nerve

Chapter 6

The Skull

1. Introduction 167

2. Views 167

3. Bones 184

4. Postnatal Development 213

1. Introduction

The skeleton of the head is a complex articulation of many bones and teeth, which are collectively referred to as the *skull* or **cranium.** On the basis of function the skull may be conveniently divided into two main areas: the (1) *neurocranium* and (2) the *facial skeleton* (*Figure 6-1*).

NEUROCRANIUM

The neurocranium is the rounded vault, or braincase, that houses and protects the brain within. The neurocranium is made up of eight bones, most of which are curved and flat. Most of the bones are united by fibrous sutures; some are united by cartilaginous synchondroses, which ultimately fuse.

The bones of the neurocranium are the **frontal bone,** the paired **parietal bones,** the paired **temporal bones,** the **occipital bone,** the **sphenoid bone,** and the **ethmoid bone.** The floor of the neurocranium consists of the ethmoid, the sphenoid, and a portion of the occipital and temporal bones. Collectively the bones making up the floor of the neurocranium are called the *cranial base.*

THE FACIAL SKELETON (VISCEROCRANIUM)

The facial portion of the cranium is suspended from the cranial base, and the face consists of several important functional areas. Two **orbits** house and protect the *organs of sight*—the eyeballs. The **nasal cavity** is associated with *respiration* and the *special sense of smell*, and the **oral cavity** is associated with *mastication, taste,* and *respiration*.

The facial skeleton consists of several irregular bones: the paired **maxillae,** including the maxillary teeth; the paired **nasal bones;** the paired **zygomatic bones;** the paired **palatine bones;** the paired **lacrimal bones;** the paired **inferior conchae;** the single **vomer;** the single **mandible,** including the mandibular teeth; and the single **hyoid bone.**

The facial skeleton includes the *upper* and *lower jaws.* The upper jaw (right and left maxillae) is fixed to the cranial base; the lower jaw (mandible) is movable and hinged to the cranial base through the *temporomandibular joint*.

2. Views

The skull is traditionally studied by rotating the skull to various views. By convention, however, the skull is described as oriented in the horizontal **Frankfort plane,** which is a plane that joins the uppermost points of the right and left external auditory meatuses (ear holes) and the lowermost points of the right and left orbits. The Frankfort plane is parallel to the floor or tabletop and approximates the anatomical position.

FRONTAL VIEW
Regions
The regions of the skull seen in this view include the *forehead*; the *zygomatic malar area* formed by the cheekbones; the *orbits*, which house the eyeballs; the *anterior nasal aperture*, to which is affixed the external nose; the *fixed upper jaw*, which houses the upper teeth; and the *lower movable jaw*, which contains the lower teeth.

167

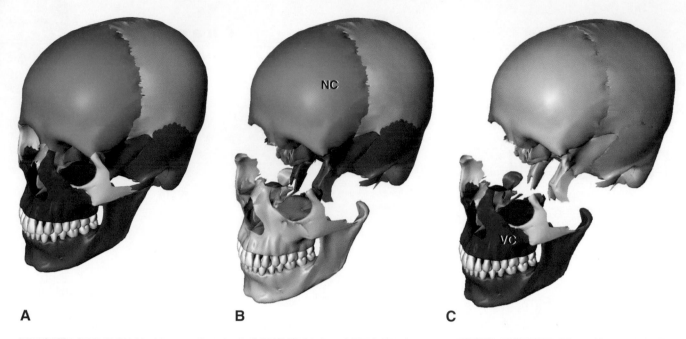

A   **B**   **C**

Figure 6-1 General plan of skull.

Bones

The bones evident in the anterior view (*Figure 6-2, A*) are the right and left maxillae, nasal bones, the right and left zygomatic bones, the right and left lacrimal bones, the right and left inferior conchae, the ethmoid bone, the vomer, the sphenoid bone, the frontal bone, and the mandible.

Features

Forehead Region. The forehead region is formed mainly by a portion of the frontal bone (*Figure 6-2, B*). The following features are found within the region of the forehead.

The **glabella** is a midline, gently rounded elevation just above the bridge of the nose. It translates as the bald spot between the eyebrows.

The **superciliary arches** (brow ridges) lie on either side of the glabella, just above the superior margins of the orbits. In men they are prominent, raised ridges of bone; in women they are less noticeable. They are absent in children, becoming prominent during adolescence when the frontal bone is ballooned out from within by the developing frontal air sinuses.

The **frontal eminences** are the gently rounded corners of the forehead. They are more prominent in the newborn skull and represent initial areas of ossification.

Zygomatic Area. The zygomatic area of the cheekbones is arranged in an arch. Three bones support the zygomatic arch: (1) the maxilla anteriorly, (2) the frontal bone superiorly, and (3) the temporal bone posteriorly. Each bone provides a buttressing zygomatic process that helps support the zygomatic arch. The *keystone* of the arch is the diamond-shaped zygomatic bone.

The **zygomaticofacial foramen** is centrally located on the prominence of the zygomatic bone and transmits the *zygomaticofacial vessels* and *nerve*.

Orbital Area. The orbits contain the eyeballs and the extraocular muscles (*see Figures 6-2 and 6-3*). Several bones contribute to the margins (rims) and to the inner walls of the bony orbit.

Margins. There are four margins in the orbital area: the superior orbital, lateral, inferior, and medial. The **superior orbital margin** is formed by the frontal bone, the **lateral margin** is formed by the zygomatic bone, and the **inferior margin** is formed by the zygomatic bone laterally and the maxilla medially.

The **medial margin** is complicated in that it exhibits an anterior aspect and a posterior aspect, which spiral in a slight corkscrew fashion. The anterior crest is formed by the frontal process of the maxilla and a portion of the frontal bone. The posterior crest is formed by the lacrimal bone.

Walls. The **roof** is formed by the frontal bone, and the **floor** is formed by the maxilla. The *lateral wall* is formed by the zygomatic bone anteriorly and the greater wing of the sphenoid posteriorly. The *medial wall* is formed by the following bones from anterior to posterior: maxilla, lacrimal bone, ethmoid bone, and the lesser wing of the sphenoid.

Orbital Openings

1. The **supraorbital notch** or **foramen** (either may be present) is located directly above the medial third of

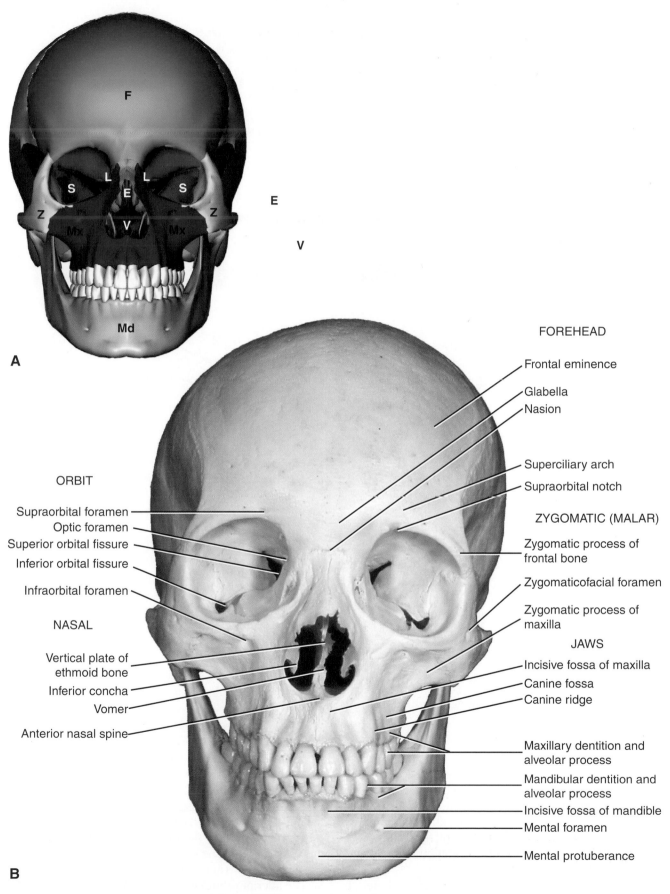

FOREHEAD

Frontal eminence

Glabella
Nasion

Superciliary arch

Supraorbital notch

ZYGOMATIC (MALAR)

Zygomatic process of
frontal bone

Zygomaticofacial foramen

Zygomatic process of
maxilla

JAWS

Incisive fossa of maxilla

Canine fossa

Canine ridge

Maxillary dentition and
alveolar process

Mandibular dentition and
alveolar process

Incisive fossa of mandible

Mental foramen

Mental protuberance

ORBIT

Supraorbital foramen

Optic foramen

Superior orbital fissure

Inferior orbital fissure

Infraorbital foramen

NASAL

Vertical plate of
ethmoid bone

Inferior concha

Vomer

Anterior nasal spine

A

B

Figure 6-2 Anterior view of skull. **A,** Bones. **B,** Features.

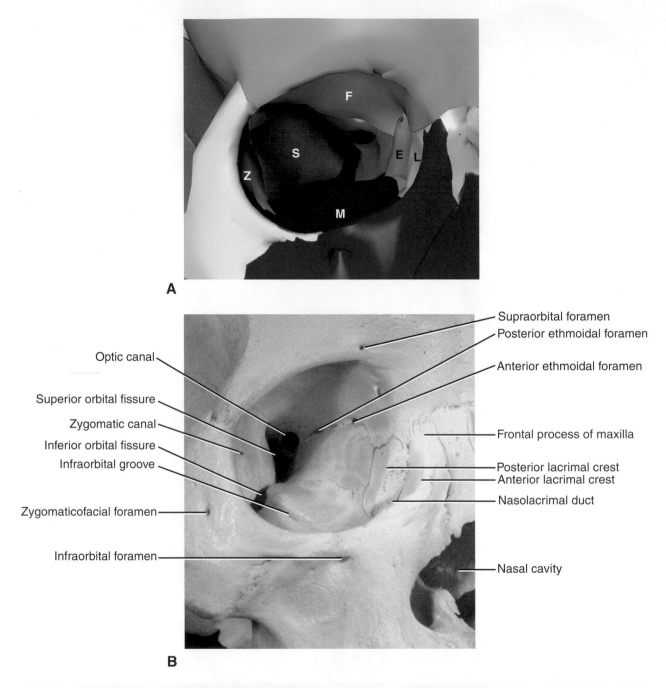

Optic canal

Superior orbital fissure

Zygomatic canal

Inferior orbital fissure

Infraorbital groove

Zygomaticofacial foramen

Infraorbital foramen

Supraorbital foramen

Posterior ethmoidal foramen

Anterior ethmoidal foramen

Frontal process of maxilla

Posterior lacrimal crest

Anterior lacrimal crest

Nasolacrimal duct

Nasal cavity

Figure 6-3 Right bony orbit. **A,** Bones that form it. **B,** Features.

the superior margin. It represents a communication between the orbit within and the forehead without and transmits the *supraorbital vessels* and *nerve*.

2. The **infraorbital foramen** is situated about 7 to 8 mm below the midpoint of the inferior margin. It communicates posteriorly with the *infraorbital canal* and *groove* in the floor of the orbit and transmits the *infraorbital vessels* and *nerve*.

3. The **optic canal** lies deep within the orbit at its posterior pole. It passes through the lesser wing of the sphenoid posteriorly to the middle cranial fossa within the skull. The optic canal transmits the *optic nerve (cranial nerve II)* and the *ophthalmic artery*.

4. The **superior orbital fissure** is a cleft between the lesser wing and the greater wing of the sphenoid. It is the superior limb of a sideways V-shaped opening and communicates posteriorly with the middle cranial fossa. It transmits the *ophthalmic veins* and *cranial nerves III, IV, V-1,* and *VI.*

5. The **inferior orbital fissure** is the lower limb of the sideways V. It is a cleft between the greater wing of the

sphenoid and the maxilla and permits communication between the posterior infratemporal region and the orbit. The inferior orbital fissure transmits the *infraorbital nerve* and *vessels* via the *infraorbital groove*.

6. The **posterior** and **anterior ethmoidal foramina** lie on the medial wall between the frontal bone above and the ethmoid bone below. The foramina transmit the *posterior* and *anterior ethmoidal nerves* and *vessels* from the orbit to the ethmoidal air sinus.

7. The **zygomatic canal** is a tiny opening in the zygomatic bone on the lateral orbital wall. The zygomatic canal divides within the bone into the zygomaticofacial and temporal canals, which convey cutaneous *zygomaticofacial* and *zygomaticotemporal nerves* and *vessels*.

8. The bony **nasolacrimal duct** is situated at the inferomedial corner of the orbital margin. It communicates with the nasal cavity and houses the *membranous nasolacrimal duct*.

Nasal Region. Several bones surround the midline, inverted pear-shaped (piriform) **anterior nasal aperture**. Fixed anteriorly to this aperture are the soft tissues, which complete the external nose.

1. The **superior margins** are formed by the rectangular paired *nasal bones*.

2. The **lateral** and **inferior margins** are formed by the paired *maxillae*.

3. The **midline bony nasal septum** is formed by the *vomer bone* inferiorly and the vertical *plate of the ethmoid bone* superiorly. The septum is usually deviated to the left.

4. The **nasal conchae** are three pairs of scroll-like, delicate shelves that hang into the nasal cavity from the lateral wall. The superior and middle conchae are part of the ethmoid; the inferior concha is a separate bone.

5. The **anterior nasal spine** is a sharp midline projection extending anteriorly from the floor of the nasal cavity, at the point where the right and left maxillae meet.

6. The **nasion** is an anthropological landmark representing the midline intersection of the nasal bones and the frontal bone.

The Jaws. The upper and lower jaws house the teeth. The upper jaw is fixed and consists of two bones; the lower jaw, or mandible, is movable and is one bone in the adult.

1. The **teeth** are the obvious features of this region. There are 32 teeth in the complete adult dentition and 20 in children's. The teeth are considered with the features of the oral cavity in Chapter 7.

2. The **alveolar processes** of the maxilla and mandible are the bony sockets that support the teeth. The facial aspect of the anterior maxillary alveolar process presents a very thin plate of bone over the roots of the anterior maxillary teeth. This is important clinically. Injected local anesthetic solution over the root

apex area diffuses readily through the thin bone to the nerves at the root apex and results in localized anesthesia. In the fabrication of dentures the ridges of bone overlying the anterior maxillary teeth roots are simulated by "festooning."

3. The **canine ridge** of the maxilla is a particularly prominent ridge of bone overlying the long and prominent maxillary canine tooth. If the maxillary canines are missing because of a previous extraction or if they fail to erupt because of a lack of space (impaction), the canine ridges are not present and the face appears flatter on the affected side. The canine ridges are important in forming the corners of the mouth.

4. The **incisive fossa** of the maxilla is the depression overlying the maxillary incisor roots. In this area, the maxillary teeth can be individually anesthetized.

5. The **canine fossa** of the maxilla, paradoxically, is the depression overlying the premolar roots distal to the canine ridge. Injections in this area anesthetize the maxillary premolar teeth.

6. The **mental protuberance** of the mandible is the triangular elevation of bone that forms the chin.

7. The **incisive fossa** of the mandible is the concavity just inferior to the mandibular incisors and above the mental protuberance.

8. The **mental foramen** of the mandible is an opening located at the level of the second mandibular premolar, midway between the alveolar crest and the inferior border of the mandible. It transmits the *mental nerve* and *vessels*. Note that the mouth of the foramen opens posteriorly and upward, rendering injections into the foramen difficult.

LATERAL VIEW

Regions

The areas seen from the lateral view are the *cranial vault region* (including the forehead, scalp, and temporal regions); the *facial region* (including the zygomatic, orbital, and nasal regions studied in the anterior view); the *infratemporal region*, which is covered and obscured by the ramus of the mandible; and the *mandible* (lateral aspect).

Bones

The bones seen from the lateral view are the frontal bone (single), parietal bones (paired), temporal bones (paired), occipital bone (single), greater wings of the sphenoid bone (paired processes of a single bone), zygomatic bones (paired), maxillae (paired), nasal bones (paired), lacrimal bones (paired), and the mandible (single). (*Figure 6-4, A*).

Features

The Cranial Vault Region. The cranial vault is formed anteriorly by the single frontal bone, laterally by the paired parietal bones, and posteriorly by the single occipital bone.

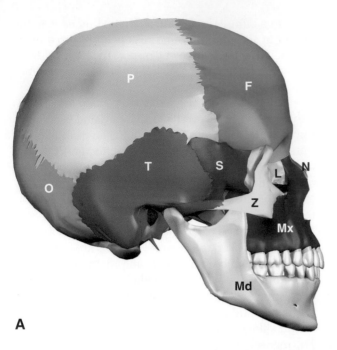

A

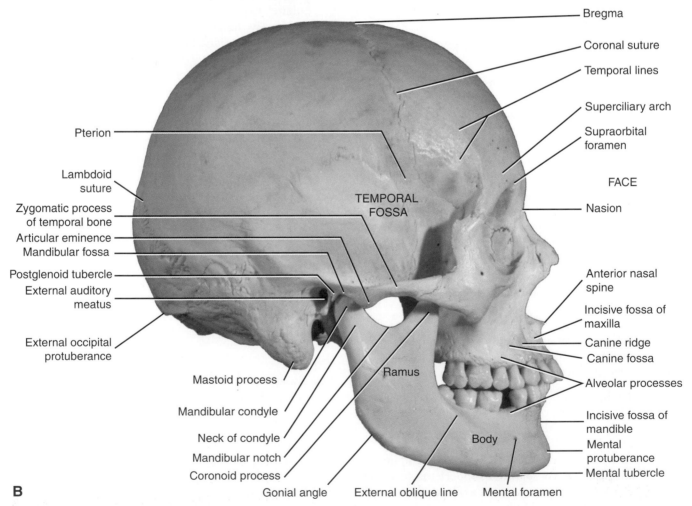

B

Figure 6-4 Lateral view of skull. **A**, Bones. **B**, Features.

Inferolaterally the walls of the vault are formed by the paired temporal bones and the paired greater wings of the single sphenoid bone. The cranial vault region presents the following features.

1. The **vertex** is the highest point on the superior margin of the cranial vault oriented in the Frankfort position.
2. **Bregma** is an anthropological landmark anterior to the vertex. It is the point where the right and left parietal bones meet the frontal bone.
3. The **temporal lines** (superior and inferior) are two curved lines that arch upward and backward from the zygomatic process of the frontal bone, travel across the frontal bone and parietal bone, and then recurve downward and forward on the parietal bone to end inferiorly on the temporal bone. They represent the superior limit of the curved origin of the temporalis muscle.
4. **Pterion** is an anthropological landmark named for the H-shaped junction of the frontal, parietal, greater wing of sphenoid, and temporal bones on the lateral aspect of the cranial vault.
5. The **temporal fossa** is the slightly depressed area on the anterolateral aspect of the skull inferior to the temporal lines. It is filled in by the temporalis muscle.
6. The **external auditory meatus** of the temporal bone forms the entrance to the middle ear within the temporal bone.
7. The **mastoid process** is a lump of bone immediately posterior and inferior to the external auditory meatus. It serves as part of the insertion of the sternomastoid muscle.
8. The **mandibular**, or **glenoid, fossa** is the depression anterior to the external auditory meatus. It houses the head, or condyle, of the mandible.
9. The **postglenoid tubercle** is a small wedge of bone that intervenes between the mandibular fossa and the external auditory meatus.
10. The **glenoid tubercle** is a small bump anterior to the mandibular fossa. It is actually the lateral aspect of the *articular eminence* on the base of the skull.
11. The **zygomatic process** of the temporal bone is a long, slender forward projection that forms the posterior root of the zygomatic arch.

The Facial Region. The bones and features of the facial region were discussed in the descriptions of the anterior view. The lateral aspect of the mandible, however, is described here.

1. The **body** of the mandible is the horizontal portion.
2. The **ramus** of the mandible is the vertical portion.
3. The **teeth** and the **alveolar process** were described with the anterior view.

4. The **gonial angle** is the junction of the posterior border of the ramus and the inferior border of the body of the mandible.
5. The **condyle**, or **condylar head,** of the mandible is a roller-shaped process that articulates with the mandibular fossa of the temporal bone above.
6. The **neck of the mandible** is the slender bony portion that supports the condyle.
7. The **coronoid process** is the sharp, bladelike, and anterosuperior process of the ramus. With the teeth occluded, the tip of the coronoid process is obscured by the zygomatic arch.
8. The **mandibular notch** is the notch between the condyle and the coronoid process.
9. The sharp anterior border of the ramus continues inferiorly onto the lateral aspect of the body of the mandible as the **external oblique line.** It continues obliquely downward and forward to end near the chin area on the inferior aspect of the body as the **mental tubercle.**
10. The **mental protuberance**, or chin, is a triangular lump of bone. Its base is directed inferiorly and its apex directed upward toward the mandibular incisive fossa.
11. The **mental foramen** is described under the anterior aspect of the skull.

The Infratemporal Region. The infratemporal region is obscured by the ramus of the mandible, which serves as the lateral wall of the region (*Figure 6-5*). With the mandible removed, the limits of the infratemporal region can be further delineated. The infratemporal region is separated from the temporal fossa above by an indistinct **infratemporal crest.**

Bones and Walls
1. The **roof** of the region is made up of the greater wing of the sphenoid **anteriorly** and the inferior portion of the temporal bone **posteriorly**.
2. The **anterior wall** is the convex posterior aspect of the maxilla.
3. The **medial wall** is the lateral pterygoid plate of the sphenoid bone.
4. The **lateral wall** is the medial surface of the mandibular ramus.
5. No inferior boundary exists.

Features
1. The **inferior orbital fissure** is a cleft between the greater wing of the sphenoid above and the maxilla below. It communicates with the orbit anteriorly. The infraorbital groove continues anteriorly from the midpoint of the lower margin of the fissure.
2. The **pterygomaxillary fissure** is a cleft between the pterygoid process of the sphenoid bone behind and the maxilla in front. The cleft communicates with the

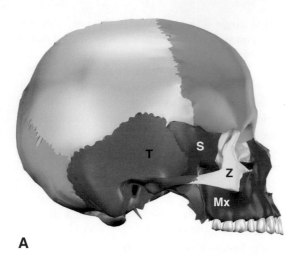

A

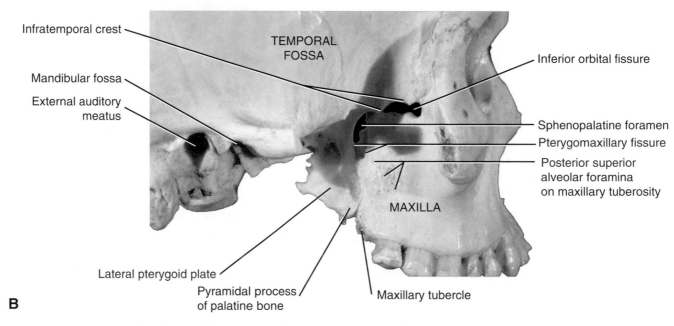

B

Figure 6-5 Lateral view of skull with mandible removed to expose infratemporal region. **A**, Bones. **B**, Features.

deeper pterygopalatine fossa, which is discussed in detail in Chapter 7.

3. The **posterior superior alveolar foramina** are centered in a grouping on the convexity (tuberosity) of the posterior or infratemporal aspect of the maxilla. They transmit the *posterior superior alveolar nerves* and *vessels*.

4. The **pyramidal process** of the palatine bone is the only portion of the palatine bone visible externally. It intervenes inferiorly between the converging pterygoid process and the maxilla.

5. The **maxillary tubercle** is the rounded elevation of bone distal to the last maxillary molar. Occasionally, the maxillary tuberosity is invaded by the maxillary air sinus from within and presents a hazard during third molar removal. Fracture of the tubercle could cause a communication between the oral cavity and the maxillary sinus (oroantral fistula).

6. The **zygomatic process of the maxilla** is the anterior continuation of the inferior border of the zygomatic arch that curves downward to end as a buttress over the roots of the maxillary first molar. It is the contribution of the maxilla to the zygomatic arch, and it considerably thickens the buccal bone overlying the roots of the maxillary first molar. This bony thickness may present a problem in achieving profound local anesthesia (see Chapter 11).

SUPERIOR VIEW

Bones

The superior aspect of the skull presents a somewhat egg-shaped outline with the small end anteriorly (*Figure 6-6*). Only four bones are seen from this view: the frontal bone anteriorly, the right and left parietal bones laterally, and the occipital bone posteriorly.

A

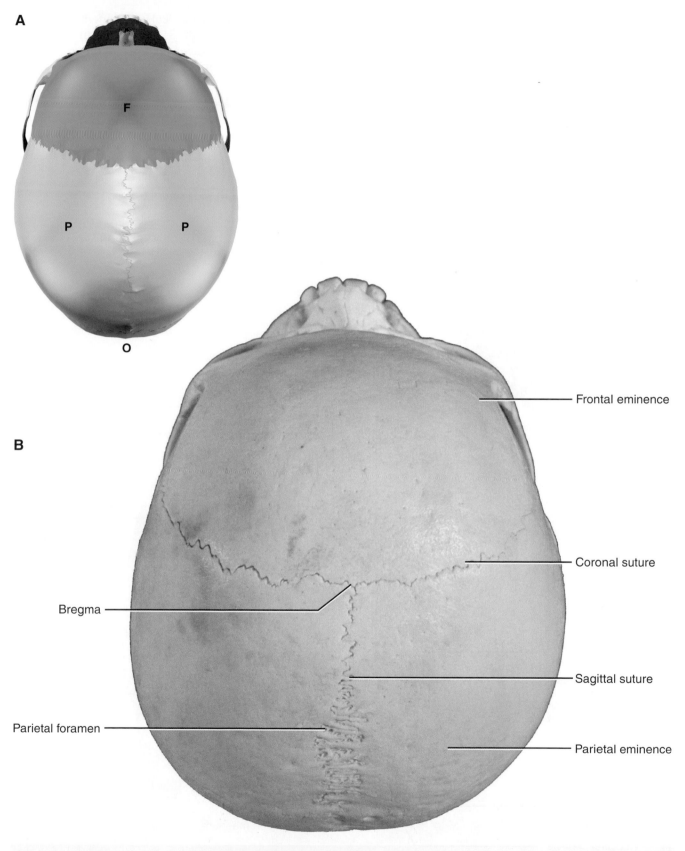

B

Frontal eminence

Coronal suture

Bregma

Sagittal suture

Parietal foramen

Parietal eminence

Figure 6-6 Superior view of skull. **A,** Bones. **B,** Features.

Features

1. The **coronal suture** separates the frontal bone anteriorly from the parietal bones posteriorly.
2. The **sagittal**, or **interparietal**, suture separates the right and left parietal bones.
3. The **lambdoidal suture** separates the parietal and temporal bones from the occipital bone (*Figure 6-7*).
4. **Bregma** is an anthropological landmark marked by the intersection of the sagittal and coronal sutures.
5. **Lambda** is an anthropological landmark located at the intersection of the lambdoid and sagittal sutures.
6. The **frontal eminences** are the anterior corners of the forehead.

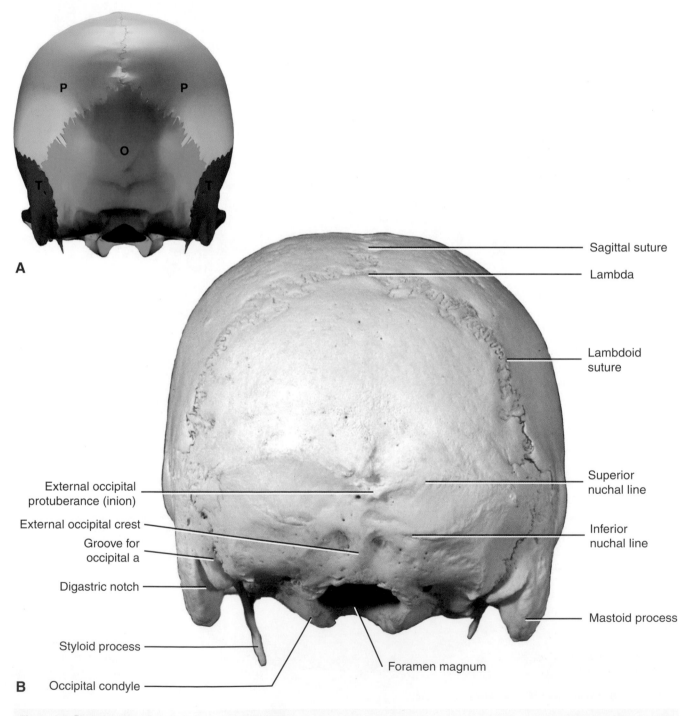

Figure 6-7 Posterior view of skull. **A**, Bones. **B**, Features.

7. The **parietal eminences** are the more prominent, posterolateral bulges. Both sets of eminences represent initial sites of ossification of the frontal and parietal bones.

8. The **parietal foramina** are paired, inconstant foramina on either side of the sagittal suture as it approaches the lambdoid suture. They transmit *emissary veins* from the scalp externally to the superior sagittal venous sinus internally.

POSTERIOR VIEW

The most prominent feature of the posterior view is the rounded posterior pole of the skull, called the *occiput* (see *Figure 6-7*). Hence, the area is often referred to as the *occipital area*.

Bones

The bones seen from this view are the **right** and **left parietal bones** superiorly and laterally, the **occipital bone** posteriorly, and the **right** and **left temporal bones** at the inferolateral aspects.

Features

1. The **inion**, or **external occipital protuberance**, is a lump of bone of varying size located in the midline between the lambda and the foramen magnum.

The posterior aspect of the skull also includes three nuchal lines, which are raised ridges that represent areas of attachment for neck muscles.

2. The **superior nuchal line** radiates laterally on either side of the inion in a curved arc ending at the mastoid process on either side.

3. The **inferior nuchal line** is a less distinct parallel line below the superior nuchal line.

4. The **highest nuchal line** is an even less distinct parallel line just above the superior nuchal line.

5. The **external occipital crest** runs down in the median plane from the inion to the foramen magnum. It provides a bony attachment for the *ligamentum nuchae*.

The following features are in a straight line traversing the base of the posterior aspect of the skull from lateral to medial.

6. The **mastoid process** of the temporal bone is a palpable bony lump that provides a site of insertion for the *sternomastoid muscle*.

7. The **digastric notch** is the site of insertion for the *posterior belly of the digastric muscle*.

8. The **occipital groove** is created by the *occipital artery* making its way onto the occiput of the skull.

9. The **occipital condyles** are the articular facets by which the skull articulates with the *atlas* below.

10. The **foramen magnum** is seen more clearly on the basal aspect of the skull. It is the opening through which the *spinal cord* enters the skull to become continuous with the brainstem.

BASAL OR INFERIOR VIEW

Bones

The bones seen from the basal aspect (*Figure 6-8, A*) are the **right** and **left maxillae** (palatal processes), the **right** and **left palatine bones** (palatal processes), the **sphenoid bone** (body, pterygoid processes, and greater wings), the **vomer**, the **right** and **left temporal bones**, and the **occipital bone**.

Regions

The study of the rather complex basal view of the skull may be simplified by defining the following areas in relation to two imaginary lines. The **anterior transverse line** joins the right and left articular eminences. The **posterior transverse line** joins the anterior aspects of the right and left mastoid processes.

The anterior and posterior lines pass through several key structures and, in addition, effectively divide the base of the skull into *anterior, intermediate*, and *posterior regions*.

Features

Anterior Region

1. The **maxillary teeth** and alveolar process lie in a U-shaped arrangement, which ends posteriorly as the maxillary tubercles (*Figure 6-8, B*).

2. The **bony palate** lies within the alveolar process and consists of two bones. The *palatal processes of the maxillae* form the anterior two thirds of the palate; the *palatal processes of the palatine bones* form the posterior third, ending as a double crescent-shaped, posterior-free border.

3. The **posterior nasal spine** is a midline posterior projection from the posterior border of the bony palate.

4. The **incisive canal** opens via the incisive foramen onto the palate distal to the central incisors. It transmits the *nasopalatine nerve* and *vessels*.

5. The **greater palatine canal** opens as the greater palatine foramen onto the palatal process of the palatine bone in line with the last maxillary molar. It transmits the *greater palatine nerve* and *vessels*.

6. The **lesser palatine canal** opens as the lesser palatine foramen posterior to the greater palatine foramen. It transmits the *lesser palatine nerve* and *vessels*.

7. The **posterior choanae**, or **posterior nasal apertures**, represent the posterior limits of the nasal cavity. The free edge of the bony nasal septum formed by the vomer divides the nasal cavity into right and left chambers.

8. The **palatinovaginal canal** runs between the body and the vaginal process of the sphenoid bone. It transmits the pharyngeal branch of the pterygopalatine ganglion posteriorly to the superior portion of the pharynx.

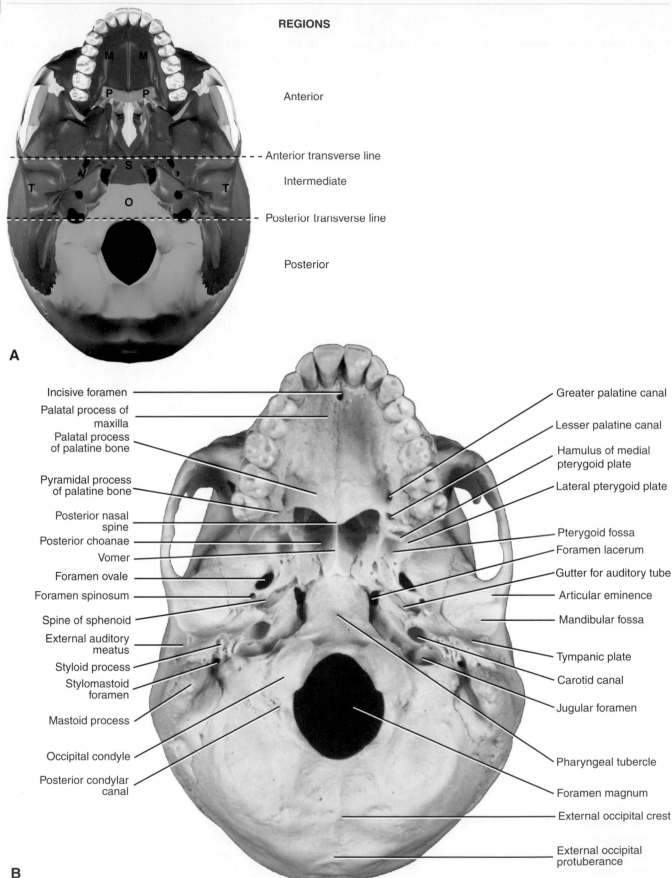

REGIONS

Anterior

– – – Anterior transverse line

Intermediate

– – – Posterior transverse line

Posterior

A

Incisive foramen

Palatal process of maxilla

Palatal process of palatine bone

Pyramidal process of palatine bone

Posterior nasal spine

Posterior choanae

Vomer

Foramen ovale

Foramen spinosum

Spine of sphenoid

External auditory meatus

Styloid process

Stylomastoid foramen

Mastoid process

Occipital condyle

Posterior condylar canal

Greater palatine canal

Lesser palatine canal

Hamulus of medial pterygoid plate

Lateral pterygoid plate

Pterygoid fossa

Foramen lacerum

Gutter for auditory tube

Articular eminence

Mandibular fossa

Tympanic plate

Carotid canal

Jugular foramen

Pharyngeal tubercle

Foramen magnum

External occipital crest

External occipital protuberance

B

Figure 6-8 Inferior view of base of skull with mandible removed. **A**, Bones. **B**, Features.

9. The **pterygoid processes of the sphenoid bone** buttress the maxillary tuberosity areas. Only the intervening wedge of the **pyramidal process of the palatine bone** prevents the maxilla and the pterygoid from contacting.

The pterygoid process consists of a **lateral** and a **medial plate.** The lateral plate provides attachment for both *lateral and medial pterygoid muscles.* The medial pterygoid plate forms the posterior limit of the lateral wall of the nasal cavity. The medial plate ends inferiorly as the **hamulus**, a small, slender hook.

Intermediate Area. From lateral to medial, the features encountered in the intermediate area are as follows (*see Figures 6-8 and 6-9*):

1. The **mandibular fossa**, which accommodates the condyle of the mandible
2. The **external auditory meatus**, which lies behind the mandibular fossa
3. The **tympanic plate**, which forms the anterior wall of the external auditory meatus and the posterior, nonfunctioning wall of the mandibular fossa
4. The **squamotympanic fissure**, which separates the mandibular fossa of the squamous portion of the temporal bone from the tympanic plate of the temporal bone. (A complicating feature within this suture is an intervening small bit of petrous temporal bone giving rise to the **petrotympanic fissure**, which transmits the *chorda tympani nerve*, a branch of cranial nerve VII.)

5. The **spine of the sphenoid**, a pointed projection medial to the mandibular fossa; a ligament joins the spine to the lingula of the mandible (*sphenomandibular ligament*)
6. The **foramen spinosum**, a small opening just anterior to the spine of the sphenoid, which transmits the *middle meningeal artery* from the base of the skull to the interior of the skull
7. The **gutter for the auditory (pharyngotympanic) tube**, which lies medial to the spine of the sphenoid. (The membranous portion of the auditory tube lies within this gutter. It runs from the middle ear deep within the temporal bone to the area of the nasopharynx.)
8. The **pharyngeal tubercle**, a small midline elevation on the basal portion of the occipital bone, that marks the superior attachment of the *pharyngeal raphé*

Structures Straddling the Posterior Line. From lateral to medial the features crossed by the posterior transverse line are as follows:

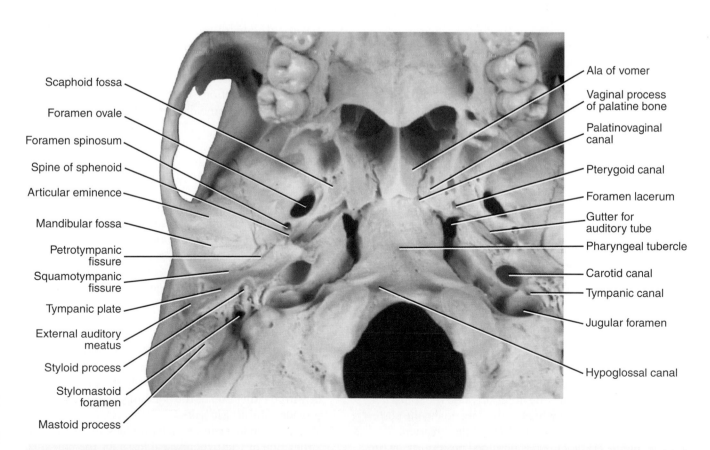

Scaphoid fossa
Foramen ovale
Foramen spinosum
Spine of sphenoid
Articular eminence
Mandibular fossa
Petrotympanic fissure
Squamotympanic fissure
Tympanic plate
External auditory meatus
Styloid process
Stylomastoid foramen
Mastoid process

Ala of vomer
Vaginal process of palatine bone
Palatinovaginal canal
Pterygoid canal
Foramen lacerum
Gutter for auditory tube
Pharyngeal tubercle
Carotid canal
Tympanic canal
Jugular foramen
Hypoglossal canal

Figure 6-9 Features of intermediate area.

179

1. The **mastoid process** of the temporal bone, which provides the site of insertion for the *sternomastoid muscle*
2. The **styloid process,** a long, slender, needlelike process that points downward, forward, and medially that is joined to the lesser horn of the hyoid bone by the *stylohyoid ligament;* also provides attachment for several muscles
3. The **stylomastoid foramen,** which lies between the styloid and mastoid processes, allowing passage of the *facial nerve (cranial nerve VII)* from within the temporal bone
4. The **jugular foramen,** a large opening through which the *internal jugular vein* and *cranial nerves IX, X, and XI* pass
5. The **entrance to the carotid canal,** which is immediately anterior to the jugular foramen and separated from the jugular foramen only by a small wedge of bone. (Passing through the canal is the *internal carotid artery* on its way to the brain within the skull.)
6. The **occipital condyles,** two convex, bean-shaped articular processes on either side of the foramen magnum that articulate below with the reciprocally shaped superior articulating facets of the *atlas*
7. The **foramen magnum,** the large, egg-shaped opening that transmits the *spinal cord, its meninges,* and the *spinal accessory portion of cranial nerve XI*

Posterior Area. All but one of the features found in this area are described with the posterior view of the skull.

The **posterior condylar canal** is a canal occasionally found passing obliquely from the skull to exit on the base of the skull just posterior to the occipital condyle. It transmits an *emissary vein.*

INTERNAL ASPECT OF THE BASE

To expose the internal features of the skull, the skullcap (calvaria) is sawn off and removed.

Bones
The bones seen in this view are the **frontal bone,** the **ethmoid bone,** the **sphenoid bone** (including the body, lesser wings, and greater wings), the **right** and **left temporal bones,** and the **occipital bone** (*Figure 6-10, A*).

Regions
The internal configuration of the base of the skull is conveniently tiered and named as three cranial fossae (*Figure 6-10, B*):

1. The **anterior cranial fossa** is bounded by the upward sweep of the frontal bone anteriorly and the sharp free borders of the lesser wings of the sphenoid bone posteriorly. It contains the *frontal lobes of the cerebrum.*
2. The **middle cranial fossa** is bounded posteriorly by the paramedian dorsum sellae and by two oblique petrous

temporal ridges, which sweep back and laterally from the dorsum sellae. The middle cranial fossa accommodates the *hypophysis cerebri* in the median plane and the *temporal lobes* of the brain laterally.
3. The **posterior cranial fossa** is bounded posteriorly by the posterior upsweep of the occipital bone and occupied by the *cerebellum,* the occipital lobes of the *cerebrum,* and the *brainstem.*

Features (*Figures 6-10,C and 6-11*)
Anterior Cranial Fossa
1. The *frontal crest* of the frontal bone is a midline bony extension into the anterior cranial fossa anteriorly. It serves as the bony attachment for the *falx cerebri.*
2. The **crista galli** ("crest of the rooster") of the ethmoid bone projects upward in the midline as a posterior extension of the frontal crest. It also provides attachment for the *falx cerebri.*
3. The cribriform plates of the ethmoid bone are perforated areas on either side of the crista galli. The small perforations communicate with the roof of the nasal cavity below and transmit the *olfactory nerve (cranial nerve I).*
4. The **foramen cecum** is a blind-ended opening between the crista galli and the frontal crest. In the fetal period this opening is patent and transmits an *emissary vein.*
5. The **orbital plates** of the frontal bone are convex elevations to either side of the cribriform plates. The orbital plates form the roof of the bony orbit below.
6. The **ethmoidal foramina** are two small openings on the anterior aspect of the cribriform plate that transmit the anterior ethmoidal nerves to the nasal cavity.

Middle Cranial Fossa. Features of the middle cranial fossa include the following:
1. The **sella turcica** (*Figure 6-11*), which translates as a "Turkish saddle."
2. The **hypophyseal (pituitary) fossa,** which is a concavity that resembles a rider's seat in the saddle and accommodates the *hypophysis cerebri,* or *pituitary gland.*
3. The **optic canals,** which pass obliquely laterally and forward to the orbits and transmit the *optic nerves (cranial nerve II)* and the *ophthalmic arteries.*
4. The **dorsum sellae,** which is literally the back of the saddle.
5. The **anterior clinoid processes,** which extend posteriorly from the lesser wing of the sphenoid bone and provide *attachments for dura.*
6. The **posterior clinoid processes,** which extend posteriorly from either end of the dorsum sellae and likewise provide *dural attachments.*
7. The **foramen lacerum,** which provides an opening on either side of the hypophyseal fossa for the entrance of the *internal carotid artery.* (If a pipe cleaner is

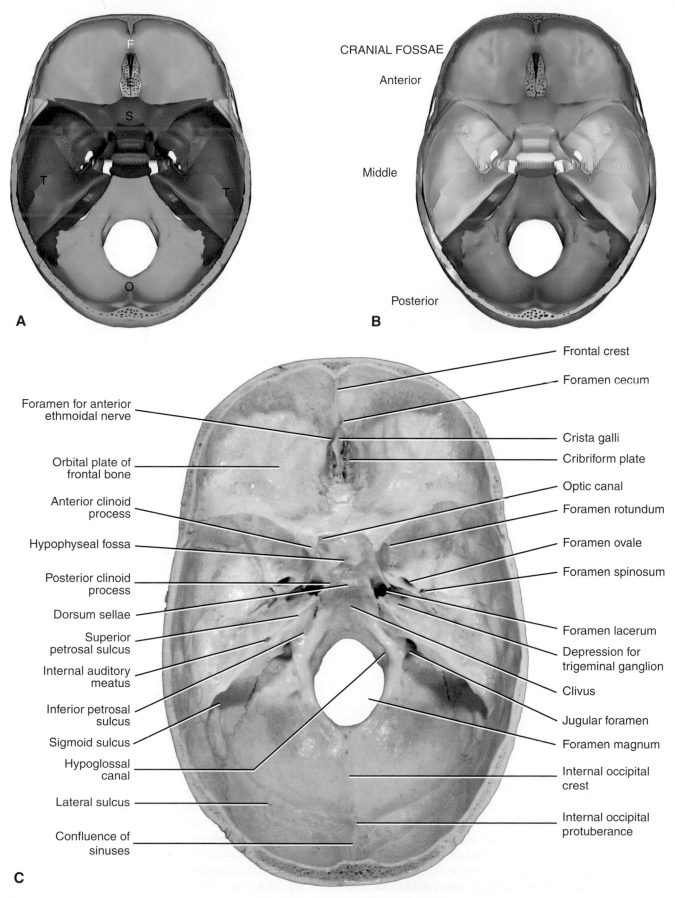

CRANIAL FOSSAE

Anterior

Middle

Posterior

A

B

Frontal crest

Foramen cecum

Foramen for anterior ethmoidal nerve

Crista galli

Orbital plate of frontal bone

Cribriform plate

Optic canal

Anterior clinoid process

Foramen rotundum

Hypophyseal fossa

Foramen ovale

Posterior clinoid process

Foramen spinosum

Dorsum sellae

Superior petrosal sulcus

Foramen lacerum

Internal auditory meatus

Depression for trigeminal ganglion

Inferior petrosal sulcus

Clivus

Sigmoid sulcus

Jugular foramen

Hypoglossal canal

Foramen magnum

Lateral sulcus

Internal occipital crest

Confluence of sinuses

Internal occipital protuberance

C

Figure 6-10 Internal view of base of skull with calvaria removed. **A,** Bones. **B,** Three tiered cranial fossae. **C,** Features.

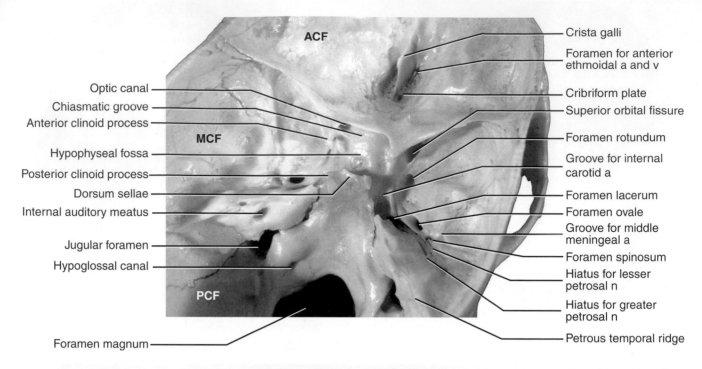

Figure 6-11 Features of middle cranial fossa as seen from a right superior oblique view.

introduced into the carotid canal, it can be seen that the carotid canal communicates with the foramen lacerum as a "T-junction." The internal carotid artery passes through the canal, continues superiorly through the upper portion of the foramen lacerum, and enters the middle cranial fossa. The artery marks a groove on the lateral aspect of the sella turcica as it travels anteriorly within the skull.)

8. The **depression for the trigeminal ganglion,** which sits near the apex of the petrous portion of the temporal bone, where it butts against the body of the sphenoid bone.

9. The **superior orbital fissure,** is an inverted, comma-shaped gap between the greater and lesser wings of the sphenoid bone found under the cover of the lesser wing that communicates with the orbit anteriorly and through which pass the *ophthalmic veins* and *cranial nerves III, IV, VI,* and *V-1.*

10. The **foramen rotundum,** a round opening posterior to the inferior orbital fissure that opens obliquely forward and inferiorly to lead to the pterygopalatine fossa; transmits the *maxillary nerve (cranial nerve V-2).*

11. The **foramen ovale,** an oval-shaped opening posterior to the foramen rotundum that leads to the infratemporal region below the skull and transmits the *mandibular nerve (cranial nerve V-3).*

12. The **foramen spinosum,** which lies immediately behind and lateral to the foramen ovale, is a small, round opening leading from the infratemporal region below that transmits the *middle meningeal artery.* (The grooves of the artery may be followed laterally and superiorly

within the skull to the point where the artery divides into an anterior and a posterior branch.)

13. The **hiatus for the greater petrosal nerve,** which exits from the anterior slope of the petrous temporal ridge (A groove can be followed to the foramen lacerum. The hiatus and groove transmit the *greater petrosal nerve* from the depths of the petrous temporal bone to the foramen lacerum of the middle cranial fossa.)

14. The **hiatus** and **groove for the lesser petrosal nerve,** which run parallel and inferior to the greater superficial hiatus and groove, which leads toward the foramen ovale and transmits the *lesser petrosal nerve.*

Posterior Cranial Fossa

1. The **superior petrosal sulcus** is a narrow, shallow groove that runs along the crest of the petrous temporal ridge and is occupied by the *superior petrosal venous sinus.*

2. The **inferior petrosal sulcus** runs from the lateral aspect of the dorsum sellae downward and backward between the petrous temporal bone and the basiocciput. It carries the *inferior petrosal venous sinus* toward the jugular foramen.

3. The **clivus** is the body of the sphenoid bone behind the dorsum sellae, which fuses to the basiocciput at the spheno-occipital synchondrosis during adolescence. The clivus slopes posteriorly and inferiorly to end as the anterior margin of the foramen magnum.

4. The **foramen magnum** is a large, oval-shaped opening through which the spinal cord is continuous with the brainstem above.

5. The **anterior condylar canal (hypoglossal canal)** is found on the lateral margin of the foramen magnum anterior to the occipital condyle. It runs obliquely anteriorly and laterally, carrying the *hypoglossal nerve (cranial nerve XII)* to the base of the skull below.

6. The **jugular foramen** is a large opening lateral to the foramen magnum that leads to the base of the skull below. It transmits the *internal jugular vein* and *cranial nerves IX, X,* and *XI*.

7. The **internal auditory meatus** lies on the posterior slope of the petrous temporal ridge just above the jugular foramen. Passing through this opening to the middle ear region within the temporal bone are *cranial nerves VII* and *VIII*.

8. The **internal occipital protuberance** is an internal projection of bone at the posterior pole of the internal aspect of the skull.

9. The **area of the confluence** is just above the internal occipital protuberance, and it represents the junction of the lateral venous sinuses.

10. The **transverse sulcus** runs laterally from the confluence, curves anteriorly, and on encountering the petrous temporal ridge, curves medially as the sigmoid sulcus. The transverse sulcus contains the *lateral venous sinus*.

11. The **sigmoid sulcus** is shaped like an S and houses the *sigmoid venous sinus*. It drains to the jugular foramen medially.

12. The **internal occipital crest** runs downward and forward from the area of the confluence to the posterior border of the foramen magnum.

KEY SECTIONS THROUGH THE SKULL

Two key cuts, sagittal and coronal, through the skull provide more insight into how individual bones contribute to the architecture of the skull and demonstrate the various cavities found within the skull (*Figure 6-12*). The cavities are of two types: (1) craniofacial (functional cavities) and (2) paranasal air sinuses.

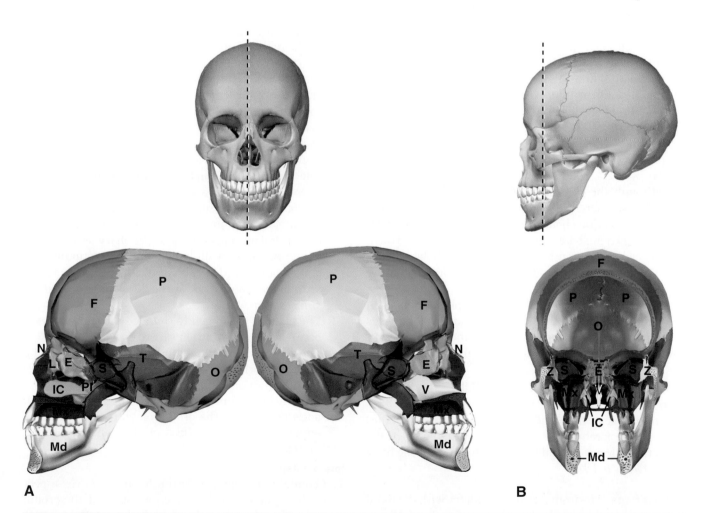

A

B

Figure 6-12 Two key sections through skull to demonstrate bony relationships and cranial cavities. **A,** Sagittal section to one side of nasal septum showing nasal septum intact on one side and removed from opposite side. **B,** Coronal section through first molar region.

Cranial Facial Cavities

Within the skull are four main functional cavities. The **neurocranial cavity** encloses and protects the *brain*, the **orbital cavities** house and protect the eyeballs, the **oral cavity** is a functional area devoted to *mastication* and *respiration*, and the **nasal cavities** are functional areas devoted to *olfaction* and *respiration*.

Paranasal Air Sinuses

Paranasal air sinuses are hollow spaces within certain bones that are clustered around the nose. In life these hollow sinuses are lined with respiratory mucosa and communicate directly with the nasal cavities. The sinuses seen in the sections include the **frontal sinuses** within the frontal bone, the **maxillary sinuses** within the right and left maxillae, the **ethmoid sinuses** within the ethmoid bone, and the **sphenoid sinuses** within the body of the sphenoid bone. The paranasal air sinuses are described in Chapter 7.

3. Bones

From a functional point of view, it seems questionable to study the individual bones of the skull. Aside from the temporomandibular joint and the interossicle joints of the middle ear, the joints of the skull are rigid sutures, or synchondroses. Therefore the skull is essentially a solid bone. In addition, soft tissues generally show little regard for interbone boundaries. The origin of the temporalis muscle, for example, spans five individual bones.

Although the skull is rigid, the individual bones do "move" in a different sense. During active growth of the skeleton the various bones of the skull grow individually and undergo remodeling. In the process each bone, in turn, is displaced in relation to the other bones. Relationships among the various bones are constantly changing during the active growth period.

A thorough knowledge of the morphology of each bone and the relationships of the various skull bones is of fundamental importance in understanding the growth and development of the craniofacial complex.

BONES OF THE NEUROCRANIUM
Frontal Bone (Single)

Contributions to the Skull. The frontal bone contributes to the entire forehead region and anterior region of the scalp, the anterior cranial fossa, and the roof of the bony orbits (*Figure 6-13*).

Articulations. The frontal bone articulates with the nasal bones, the maxillae, the lacrimal bones, the ethmoid bone, the sphenoid bone, the zygomatic bones, and the parietal bones.

Parts and Features
Anterior (External) Aspect

1. The **squamous portion** of the anterior aspect is the convex, curved portion that forms the vault of the forehead externally (*Figure 6-14, A*).
2. The **orbital plates** are two plates of thin bone that project posteriorly from the anteroinferior border of the frontal bone. The orbital plates form the roof of the orbital cavities and the floor of the anterior cranial fossa.
3. The **ethmoidal notch** is a roughly rectangular deficiency between the orbital plates. The notch represents the area of articulation with the ethmoid bone.
4. The **supraorbital margin** is a concave ridge between the external aspect of the orbital plate and the squamous portion.
5. The **medial angular process** represents the medial termination of the supraorbital margin.
6. Between the medial angular processes is the **nasal margin**, which represents the jagged articulation with the nasal bone.
7. Projecting anteriorly from the median aspect of the nasal margin is the **nasal spine**. The inferior surface of the nasal spine forms a tiny portion of the roof of the nasal cavity.
8. The **zygomatic process** of the frontal bone is the lateral limit of the superior orbital margin and is one of the supporting buttresses of the zygomatic arch and articulates with the zygomatic bone. The posterior aspect of the zygomatic process sweeps upward and backward as the inferior temporal line.
9. The **supraorbital notch,** or **foramen,** transmits the *supraorbital nerve* and *vessels.* It is located in the medial third of the superior orbital margin.
10. Slight elevations just above and parallel to the superior orbital margins are the **superciliary arches**. They are pronounced in adult men, are less pronounced in adult women, and are absent in children. They represent the ballooning out of the developing *frontal air sinuses* from within.
11. The **glabella** is the gently rounded median elevation between the right and left superciliary arches.
12. The **lacrimal fossa** is a slight lateral depression on the inferior, or orbital, aspect of the orbital plate. It lodges the deep portion of the *lacrimal gland.*
13. The **trochlear depression** is a small pit at the medial anterior angle of the orbital plate. It represents the attachment of the *trochlea* of the superior oblique muscle of the eye.

Internal Aspect

1. **Cerebral markings** appear on the inner convex aspect of the squama and the superior aspect of the orbital plates (*Figure 6-14, B*). They represent the various sulci and *gyri of the frontal lobes* of the cerebral hemispheres.

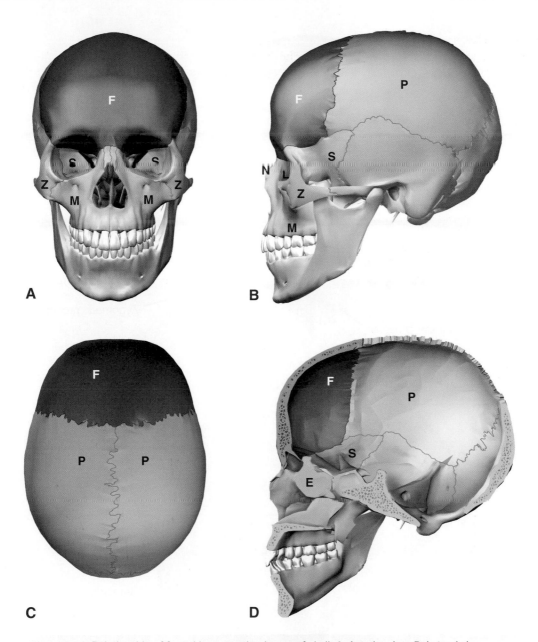

Figure 6-13 Relationship of frontal bone to other bones of skull. **A**, Anterior view. **B**, Lateral view. **C**, Superior view. **D**, Sagittal section with nasal septum intact.

2. The **frontal crest** is a midline ridge of bone on the internal aspect. It sweeps forward and up on the inner squama in the midline and serves as the anterior anchor for the *falx cerebri.*

3. The **superior sagittal sulcus** is the upward continuation of the frontal crest that splits to form the lips of the groove. The superior sagittal sulcus houses the *superior sagittal venous sinus* at the base of the falx cerebri.

Development. The frontal bone develops from two membranous ossification centers at the future sites of the fron-

tal eminences during the seventh fetal week. At birth, right and left frontal bones are present, separated by a midline metopic, or interfrontal, suture. The suture begins to fuse during the first year of life and is usually obliterated at 6 years of age. Remnants of the metopic suture generally persist just below the glabella. The entire suture occasionally remains unossified.

The Parietal Bone (Paired)

Contributions. The parietal bones form portions of the superior, lateral, and posterior aspects of the cranial vault (*Figure 6-15*).

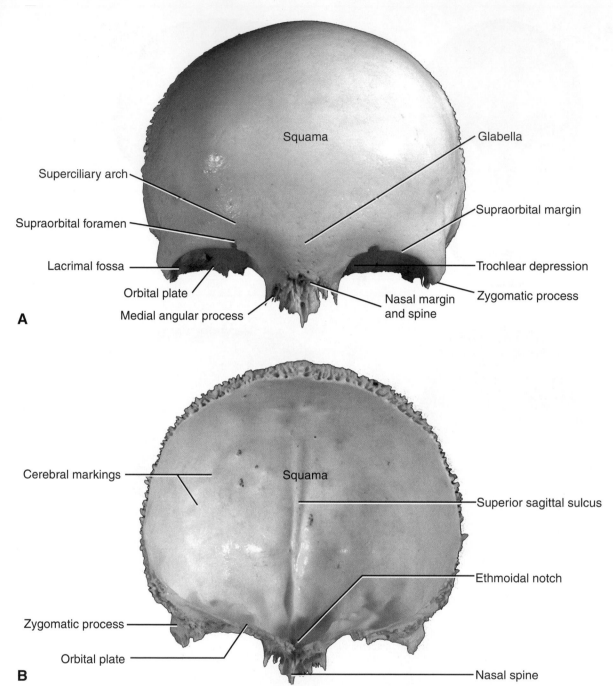

Figure 6-14 Feature of the frontal bone. **A**, Anterior view. **B**, Internal view.

Articulations. The parietal bone articulates with the opposite parietal bone, the frontal bone, the occipital bone, the temporal bone, and the sphenoid bone (greater wing).

Parts and Features. The parietal bone is a relatively simple, curved bone with a convex outer surface, a concave inner surface, four borders that articulate with the remaining calvaria, and four angles. For orientation the superior border presents extremely sharp projections; the inferior border is smooth, concave, and sharp, to overlap the squama of the temporal bone below. The anteroinferior (sphenoid) angle is sharp and acute; the posteroinferior angle (mastoid angle) is obtuse.

Lateral (External) Aspect
1. **Temporal lines** are found on the outer surface as two faint, parallel, curved, linear elevations that sweep across the lateral surface as an arc. They mark the site

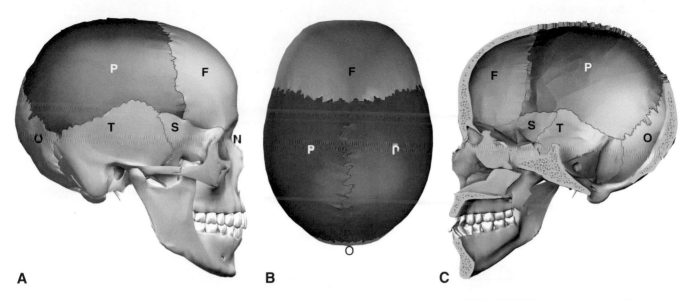

Figure 6-15 Relationship of right parietal bone to the other bones of skull. **A,** Lateral view. **B,** Superior view. **C,** Sagittal section with nasal septum removed.

of origin of the *temporalis muscle* and provide attachment for temporalis fascia and muscle (*Figure 6-16, A*).

2. The **parietal eminence** is the highest point of contour on the external surface. It is the site of initial ossification of the parietal bone.

Internal Aspect

1. **Cerebral markings** are found on the internal aspect and reflect underlying sulci and *gyri of the parietal lobes* of the cerebral hemisphere (*Figure 6-16, B*).
2. **Depressions for arachnoid granulations** parallel the superior border along the internal aspect.
3. **Middle meningeal grooves** mark the route of the posterior and anterior branches of the *middle meningeal artery* as they track along the inner surface.
4. The **transverse sulcus** containing the *transverse venous sinus* cuts across the internal aspect of the posteroinferior angle.

Development. The parietal bone develops in membrane at the site of the future parietal eminence during the seventh week of fetal life. Unlike the frontal bone the parietal bones do not fuse after birth. They may, however, begin to fuse as one bone in the third decade of life.

Occipital Bone (Single)

Contributions. The occipital bone forms the posteroinferior aspect of the cranial vault and the posterior aspect of the posterior cranial fossa (*Figure 6-17*).

Articulations. The occipital bone articulates with the right and left parietal bones, the right and left temporal bones, and the sphenoid bone. The occipital bone and sphenoid bone fuse after adolescence.

Parts and Features. The occipital bone can be divided into four parts, based on development. The four parts develop separately around the future foramen magnum and eventually fuse to form one single adult bone.

1. The **squama** is the curved, thin, saucer-shaped portion posterior to the foramen magnum.
2 and 3. The **right** and **left condylar portions** bear the occipital condyles and lie laterally to the foramen magnum.
4. The **basilar portion** is anterior to the foramen magnum.

External Aspect

1. The **external occipital protuberance**, or **inion**, occupies the central external aspect of the squama (*Figure 6-18, A*). It may be a prominent lump of bone or may be inconspicuous.
2. The **superior nuchal lines** arch to the right and left from the central inion. They provide attachments for **neck**, or **nuchal**, **muscles**.
3. The **inferior nuchal lines** run parallel to the superior set and represent insertions of *nuchal muscles*.
4. Running in a parallel arc above the superior nuchal lines are the **highest nuchal lines**, which are less distinct.
5. The **external occipital crest** extends from the inion to the posterior lip of the foramen magnum. Attached to it is the *ligamentum nuchae*.
6. The **foramen magnum** is a large, oval-shaped foramen on the inferior aspect of the occipital bone. As the spinal cord passes upward through the foramen magnum, it becomes the brainstem.

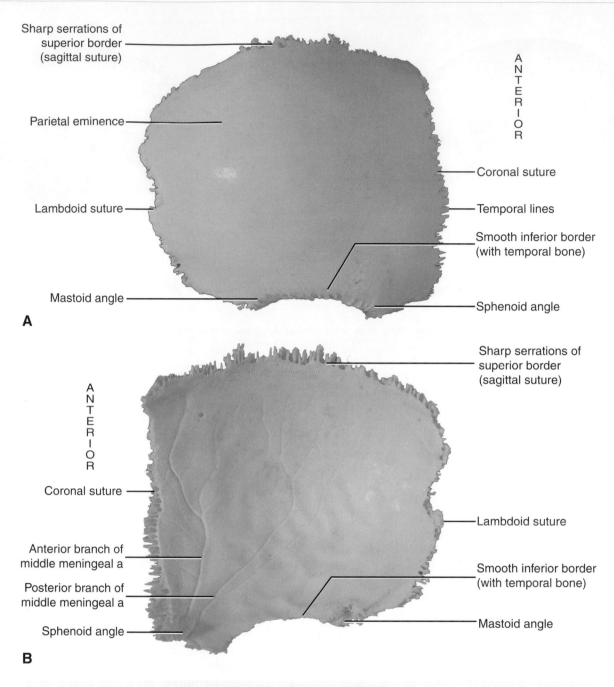

Sharp serrations of
superior border
(sagittal suture)

Parietal eminence

Lambdoid suture

Mastoid angle

A

ANTERIOR

Coronal suture

Temporal lines

Smooth inferior border
(with temporal bone)

Sphenoid angle

Sharp serrations of
superior border
(sagittal suture)

ANTERIOR

Coronal suture

Anterior branch of
middle meningeal a

Posterior branch of
middle meningeal a

Sphenoid angle

B

Lambdoid suture

Smooth inferior border
(with temporal bone)

Mastoid angle

Figure 6-16 Features of right parietal bone. **A**, External view. **B**, Internal view.

7. The **occipital condyles** are bean-shaped articular processes on the external aspect, perched on the lateral margins of the foramen magnum. The condyles articulate with the reciprocally shaped *superior articular processes of the atlas*.

Internal Aspect

1. The **internal occipital protuberance** is the internal median projection at the midpoint of the internal squamosal surface (*Figure 6-18, B*).

2. The **superior sagittal sulcus** sweeps upward from the internal occipital protuberance. It houses the posterior aspect of the *superior sagittal venous sinus* and is the base of attachment for the *falx cerebri*.

3. The **right** and **left transverse sulci** radiate out to either side of the internal occipital protuberance. They house the right and left *transverse venous sinuses* and form the base for the *tentorium cerebelli*.

4. The **internal occipital crest** slopes downward and forward from the internal occipital protuberance to the posterior margin of the foramen magnum. It marks the attachment of the *falx cerebelli*.

5. *Cerebral* and *cerebellar markings* disclose the presence of sulci and *gyri of the occipital lobes of the*

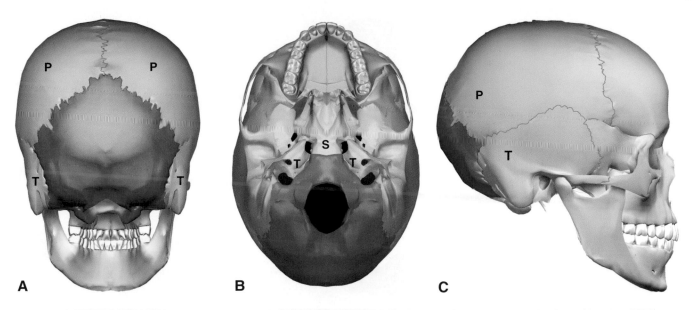

Figure 6-17 Relationship of occipital bone to the other bones of the skull. **A,** Posterior view. **B,** Inferior view. **C,** Lateral view.

cerebral hemispheres above the transverse sulci and of the *cerebellum* below the transverse sulci.

6. The **jugular processes** project as bony bars laterally from the foramen magnum.

7. The **jugular foramen** is formed posteriorly by the jugular process of the occipital bone and anteriorly by the petrous portion of the temporal bone. The internal aspect of the foramen exhibits a fossa for the funnel-like jugular bulb to which all the cranial venous sinuses ultimately drain to form the *internal jugular vein*. The foramen also transmits *cranial nerves IX, X,* and *XI.*

8. The **anterior condylar (hypoglossal) canal** is an opening that originates from the lateral margin of the foramen magnum and runs obliquely forward to end on the anterior aspect of the base of the occipital condyle. The canal is traversed by the *hypoglossal nerve (cranial nerve XII).*

9. The **posterior condylar canal** originates from the internal aspect of the occipital bone near the jugular foramen and passes obliquely through the base of the occipital condyle to end on the external aspect of the skull behind the condyle. An *emissary vein* passes through it.

10. The **basiocciput** is a block of bone that extends anteriorly from the foramen magnum. It ends as a butt-end against the body of the sphenoid bone anteriorly at the *spheno-occipital synchondrosis.* The synchondrosis fuses during adolescence, uniting the basiocciput and the body of the sphenoid as the clivus.

Development. The occipital bone begins to develop in the eighth week of life. The squama above the superior nuchal line begins to form in membrane. The squama below this region, the condylar portions, and the basiocciput develop within cartilage. At birth the occipital bone is in four parts surrounding the foramen magnum: the squama, the right and left condylar portions, and the basiocciput. At age 4 years the squamous and condylar portions fuse, and at age 6 years the basilar and condylar portions fuse.

At approximately 16 years of age the spheno-occipital synchondrosis fuses, thus joining the basiocciput and the body of the sphenoid.

Temporal Bone (Paired)

Contribution to the Skull. The temporal bones contribute to the lower lateral aspects of the cranial vault and the cranial base (*Figure 6-19*). The temporal bones form the posterolateral aspect of the middle cranial fossa and the anterolateral aspect of the posterior cranial fossa.

Articulations. The temporal bone articulates with the occipital bone, the parietal bone, the sphenoid bone (greater wing and body), and the zygomatic bone. In addition, it articulates with the mandible through the movable temporomandibular joint.

Parts. The temporal bone forms initially as three separate components that ultimately fuse. The names of the components are retained, however, in the adult bones as three areas. Each portion of the temporal bone is centered on the external auditory meatus.

1. The **squamous portion**, or **squama**, is the flattened portion of the bone. It includes the slender zygomatic process of the temporal bone. The squama presents an external surface on the lateral aspect of the cranial vault and an internal, or cerebral, surface.

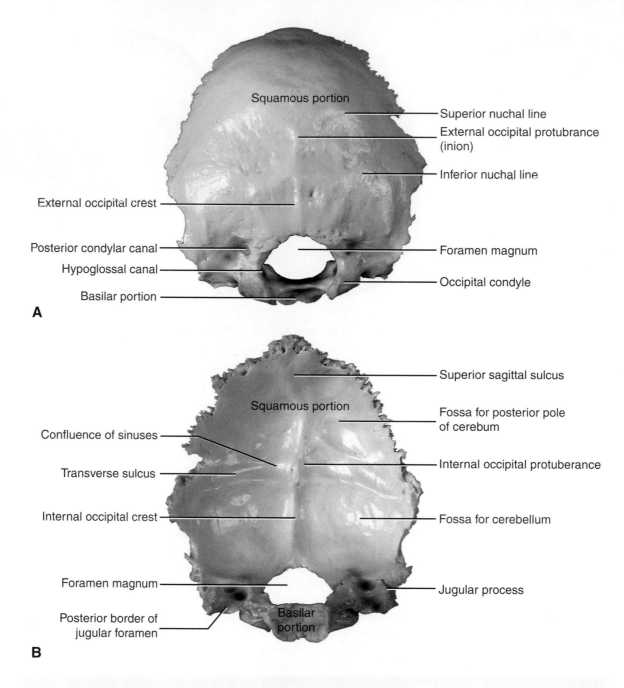

Figure 6-18 Features of the occipital bone. **A,** External view. **B,** Internal view.

2. The **petromastoid portion** (*petrous*, meaning "like a rock") more or less describes the substantially thicker, pyramid-shaped portion of the temporal bone. The mastoid process is visible from the lateral aspect as a large, inferior elevation. The remainder of the petrous portion forms the large, thick ridge that separates the middle and posterior cranial fossae within the skull. The petrous portion also contributes to the external base of the skull.

Within the petrous temporal bone lie the middle ear chamber with its three ossicles and the inner ear with its cochlea and semicircular canals.

3. The **tympanic portion** is present at birth as a ring of bone deficient superiorly. The ring extends medially to form the floor, anterior wall, and a portion of the posterior wall of the external auditory meatus. The tympanic portion extends medially and downward as a plate of bone to form the posterior wall of the mandibular fossa.

Features

Lateral Aspect

1. The **zygomatic process** is a long, slender process that projects anteriorly from the lateral aspect (*Figure 6-20, A*)

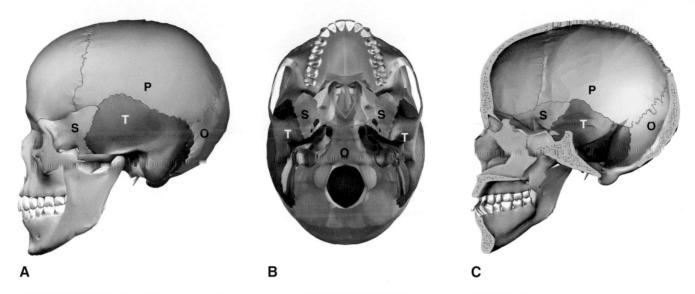

Figure 6-19 Relationship of the right temporal bone to the other bones of the skull. **A,** Lateral view. **B,** Inferior view. **C,** Sagittal section with nasal septum removed.

of the squama. The zygoma forms the *posterior root of the zygomatic arch.*

2. The **mastoid process** is a large lump of bone on the posterolateral surface. It forms in the first year of life in response to the muscle pull of the *sternocleidomastoid muscle.* Within, it contains many air-filled spaces (*mastoid antrum*) that communicate with the middle ear.

3. The **external auditory meatus** is an oval-shaped opening and canal anterior to the mastoid process. It leads to the chamber of the middle ear within the petrous portion.

4. The **supramastoid crest** follows the superior border of the zygomatic process backward above the mastoid process. It then sweeps upward as the posteroinferior portion of the temporal lines.

5. The **suprameatal triangle** lies between the superior border of the external auditory meatus and the supramastoid crest. The triangle marks the surgeon's approach to the mastoid antrum within.

6. The **mandibular fossa** is seen from the lateral aspect as a concavity anterior to the external auditory meatus.

7. The **glenoid tubercle** is the lateral aspect of the *articular eminence.* It gives rise to the *temporomandibular ligament.*

8. The **postglenoid tubercle** is a small wedge of bone between the tympanic plate of the external auditory meatus and the mandibular fossa.

Internal Aspect

1. **Cerebral fossae** and **ridges** on the inner aspect of the squama are marked by the *gyri* and *sulci of the temporal lobes* of the brain (*Figure 6-20, B*).

2. The **groove for the middle meningeal artery** marks the path of the artery on the inner aspect of the squama.

3. The **petrous temporal ridge** is a prominent feature of the internal aspect of the skull. It runs laterally and posteriorly from the body of the sphenoid and effectively separates the middle cranial fossa anteriorly from the posterior cranial fossa posteriorly.

4. The **anterior slope**, or cerebral surface, is in contact with the temporal lobes of the brain.

5. The **posterior slope**, or cerebellar surface, is in contact with the cerebellum.

6. The **superior petrosal sulcus** runs along the crest of the petrous ridge and houses the *superior petrosal venous sinus.*

7. The **sigmoid sulcus** is a wide depression on the lateral aspect of the posterior slope. It contains the *sigmoid venous sinus,* which empties toward the jugular foramen. The *mastoid foramen* is an opening within the sulcus that transmits an *emissary vein.*

8. The **jugular foramen** is formed anteriorly by the posterior slope of the petrous portion; posteriorly, it is formed by the occipital bone. Passing through the jugular foramen are the *internal jugular vein* and *cranial nerves IX, X,* and *XI.*

9. The **internal auditory meatus** is an opening on the posterior petrous slope. The meatus passes into the petrous bone and transmits two *cranial nerves: VII* and *VIII.* The *facial nerve* enters the meatus, passes through the petrous bone via the facial canal, and exits inferiorly through the stylomastoid foramen at the external base of the skull. The *vestibulocochlear nerve* enters the meatus to supply the cochlea and the semicircular canals of the inner ear.

10. The **greater petrosal hiatus** opens onto the anterior slope of the petrous ridge as a tiny slit. It transmits the

191

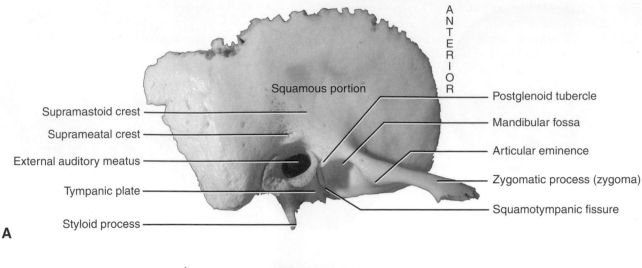

Supramastoid crest

Suprameatal crest

External auditory meatus

Tympanic plate

Styloid process

Squamous portion

ANTERIOR

Postglenoid tubercle

Mandibular fossa

Articular eminence

Zygomatic process (zygoma)

Squamotympanic fissure

A

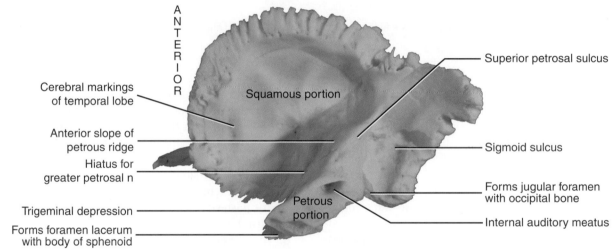

ANTERIOR

Cerebral markings
of temporal lobe

Anterior slope of
petrous ridge

Hiatus for
greater petrosal n

Trigeminal depression

Forms foramen lacerum
with body of sphenoid

Squamous portion

Petrous
portion

Superior petrosal sulcus

Sigmoid sulcus

Forms jugular foramen
with occipital bone

Internal auditory meatus

B

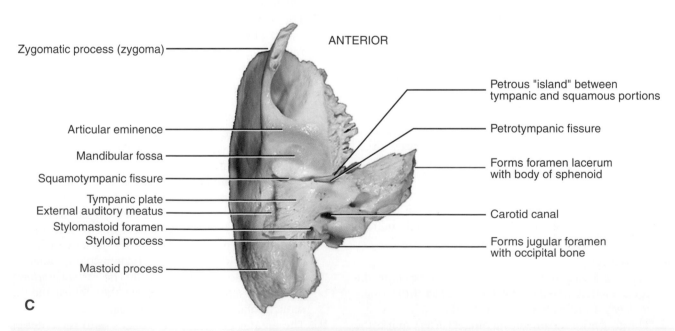

Zygomatic process (zygoma)

ANTERIOR

Articular eminence

Mandibular fossa

Squamotympanic fissure

Tympanic plate

External auditory meatus

Stylomastoid foramen

Styloid process

Mastoid process

Petrous "island" between
tympanic and squamous portions

Petrotympanic fissure

Forms foramen lacerum
with body of sphenoid

Carotid canal

Forms jugular foramen
with occipital bone

C

Figure 6-20 Right temporal bone. **A,** External view. **B,** Internal view. **C,** Inferior view.

greater petrosal branch of cranial nerve VII to the middle cranial fossa from the facial canal.

11. The **lesser petrosal hiatus** opens onto the anterior petrous slope just below the greater hiatus. It transmits the *lesser petrosal branch of cranial nerve IX* to the middle cranial fossa from the middle ear.

12. The **trigeminal depression** is a rounded, depressed area on the anterior petrous slope near the apex. The depression accommodates the *trigeminal ganglion.*

13. The **posterior and lateral margins of the foramen lacerum** are formed by the blunted apex of the petrous temporal. The upper portion of the foramen lacerum transmits the *internal carotid artery.*

Inferior Aspect

1. The **mandibular fossa** is an oval depression on the inferior aspect. The anterior walls and roof belong to the squama and are lined with articular cartilage. The posterior wall is formed by the flat tympanic plate, which is not an articular portion of the temporomandibular joint (*Figure 6-20, C*).

2. The **squamotympanic fissure** marks the separation of the roof and posterior wall of the mandibular fossa. A small island of petrous bone appears within the medial half of the suture and complicates the nomenclature. The medial half of the fissure becomes the *petrotympanic* and the *petrosquamous sutures* on either side of the small wedge of petrous temporal bone. The *chorda tympani,* an important branch of the facial nerve, passes through the *petrotympanic fissure.*

3. The **articular eminence** is a rounded ridge of bone that runs transversely across the anterior limit of the mandibular fossa. The articular eminence is a functional and articular portion of the temporomandibular joint.

4. The **carotid canal** is found on the inferior aspect anterior to the jugular foramen. The canal curves superiorly and medially to join the foramen lacerum.

5. The **digastric notch** represents the origin of the *posterior belly of the digastric muscle.* The notch is immediately deep to the mastoid process.

6. The **styloid process** is a sharp, slender process that angles inferiorly, medially, and anteriorly. It provides attachment for a number of muscles and two ligaments. A portion of the tympanic plate wraps itself around the base of the styloid like a scroll. This is the *vaginal process* of the temporal bone.

7. The **stylomastoid foramen** is a small opening between the styloid and mastoid processes. It marks the end of the facial canal; issuing from the foramen is the *facial nerve* (cranial nerve VII).

8. The **auditory (pharyngotympanic) canal** is found on the inferior surface, running medially from under the cover of the medial border of the tympanic plate. It leads laterally to the middle ear cavity within the petrous bone. Medially it opens into a gutter, or trough, bordered by the sphenoid bone anteriorly and the petrous temporal bone posteriorly. The trough heads medially toward the area of the nasopharynx and, in life, houses the cartilaginous and membranous components of the *auditory tube.*

9. The **tympanic canal** is a small opening located inferiorly on the wedge of bone separating the carotid canal and the jugular foramen. The tympanic canal transmits the *tympanic branch of the glossopharyngeal nerve (cranial nerve IX).*

10. The **middle** and **internal ear** within the petrous temporal bone are discussed in Chapter 7.

Development. The squamous and tympanic portions of the temporal bone begin to develop in membrane during the eighth fetal week. The petromastoid portion develops in cartilage. At birth the three separate elements begin to unite during the first year of life.

The ossicles and the styloid process develop from the first two branchial arches. The middle ear cavity forms from the first pharyngeal cleft.

The Sphenoid Bone (Single)

Contributions. The sphenoid bone contributes to the following regions of the skull: anterior cranial fossa, middle cranial fossa, orbit, infratemporal roof, pterygopalatine fossa, roof and lateral wall of the nasal cavity, and lateral wall of the cranial vault (*Figure 6-21*).

Articulations. The sphenoid bone articulates with the ethmoid bone, the frontal bone, the temporal bones, the parietal bones, the zygomatic bones, the palatine bones, the vomer, and occipital bone.

Parts. The sphenoid bone is a key bone in understanding the architecture of the skull (*Figure 6-22*); however, it is also a complicated bone, and to understand its form takes a bit of fanciful imagination.

The sphenoid bone, when viewed anteriorly, resembles an owl complete with body, face, ears, wings, and legs.

1. The **body** is a hollow, cube-shaped structure that supports three pairs of processes.
2. The **lesser wings** are the ears of the owl and protrude from the superoanterior aspect of the body.
3. The **greater wings** are the wings of the owl, protruding from the lateral aspects of the body.
4. The **pterygoid processes** are the legs of the owl and descend from the inferior aspect of the body.

At the base of each process, where it is fixed to the body, is an opening.

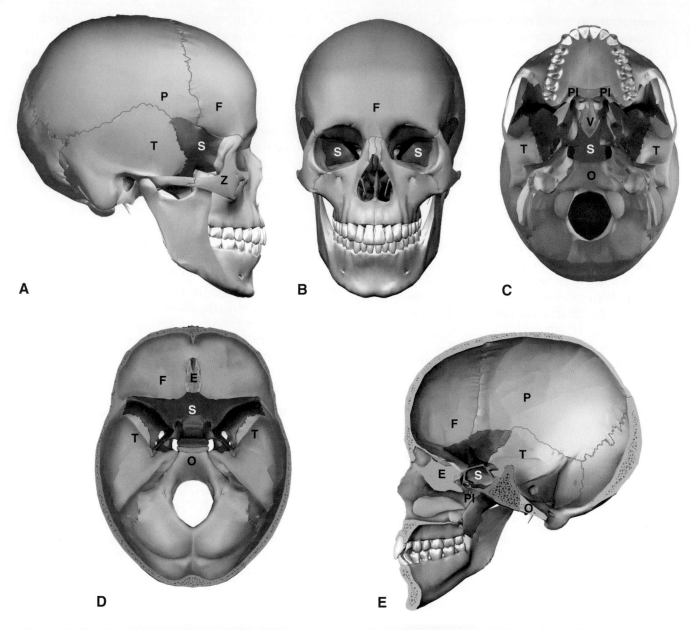

Figure 6-21 Relationship of sphenoid bone to the other bones of the skull. **A**, Lateral view. **B**, Anterior view. **C**, Inferior view. **D**, Internal aspect of cranial base. **E**, Sagittal section with nasal septum removed.

Features

Body

1. The **ethmoidal spine** is an anterior sharp projection from the superoanterior aspect of the midline.
2. Continuing downward from the ethmoidal spine as a midline sharp ridge of bone is the **sphenoidal crest**.
3. The **rostrum**, or beak of the owl, is the inferior spiny ending of the sphenoidal crest.
4. **Ostia**, or openings, of the sphenoidal air sinuses are the eyes of the owl. They are on either side of the sphenoidal crest, about two thirds of the way up from the inferior aspect.

5. The ostia lead to the **paranasal air sinuses** of the sphenoid within the body. The size of the sinuses is variable.
6. The **sella turcica** occupies the superior aspect of the body. *Sella turcica* means "Turkish saddle," complete with pommel, seat, and back.
7. The **tuberculum sellae** is the pommel, a transverse ridge of bone marking the anterior limit of the saddle.
8. The **chiasmatic groove** runs anterior to the tuberculum sellae. It accommodates the *optic nerve* and *chiasma.*
9. The **dorsum sellae** is the back of the saddle.
10. The **hypophyseal fossa** is the seat of the saddle and houses the *hypophysis cerebri* (*pituitary gland*).

11. Lateral and posterior to the hypophyseal fossa lies the **foramen lacerum**. The sphenoid bone contributes to its anterior border; the petrous temporal bone contributes to its posterior border. Passing through the upper portion of the foramen lacerum is the *internal carotid artery*. A groove on either side of the hypophyseal fossa indicates the anterior course of the artery within the skull.

12. The **anterior** and **posterior clinoid processes** are four corners of the saddle, which project posteriorly. They represent the pull of *dural attachments*.

13. The **optic canals** are round openings on either end of the optic groove at the point where the lesser wings attach to the body. Passing through the canals from the middle cranial fossa to the orbits are the *optic nerves (cranial nerves II)* and the *ophthalmic arteries*.

The Greater and Lesser Wings

14. The **lesser wings** of the sphenoid bone are triangular plates of bone. The posterior borders represent the posterior limits of the anterior cranial fossa. The superior surface contributes to the *anterior cranial fossa*,

and anteriorly the lesser wings articulate with the orbital plates of the frontal bone.

15. The **greater wings** fan out on either side of the body. They present internal aspects that contribute to the middle cranial fossae and outer aspects that contribute to the lateral wall of the cranial vault and the roof of the infratemporal region. Two foramina are found at the basal attachment of the greater wings to the body.

16. The **foramen rotundum**, or round hole, joins the middle cranial fossa and the pterygopalatine fossa. It transmits the *maxillary nerve (cranial nerve V-2)*.

17. The **foramen ovale**, or oval hole, is posterior to the foramen rotundum. It transmits the *mandibular nerve (cranial nerve V-3)* from the middle cranial fossa above to the infratemporal region below.

18. The **spine of the sphenoid** is a sharp projection on the inferior aspect at the posterolateral angle of the greater wing. Attached to it is the *sphenomandibular ligament*.

19. The **foramen spinosum** pierces the spine of the sphenoid and allows passage of the *middle meningeal artery*

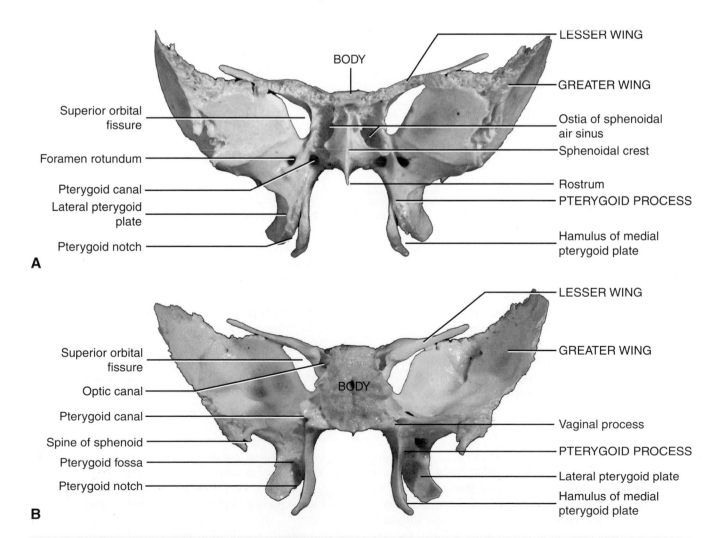

Figure 6-22 Features of the sphenoid bone. **A**, Anterior view. **B**, Posterior view.

195

Continued

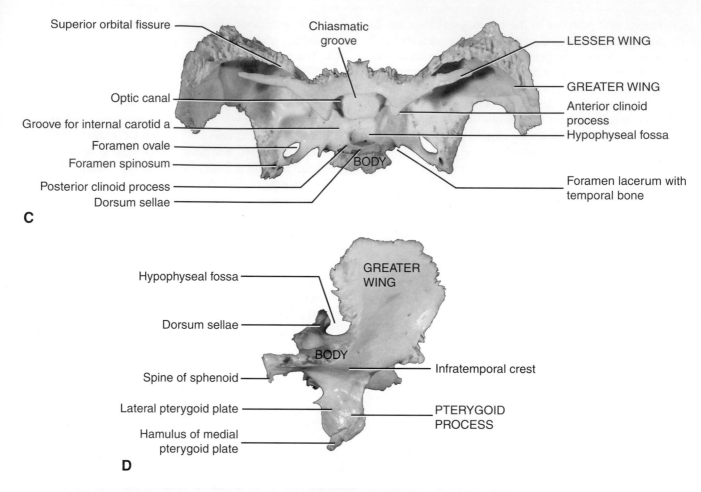

Superior orbital fissure
Chiasmatic groove
LESSER WING
Optic canal
GREATER WING
Anterior clinoid process
Groove for internal carotid a
Hypophyseal fossa
Foramen ovale
Foramen spinosum
BODY
Posterior clinoid process
Dorsum sellae
Foramen lacerum with temporal bone

C

Hypophyseal fossa
GREATER WING
Dorsum sellae
BODY
Spine of sphenoid
Infratemporal crest
Lateral pterygoid plate
PTERYGOID PROCESS
Hamulus of medial pterygoid plate

D

Figure 6-22 Cont'd. **C**, Lateral view. **D**, Superior view.

from the infratemporal region of the middle cranial fossa.

20. The **superior orbital fissure** is the cleft between the lesser and greater wings. It transmits *cranial nerves III, IV, VI,* and *V-1* and ophthalmic veins between the orbit and the middle cranial fossa.

21. The **inferior orbital fissure** is a cleft between the antero-inferior border of the greater wing and the body of the maxilla. It transmits the *infraorbital nerve* and *vessels.*

22. The **infratemporal crest** is the sharp ridge on the inferior aspect of the greater wing. It separates the temporal fossa above from the infratemporal region below.

The Pterygoid Processes. The pterygoid processes consist of *two plates,* or *laminae,* which converge anteriorly as a V.

23. The **lateral pterygoid plate** is a thin, roughly rectangular plate that angles backward and laterally. Attached to the medial and lateral aspects of the plate are the origins of the *medial* and *lateral pterygoid muscles,* respectively.

24. The **medial pterygoid plate** is triangular and ends inferiorly as a slender hook, or **hamulus.** It forms the posterior aspect of the lateral wall of the nasal cavity.

25. The **pterygoid fossa** is the posterior depression between the medial and lateral pterygoid plates.

26. The **scaphoid fossa** is a canoe-shaped shallow depression at the base of the medial pterygoid plate. The *tensor veli palatini muscle* originates from this area.

27. The **pterygoid notch** is an inferior V-shaped deficiency between the medial and lateral pterygoid plates, which articulates with and is filled in by the *pyramidal process of the palatine bone.*

28. The **pterygoid canal** passes through the base of the pterygoid process. The mouth of the canal is immediately medial to the scaphoid fossa, passing into the anterior margin of the foramen lacerum. In the articulated skull a thin wire passed through the canal ends in the pterygopalatine fossa. The canal transmits the *nerve* and *artery of the pterygoid canal.*

29. The **vaginal process** of the sphenoid is a plate of bone that extends perpendicularly from the base of the medial pterygoid plate to the midline vomer.

Development. Ossification begins in the eighth week of intrauterine life from a number of centers. The body and lesser wing, the bases of the greater wings, and the lateral pterygoid processes develop in cartilage. The remainder of the greater wings and the medial pterygoid plates develop in membrane.

At birth the sphenoid bone is in three parts: the body and lesser wings, the greater wings, and the pterygoid processes. Union of the three parts begins in the first year of life. At 3 years of age, nasal mucous membrane invades the body via the future ostia and balloons out within the body to form the right and left sphenoidal air sinuses, separated by a midline septum. The sinuses are lined with respiratory mucosa and maintain communication with the nasal cavity via the two ostia.

The Ethmoid Bone (Single)

The ethmoid bone is another key bone, that is vital to the understanding of craniofacial architecture.

Contributions. The ethmoid bone contributes to the anterior cranial fossa; the roof, lateral wall, and median septum of the nasal cavity; and the medial wall of the orbit (*Figure 6-23*).

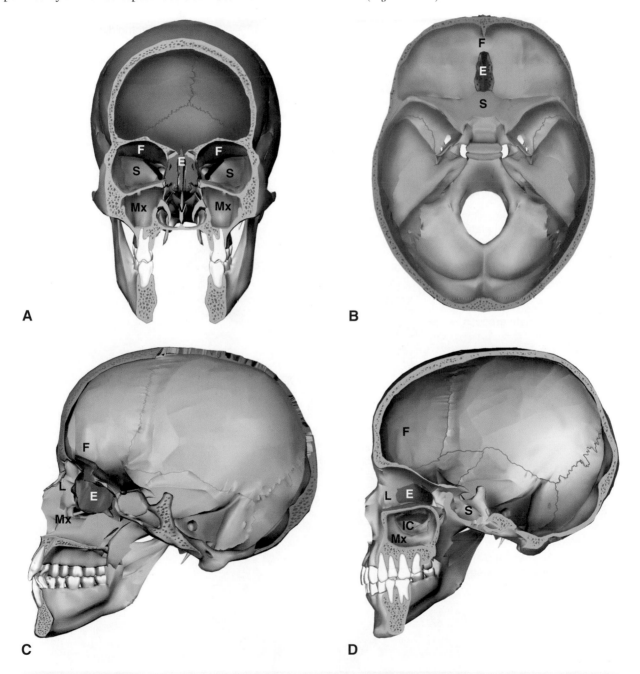

Figure 6-23 Relationship of ethmoid bone to the other bones of the skull. **A,** Coronal section. **B,** Internal aspect of cranial base. **C,** Sagittal section through orbit and maxillary sinus. **D,** Sagittal section through nasal cavity with nasal septum removed.

Articulations. The ethmoid bone articulates with the frontal bone, the body of the sphenoid, the lacrimal bones, the palatine bones, the vomer, the inferior concha, and both maxillae.

Parts and Features. The ethmoid bone consists of a vertical plate and a horizontal plate. Suspended from the horizontal plate, like two saddlebags, are the ethmoid labyrinths (*Figure 6-24*).

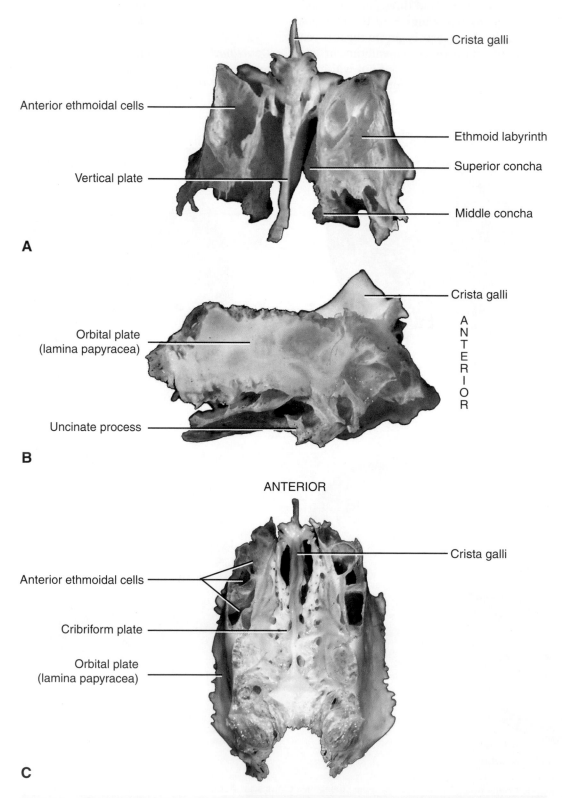

A

Crista galli

Anterior ethmoidal cells

Ethmoid labyrinth

Superior concha

Vertical plate

Middle concha

B

Crista galli

Orbital plate (lamina papyracea)

ANTERIOR

Uncinate process

C

ANTERIOR

Crista galli

Anterior ethmoidal cells

Cribriform plate

Orbital plate (lamina papyracea)

Figure 6-24 Features of the ethmoid bone. **A,** Anterior view. **B,** Lateral view. **C,** Superior view.

Vertical Plate. The **crista galli** is a ridge of bone that peaks upward in the median plane into the anterior cranial fossa. The *falx cerebri* is attached to it.

The **septal plate** is the inferior extension of the vertical plate into the nasal cavity. It forms the anterosuperior aspect of the bony septum and articulates with the vomer behind and below. Anteriorly it articulates with the cartilaginous portion of the nasal septum.

Horizontal Plate. The **cribriform plates** project laterally from the crista galli. They are sievelike plates in the floor of the anterior cranial fossa above and form the perforated roof of the nasal cavity below. Passing through the perforations are the several branches of the *olfactory nerve (cranial nerve I)*.

Ethmoid Labyrinth. The **ethmoidal air cells** are formed by a honeycomb network of interconnecting septa of extremely thin bone. The cells are lined with respiratory mucosa, and each cell communicates directly or indirectly with the nasal cavity via tiny openings in the lateral wall. The paper-thin lateral aspects of the ethmoid labyrinth form a portion of the medial wall of the orbit termed the *orbital plate*, or **lamina papyracea.**

The **superior concha** is a scroll-like projection of bone that hangs from the posteromedial aspect of the labyrinth into the nasal cavity. The **middle concha** is a larger scroll that is really an inferior continuation of the medial labyrinth wall. The **uncinate process** is a bony hook that curves posteriorly from the middle concha to meet the *ethmoid process of the inferior concha.*

Formation. The ethmoid bone forms in the cartilage of the cranial base and the cartilage of the nasal capsule. The labyrinths ossify initially in the fifth intrauterine month and are completely ossified at birth. The vertical portion begins to ossify within the cartilaginous septum during the first year of life. The horizontal and vertical components fuse as one bone between 2 and 5 years of age.

BONES OF THE FACE
Maxilla (Paired)
The right and left maxillae contribute to the greater part of the upper facial skeleton.

Contributions to the Skull. The maxillae help form the upper face, the infratemporal region, the orbital floor, the lateral wall of the nasal cavity, the floor of the nasal cavity, and the roof of the oral cavity (*Figure 6-25*).

Articulations. The maxilla articulates with the opposite maxilla, the nasal bone, the lacrimal bone, the ethmoid bone, the palatine bone, the frontal bone, the vomer, the zygomatic bone, and the inferior concha. In addition, the maxillary teeth articulate with the teeth of the mandible through the temporomandibular joint.

Parts and Surfaces. In simple terms the maxilla may be thought of as a hollow, pyramidal body presenting four sides, or surfaces, and possessing four attached processes.

Surfaces
1. The **facial,** or **anterior, surface** helps form the upper face.
2. The **infratemporal,** or **posterior, surface** forms the anterior wall of the infratemporal region.
3. The **orbital surface** is the superior aspect. It forms the floor of the orbit.
4. The **nasal,** or **medial, surface** is the base of the pyramid. It helps form the bulk of the lateral wall of the nasal cavity.

Processes
1. The **alveolar process** of the maxilla forms the sockets and supporting bone for the maxillary teeth. The alveolar processes of both maxillae form the upper dental arch.
2. The **zygomatic process** of the maxilla is on the lateral aspect and is the buttressing maxillary contribution to the zygomatic arch. The zygomatic process is the apex of the pyramid.
3. The **frontal process** of the maxilla is a bar of bone that projects upward from the anterosuperior aspect to contact the frontal bone above.
4. The **palatal process** of the maxilla is a horizontal shelf projecting from the medial aspect of the maxilla toward the midline and its opposite counterpart. The palatal process helps form the roof of the oral cavity and the floor of the nasal cavity.

Features
Facial (Anterior) Surface
1. The **orbital margin** forms a portion of the inferior and medial margins of the orbit (*Figure 6-26, A*).
2. The **anterior lacrimal crest** is a ridge of bone that extends upward on the surface of the frontal process. Together with the posterior lacrimal crest of the lacrimal bone behind, the two bones form the depression for the *nasolacrimal duct.*
3. The **infraorbital foramen** opens onto the facial surface about 7 mm below the midpoint of the inferior orbital margin. It is the mouth of the infraorbital canal and transmits to the face the *infraorbital nerves* and *vessels.*
4. The **nasal margin** forms the lateral and inferior borders of the *anterior nasal aperture*, or piriform aperture.
5. The **anterior nasal** spine is a sharp, midline, anterior projection of the inferior nasal border.
6. The **incisive fossa** of the maxilla is a shallow concavity overlying the roots of the incisor teeth just below the nasal cavity. It is the site of injection for local anesthesia of the maxillary incisors (see *Figure 6-2*).
7. The **canine ridge** is a pronounced, elongated elevation of alveolar bone overlying the large maxillary canine root.
8. The **canine fossa** is the concavity distal to the canine ridge overlying the maxillary premolar roots. It extends

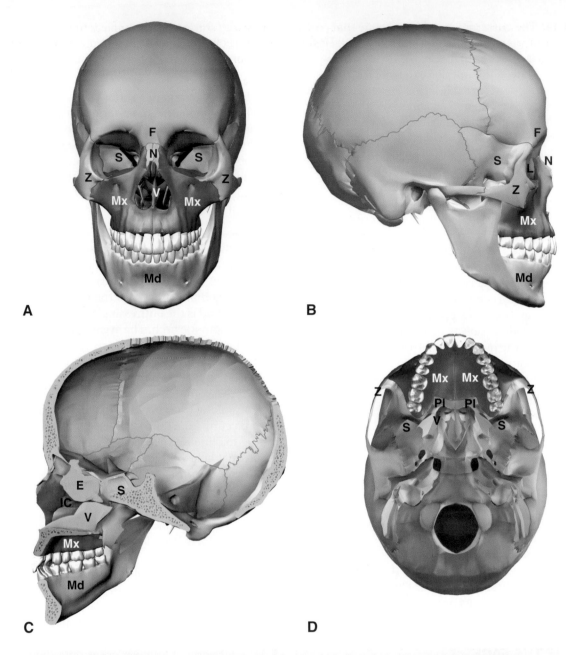

Figure 6-25 Relationship of the maxillae to the other bones of the skull. **A,** Anterior view. **B,** Lateral view. **C,** Sagittal section with nasal septum intact. **D,** Inferior view of base.

upward to the infraorbital foramen. It is the site of injection for local anesthesia of the premolar maxillary teeth.

9. The **buttress of the zygomatic process** of the maxilla limits the facial aspect of the maxilla posteriorly. The supporting buttress spills down onto the buccal alveolar surface of the first molar, creating a thick buccal plate of bone.

Infratemporal (Posterior) Surface. The infratemporal, or posterior, surface presents a gently rounded convex contour termed the *maxillary tuberosity*.

1. The **posterior superior alveolar foramina** are several small perforations at the apex of the convexity through which the *posterior superior alveolar nerves* and *vessels pass*.

2. The **maxillary tubercle** is a smaller convexity immediately distal to the last maxillary molar. It occasionally is hollowed from within by the encroaching maxillary sinus.

The area superior to the maxillary tubercle is roughened for the attachment of the *pyramidal process of the palatine bone*. The pyramidal process intervenes between the maxilla and the buttressing pterygoid processes.

3. The superior aspect of the infratemporal surface ends abruptly as the inferior margin of the **inferior orbital fissure**. In the intact skull it is a cleft between this area of the maxilla and the greater wing of the sphenoid bone.

Orbital (Superior) Surface. The orbital, or superior, surface is a thin plate of bone that forms the floor of the orbit and sweeps upward and medially to help form the medial orbital wall (see *Figure 6-26, A*). Immediately deep to this thin plate is the maxillary sinus.

The **infraorbital sulcus** or **groove** runs anteriorly along the orbital floor from the inferior orbital fissure. At the midpoint of its course, it angles slightly but deeply as the **infraorbital canal.** The canal, in turn, opens onto the facial surface as the **infraorbital foramen.**

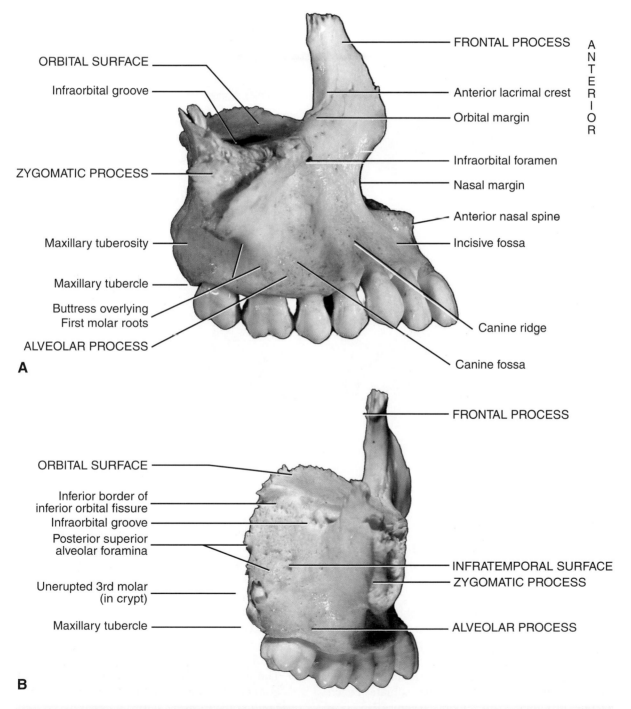

Figure 6-26 Features of right maxilla. **A,** Lateral view. **B,** Posterior view.

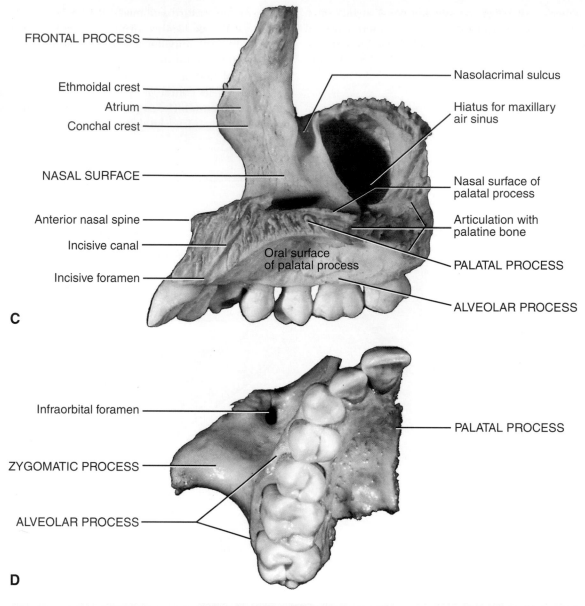

FRONTAL PROCESS

Ethmoidal crest

Atrium

Conchal crest

NASAL SURFACE

Anterior nasal spine

Incisive canal

Incisive foramen

Oral surface
of palatal process

Nasolacrimal sulcus

Hiatus for maxillary
air sinus

Nasal surface of
palatal process

Articulation with
palatine bone

PALATAL PROCESS

ALVEOLAR PROCESS

C

Infraorbital foramen

ZYGOMATIC PROCESS

ALVEOLAR PROCESS

PALATAL PROCESS

D

Figure 6-26 Cont'd. **C**, Medial view. **D**, Inferior view.

Nasal (Medial) Surface

1. The **maxillary hiatus** is a large (1 to 1.5 cm wide) opening to the maxillary sinus within (*Figure 6-26, C*).
2. The **maxillary sinus** is variable in size but generally extends anteriorly to the facial surface, laterally into the zygomatic process, posteriorly to the infratemporal wall, superiorly to the orbital floor, and inferiorly down into the alveolar process. Running across the roof of the sinus is the bony infraorbital canal extending into the sinus like a ridge. Occasionally the roots of the maxillary molar teeth may approximate or even protrude through the sinus floor (see Figure 7-57).
3. The **nasolacrimal sulcus** anterior to the maxillary hiatus runs in a vertical direction. Along with the lacrimal bone it forms the *nasolacrimal canal*, which transports tears from the orbit to the nasal cavity.
4. The **ethmoidal crest** is a transverse ridge that runs across the nasal surface of the frontal process. Attached to it in the articulated skull is the *middle concha* of the ethmoid bone.
5. The **conchal crest** is a parallel ridge about 1.5 cm below the ethmoidal crest. It provides attachment for the *inferior concha*.
6. The **atrium** is the shallow depression between the ethmoidal and conchal crests. It is part of the *middle meatus* of the nasal cavity.
7. The area posterior and inferior to the maxillary ostium is roughened for articulation with the **palatine bone**.

8. The **palatal process** of the maxilla forms the *anterior two thirds of the bony palate*.
9. The **nasal crest** is a raised median ridge extending the length of the superior medial aspect of the palatal process. With its counterpart, it contributes to the bony nasal septum.
10. The **incisive crest** is the more prominent anterior portion of the nasal crest.
11. The **incisive canal** runs downward and anteriorly just off the midline from the midpoint of the nasal surface of the palatal process to the oral surface behind the central incisor.
12. The **incisive foramen** is the mouth of the incisive canal behind the central incisor. The foramen is a common opening for the right and left incisive canals. The canal and foramen transmit the *nasopalatine nerve* and the *sphenopalatine artery*.
13. The **superior nasal surface** of the palatal process presents a smooth surface.
14. The **inferior oral surface** of the palatal process is roughened for attachment of the dense palatal mucosa (*Figure 6-26, D*).

Development. The maxillae develop during fetal life in membrane. The initial site of ossification is at the junction of the infraorbital nerve and the anterior superior alveolar nerve. Separate centers of ossification develop in the "premaxillary" area, or primary palate, anterior to the incisive foramen. This area includes the future site of the incisor teeth and associated alveolar process. The centers of ossification coalesce during later fetal life.

At birth the maxillary sinus is rudimentary or nonexistent. Invading nasal mucosa enters at the future site of the maxillary ostium and gradually hollows out the developing maxilla.

The Palatine Bone (Paired)

Contributions to the Skull. The palatine bones help form the nasal cavity (lateral wall and floor), the oral cavity (posterior third of hard palate), the pterygopalatine fossa (medial wall), and the orbit (a small portion of posterior wall) (*Figure 6-27*).

Articulations. The palatine bone articulates with the maxilla, the sphenoid bone, the ethmoid bone, the vomer, the inferior concha, and the opposite palatine bone.

Parts. The palatine bone is shaped like an L, and it meets its opposite counterpart as a mirror image. Therefore it has a vertical, or ascending, portion and a horizontal, or palatal, portion. In addition, it features three processes.

Features

Vertical Plate. The vertical plate presents a medial, or nasal, surface and a roughened, lateral surface for articulation with the maxilla (*Figure 6-28*). Its superior aspect carries an anterior and posterior process separated by a notch.

1. The **orbital process** is the anterior process. It projects forward to articulate with the sphenoid and ethmoid bones on the posteromedial orbital wall. The orbital process is generally hollow, containing a small air cell.

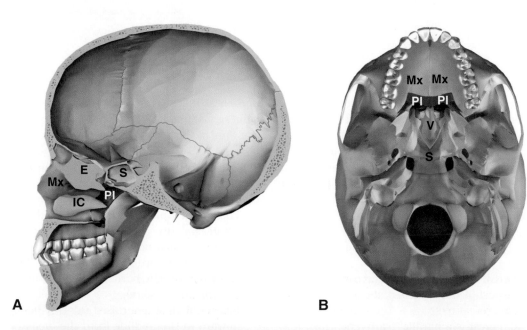

A　　　　**B**

Figure 6-27 Relationship of right palatine bone to the other bones of the skull. **A**, Sagittal section with nasal septum removed. **B**, Inferior view.

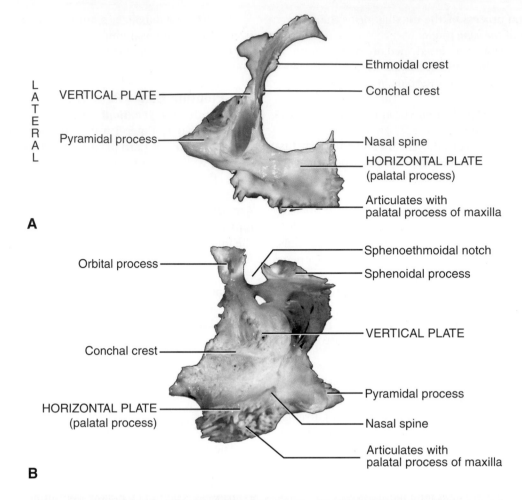

L
A
T
E
R
A
L

VERTICAL PLATE

Pyramidal process

Ethmoidal crest

Conchal crest

Nasal spine

HORIZONTAL PLATE
(palatal process)

Articulates with
palatal process of maxilla

A

Orbital process

Conchal crest

HORIZONTAL PLATE
(palatal process)

Sphenoethmoidal notch

Sphenoidal process

VERTICAL PLATE

Pyramidal process

Nasal spine

Articulates with
palatal process of maxilla

B

Figure 6-28 Features of the right palatine bone. **A,** Anterior view. **B,** Medial view.

2. The **sphenoidal process** is the posterior projection. It articulates with the body of the sphenoid above.
3. The **sphenoidal notch** separates the two processes, and when the palatine bone is articulated with the body of the sphenoid, the notch becomes the **sphenopalatine foramen.** Passing through this foramen are **nasal** and **pharyngeal branches** of the **pterygopalatine ganglion** and maxillary artery.
4. The **pyramidal process** is a posterior inferior extension of the vertical plate. It intervenes between the pterygoid process posteriorly and the maxillary tubercle anteriorly.
5. The **conchal crest** runs transversely across the middle of the nasal aspect of the vertical plate. It supports the **inferior concha.**
6. The **ethmoidal crest** is a parallel transverse ridge just below the sphenopalatine notch. It marks the articulation with the **middle concha** of the ethmoid bone.

Horizontal Plate. The horizontal plate features an *upper nasal surface* and an *inferior oral surface*. It forms the posterior *third* of the bony *palate*.

1. The **lesser palatine foramen** is the mouth of the lesser palatine canal of the vertical plate. It transmits the *lesser palatine nerve* and *vessels* (see also *Figure 6-8*).
2. The **greater palatine foramen** is the mouth of the greater palatine canal on the oral surface. It transmits the *greater palatine nerve* and *vessels*.
3. The posterior border of the **horizontal plate** is smooth and concave. The border ends medially as the pointed **posterior nasal spine.**
4. The **nasal crest** is a raised ridge of bone that projects upward in the midline from the medial border of the horizontal plate. The crest helps form the bony nasal septum and articulates with the vomer above.

Development. During fetal development the vertical plate ossifies in membrane. The horizontal plate develops subsequent to the vertical plate during the formation of the secondary palate.

The Zygomatic Bone (Paired)

The zygomatic bone is a roughly diamond-shaped bone in outline, with four borders, four angles, three surfaces, and three foramina.

Contributions. The zygomatic bone helps form the zygomatic arch (the "keystone"), the lateral wall of the orbit, and the anterior wall of the infratemporal region (*Figure 6-29*).

Articulations. The zygomatic bone articulates with the frontal bone, the greater wing of the sphenoid, the maxilla, and the temporal bone.

Parts and Features

Surfaces
1. The **facial surface** is the smooth lateral aspect of the bone. It forms the *prominence of the cheek (Figure 6-30)*.
2. The **temporal surface** is the curved medial aspect of the bone.
3. The **orbital surface** is almost perpendicular to the facial surface. It helps form the lateral and inferior orbital margins and a portion of the lateral orbital wall. The posterior aspect of the orbital surface separates the orbital cavity anteriorly from the temporal fossa behind.

Processes
1. The **frontal process** articulates superiorly with the frontal bone.
2. The **maxillary process** of the zygomatic bone articulates with the maxilla inferiorly.
3. The **temporal process** of the zygomatic bone articulates posteriorly with the zygomatic process of the temporal bone.

Foramina. The zygomatic bone contains a Y-shaped canal that transmits the *zygomatic nerve* and *artery*. The nerve and vessels enter the zygomatic bone from the orbital side and penetrate the bone as a canal. Within the bone the canal divides into two canals, each carrying with it the branches of the zygomatic nerve and artery. The canals continue to open onto the facial and temporal aspects as foramina of the same name.

1. The **zygomatico-orbital foramen** is the beginning of the zygomatic canal on the orbital surface.
2. The **zygomaticofacial foramen** is the exit onto the facial surface and transmits the *zygomaticofacial nerve* and *artery*.
3. The **zygomaticotemporal foramen** is the exit onto the temporal surface, and it transmits the *zygomaticotemporal nerve* and *artery*.

Development. The zygomatic bone develops early in fetal life from a single center of ossification within membrane.

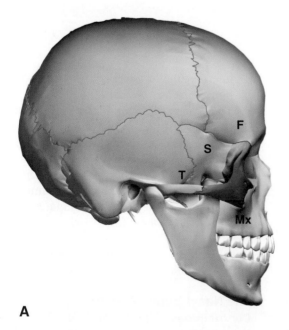

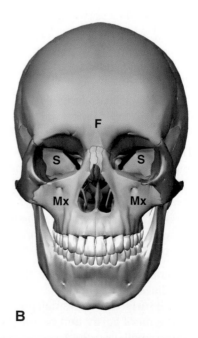

A **B**

Figure 6-29 Relationship of right zygomatic bone to the other bones of the skull. **A**, Lateral view. **B**, Anterior view.

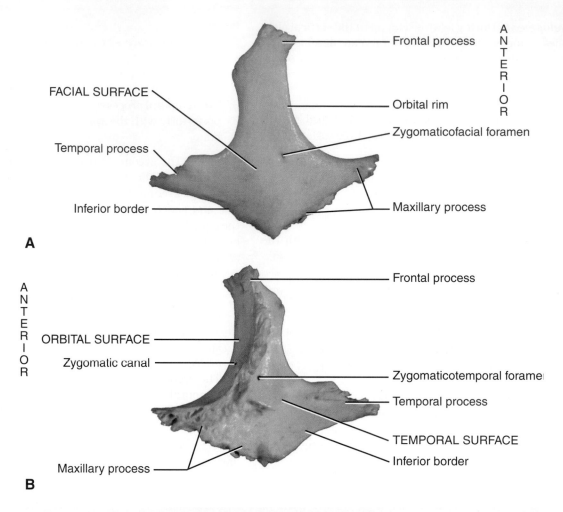

Figure 6-30 Features of right zygomatic bone. **A,** Lateral view. **B,** Medial view.

The Lacrimal Bone (Paired)

Contributions. The lacrimal bone forms part of the orbit (medial wall) and the nasal cavity (lateral wall) (*Figure 6-31*).

Articulations. The lacrimal bone articulates with the maxilla, the ethmoid bone, the frontal bone, and the inferior concha.

Parts and Features. The lacrimal bone is a small, thin, fragile bone with two surfaces and four borders, which articulate with surrounding bones (*Figure 6-32*).

1. The **orbital (lateral) surface** forms the thin anterior aspect of the medial orbital wall.
2. The **nasal (medial) surface** forms a small portion of the lateral wall of the nasal cavity and partially overlaps and obstructs the maxillary ostium.
3. The lacrimal bone and frontal process of the maxilla share in forming the **lacrimal sulcus**, a groove at the

inferomedial anterior corner of the orbit. The groove houses the *lacrimal sac.*

4. The **posterior lacrimal crest** is the posterior lip of the sulcus. The anterior lip is on the frontal process of the maxilla. The posterior lacrimal crest provides attachment for the *orbital septum.*
5. The posterior lacrimal crest sweeps inferiorly and anteriorly as the hooklike **lacrimal hamulus**, which helps form part of the posterior and lateral wall of the *bony nasolacrimal duct.*

Development. The lacrimal bone ossifies in membrane during fetal life.

The Nasal Bone (Paired)

Contributions. The nasal bone helps form part of the bony external nose, the lateral wall of the nasal cavity, and a small contribution to the bony nasal septum (*Figure 6-33*).

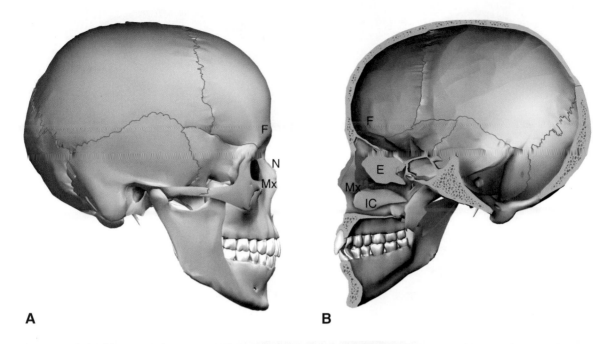

A   **B**

Figure 6-31 Relationship of right lacrimal bone to other bones of skull. **A**, Lateral view. **B**, Sagittal section with nasal septum removed.

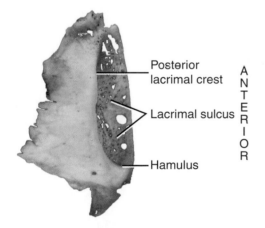

Figure 6-32 Features of lateral aspect of right lacrimal bone.

Articulations. The nasal bone articulates with the opposite nasal bone, the frontal bone, the maxilla, and the ethmoid bone.

Parts and Features. The nasal bone is a thin, flat, rectangular bone with two surfaces and four borders (*Figure 6-34*). Each of the borders articulates with other facial bones, except for the free, notched, inferior border.

1. The **facial (lateral) surface** is slightly concave in a super inferior direction. At the facial midpoint may be a tiny foramen, which transmits a *small emissary vein* from the nasal mucosa within the nasal cavity.

2. The **nasal (inner) surface** features a sharp median crest that contributes in a small way to the nasal septum. At this point it articulates with the nasal spine of the frontal bone and the vertical plate of the ethmoid bone. A shallow groove runs along the long axis and transmits the *anterior ethmoidal nerve inferiorly*.

3. The **superior borders** of the right and left nasal bones articulate superiorly with the *nasal notch of the frontal bone*.

4. The **inferior border** articulates with the lateral nasal cartilage of the external nose.

Development. A single center of ossification develops in membrane early in fetal life.

The Inferior Concha (Paired)

Contributions. The inferior concha is a *separate bone*, unlike the superior and middle conchae, which belong to the ethmoid bone (*Figure 6-35*). The inferior concha helps form the lateral wall of the nasal cavity. Because it covers part of the deficiency of the maxillary ostium, it helps form part of the medial wall of the maxillary sinus.

Articulations. The inferior concha hangs from the lateral wall of the nose down into the nasal cavity like a scroll. Its superior border is attached to the conchal crests of the maxilla and the palatine bone. It articulates with the maxilla, the lacrimal bone, the ethmoid bone, and the palatine bone.

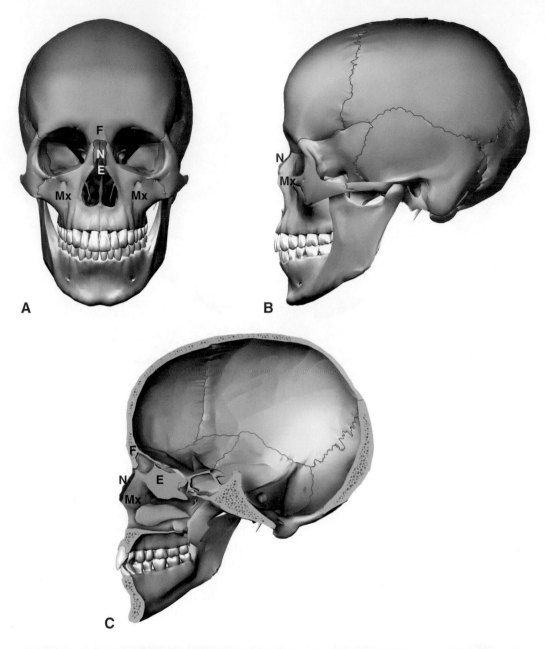

A

B

C

Figure 6-33 Relationship of right nasal bone to other bones of skull. **A,** Anterior view. **B,** Left lateral view. **C,** Sagittal section with vomer removed.

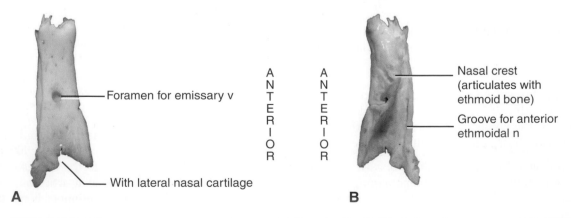

— Foramen for emissary v

— With lateral nasal cartilage

A

ANTERIOR

ANTERIOR

Nasal crest (articulates with ethmoid bone)

Groove for anterior ethmoidal n

B

Figure 6-34 Features of right nasal bone. **A,** Anterior (facial) view. **B,** Internal (nasal) view.

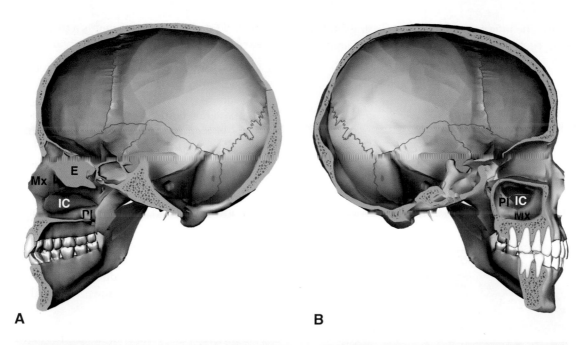

Figure 6-35 Relationship of right inferior concha to other bones of the skull. **A,** Sagittal section with nasal septum removed. **B,** Sagittal section through orbit and maxillary sinus.

Parts and Features. The inferior concha is like a delicate half-shell, with two surfaces and three processes (*Figure 6-36*).

1. The **lateral surface** is concave. The superior border fixes the bone to the lateral wall of the nasal cavity; the inferior border is free and thickened.
2. The **maxillary process**, a triangular thin plate of bone, extends over part of the maxillary ostium and forms part of the medial wall of the sinus.

3. The **medial surface** is convex and roughened.
4. The **lacrimal process** is an anterior vertical extension from the superior border. It helps form the medial wall of the bony nasolacrimal canal.
5. The **ethmoidal process** angles upward and backward from the superior border to articulate with the uncinate process of the ethmoid bone; these processes form the inferior border of the hiatus semilunaris.

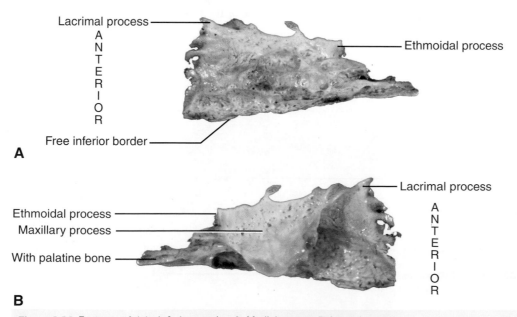

Figure 6-36 Features of right inferior concha. **A,** Medial aspect. **B,** Lateral aspect.

Development. The inferior concha forms during fetal life from a single center of ossification in the cartilaginous nasal capsule.

The Vomer (Single)

Contributions. The vomer provides a major contribution to the bony nasal septum (*Figure 6-37*).

Articulations. The vomer articulates with the sphenoid body, the maxilla (palatal process), the palatine bone (palatal process), the vertical plate of the ethmoid bone, and the cartilaginous nasal septum.

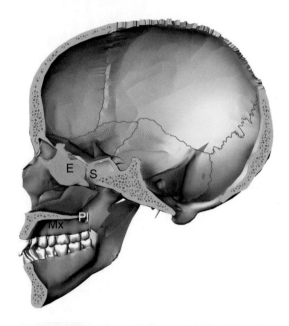

Figure 6-37 Relationship of vomer to other bones of the skull. Sagittal section with nasal septum intact.

Parts and Features. The vomer is a thin, flat bone that appears trapezoidal in outline (*Figure 6-38*).

1. The superior aspect flares out laterally as two wings, or **alae**, that articulate with the body of the sphenoid bone above.
2. The **posterior border** is sharp, smooth, and concave. It forms the entire posterior free border of the nasal septum.
3. The **anterior border** slopes downward and forward. The superior half articulates with the *vertical plate of the ethmoid bone*. The inferior half is grooved to articulate with the *cartilaginous septum*.
4. The **inferior border** articulates posteriorly with the nasal crest of the palatine bone and anteriorly with the nasal crest of the maxilla.
5. The **groove for the nasopalatine nerve** and **sphenopalatine artery** descends downward and forward on either side of the vomer. In the articulated skull it leads toward the incisive canal.

Development. The vomer develops in membrane on either side of the primitive cartilaginous nasal septum. The developing bone initially forms a sandwich on either side of the cartilage but gradually displaces the intervening cartilage and fuses from either side as one bone. Occasionally deep clefts within the vomer betray its original bilateral origin.

The Mandible (Single)

Contributions. The mandible forms the entire lower jaw and facial area (*Figure 6-39*).

Articulations. The mandible articulates with the temporal bone of the skull through a movable synovial joint. The occlusal aspects of the mandibular teeth articulate with those of the maxillary teeth.

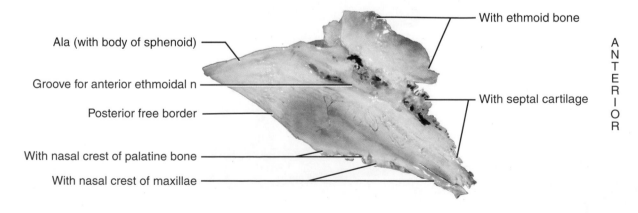

Ala (with body of sphenoid)

Groove for anterior ethmoidal n

Posterior free border

With nasal crest of palatine bone

With nasal crest of maxillae

With ethmoid bone

With septal cartilage

ANTERIOR

Figure 6-38 Features of right side of vomer.

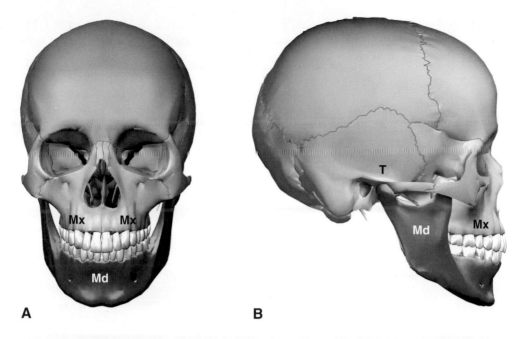

Figure 6-39 Relationship of mandible to other bones of the skull. **A**, Anterior view. **B**, Lateral view.

Parts. The mandible consists of two parts: the body and the ramus. The **body** is the horizontal portion. Anteriorly the right and left bodies are fused in the midline to form a U-shaped bone.

The **ramus** ascends vertically on each side from the posterior aspects of the bodies. The ramus is topped by two processes: an anterior sharp coronoid process and a posterior roller-shaped condylar process.

Features

Lateral Aspect

1. In the adult the **alveolar process** houses eight teeth on each side (*Figure 6-40, A*). The alveolar process consists of two plates of bone: a facial, or lateral, plate and a lingual, or medial, plate. Joining the plates transversely are septa of bone. *Interalveolar septa* form sockets between the roots of adjacent teeth. *Interradicular septa* form individual sockets for the multirooted teeth. As in the maxilla the facial plate of bone is thin anteriorly and the contours of the roots of the anterior teeth are obvious.

2. The **inferior** border is thick, smooth, and rounded and extends from the midline anteriorly to the angle of the mandible posteriorly. In a living person it can be palpated in its entirety just deep to the skin.

3. The **midline symphysis menti** is present at birth and begins to fuse in the first year of life, resulting in one mandible. In the adult, no symphysis is present, yet the term persists as a radiological phenomenon created by the superimposition of the right and left sides in the region of the chin.

4. The **incisive fossa** is a shallow depression immediately overlying the incisor roots.

5. The **mental protuberance** (chin) is a triangular elevation of bone immediately inferior to the incisive fossa. The apex of the triangle is directed superiorly; the base is the inferior border.

6. The **mental tubercles** are small elevations on either side of the triangular base.

7. The **external oblique line** is a ridge of bone that originates at the mental tubercle and sweeps upward and posteriorly to become the sharp anterior border of the vertical ramus.

8. The **mental foramen** is located at the midpoint of the inferior border and the alveolar crest in the region of the second premolar. The opening is angled upward and posteriorly. It transmits the *mental nerve* and *artery*.

9. The **(gonial) angle** of the mandible is the rounded corner where the inferior border sweeps upward as the posterior border of the ramus. The lateral and medial aspects of the angle are roughened for the insertions of the *masseter muscle* laterally and the *medial pterygoid muscle* medially.

10. The **antegonial notch** is a slight concavity on the inferior border anterior to the angle. Slightly anterior to this notch, in the living person, the pulsations of the *facial artery* may be felt.

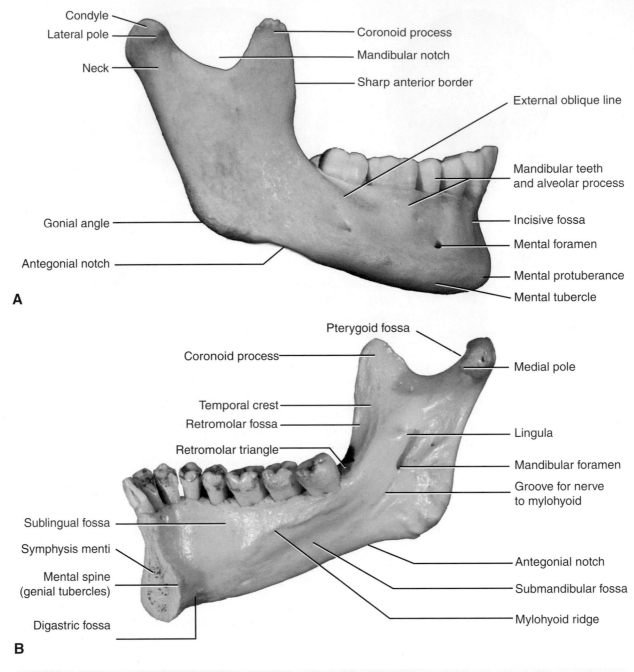

Figure 6-40 Features of mandible. **A**, Right lateral view. **B**, Medial view of right side.

11. The **condyle** is a roller-shaped process. It articulates with the reciprocally shaped *mandibular fossa* of the temporal bone.

12. The **neck of the condyle** is the bar of bone that supports the condyle atop the ramus.

13. The **pterygoid fossa** is an anterior depression on the neck of the condyle for insertion of the *lateral pterygoid muscle*.

14. The **coronoid process** is a sharp, beaklike process anterior to the condyle. It is a traction process produced by the pull of the inserted *temporalis muscle*.

15. The **mandibular notch** is the sharp concave superior border between the condyle and the coronoid process.

16. The **anterior border** of the ramus is sharp and continues downward to the body, where it becomes continuous with the *external oblique line*.

Internal Aspect

1. The **digastric fossae** are found on the anterior internal aspect just above the inferior border (*Figure 6-40, B*). They are small depressions on either side of the midline and reflect the bony origins of the *anterior belly of the digastric muscle.*

2. The **mental spine (genial tubercles)** lies in the midline superior to the digastric fossae. There may be four separate spines or a single fused spine. Attached to the upper aspect of the spine is the origin of the *genioglossus muscle.* Attached to the lower aspect is the origin of the *geniohyoid muscle.*

3. The **mylohyoid ridge** is a raised line that runs obliquely from the lateral aspect of the digastric fossa to the area below the lingual alveolar crest of the last mandibular molar. It is the origin of the *mylohyoid muscle.*

4. The **submandibular fossa** is a shallow concavity below the mylohyoid line that accommodates the superficial portion of the *submandibular gland.*

5. The **sublingual fossa** is a shallow concavity above the mylohyoid line that accommodates the *sublingual gland.*

6. The **mandibular foramen** is an oblique opening at the midpoint of the rectangular ramus of the mandible. If the occlusal plane of the mandibular teeth were extended posteriorly, the mandibular foramen would be a few millimeters below this line.

7. The **mandibular canal** is the continuation of the mandibular foramen deep into the mandible. The canal runs inferiorly and anteriorly through the ramus and body just below the roots of the mandibular teeth and ends at the midline. It carries the *inferior alveolar nerve* and *artery* to the mandibular teeth. Cutaneous branches of the nerve and artery pass to the facial aspect of the mandible through the **mental foramen.**

8. The **lingula** is a tonguelike projection of bone guarding the superoanterior border of the mandibular foramen. Attached to it is the *sphenomandibular ligament.* The lingula may interfere with anesthetic injections of the inferior alveolar nerve at the mouth of the mandibular foramen.

9. The **mylohyoid sulcus** is a narrow groove that runs downward and forward from the inferior border of the mandibular foramen. Occupying this groove is the *nerve to the mylohyoid muscle.*

The following terminology is not found in the *Terminologia Anatomica,* but it is used widely by dental practitioners.

1. The **internal oblique line,** or **temporal crest,** is a buttressing ridge of bone on the internal surface of the ramus. It begins indistinctly on the coronoid process and slopes downward and forward. As it approaches the last molar, the ridge divides to pass around the last molar, the divisions becoming continuous with the buccal and lingual alveolar crests.

2. The **coronoid notch** (not to be confused with the mandibular notch between the coronoid and condylar processes) is the concavity on the anterior border of the ramus as it approaches the body below.

3. The **retromolar fossa,** or **triangle,** is the depression between the anterior border of the ramus and the temporal crest.

These three landmarks are extremely important in locating the site of injection for an anesthetic block of the inferior alveolar nerve.

Development. The mandible begins to ossify in membrane during the sixth fetal week. The ossification center develops lateral to Meckel's cartilage at the junction of the mental and incisive branches of the inferior alveolar nerve. A secondary center in the ramus ossifies in cartilage, and some cartilage persists as the articular cartilage of the condyle. At birth the mandible consists of two fragile halves. The symphysis menti, which separates the bodies in the midline, begins to ossify in the first year of life and fuses as one bone by about the second year.

The Hyoid Bone (Single)

The hyoid bone is described with the skeleton of the larynx in Chapter 5.

The Ossicles of the Middle Ear (Paired)

Three ossicles are found within the petrous temporal bone in the cavity of the middle ear. They are the malleus, the incus, and the stapes. These bones are discussed, along with a complete description of the middle ear, in Chapter 7.

SKULL FORAMINA

A summary of the foramina of the skull is presented in *Table 6-1.*

4. Postnatal Development

GROWTH

The cranial vault and orbits are large at birth and follow a neural growth pattern (*Figures 6-41 and 6-42*). The vault, like the underlying brain, is almost adult in size at 8 to 10 years of age. Further growth in the cranial vault results from bony apposition and the development of the frontal air sinuses. The cranial base and face are small at birth and follow a general growth pattern. The face is lacking in vertical dimension because the teeth are not yet erupted, and the maxillary air sinuses are still rudimentary. At birth the vault-to-face ratio is 8:1, which decreases in the adult to 2:1.

TABLE 6-1

Summary of Cranial Foramina

Region of Skull	Foramen	Bone(s)	Position	Areas Connected	Contents
Face	Supraorbital notch or foramen	Frontal	Superior orbital margin	Orbit and forehead	Supraorbital n, a, v
	Infraorbital foramen and canal	Maxilla	7 mm below inferior orbital margin	Pterygopalatine fossa and face	Infraorbital n, a, v
	Zygomaticofacial foramen	Zygomatic	Facial aspect of zygomatic bone	Orbit and face	Zygomaticofacial n, a, v
	Zygomaticotemporal foramen	Zygomatic	Temporal aspect of orbital process	Orbit and temporal fossa	Zygomaticotemporal n, a, v
	Mental foramen	Mandible	Facial aspect of body below apex of second premolar tooth	Mandibular canal and face	Mental n, a, v
Cranial vault	Mastoid foramen	Temporal	Behind base of mastoid process	Transverse venous sinus of posterior cranial fossa and exterior of skull	Emissary v
	Parietal foramen	Parietal	Either side of posterior third of sagittal suture	Superior sagittal venous sinus within skull and exterior of skull	Emissary v
Cranial base (external)	Foramen ovale	Sphenoid	Base of lateral pterygoid plate	Middle cranial fossa and infratemporal region	Mandibular n (cranial nerve V-3)
	Foramen spinosum	Sphenoid	Base of spine of sphenoid	Middle cranial fossa and infratemporal region	Middle meningeal a
	Foramen lacerum	Temporal, sphenoid	Between apex of temporal and body of sphenoid	Inferior aspect is obliterated with cartilage	Internal carotid a; nervus spinosus Sympathetic plexus
				Superior aspect connects middle cranial fossa and carotid canal	Nerve of pterygoid canal
	Pterygoid canal	Sphenoid	Base of medial pterygoid plate, anterior margin of foramen lacerum	Foramen lacerum and pterygopalatine fossa	N and a of pterygoid canal
	Palatinovaginal canal	Sphenoid, vomer	Junction of alar plate of vomer and vaginal process of sphenoid	Mouth of sphenopalatine foramen and roof of nasopharynx	Pharyngeal n, a
	Bony auditory (pharyngotympanic) tube	Temporal, sphenoid	Issues medially from under cover of tympanic plate	Middle ear and nasopharynx	Air
	Petrotympanic fissure	Temporal	Between petrous wedge inferiorly and tympanic plate	Middle ear and infratemporal region	Chorda tympani
	Carotid canal	Temporal	Posterior to tympanic plate on petrous portion	External base of skull and middle cranial fossa via foramen lacerum	Internal carotid a and sympathetic plexus
	Jugular foramen	Temporal, occipital	Posterior to carotid canal opening	External base of skull and posterior cranial fossa	Internal jugular v and cranial nerves IX, X, and XI

	Opening	Bone	Location	Communication	Transmits
	Tympanic canal	Temporal	Between carotid and jugular openings	Base of skull and middle ear	Tympanic branch of cranial nerve IX
	Stylomastoid foramen	Temporal	Between styloid and mastoid processes	Internal auditory meatus of posterior cranial fossa via facial canal to external base of skull	Facial n (cranial nerve VII)
	Hypoglossal canal	Occipital	Lateral to foramen magnum anterior to condyle	Posterior cranial fossa to external base of skull	Hypoglossal n (cranial nerve XII)
	Foramen magnum	Occipital	Junction of squamous, condylar, and basal portions of occipital	Posterior cranial fossa and vertebral canal	Spinal cord, vertebral arteries, spinal accessory nerves, meninges
Cranial base (internal)	Foramen cecum	Frontal and ethmoid	Anterior to crista galli	A blind opening	Emissary v in fetal life
	Olfactory foramina	Ethmoid	Cribriform plates on either side of crista galli	Anterior cranial fossa and roof of nasal cavity	Olfactory nerves (cranial nerve I)
	Optic foramen and canal	Sphenoid	Base of lesser wing of sphenoid	Middle cranial fossa and orbit	Optic n (cranial nerve II); ophthalmic a
	Superior orbital fissure	Sphenoid	Between greater and lesser wings of sphenoid	Middle cranial fossa and orbit	Cranial nerves III, IV, V-1, and VI; ophthalmic vv
	Foramen rotundum	Sphenoid	Base of greater wing of sphenoid	Middle cranial fossa and pterygopalatine fossa	Maxillary n (cranial nerve V-2)
	Foramen ovale	Sphenoid	Base of greater wing of sphenoid behind foramen rotundum	Middle cranial fossa and infratemporal region	Mandibular n (cranial nerve V-3); accessory meningeal a
	Foramen spinosum	Sphenoid	Behind foramen ovale	Middle cranial fossa and infratemporal region	Nervus spinosus; middle meningeal a
	Superior petrosal hiatus and sulcus	Temporal	Anterior aspect of petrous temporal in middle cranial fossa	Facial canal within petrous temporal and middle cranial fossa	Greater (superficial) petrosal nerve of cranial nerve VII
	Inferior petrosal hiatus and sulcus	Temporal	Below and parallel to superior hiatus	Middle ear and middle cranial fossa	Lesser (superficial) petrosal n of cranial nerve IX
	Internal auditory meatus	Temporal	Posterior aspect of petrous ridge	Posterior cranial fossa and inner ear; facial canal	Vestibulocochlear n, facial n, internal auditory a
	Jugular foramen	Temporal and occipital	Posterior cranial fossa at base of petrous ridge	Posterior cranial fossa and external base of skull	Internal jugular v and cranial nerves IX, X, and XI
	Hypoglossal canal	Occipital	Superior to anterolateral margin of foramen magnum	Posterior cranial fossa and external base of skull	Hypoglossal n (cranial nerve XII)

Continued

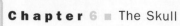

TABLE 6-1

Summary of Cranial Foramina—cont'd

Region of Skull	Foramen	Bone(s)	Position	Areas Connected	Contents
	Foramen magnum	Occipital	Middle of posterior cranial fossa	Posterior cranial fossa and vertebral canal	Spinal cord, vertebral arteries, meninges
Orbital cavity	Optic foramen	Sphenoid	Posterior pole of orbit	Middle cranial fossa and orbit	Optic n (cranial nerve II) and ophthalmic a
	Superior orbital fissure	Sphenoid	Posterior pole of orbit	Middle cranial fossa and orbit	Cranial nerves III, IV, V-1, and VI; ophthalmic v
	Inferior orbital fissure	Sphenoid and maxilla	Posterior aspect of orbital floor	Infratemporal region and orbit	Infraorbital n, a, v, via infraorbital groove and canal; zygomatic nerves
	Anterior ethmoidal canal	Ethmoid and frontal	Medial wall of orbit	Orbit and anterior ethmoidal cells and then to roof of nasal cavity	Anterior ethmoidal n, a
	Posterior ethmoidal canal	Ethmoid and frontal	Medial wall of orbit posterior to the anterior canal	Orbit and posterior ethmoidal cells	Posterior ethmoidal n, a, v
	Supraorbital notch or foramen	Frontal	Superior orbital margin	Orbit and forehead	Supraorbital n, a, v
	Nasolacrimal duct	Maxilla, lacrimal, and inferior concha	Inferomedial margin of orbit	Orbit and inferior meatus of nasal cavity	Membranous nasolacrimal duct, tears
Oral cavity	Incisive foramen and canal	Maxilla	Anterior aspect of midpalatal suture	Nasal cavity and oral cavity	Nasopalatine n and sphenopalatine a, v
	Greater palatine foramen and canal	Maxilla and palatine	Posterior of hard palate opposite last molar	Pterygopalatine fossa and oral cavity	Greater palatine n, a, v
	Lesser palatine foramen and canal	Palatine	Posterior to greater palatine foramen in pyramidal process	Pterygopalatine fossa and oral cavity	Lesser palatine n, a, v
	Posterior superior alveolar foramina	Maxilla	Infratemporal surface of maxilla	Infratemporal region and maxillary sinus	Posterior superior alveolar n, a, v
	Mandibular foramen and canal	Mandible	Internal aspect of ramus at midpoint	Infratemporal fossa and via mandibular canal to teeth	Inferior alveolar n, a, v
Nasal cavity	Ethmoidal foramen and sulcus	Nasal, ethmoid	Anterior roof of nasal cavity	Anterior cranial fossa and roof of nasal cavity	Anterior ethmoidal n, a
	Sphenopalatine foramen	Sphenoid, palatine	Lateral wall of nasal cavity	Pterygopalatine fossa and nasal cavity	Sphenopalatine n, a, v
	Incisive canal	Maxilla	Floor of nasal cavity	Floor of nasal cavity and oral cavity	Nasopalatine n and sphenopalatine a, v

n, Nerve; *a,* artery; *v,* vein.

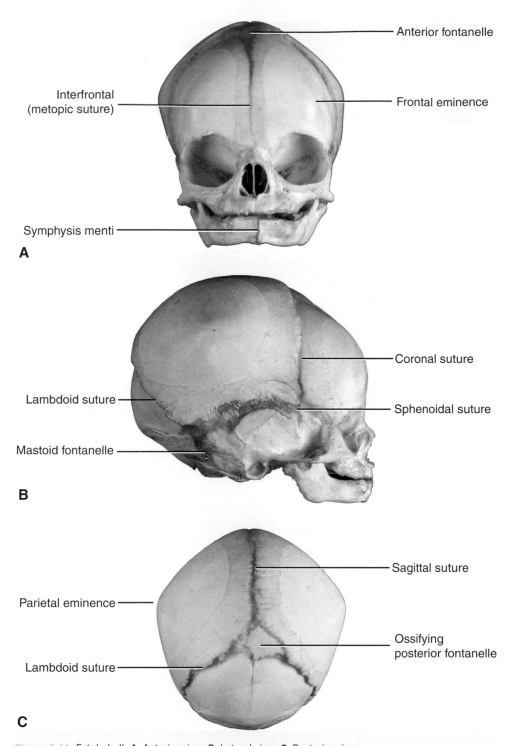

Figure 6-41 Fetal skull. **A**, Anterior view. **B**, Lateral view. **C**, Posterior view.

FUSION OF BONES

Several bones of the neonatal skull have not yet fused as single bones. At birth the frontal bone is separated by the midline metopic or interfrontal suture, which ossifies in the first year of life. The symphysis menti separates the mandible into two equal halves at birth; these halves fuse in the first year. In addition, the various components of the temporal, occipital, sphenoid, and ethmoid bones have not yet fused as single bones at birth. These fuse over time during infancy and early childhood. The spheno-occipital synchondrosis, an important growth site, fuses at some time after adolescence and unites the bodies of the sphenoid and occipital bones as the single clivus.

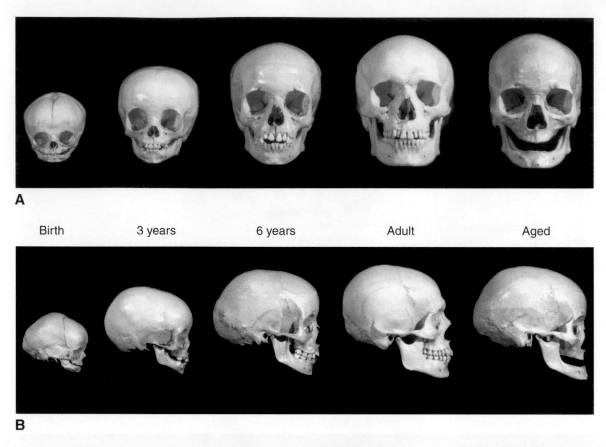

Birth 3 years 6 years Adult Aged

Figure 6-42 Stages of postnatal development of human skull. **A**, Anterior view. **B**, Lateral view.

SUTURES AND FONTANELLES

In contrast to the sutures of the adult, those of the infant are smooth and wide, allowing for birth molding of the skull during delivery. Within the suture lines are areas of membrane that have not yet been replaced by bone. These are termed *fontanelles* (*soft spots*). Two major fontanelles are seen on the superior aspect of the infant skull. The *anterior fontanelle* is at the intersection of the interfrontal, coronal, and sagittal sutures. The fontanelle is diamond-shaped and disappears at about 1½ years of age. Venipuncture is a fairly difficult procedure in the neonate, but the superior sagittal venous sinus may be conveniently entered through the membranous anterior fontanelle. The *posterior fontanelle* lies at the intersection of the sagittal and lambdoid sutures and is triangular. It fuses in the first year of life. Other small fontanelles are seen on the lateral aspect of the infant skull.

DEVELOPMENT OF KEY FACIAL BONES

Maxilla

At birth the body of the maxilla is entirely filled with the developing tooth crypts. These crypts occupy a superior crowded position just below the orbital floor. The maxillary sinus is rudimentary, and as the developing dentition moves downward, nasal mucosa invades the body and gradually renders it hollow. Vertical growth of the upper face is largely caused by dentoalveolar development and the formation of the maxillary air sinus.

Mandible

The mandible, at birth, is in two delicate halves separated at the chin by the **symphysis menti**. The mandibular body is merely a shell containing the developing tooth crypts. The condylar and coronoid processes are short. During the first year the symphysis menti fuses from below upward, and childhood development produces further changes. The condylar process lengthens, and the gonial angle and coronoid process develop in response to increased muscular function. The chin (mental protuberance) begins to develop in the second year and reaches full development after puberty. Chin development is more pronounced in males. The alveolar process grows in height and length to accommodate the developing dentition.

Detailed descriptions of the **developing dentition** may be found in textbooks of dental anatomy. The mandibular incisors generally erupt first at 6 months of age. The complete primary dentition is usually present at 2 years of age. Permanent teeth begin to erupt at 6 years of age, with the intraoral appearance of the mandibular first molars behind the primary dentition. Thereafter each of the primary teeth is replaced by succeeding permanent teeth, the last primary tooth replacement occurring at 11 to 12 years of age. The second molars erupt distally to the first molars at age 12 years, and the *third molars (if present) erupt toward the end of adolescence.*

Temporal Bone

The components of the temporal bone have not yet fused at birth. The mastoid process is rudimentary, which exposes the facial nerve as it issues from the stylomastoid foramen. The facial nerve may be damaged as a result of a forceps delivery, which may cause facial paralysis. The bony tympanic ring has not yet developed, resulting in a more superficial and vulnerable tympanic membrane. The ossicles and middle ear cavity are adult in size within the petrous temporal bone.

The mandibular fossa is considerably flatter and exhibits no articular eminence. As the child changes from sucking to mastication and as the dentition develops, the mandibular fossa deepens and the articular eminence forms concurrently with the growing condyle of the developing mandible.

SEXUAL DIMORPHISM

Within a homogeneous population, female skulls tend to be smaller, lighter, thinner-walled, and generally more like the developing juvenile skull. The forehead retains its childlike rounded anterior contour, and the teeth are smaller, with rounded incisal angles. Male skulls, on the other hand, are larger and heavier and exhibit more rugged muscle markings and prominences. The teeth are larger and squared incisally, and the forehead is beetle-browed as a result of the developing frontal sinuses, which are larger in men and form more prominent superciliary arches externally.

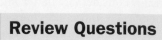
Review Questions

1. All of the following bones contribute to the floor of the neurocranium (cranial base) EXCEPT the _____.
   a. temporal bones
   b. occipital bone
   c. sphenoid bone
   d. parietal bones
   e. ethmoid bone

2. The medial opening of the pterygopalatine fossa that communicates with the nasal cavity is the _____.
   a. sphenopalatine foramen
   b. nasopalatine foramen
   c. foramen lacerum
   d. greater palatine foramen
   e. foramen spinosum

3. The inferior margin of the bony orbit is formed by the _____.
   a. ethmoid bone
   b. lacrimal bone
   c. maxilla
   d. zygomatic bone
   e. maxilla and zygomatic bone

4. Pterion is the landmark found at the _____.
   a. junction of frontal, temporal, and parietal bones and the greater wing of the sphenoid
   b. junction of sagittal and coronal sutures
   c. junction of sagittal and lamdoidal sutures
   d. junction of internasal suture and frontal bone
   e. vertex of the skull

5. The inferior orbital fissure is a cleft between the maxilla and the _____.
   a. vertical plate of palatine bone
   b. greater wing of sphenoid
   c. lesser wing of sphenoid
   d. frontal bone
   e. ethmoid bone

6. The canine fossa is a bony depression _____.
   a. overlying the maxillary incisors' roots
   b. overlying the maxillary canine root
   c. overlying the maxillary premolar roots
   d. posterior to the zygomatic process of the maxilla
   e. surrounding the infraorbital foramen

7. The articular eminence is a feature of the _____.
   a. mandible
   b. maxilla
   c. sphenoid bone
   d. palatine bone
   e. temporal bone

8. The internal carotid artery passes through the carotid canal and enters the internal aspect of the skull through the _____.
   a. foramen lacerum
   b. foramen ovale
   c. foramen spinosum
   d. jugular foramen
   e. internal auditory meatus

9. Paranasal air sinuses are hollow spaces found in each of the following bones EXCEPT the _____.
   a. frontal bone
   b. ethmoid bone
   c. maxilla
   d. sphenoid bone
   e. inferior concha

10. All of the following pass through the jugular foramen EXCEPT _____.
    a. CN IX
    b. CN VIII
    c. CN X
    d. CN XI
    e. the internal jugular vein

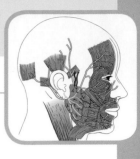

Chapter **7**

The Head by Regions

1. The Face and Scalp 221

2. The Contents of the Neurocranium.................. 238

3. The Orbital Cavity.. 256

4. The Parotid Region... 265

5. The Masticator Region 269

6. The Pterygopalatine Fossa 291

7. The Nasal Cavity and Paranasal Air Sinuses 297

8. The Oral Cavity 308

9. Structures and Areas of the Oral Cavity 314

10. The Pharynx.. 333

11. The Larynx.. 340

12. The Ear 349

1. The Face and Scalp

The face is that part of the head visible in a frontal view, that is, all that is anterior to the external ears and all that lies between the hairline and the chin. Clustered in this region are the various facial openings and their associated sensory structures.

The scalp covers the forehead, the superior aspect of the cranial vault, and the occipital region above the superior nuchal line. Laterally, the scalp blends in with the temporal area.

REGIONS OF THE FACE

The **facial region** may be subdivided into a number of areas (*Figure 7-1*): (1) the *forehead*, extending from the eyebrows to the hairline; (2) the *temples* or *temporal area* anterior to the ears; (3) the *orbital area* containing the eye and covered by the eyelids; (4) the *external nose*; (5) the *zygomatic* (*malar*) *area* (prominence of the cheek); (6) the *mouth* and *lips*; (7) the *cheeks*; (8) the *chin*; and (9) the *external ear*.

SKELETON

The anterior, superior, lateral, and posterior aspects of the skull are discussed in Chapter 6.

SKIN AND FASCIA

Skin

The **skin** of the face is medium to thin in relative thickness. It is pliable and movable over a layer of loose areolar connective tissue except in the external ear and the ala of the nose, where the skin is fixed to underlying cartilage. Facial skin contains numerous sweat and sebaceous glands.

Superficial Fascia

The superficial fascia or subcutaneous connective tissue contains variable amounts of fat that smooth out the contours of the face, particularly between the muscles of facial expression. In some areas the fat is extensive. The buccal (sucking) fat pad fills out the cheeks and extends upward to the scalp behind the bony orbit. Located within the subcutaneous tissue are facial vessels, sensory and motor nerves, and the superficial muscles of facial expression.

Deep Fascia

There is no discrete layer of deep fascia in the face.

SENSORY (CUTANEOUS) NERVES OF THE FACE

The facial cutaneous nerve supply is principally derived from the trigeminal nerve (cranial nerve V) (*Figure 7-2*). Within the skull, the trigeminal nerve divides into three

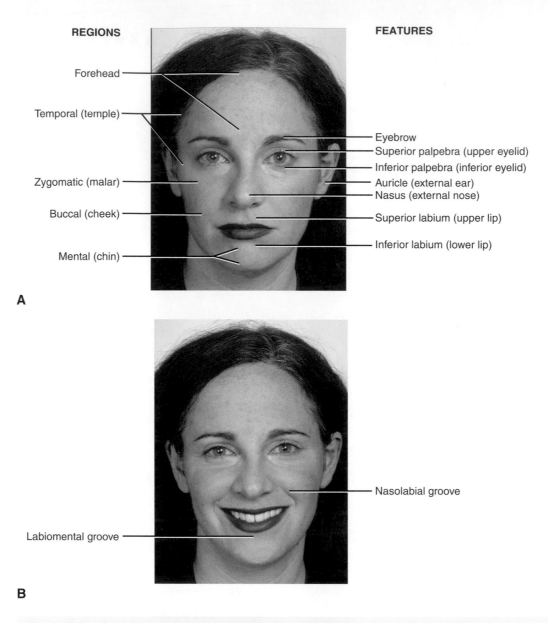

REGIONS

Forehead

Temporal (temple)

Zygomatic (malar)

Buccal (cheek)

Mental (chin)

A

FEATURES

Eyebrow
Superior palpebra (upper eyelid)
Inferior palpebra (inferior eyelid)
Auricle (external ear)
Nasus (external nose)
Superior labium (upper lip)

Inferior labium (lower lip)

Nasolabial groove

Labiomental groove

B

Figure 7-1 Regions of the face. **A,** At rest. **B,** Smiling.

parts: (1) the **ophthalmic nerve (cranial nerve V-1),** a sensory nerve associated mainly with the orbit and its contents; (2) **the maxillary nerve (cranial nerve V-2),** a sensory nerve associated with the nasomaxillary complex; and (3) the **mandibular nerve (cranial nerve V-3),** a sensory and motor nerve associated with the lower jaw and the muscles of mastication. Only the mandibular nerve contains motor as well as sensory fibers. Each division of the trigeminal nerve contributes sensory cutaneous branches to the face.

Facial Branches of the Ophthalmic Nerve

The ophthalmic nerve contributes several branches to the upper eyelid, the forehead and scalp, and the external nose.

Supraorbital Nerve. The supraorbital nerve emerges from the roof of the orbit through the supraorbital foramen, or notch. It travels to and supplies a small portion of the frontal sinus, a large portion of the upper eyelid, and a large portion of the forehead and scalp.

Supratrochlear Nerve. The supratrochlear nerve within the orbit passes over the pulley, or trochlea, of the superior oblique muscle. It emerges from the medial aspect of the superior orbital margin to supply the medial portion of the upper eyelid and adjacent forehead.

Infratrochlear Nerve. The infratrochlear nerve passes under the trochlea in the orbit and emerges near the

On the face, it immediately breaks up into three sets of branches.

1. **Inferior palpebral branches,** which convey sensation from the skin and conjunctivum of the lower lid
2. **Lateral nasal branches,** which convey sensation from the lateral aspect of the external nose
3. **Superior labial branches,** which convey sensation from the skin and mucous membrane of the upper lip.

Zygomaticofacial Nerve. The zygomaticofacial nerve is a small branch of the zygomatic nerve, which, in turn, is a branch of the maxillary nerve. It emerges onto the face through the zygomaticofacial foramen to supply skin of the zygomatic prominence.

Zygomaticotemporal Nerve. The zygomaticotemporal nerve is another branch of the zygomatic nerve, which passes through the zygomaticotemporal foramen and ascends to supply skin of the anterior aspect of the temporal fossa and scalp.

Facial Branches of the Mandibular Nerve
The cutaneous contribution of cranial nerve V-3 to the face is fairly widespread, ranging from the temples to the chin.

Auriculotemporal Nerve. The auriculotemporal nerve surfaces between the temporomandibular joint and the tragus of the ear. It ascends to supply the skin of a portion of the external ear and ear canal, the temporal region, and the lateral aspect of the scalp.

Buccal Branch of Cranial Nerve V-3. The buccal branch of cranial nerve V-3 appears on the face from under the cover of the ramus of the mandible. It spreads over the cheek and conveys sensation from the skin and mucous membrane of the cheek. In addition, it conveys sensory information from the vestibular (buccal) gingiva of the mandibular molars.

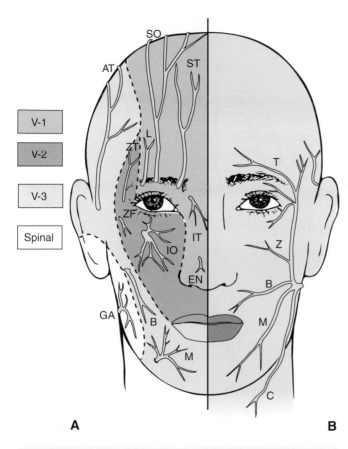

Figure 7-2 **A,** Cutaneous nerves of the face. *V-1 (ophthalmic nerve):* SO, Supraorbital nerve; ST, supratrochlear nerve; L, lacrimal nerve; IT, infratrochlear nerve; EN, external nasal nerve. *V-2 (maxillary nerve):* IO, Infraorbital nerve. *V-3 (mandibular nerve):* AT, Auriculotemporal nerve; B, buccal nerve; M, mental nerve. *Spinal nerve:* GA, Great auricular nerve. **B,** Motor nerves to the muscles of facial expression. *Facial branches of CN VII:* T, Temporal branches; Z, zygomatic branches; B, buccal branches; M, mandibular branches; C, cervical branches.

medial angle of the eye; this nerve supplies the medial angle of the upper lid and the lacrimal sac.

Lacrimal Nerve. The lacrimal nerve is a tiny branch that emerges from the lateral aspect of the superior margin of the orbit to supply a small, lateral portion of the upper eyelid.

External Nasal Nerve. The external nasal nerve surfaces on either side of the midline at the junction of the nasal bone and nasal cartilages. It supplies a median strip of external nose below the nasal bones.

Facial Branches of the Maxillary Nerve
Infraorbital Nerve. The infraorbital nerve is the large, terminal branch of the maxillary nerve. The infraorbital nerve passes through a bony canal in the orbital floor to emerge onto the face through the infraorbital foramen.

CLINICAL NOTES

Dental Anesthesia
Various facial branches of the trigeminal nerve are anesthetized following routine local anesthetic injections for dental procedures. Anesthesia of the mandibular teeth will also result in anesthesia of the mental nerve supplying the chin and lower lip. Anesthesia of the maxillary anterior teeth will also block sensation from the lower eyelid, lateral nose, and the upper lip. Numbness in these areas indicates successful local anesthesia.

Trigeminal Neuralgia (Tic Douloureux)

Disorders of the trigeminal ganglion, within the skull, can give rise to paroxysms (sudden, severe bouts of pain) along the pathways of the sensory facial branches of the trigeminal nerve. Trigeminal neuralgia occurs more often in territories supplied by the maxillary (cranial nerve V-2) or mandibular (cranial nerve V-3) nerves. These episodes of pain can be triggered by just a light touch to the face or hot or cold foods in the mouth. Treatment sometimes consists of resection of the maxillary or mandibular division. Following resection, patients must chew very carefully to prevent biting the cheek. Patients who have undergone such a resection should visit their dentists frequently to monitor possible intraoral problems that the patient can no longer detect because intraoral pain is no longer a warning that something is wrong.

Mental Nerve. The mental nerve is a cutaneous branch of the inferior alveolar nerve. The mental nerve leaves the mandibular canal through the mental foramen and exits onto the face lateral to the chin. It immediately breaks up into three sets of branches.

1. **Mental branches** supply the skin of the chin.
2. **Inferior labial branches** supply the skin and mucous membrane of the lower lip.
3. **Gingival branches** supply the vestibular (labial) gingiva of the mandibular anterior teeth.

ARTERIES OF THE FACE

The face is richly supplied with blood from various arteries, and the terminal branches of these various arteries anastomose freely (*Figure 7-3*). The entire blood supply is derived from either the internal or the external carotid arteries. Their facial branches travel as companion arteries to the sensory facial nerves described previously and, in general, carry the same names as the facial sensory nerves.

Facial Branches of the Ophthalmic Artery

The facial branches arise directly or indirectly from the ophthalmic artery of the orbit and stream out of the orbit as five branches.

Supraorbital Artery. The supraorbital artery, along with its companion cutaneous nerve, leaves the orbit through the supraorbital notch, or foramen, to supply the upper eyelid, forehead, and scalp.

Supratrochlear Artery. The supratrochlear artery emerges medial to the supraorbital artery and supplies the upper lid, forehead, and scalp.

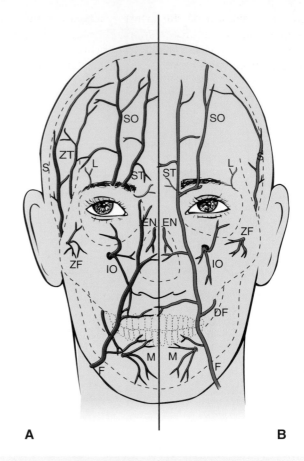

A   **B**

Figure 7-3 **A,** Superficial arteries of face. *SO,* Supraorbital artery; *ST,* supratrochlear artery; *L,* lacrimal artery; *EN,* external nasal artery; *ZF,* zygomaticofacial artery; *ZT,* zygomaticotemporal artery; *IO,* infraorbital artery; *S,* superficial temporal artery; *M,* mental artery; *F,* facial artery. **B,** Superficial veins of face. *SO,* Supraorbital vein; *ST,* supratrochlear vein; *L,* lacrimal vein; *EN,* external nasal vein; *ZF,* zygomaticofacial vein; *IO,* infraorbital vein; *S,* superficial temporal vein; *M,* mental vein; *F,* facial vein; *DF,* deep facial vein.

Dorsal Nasal Artery. The dorsal nasal artery is the companion artery to the infratrochlear nerve. It emerges from the medial-superior angle of the orbit to supply the medial upper lid, the lacrimal sac, and the bridge of the nose.

Lacrimal Artery. The lacrimal artery is the small terminal portion of the ophthalmic artery, which emerges at the lateral aspect of the supraorbital margin to supply the lateral aspect of the upper lid.

External Nasal Artery. The external nasal artery surfaces on either side of the midline at the junction of the nasal bone and nasal cartilages. It supplies a median strip of external nose below the nasal bones.

Zygomatic Artery. The zygomatic artery passes through the zygomatic canal in the lateral wall of the orbit and divides into two terminal branches that emerge on the face. The **zygomaticofacial artery** emerges through the zygomaticofacial foramen to supply the skin of the prominence of the cheek. The **zygomaticotemporal artery** emerges through the zygomaticotemporal foramen to supply the skin of the anterior temporal region.

Facial Branches of the Maxillary Artery

Infraorbital Artery. The infraorbital artery issues from the infraorbital foramen below the orbit and immediately breaks up into (1) **inferior palpebral branches** to the lower eyelid, (2) **nasal branches** to the lateral aspect of the nose, and (3) **superior labial branches** to the upper lip.

Buccal Artery. The buccal artery appears from under the cover of the ramus and masseter muscle. It spills onto the cheek, supplying the skin and mucous membrane of the cheek and vestibular gingiva of the mandibular molar area.

Mental Artery. The mental artery branches from the inferior alveolar artery within the mandibular canal of the mandible. It exits through the mental foramen, along with the mental nerve, to supply the chin, lower lip, and vestibular gingiva of the mandibular anterior teeth.

Branches of the Facial Artery

The facial artery, a collateral branch of the external carotid artery, leaves the submandibular region of the neck and ascends over the inferior border of the mandible through the antegonial notch. As the facial artery ascends obliquely on the face, it follows a somewhat tortuous route toward the medial angle of the eye. It passes between the more superficial and the deeper muscles of facial expression and supplies several branches to the face that anastomose freely with terminal branches of the maxillary and ophthalmic arteries.

Superior and Inferior Labial Branches. As the facial artery travels diagonally toward the medial angle of the mouth, it gives off the **inferior labial artery** to the lower lip and the **superior labial artery** to the upper lip. The pulsations of the labial arteries may be felt in your own lip by grasping the lip between the thumb and forefinger.

Lateral Nasal Branches. Lateral nasal branches are given off to the side of the nose; these anastomose with nasal branches of the infraorbital artery and the external nasal artery.

Angular Artery. The facial artery ends at the medial angle of the eye as the angular artery. It provides branches to the nose and medial aspect of the lids.

Facial Branches of the Superficial Temporal Artery

The superficial temporal artery is a terminal branch of the external carotid artery that emerges onto the face between the jaw joint and the ear to ascend on the scalp. Just below the ear, it sends a branch forward as the transverse facial

artery immediately below the zygomatic arch. It accompanies the auriculotemporal nerve on the side of the head.

VEINS OF THE FACE

The veins of the face follow somewhat the same pattern of distribution as the arterial supply, except for a few small but important differences (see *Figures 7-3* and *7-4*). Veins generally show more variability in their distribution than do arteries.

Veins that Accompany Cutaneous Nerves and Arteries

For each of the named arteries described previously as facial branches of the ophthalmic artery or maxillary artery, there are corresponding veins of the same name that flow in the opposite direction. The veins of the forehead, scalp, and upper lid flow to the **superior ophthalmic vein** in the orbit; the veins of the upper lip, lateral nose, and lower lid flow via the infraorbital vein to the **pterygoid plexus of veins** in the infratemporal region.

The Facial Vein. The facial vein roughly parallels the route of the facial artery. However, it is more posterior, takes a straighter and less tortuous course, and travels in the opposite direction. The facial vein originates and gathers tributaries in the following manner:

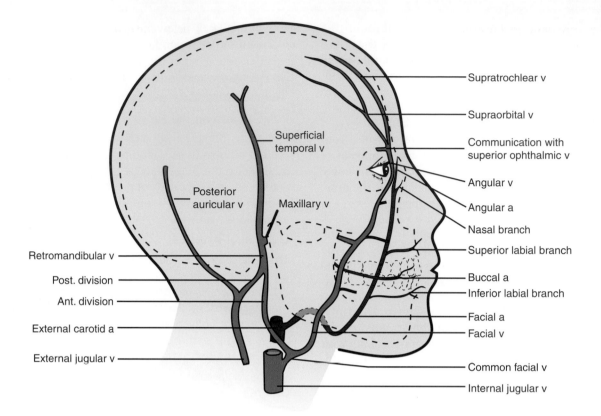

Figure 7-4 Lateral view of the facial artery and vein.

1. The **angular vein** forms at the medial angle of the eye by the union of the *supraorbital* and *supratrochlear* veins. The angular vein divides, and one division passes into the orbit to drain to the superior ophthalmic vein. The other division remains superficial and passes inferiorly as the facial vein.
2. The **facial vein** angles posteriorly toward the angle of the jaw and, as it descends, picks up several tributaries.
3. **Nasal veins** drain the side of the nose and communicate with tributaries of the infraorbital vein.
4. The **deep facial vein** communicates with the pterygoid plexus of veins deep within the infratemporal region.
5. **Labial veins** drain the upper and lower lips: the superior labial vein communicates with the infraorbital vein; the inferior labial vein communicates with the mental vein.

The facial vein then descends over the inferior border near the antegonial notch to enter the submandibular region of the neck. Unlike the facial artery, the vein takes a superficial course through the submandibular region.

The Retromandibular Vein. The **retromandibular vein** is formed from two sources. The **superficial temporal vein** drains the scalp and side of the head. It descends anterior to the ear and plunges into the substance of the parotid gland. Here it unites with the **maxillary vein** from the infratemporal region.

The retromandibular vein continues inferiorly, picking up glandular tributaries, and leaves the gland at its inferior border. At the angle of the mandible, the retromandibular vein divides into an anterior and a posterior division in the neck. The posterior division of the retromandibular vein unites with the **posterior auricular vein** from behind the ear to form the **external jugular vein**.

The **anterior division** of the retromandibular vein joins the **facial vein** in the neck to form the short common facial vein. The **common facial vein** drains deep to the **internal jugular vein** (see Chapter 5).

CLINICAL NOTES

Spread of Infection

Infections arising from the face or the orbit can spread through these venous communications to the cavernous sinus and cause an infective intracranial thrombus (clot). The condition is termed ***cavernous sinus thrombosis,*** is difficult to eradicate even with extensive antibiotic therapy, and may be fatal. Organisms in the blood from infections on the face could, therefore, be swept through the orbit to the cavernous sinus, where a secondary, more dangerous site of infection could develop.

Venous Communications

The facial vein contains no valves and communicates with relatively small tributaries of the infraorbital, zygomatic, and mental veins. In addition, two major communications are highly significant.

1. The facial vein communicates directly with the *superior ophthalmic vein via the angular vein*. Venous drainage from the angle of the eye may travel down the facial vein to the neck or may track into the orbit via the superior ophthalmic vein. The superior ophthalmic vein, in turn, drains to the **cavernous sinus** within the skull, where venous blood pools and flow is sluggish.
2. Venous drainage may back along the *deep facial vein to the pterygoid plexus of veins* in the infratemporal region. The plexus, in turn, communicates with the cavernous sinus within the skull.

MUSCLES OF THE FACE

The muscles of the face, or muscles of facial expression, are derived from the second branchial arch and are supplied by the cranial nerve of the second arch, the facial nerve (cranial nerve VII) (*Figure 7-5* and *Table 7-1*). The muscles of the scalp and the platysma muscle of the neck belong to the same muscle group.

In general, the muscles are found within the superficial fascia around the facial orifices. They perform two functions: (1) *as dilators and sphincters* they control the openings of the orifices, and (2) *as movers of overlying skin* they reflect the various *facial expressions*.

Most facial muscles originate from bone or from fascia, and all insert into the skin of the face. Upon contraction, therefore, they move the facial skin into various attitudes that reflect emotions, such as smiling, grinning, frowning, and forehead wrinkling of puzzlement. The muscles are grouped by regions.

Mouth

Orbicularis Oris. The orbicularis oris muscle is the *sphincter of the oral aperture* and lies within the upper and lower lips, encircling the mouth. Its fibers originate mainly from contributions of other facial muscles that converge on the mouth. A few intrinsic fibers arise from labial alveolar bone overlying the upper and lower incisors.

The orbicularis oris muscle closes the oral aperture, presses the lips against the teeth, and protrudes the lips.

Levator Anguli Oris. The levator anguli oris muscle originates from the canine fossa of the maxilla immediately inferior to the infraorbital foramen. It inserts into the angle of the mouth, blending with fibers of the orbicularis oris muscle. The function is self-descriptive; the muscle lifts the angles of the mouth.

Depressor Anguli Oris. The depressor anguli oris is a triangular muscle, the base of which originates from the external oblique line of the mandible. The ascending fibers converge at the apex to insert into the angle of the mouth from below and blend with the fibers of the orbicularis oris muscle. The depressor anguli oris muscle pulls the angles of the mouth downward.

Zygomaticus Major. The zygomaticus major muscle arises from the facial aspect of the zygomatic bone. Its fibers angle downward and medially to insert into the angle of the mouth and blend with the orbicularis oris muscle. It is the "laughing" muscle of the face, drawing the angle of the mouth upward and backward.

Risorius. The risorius muscle is a thin, wispy muscle that arises from parotid and masseteric fascia, plus a small contribution from upper fibers of platysma muscle sweeping up from the neck. Risorius muscle inserts transversely into the angle of the mouth and retracts the angle posteriorly, as in grinning.

Lips

Levator Labii Superioris. The levator labii superioris muscle has three origins that blend and pass into the upper lip.

1. The *angular head* (levator labii superioris alaeque nasi) arises from the frontal process of the maxilla.
2. The *infraorbital head*, the largest component, originates from the inferior orbital margin.
3. The *zygomatic head* (zygomaticus minor) originates from the facial aspect of the zygomatic bone.

All three origins insert as one into the upper lip and, upon contraction, raise the upper lip. A slip of the angular head inserts into the ala of the nose and helps to dilate the nostril.

Depressor Labii Inferioris. The depressor labii inferioris muscle arises from the lowest portion of the oblique line of the mandible, inserts into the lower lip, and depresses the lower lip.

Cheek

Buccinator

Origin. The buccinator muscle arises from three areas (*Figure 7-6*).

1. The **pterygomandibular raphé** is a thin, fibrous band running from the hamulus of the medial pterygoid plate down to the mandible, just behind the last mandibular molar. The raphé is actually a shared attachment with the **superior constrictor muscle** of the pharynx, the fibers of which interdigitate with those of the buccinator muscle as a common origin. The buccinator sweeps

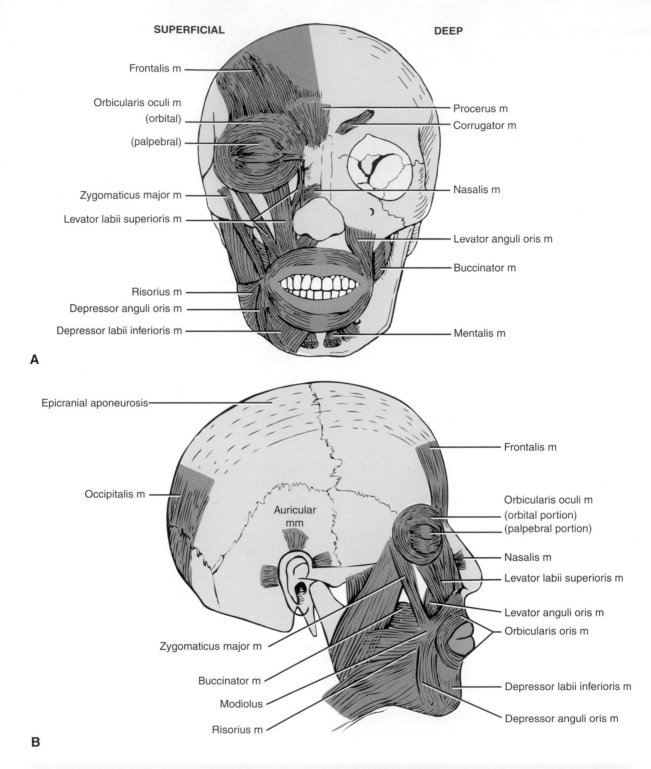

Figure 7-5 Muscles of facial expression. **A,** Anterior view. Superficial muscles are shown on right; deeper muscles are shown on left. **B,** Lateral view.

anteriorly into the wall of the cheek; the superior constrictor sweeps posteriorly into the wall of the pharynx.

2. The **lateral aspect of the maxillary alveolar process** in the molar region provides attachment for the superior muscle fibers of the buccinator muscle.

3. The **lateral aspect of the mandibular alveolar process** in the molar region provides attachment for the inferior muscle fibers of the buccinator muscle along the posterior half of the external oblique line.

TABLE 7-1

Muscles of the Face

Muscle	Origin	Insertion	Action	Cranial Nerve
Muscles of the Mouth				
Orbicularis oris	Extrinsic fibers: from insertions of circumoral muscles	Extrinsic fibers pass around mouth within the lips as a sphincter	Compresses lips against anterior teeth, closes mouth, protrudes lips	VII—zygomatic, buccal, and mandibular branches
	Intrinsic fibers: from incisive fossae of mandible and maxilla	Intrinsic fibers pass obliquely forward and insert into the skin of the lip		
Depressor anguli oris	Oblique line of mandible	Angle of mouth	Depresses angle of mouth	VII—buccal and mandibular branches
Levator anguli oris	Canine fossa of maxilla, below infraorbital foramen	Angle of mouth	Elevates angle of mouth	VII—zygomatic and buccal branches
Zygomaticus major	Zygomatic bone	Angle of mouth	Draws angle of mouth up and back	VII—zygomatic and buccal branches
Risorius	Contributions of platysma fibers, fascia of parotid and masseteric regions	Angle of mouth	Draws angle of mouth laterally	VII—zygomatic and buccal branches
Muscles of the Lips				
Levator labii superioris	Angular head: frontal process of maxilla	Alar cartilage and skin of nose	Elevates upper lip, flares nostril	VII—zygomatic and buccal branches
	Infraorbital head: inferior margin of orbit	Upper lip		
	Zygomatic head (zygomaticus minor): zygomatic bone	Nasolabial groove and upper lip		
Depressor labii inferioris	Oblique line of mandible	Lower lip	Depresses lower lip	VII—mandibular branches
Muscle of the Cheek				
Buccinator	Pterygomandibular raphé, buccal alveolar processes of maxilla and mandible	Upper fibers cross to insert into lower lip; lower fibers cross to insert into upper lip	Compresses cheeks against molar teeth; sucking and blowing	VII—buccal branches
Muscle of the Chin				
Mentalis	Incisive fossa mandible	Skin of chin	Puckers skin of chin, protrudes lower lip	VII—mandibular branches
Muscle of the Nose				
Nasalis	Compressor nares: canine eminence of maxilla	Midline aponeurosis overlying lateral nasal cartilages	(a) Compresses nostrils	VII—zygomatic and buccal branches
	Dilator nares: nasal notch of maxilla	Skin of margin of nostril	(b) Dilates or flares nostrils	
Muscle of the Eye				
Orbicularis oculi	Orbital: bone of upper medial orbital margin	Fibers encircle margins of orbit and insert into medial palpebral ligament	(a) Closes eye forcefully	VII—temporal and zygomatic branches
	Palpebral: medial palpebral ligament	Fibers arch laterally through lids and interdigitate laterally in a raphé	(b) Closes eye gently	
	Lacrimal: lacrimal bone behind lacrimal sac	Medial aspect of lids	(c) Squeezes lubricating tears against eyeball	

Continued

TABLE 7-1

Muscles of the Face—cont'd

Muscle	Origin	Insertion	Action	Cranial Nerve
Muscles of the Forehead				
Procerus	Nasal bone and lateral nasal cartilage	Skin of glabella	Transverse wrinkling of bridge of nose	VII—temporal and zygomatic branches
Corrugator	Medial aspect of supraorbital margin	Skin underlying eyebrow	Vertical wrinkling of bridge of nose	VII—temporal branches
Frontalis	Aponeurosis of scalp	Skin of forehead	Pulls scalp up and back	VII—temporal branches
Occipitalis	Lateral two thirds of superior nuchal line, mastoid process	Skin of occipital area	Pulls scalp backward and forward along with occipitalis	VII—posterior auricular branches
Muscles of the External Ear				
Anterior auricular	Aponeurosis of scalp, temporal fascia	Anterior medial aspect of helix of auricle	Pulls ear forward	VII—temporal branches
Posterior auricular	Superior lateral aspect of mastoid process	Inferior medial aspect of auricle	Pulls ear backward	VII—temporal branches
Superior auricular	Aponeurosis of scalp, temporal fascia	Superior medial aspect of auricle	Pulls ear superiorly	VII—posterior auricular branches

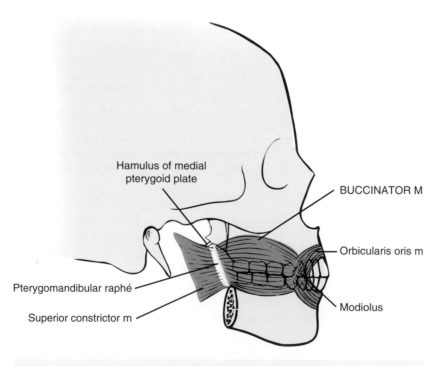

Figure 7-6 Attachments of the buccinator muscle.

Insertion. The muscle fibers sweep anteriorly through the cheek as a flattened sheet. On approaching the angles of the mouth, the upper fibers sweep inferiorly and the lower fibers sweep superiorly to blend with the orbicularis oris muscle.

Function. The buccinator muscle presses the cheek against the vestibular surfaces of the molar teeth. In doing so, it aids in *mastication* by pushing food onto the occlusal surfaces of the teeth in opposition to the tongue, which pushes the food in the opposite direction. The buccinator muscle also prevents the cheeks from expanding when forcefully *expelling air* from the oral cavity against resistance, as in playing wind or brass musical instruments.

Eye Region

Orbicularis Oculi. The orbicularis oculi muscle is contained within the upper and lower eyelids (palpebrae). It is a sphincteric muscle and helps close the eyelids. The orbicularis oculi muscle originates as three components.

Attachments. The **orbital portion** originates from bone of the upper medial orbital margin, encircles the orbital margin, and inserts from below into the prominent medial palpebral ligament. The ligament, in turn, is anchored to the anterior lacrimal crest of the maxilla.

The **palpebral portion** arises from the medial palpebral ligament and arches laterally within the upper and lower eyelids. The fibers of the upper and lower lids interdigitate laterally at the less prominent lateral palpebral ligament.

The **lacrimal portion** is small and originates from the lacrimal bone deep behind the lacrimal sac. It inserts into the medial portions of the lids.

Actions. The **palpebral portion** lightly approximates the lids, as in light blinking or during sleep. The **orbital portion**, because of its attachment to bone of the orbital periphery, is in a good mechanical position to forcibly squeeze the lids tightly to block out foreign objects or intense light. The **lacrimal portion** holds the lids against the globe of the eyeball for more even distribution of moistening tears and guiding tears to the small openings, or puncta, of the nasolacrimal apparatus for tear removal to the nasal cavity.

Chin: Mentalis

The mentalis muscle is a conical muscle, the apex of which arises from the mandibular incisive fossa. The fibers converge as the base to insert into the skin of the chin superficially. Contraction of the fibers puckers the skin overlying the chin and helps the orbicularis oris muscle in clearing food from the mandibular labial vestibule.

Nose: Nasalis

The nasalis muscle is the main muscle of the nose, and it arises as two parts.

The **transverse portion** (compressor nares) arises from the upper portion of the canine ridge of the maxilla. It arches upward and medially to insert along with its counterpart in a midline aponeurosis overlying the nasal cartilages.

The **alar portion** (dilator nares) arises from the nasal margin of the maxilla and inserts into the skin of the nostril. It acts to "flare" the nostrils. Some alar fibers sweep up to the ala and septum as the *depressor septi muscle*. These fibers tend to pull down on the septum and ala during nostril dilation.

Forehead

Procerus. The procerus muscle arises as small slips from fascia overlying the dorsum of the nose. The fibers sweep upward to insert into the skin overlying the glabella. Contraction produces transverse wrinkles over the bridge of the nose.

Corrugator. The corrugator is a small muscle slip that originates from the medial supraorbital margin. The fibers travel laterally to insert into the skin underlying the eyebrow. It produces vertical wrinkles over the glabella in certain individuals.

Frontalis. The frontalis muscle is the anterior component of the **occipitofrontalis** muscle of the scalp. It originates from a membranous sheet, or aponeurosis, on the scalp and inserts into the skin of the frontal region above the eyebrows. Contraction produces transverse wrinkling of the brow, as in worrying, or raising of the eyebrows, as in surprise.

MOTOR NERVES OF THE FACE: THE FACIAL NERVE

The facial nerve exits from the skull through the stylomastoid foramen at the base of the skull (see *Figure 7-2*). It passes inferiorly and anteriorly for several millimeters, enters the substance of the parotid gland, and here breaks up into five main groups of branches that radiate from the anterior margin of the gland and travel to various areas of the face.

Superficial Branches

Many facial muscles are supplied by more than one of the five branches of the facial nerve.

CLINICAL NOTES

Facial Muscles and Orthodontics

The actions of the nasalis muscle are insignificant, yet to the observant clinician, they are of diagnostic value. A true nasal breather can quite visibly flare the nostrils. Habitual mouth breathing caused by nasal obstruction decreases, if not eliminates, the ability to flare the nostrils. Mouth breathing is a cause of some dental malocclusions in children.

In children with class II malocclusions (small mandible in relation to the maxilla), the mentalis muscles are hyperactive when the lips are closed. The dimpling of the chin indicates hyperactive mentalis muscles.

Temporal Branches. The temporal branches travel superiorly and anteriorly to supply facial muscles situated above the zygomatic arch, including the orbit and forehead. They innervate the anterior and superior auricular muscles, the frontalis muscle, and the superior portion of the orbicularis oculis muscle.

Zygomatic Branches. The zygomatic branches travel transversely across the face to supply facial muscles in the zygomatic, orbital, and infraorbital areas. They supply the inferior portion of the orbicularis oculis muscle, and the superior portions of the zygomaticus major, levator labii superioris, levator anguli oris, nasalis and orbicularis oris muscles.

Buccal Branches. Buccal branches supply muscles of the cheek and circumoral muscles. They innervate the buccinator and orbicularis oris muscles, and the inferior portions of the zygomaticus major, levator labii superioris, levator anguli oris, nasalis, and orbicularis oris muscles.

Mandibular Branches. The mandibular branches supply muscles of the chin and lower lip. Specifically they pass to the depressor anguli oris, depressor labii inferioris, and to the mentalis muscle.

Cervical Branches. Cervical branches descend to the neck to supply platysma, posterior belly of the digastric, and stylohyoid muscles. Cervical branches also pass posteriorly to supply the occipitalis and posterior auricular muscles.

Sensory Nerve Communications

The motor branches of the facial nerve communicate with *cutaneous branches of the trigeminal nerve* on the face and cutaneous branches of spinal nerves in the neck. It is likely that these communications represent sensory proprioceptive contributions, which distribute with the facial nerve branches to the various facial muscles.

CLINICAL NOTES

Facial Paralysis

Damage to the facial nerve results in some form of facial paralysis (*Figure 7-7*). The type of paralysis is dependent upon where the lesion (damage) occurs.

Lesions of the upper motor neuron

Axons of the upper motor neurons of the facial nerve cross the midline of the brainstem to supply facial muscles of the contralateral side. The upper facial muscles (frontalis and orbicularis oculi) also receive axons from the same or ipsilateral side. Damage to the upper motor neurons of the facial nerve results in *paralysis of the lower facial muscles on the contralateral side*. The upper facial muscles continue to receive an ipsilateral nerve supply. Strokes are the most common cause of this type of facial paralysis.

Lesions of the lower motor neuron

Damage to the lower motor neurons at any point along their path results in *paralysis of the upper and lower facial muscles on the ipsilateral side*. The causes of lower motor neuron damage are varied.

The mastoid process, at birth, is small and offers little protection to the facial nerve that emerges through the stylomastoid foramen. The nerve can be crushed in a forceps delivery.

Viral infections can cause inflammation of the facial nerve as it passes through the facial canal. Swelling of the nerve in the enclosed bony canal causes pressure and a temporary facial paralysis or **Bell's palsy**.

A local anesthetic mistakenly injected into the parotid gland anesthetizes the facial nerve within the gland and results in a temporary facial paralysis. (See page 269.)

Effects of facial paralysis

Each muscle of facial expression can be affected but the most disabling and distressing effects are those on eyelids and those on the mouth and oral cavity.

The eyelids cannot close to lubricate the eye because the orbicularis oculi muscle is inactive and the levator palpebrae muscle, the opener of the upper eyelid acts unopposed. Tears fall onto the face because the punctum of the lower eyelid (hole that drains tears) is no longer applied closely to the eye (paralysis of the lacrimal portion of the orbicularis oculi).

Saliva may dribble from the mouth, and food cannot be chewed properly on the affected side because of paralysis of the buccinator and orbicularis oris muscles. In addition, expressive lines produced by facial muscles are obliterated, and facial distortion may occur because of contractions of unopposed contralateral facial muscles.

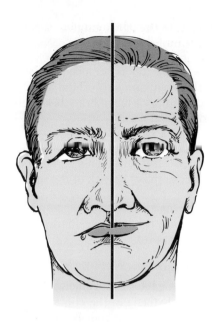

Figure 7-7 Facial paralysis resulting from damage to lower motor neurons of the facial nerve (cranial nerve VII). (Redrawn from Wilson-Pauwels L, Akesson EJ, Stewart PA: *Cranial Nerves: Anatomy and Clinical Comments.* Toronto, 1998, BC Decker).

FEATURES OF THE FACE

Lips (Labia)

The upper and lower lips surround the mouth, or entrance to the oral cavity (*Figure 7-8*). The upper lip lies between the nose above and the opening of the mouth below. Laterally, the lips are separated from the cheeks by the nasolabial groove, a furrow extending from the ala of the nose to approximately 1 cm lateral to the angle of the mouth. The **philtrum** is a wide (6 to 7 mm), shallow trough extending from the nose to the red (vermilion) border of the upper lip. Superiorly, the philtrum ends at the **columella**, the fleshy external partition between the nostrils.

The lower lip lies between the mouth above and the **labiomental groove** below. This groove separates the lower lip from the chin below.

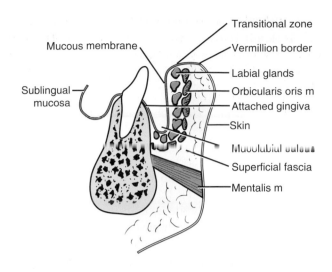

Figure 7-9 Sagittal section through the lower lip to demonstrate layers.

The upper and lower lips are continuous at the angles of the mouth and blend laterally with the cheeks.

Layers. The lip consists of several layers sandwiched between the skin externally and oral mucous membrane internally (*Figure 7-9*).

Skin. The skin of the lip exhibits all the general features of thin skin, such as hair, sweat, and sebaceous glands. As the skin of the lip approaches the mouth, it changes color abruptly to red. The point at which this change occurs is the **vermilion border** and marks the beginning of the red transitional zone between the external skin and the internal mucous membrane. The skin of the transitional zone is extremely thin and hairless, allowing the redness of the underlying capillary bed to show through.

Muscle. The muscle of the lip is the **orbicularis oris** muscle, the sphincter of the mouth. In addition, the circumoral muscles, which contribute to the orbicularis oris muscle, occupy this layer. The muscles lie within the superficial fascia.

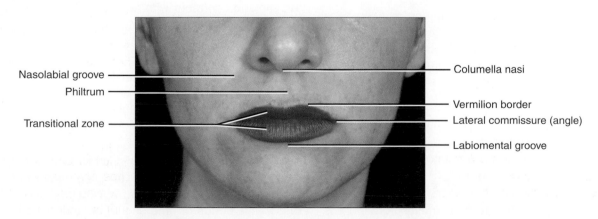

Figure 7-8 External features of the lips.

Glands. Within the submucosa lie numerous **labial mucous glands,** or labial glands. These can be felt by running the tongue against the bumpy internal surface of your own lips. These glands open directly through tiny duct openings to the vestibule of the mouth.

Mucous Membrane. The transitional zone sweeps into the mouth and is transformed into true, moist, nonkeratinizing mucous membrane. The mucous membrane coats the intraoral vestibular portion of the lip and then reflects down from the upper lip or up from the lower lip onto the alveolar process. The fold is the **vestibular,** or **mucolabial, fold.** The mucous membrane ascends on the alveolar process and turns abruptly to gingiva (gums). The demarcation is abrupt, with the gingiva assuming a lighter color and a stippled surface. The gingiva is firmly attached to the underlying alveolar bone. The gingiva is described in greater detail in section 8 of this chapter.

Labial Frenula. These are folds of mucous membrane that run in the midline of the upper lip and the lower lip

from the mucosa to the labial gingiva. Secondary frenula are found in the molar and premolar areas as well.

Arteries. The upper lip is supplied by superior labial branches of the facial and infraorbital arteries. The lower lip is supplied by inferior labial branches of the facial and mental arteries.

Sensory Nerves. The upper lip is supplied by the superior labial branch of the infraorbital nerve. The lower lip is supplied by the inferior labial branch of the mental nerve.

Functions. The lips are used for grasping food, sucking liquids, clearing the labial vestibule of food, forming speech, and osculation.

Cheeks (Buccae)

The cheeks form the lateral movable walls of the oral cavity (*Figure 7-10*). Externally, the cheek includes not only the movable portion but also the prominence of the cheek over the zygomatic arch. This terminology, however, is from common usage, and our definition of *cheek* is confined to the movable portion.

Layers. The cheek layers are similar to those of the lip and from superficial to deep are (1) skin, (2) the **buccinator muscle,** (3) **molar glands** within the submucosa, and (4) **buccal mucous membrane**.

The mucosa of the cheek ends in a **mucobuccal fold** superiorly and inferiorly, that sweeps onto the alveolar process. As the mucosa ascends to the alveolar crest, it becomes firmly attached to the bone as the gingiva.

CLINICAL NOTES

Labial Frenectomy

Occasionally, an overly large frenulum must be resected. Excessively large frenula may cause spacing between the central incisors in children. In adults, large frenula may contribute to gingival recession.

CLINICAL NOTES

Lesions of the Lips

Even before the dentist examines the oral cavity, the lips are examined because they are targets for many types of lesions and diseases.

Angular cheilosis is an inflammation and cracking of the skin and transition zone at the angles of the mouth. It is a condition that is usually associated with a B vitamin deficiency. It may also be infected with bacteria and/or fungi and is called *perlèche.* Treatment consists of a regimen of antibacterial and antifungal medication. This condition is common in older edentulous patients with angular wrinkling and leakage of saliva contributing to irritation and inflammation. Restoration of facial contours with dentures helps rectify this problem.

Herpes labialis, or cold sores, are painful vesicular lesions (watery blisters) at the vermilion border of the lip that are caused by the herpes simplex virus. The

vesicles rupture and form yellow crusted lesions that last about 10 days. Primary infections occur in early childhood and, after remission, the virus remains dormant in the trigeminal ganglion. The virus is opportunistic and can recur with fever-producing diseases, onset of menstruation, anxiety, exposure to sun, and occasionally dental treatment.

A **labial mucocele** or mucous retention cyst is a labial mucous gland with a blocked secretory duct that causes the gland and the overlying epithelium to bulge and assume a bluish tinge. Mucoceles usually occur on the lower lip. Large or noticeable cysts can be surgically removed.

Squamous cell carcinoma is a type of cancer. An ulcerated (cratered) lesion on the vermilion border of usually the lower lip that does not appear to heal over a reasonable period of time should be under suspicion and investigated.

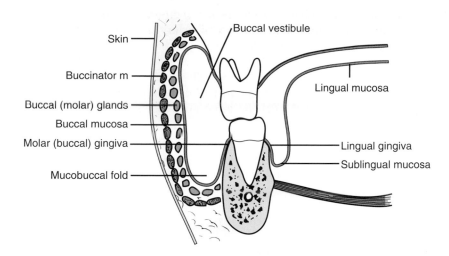

Figure 7-10 Coronal section through the cheek to demonstrate layers.

Occupying the space superficial to the buccinator muscle is a collection of fat, that is continuous with fat deposits deep to the ramus of the mandible and deep to the zygomatic arch lateral to the orbit. This fat depot is relatively larger in the infant, presumably to reinforce the cheeks and keep them from collapsing during sucking actions. Hence its name—the **buccal sucking fat pad**.

The **parotid duct** opens intraorally through the mucosa of the cheek at the occlusal level of the second maxillary molar.

Blood Supply. The cheek is supplied by the buccal branch of the maxillary artery.

Nerve Supply (Sensory). The cheek is innervated by the **buccal branch of the mandibular nerve** (long buccal nerve).

Functions. The cheeks and lips really function as a single unit and act as an oral sphincter to push food from the vestibular area to the oral cavity proper. In addition, they act together with the lips during sucking and blowing actions.

External Nose

Framework. The framework of the external nose consists of the paired nasal bones superiorly and a movable hyaline cartilage and fibroareolar portion below (*Figure 7-11*).

1. The **nasal bones** are described with the skull in Chapter 6.
2. The **septal cartilage** is a midline plate of hyaline cartilage that posteriorly forms a portion of the movable nasal septum.
3. The **lateral cartilages** are winglike anterior extensions of the **septal cartilage**; they flare to the right and left and are firmly attached to the nasal bones superiorly and the nasal notch of the maxilla laterally.

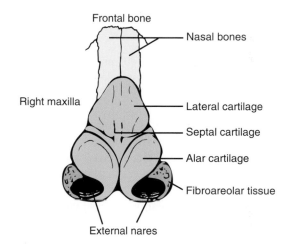

Figure 7-11 Skeleton of external nose.

4. The **alar cartilages** lie below the lateral cartilages like backward **C**s. They are anchored to the lateral cartilages above by areolar tissue. Fibroareolar tissue completes the deficiency of the **C** laterally to create the oval openings of the external nares.

Skin. The skin of the nose continues beyond the opening of the external nares into the vestibule of the nose. Within the vestibule, the skin is less keratinized but contains hair follicles and sebaceous glands. Nasal hairs are long (more prominent in the adult male) and act to filter larger particles of dust from the inhaled air.

The bulge of the alar cartilages into the floor and lateral wall of the vestibule marks the transition of skin to the respiratory nasal mucosa of the nasal cavity within.

Muscles. The muscle of the nose is the nasalis muscle, consisting of two sets of fibers: (1) the **dilator nares,** which flare the nostrils, and (2) the **compressor nares,** which flatten the nostrils (see *Figure 7-5*).

Blood Supply. The external nose is supplied by (1) the dorsal nasal branch of the ophthalmic artery, (2) the external nasal branch of the anterior ethmoidal artery, (3) the nasal branch of the infraorbital artery, and (4) the nasal branch of the facial artery.

Sensory Nerve Supply. The external nose is supplied by (1) the external nasal nerve (cranial nerve V-1), (2) the infratrochlear nerve (cranial nerve V-1), and (3) the nasal branches of the infraorbital nerve (cranial nerve V-2).

External Ear (Auricle)

Cartilage. A single elastic cartilage provides support for the external ear (*Figure 7-12*). The pendulous lower portion, or **earlobe**, contains no cartilage but does contain fibroareolar tissue. The cartilage of the ear is continuous with the cartilage of the external auditory meatus (canal), leading within the petrous temporal bone to the middle ear.

Muscles. The muscles of the ear are the **superior, anterior**, and **posterior auricular muscles**, which wiggle the ear (see *Figure 7-5*).

Skin. The skin of the auricle is tightly bound to the cartilage, with no intervening subcutaneous layer. The skin funnels into the opening of the external auditory meatus and lines the canal and the lateral aspect of the tympanic membrane (eardrum).

Ceruminous glands resembling sweat glands lie within the skin of the ear canal. These glands, along with secretions of sebaceous glands, produce cerumen, or earwax.

Prominent hair is not generally visible on the auricle. In older men, however, coarse tufts of hair appear on the tragus of the ear, guarding the entrance of the meatus.

Features. The cartilage and skin of the ear are thrown into several folds. The names of these resulting ridges and depressions are found in *Figure 7-12*.

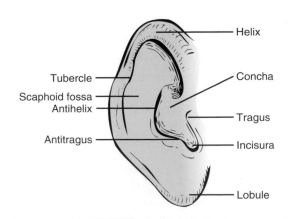

Figure 7-12 Features of the right external ear (auricle).

Blood Supply. The external ear is supplied by (1) branches of the **superficial temporal artery** and (2) branches of the **posterior auricular artery**.

Sensory Nerve Supply. The sensory innervation of the ear is from (1) the **auriculotemporal nerve** (from cranial nerve V-3), (2) the **great auricular nerve** (from anterior primary rami [APR] of C2 and C3), and (3) the **lesser occipital nerve** (from APR of C2 and C3).

In addition, small sensory contributions arise from the vagus (cranial nerve X) and the facial (cranial nerve VII) nerves.

Eyelids (Palpebrae)

The upper and lower lids form a curtain for the ocular globe, or eyeball. When closed, the lids protect the eye from light and harmful objects.

External Features (Figure 7-13)

1. The **palpebral fissure** is the transverse, elliptical opening between the upper and lower lids.
2. The **palpebral commissures** are the lateral and medial junctions of the upper and lower lids.
3. The **superior palpebral margin** covers the superior one fifth of the iris when the lids are open.
4. The **inferior palpebral margin** cuts across the lower border of the iris when the lids are open.
5. **Cilia**, or **eyelashes**, project from the palpebral margins in two or three irregular rows; the medial one sixth of each palpebral margin is devoid of cilia.
6. The **plica semilunaris** is a crescent fold at the medial angle of the eye that separates the white of the eye from the medial, reddish-colored lacus lacrimalis.
7. The **lacus lacrimalis** (lake of tears) is a small, raised, triangular area bordered by the plica semilunaris and the medial converging margins of the lid; a raised, reddish area within the lacus is the *caruncle*.
8. **Superior** and **inferior papillae** appear as small, raised bumps at the junction of the ciliated and hairless margins of the lids; the apex of the papilla presents a small opening, or punctum, which sucks up excess tears.
9. A mucous membrane inner lining of the eyelid, the **conjunctivum**, is seen when the eyelid is everted; the conjunctivum reflects up onto the eyeball to cover its anterior aspect. The conjunctival layer of the eyeball is reduced to a single layer of cuboidal epithelium, which is transparent. The space between the red conjunctivum of the lid and the transparent conjunctivum of the eyeball is termed the ***conjunctival sac***.

Layers

Skin. Extremely thin skin covers the lids of the eye (*Figure 7-14*). At the margins of the eye, prominent hairs, or cilia, form two or three irregular rows along the lateral

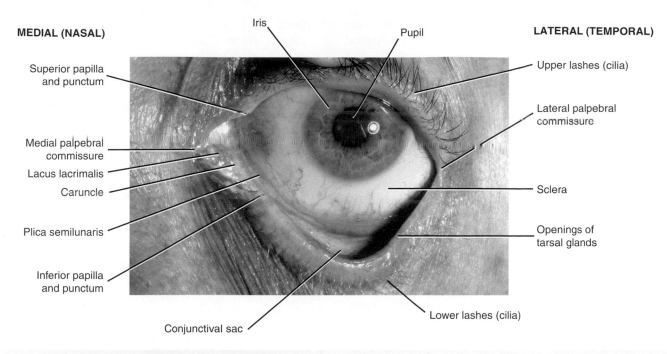

MEDIAL (NASAL)

Iris

Pupil

LATERAL (TEMPORAL)

Superior papilla and punctum

Upper lashes (cilia)

Lateral palpebral commissure

Medial palpebral commissure

Lacus lacrimalis

Caruncle

Plica semilunaris

Sclera

Openings of tarsal glands

Inferior papilla and punctum

Lower lashes (cilia)

Conjunctival sac

Figure 7-13 Surface features of the left eye and eyelids.

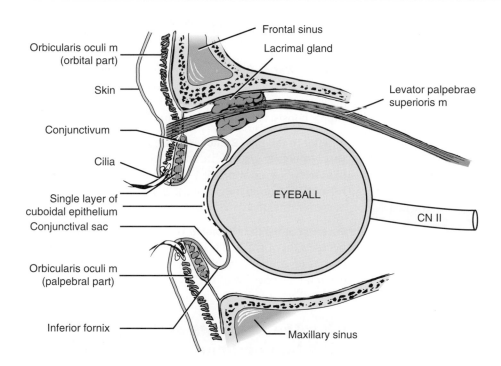

Orbicularis oculi m (orbital part)

Frontal sinus

Lacrimal gland

Skin

Levator palpebrae superioris m

Conjunctivum

Cilia

EYEBALL

Single layer of cuboidal epithelium

CN II

Conjunctival sac

Orbicularis oculi m (palpebral part)

Inferior fornix

Maxillary sinus

Figure 7-14 Sagittal section through eyelids and orbit to demonstrate layers of eyelids.

five sixths of the margin. Associated with the cilia are large sebaceous glands, or **ciliary glands** (glands of Zeis). Infected ciliary glands result in the common stye.

Muscular Layer. The palpebral portion of the **orbicularis oculi muscle** occupies the muscular. The fibers act as a sphincter and approximate the lids.

Fibers of the **levator palpebrae superioris** muscle pass through the orbicularis oculi muscle to insert superficially into the skin of the upper lid. This muscle opens the lid.

The motor nerve of the orbicularis oculi is the facial nerve; the motor nerve to the levator palpebrae superioris consists of the oculomotor nerve and some sympathetic fibers.

Orbital Septum and Tarsi. The orbital septum and tarsi form the "skeleton" of the eyelid (see *Figure 7-14* and also *Figure 7-34* later in this chapter). The orbital septum is a membranous connective tissue sheet that attaches to the periphery of the orbital margin. Medially, it attaches

237

to the posterior lacrimal crest. The septum forms a curtain with an elliptical transverse opening, the **palpebral fissure**.

The margins of the septum around the palpebral fissure are thickened as **tarsal plates**, or **tarsi**. The tarsi are half-moon in outline, and the lower tarsus is not as large as the upper one. Medially, the tarsi attach to the anterior lacrimal crest via the stout medial palpebral ligament. The lateral anchorage is weaker via the less prominent lateral palpebral ligament to the lateral margin of the orbit.

The tarsi contain large **tarsal glands**, seen as yellowish streaks shining through the conjunctivum in the everted lid. The ducts open to the margins of the lids and secrete an oily substance.

Conjunctiva. The *conjunctiva* is the special name given to the mucous membrane of the lids. It lines the inner aspect of the lid as *palpebral conjunctiva* and then at the base of the conjunctival sac reflects back onto the eyeball as *transparent bulbar conjunctiva*.

Lacrimal Apparatus. The lacrimal gland, which produces tears, and the duct system, which conveys excess tears away from the conjunctival sac, are discussed with the orbit and its contents in section 3 of this chapter.

Sensory Nerve Supply. The upper lid is supplied by branches of cranial nerve V-1: (1) the supraorbital nerve, (2) the supratrochlear nerve, (3) the infratrochlear nerve, and (4) the lacrimal nerve.

The lower lid is supplied entirely by palpebral branches of the infraorbital nerve (cranial nerve V-2).

Blood Supply. The upper lid is supplied by arteries that accompany the above nerves. In addition, the angular branch of the facial artery provides "twigs" to the lids.

The Scalp

The forehead, the anterior portion of the scalp, was considered with the face. The posterior portion of the scalp was considered with the suboccipital region.

As a unit, the scalp extends from the supraorbital margins back to the superior nuchal line posteriorly. Laterally, the scalp extends down into the temporal fossae.

Layers. The five layers of the scalp are easily learned by using the time-honored mnemonic *S-C-A-L-P*. From superficial to deep:

1. *Skin.* A layer of thin skin containing numerous hair follicles, sweat glands, and sebaceous glands covers the scalp.
2. *Connective tissue.* A thick, dense, subcutaneous connective tissue is anchored firmly to the skin above and the membranous layer below.
3. *Aponeurosis.* The membranous aponeurosis (galea aponeurotica) is an intermediate tendon for the two

fleshy bellies of the **occipitofrontalis (epicranius)** muscle (see *Figure 7-5, B*). The **occipitalis portion** originates just above the superior nuchal line and inserts into the aponeurosis. It pulls the scalp and the attached superficial layers back. The **frontalis portion** originates from the aponeurosis and inserts into skin above the eyebrows. It pulls the scalp forward and produces transverse wrinkling of the brow.
4. *Loose connective tissue.* The fourth layer consists of loose areolar tissue and allows freedom of movement of the superficial three layers over the top of the skull.
5. *Periosteum.* The periosteum is firmly anchored to the underlying bone.

Blood and Nerve Supply. The blood supply to the scalp arises from various sources but basically arises from branches of the ophthalmic and external carotid arteries (Figure 7-15). The arteries ascend to the scalp from the face below in a semicircle.

Anterior to the Ear. (1) The supratrochlear artery, (2) the supraorbital artery, (3) the zygomaticotemporal artery, (4) the superficial temporal artery.

Posterior to the Ear. (5) The posterior auricular artery, and (6) the occipital artery.

Sensory Nerve Supply. The cutaneous nerve supply to the scalp arises from the three divisions of the trigeminal nerve anterior to the ear. Posterior to the ear, the nerve supply consists of spinal cutaneous nerves from the neck.

Anterior to the Ear (Branches of Trigeminal Nerve). (1) The supratrochlear nerve (cranial nerve V-1), (2) the supraorbital nerve (cranial nerve V-1), (3) the zygomaticotemporal nerve (cranial nerve V-2), (4) the auriculotemporal nerve (cranial nerve V-3).

Posterior to the Ear (Spinal Nerves). (5) The lesser occipital nerve (APR of C2 and C3), (6) the greater occipital nerve (posterior primary rami [PPR] of C2), and (7) the third occipital nerve (PPR of C3).

2. The Contents of the Neurocranium

When the vault of the neurocranium is removed with a horizontal saw cut, the following structures are encountered within: (1) the meninges of the brain, (2) the dural venous sinuses, (3) the brain, (4) the cranial nerves, and (5) the blood supply to the brain.

SKELETON

Review the superior aspect of the skull and the internal aspect of the cranial base (see Chapter 6).

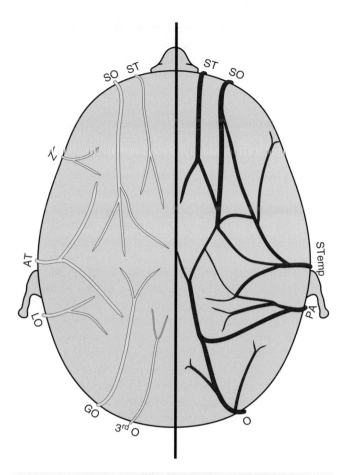

Figure 7-15 Superior view of the scalp to show the nerves and arteries. **Left:** *ST*, Supratrochlear nerve; *SO*, supraorbital nerve; *ZT*, zygomaticotemporal nerve; *AT*, auriculotemporal nerve; *LO*, lesser occipital nerve; *GO*, greater occipital nerve; *3rd O*, third occipital nerve. **Right:** *ST*, Supratrochlear artery; *SO*, supraorbital artery; *STemp*, superficial temporal artery; *PA*, posterior auricular artery; *O*, occipital artery.

CLINICAL NOTES

Detachment of the Scalp

Long hair caught in machinery is a potential industrial hazard, for it can result in the tearing of the scalp along the plane of loose connective tissue (layer 4). Scalp detachment is also common in automobile accidents in which victims are hurled forward through the windshield. The excellent anastomoses and collateral arterial supply ensure a good prognosis following reattachment.

Lacerations

Lacerations to the scalp are a common head injury that generally require surgical attention. The blood supply to the scalp is profuse and, to complicate matters, the arterial walls are fixed within layer 2 and cannot retract to allow clotting. To stem the continuous bleeding, direct pressure must be applied.

Infections

Infections within layer 4 tend to spread readily through the space. Infection may spread deeper via emissary veins to infect dural venous sinuses within the cranial cavity.

MENINGES

The meninges consists of three layers, each called *mater* ("mother"): (1) dura mater externally, (2) arachnoid mater, the intermediate layer, and (3) pia mater internally (*Figure 7-16*).

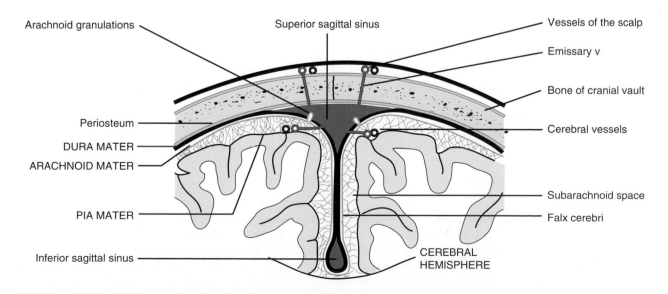

Figure 7-16 Coronal section through the falx cerebri to show meninges and superior and inferior sagittal sinuses.

Dura Mater

Dura mater is a tough, membranous outer lining of the meninges. Within the skull, dura is traditionally described as consisting of two layers, the inner layer of dura proper and an outer layer that is actually the periosteum of the internal cranial vault. The two layers of dura are closely adherent.

Dura mater coats the internal aspect of the cranial vault and the cranial base. Its inner surface is smooth and glistening.

Dural Folds. In four areas, the dura proper folds upon itself and projects into the cranial cavity, interposed between various portions of the brain. There are two vertical folds and two horizontal folds.

Vertical Folds. The **falx cerebri** is a large, sickle-shaped fold (*Figure 7-17*). Its base is attached in the median plane to the internal aspect of the skull. It hangs down into the cranial cavity like a knife slicing the right and left cerebral hemispheres in two. It has an inferior free edge. Running through the base of the falx cerebri and through the inferior free edge are venous dural channels, or sinuses, described later.

The base of the falx cerebri is attached anteriorly to the crista galli, the frontal crest, and then sweeps upward and backward attached to the lips of the superior sagittal sulcus on the internal aspect of the skull vault. The attached base ends posteriorly at the internal occipital protuberance. The anterior two thirds of the inferior border is free-edged; the posterior third is attached to the horizontal tentorium cerebelli.

The **falx cerebelli** is a small, crescent midline fold interposed between the right and left cerebellar hemispheres. Its attached base runs downward from the internal occipital crest toward the posterior margin of the foramen magnum. Its anterosuperior border is free-edged.

Horizontal Folds. The **tentorium cerebelli** is a somewhat horizontal fold stretching across the posterior third of the *internal skull* to separate the cerebral hemispheres above from the cerebellum below (*Figure 7-18*). Its attached border is to bone beginning at the margins of the internal occipital protuberance and arching laterally on each side adherent to the margins of the bony transverse sulcus within the skull. On reaching the petrous temporal ridge, the dura attaches to the margins of the superior petrosal sulcus and ends medially at the posterior clinoid process.

The tentorium cerebelli presents a U-shaped, free-edged border, which permits passage of the brainstem. Anteriorly, the free edges attach to the anterior clinoid processes. The three-point attachment of dura running from the petrous temporal ridge to the posterior clinoid process and to the *anterior clinoid process* is termed the *triangular field* and is noted solely because two cranial nerves pierce the dura of the triangular field en route to leaving the skull. The superior median aspect of the tentorium provides attachment for the posteroinferior portion of the falx cerebri.

The **diaphragma sellae** is a small, horizontal fold stretched between the anterior and posterior clinoid

---

CLINICAL NOTES

Intracranial Hemorrhage

Intracranial hemorrhages are leakages of blood into the meningeal spaces described previously. **Extradural hemorrhage** in the skull is caused by a rupture of the middle meningeal artery or one of its branches. The middle meningeal artery is closely applied to the inner aspect of the skull and is particularly vulnerable in the temple region, where the skull vault is very thin and susceptible to fracture accompanied by laceration of the underlying artery. The escaping blood exerts enough pressure to strip the dura from the skull and form a pool of blood (hematoma) that exerts pressure on the brain. If the intracranial pressure is not relieved, unconsciousness and death can ensue.

A **subdural hemorrhage** is caused by a rupture of cerebral veins as they enter the superior sagittal sinus. The blood escapes, separates the dura and arachnoid layers, and forms a hematoma in the newly created subdural space, creating pressure on the underlying brain. Venous hemorrhage is not as rapid as arterial

so that the condition takes longer to unfold in comparison to extradural hemorrhage.

Subarachnoid hemorrhage is usually the result of a rupture in the arterial circle of Willis at the base of the brain. The ruptures, in turn, are generally caused by a congenital weakness in the arterial wall. Arterial pressure can cause the weakened wall to bulge (berry aneurysm) and rupture into the subarachnoid space, allowing blood to mix with the cerebrospinal fluid and increasing pressure on the brain below. Leakage of blood into this space is revealed by a diagnostic spinal tap, which is a search for blood cells not normally present in the fluid (see Chapter 1, Section 7).

Meningitis

Meningitis is an inflammation of the meningeal coverings of the brain and spinal cord caused by bacterial, viral, or fungal infections. Infective toxins not only inflame the meninges but the underlying brain as well (encephalitis). Inflammation of both sets of tissues is termed *meningo-encephalitis*. The condition is characterized by stiffness in the neck and movement-associated pain.

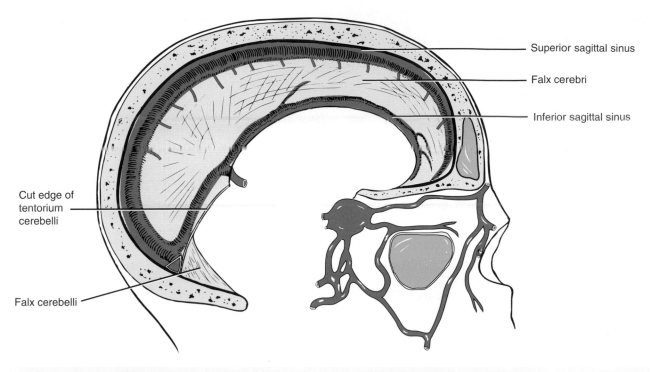

Superior sagittal sinus

Falx cerebri

Inferior sagittal sinus

Cut edge of
tentorium
cerebelli

Falx cerebelli

Figure 7-17 Two vertical folds of dura and deep venous drainage of the face.

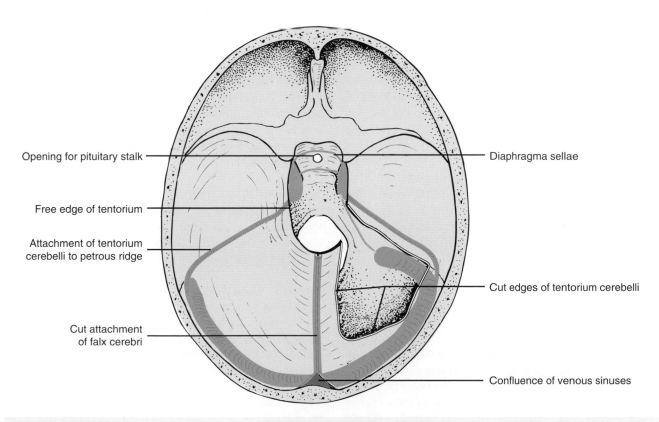

Opening for pituitary stalk

Free edge of tentorium

Attachment of tentorium
cerebelli to petrous ridge

Cut attachment
of falx cerebri

Diaphragma sellae

Cut edges of tentorium cerebelli

Confluence of venous sinuses

Figure 7-18 Two horizontal folds of dura.

processes of the sella turcica like a tiny trampoline. A small opening through the center permits passage of the stalk of the hypophysis cerebri (see also *Figure 7-27, B*).

Arachnoid Mater

The arachnoid mater lies immediately deep to the dura mater (*Figure 7-18*). It sends fine, weblike filaments deep to the layer of pia mater below. The arachnoid does not follow the folds of the brain but rather bridges across them.

Pia Mater

Pia mater is a thin, delicate layer that intimately adheres to the gyri and sulci of the cortical surface.

Meningeal Spaces

Extradural (Epidural) Space. The dura is fused to the periosteum lining the internal aspect of the skull so the subdural space between the skull and the dura is a potential space only (see *Figure 7-16*).

Subdural Space. This is another potential space immediately below the dura. It is normally obliterated by pressure of the underlying arachnoid layer.

Subarachnoid Space. Below the arachnoid layer, in the space occupied by the fine arachnoid filaments, is the subarachnoid space. It is filled with cerebrospinal fluid.

Blood Supply to the Meninges

Only the dura mater is supplied with an external source of blood. The supply is through so-called meningeal arteries, which, in addition to dura, supply the inner table and the diploë (middle spongy layer) of the skull bones.

The dura of the anterior and middle cranial fossae is supplied by the middle meningeal artery. Dura of the posterior cranial fossa is supplied by meningeal branches arising from the vertebral artery.

Sensory Nerve Supply to the Meninges

The dura mater of the anterior and middle cranial fossae receives sensory nerves from all three divisions of the trigeminal nerve. Dura of the posterior cranial fossa receives sensory nerves from branches of cervical spinal nerves.

CRANIAL VENOUS SINUSES

Blood return from the brain flows via cerebral veins to special channels within the skull called *venous sinuses* (*Figure 7-19*). Cranial venous sinuses contain no valves and, aside from an endothelial lining, do not have regular venous walls. The venous sinuses occupy spaces where the inner layer of dura separates from the outer periosteal layer, such as at the base of dural folds (see *Figure 7-16*).

All venous blood within the skull is collected by venous sinuses, which ultimately carry the venous blood to the jugular foramina. A small amount of venous blood exits directly through small *emissary veins*, which pierce the cranial bones and drain to the external veins of the scalp (see *Figure 7-16*). Only the major cranial venous sinuses are described in the following section.

Superior Sagittal Sinus

The superior sagittal sinus forms by receiving contributions from several **cerebral veins**, which drain the brain. It occupies the attached base of the falx cerebri in the space created by the separation of the dura proper and the periosteal layer of dura (see *Figure 7-16*).

Arachnoid granulations are small, cauliflower-like extensions that protrude into the lateral aspects of the superior sagittal sinus (see *Figure 7-16*). Cerebrospinal fluid leaks back across the arachnoid membrane through these arachnoid granulations to enter the venous blood of the superior sagittal sinus.

The superior sagittal sinus forms anterior to the crista galli and sweeps upward and backward in the base of the falx cerebri. It ends posteriorly at the **confluence**, which then leads to the right and left as the right and left transverse venous sinuses.

Inferior Sagittal Sinus

The inferior sagittal sinus starts anteriorly in the region of the crista galli and follows the inferior border within the falx cerebri upward and backward. It receives blood from small cerebral veins. As it approaches the tentorium cerebelli posteriorly, it joins with the large great cerebral vein (of Galen) to form the straight sinus.

Straight Sinus. The straight sinus occupies the hollow interval between the inferior base of the falx cerebri and the tentorium cerebelli. The straight sinus passes posteriorly to the internal occipital protuberance, where it ends at the **confluence**, which leads to the right and left transverse sinuses.

Transverse Sinus (Paired). The transverse sinus passes laterally and anteriorly within the attached base of the tentorium cerebelli from the confluence. As the sinus approaches the petrous temporal ridge, it takes a deeper S-shaped course medially as the sigmoid sinus.

Sigmoid Sinus (Paired). The sigmoid sinus continues medially from the transverse sinus at the base of the petrous ridge. It ends at the mouth of the jugular foramen. *Thus, all the venous blood ultimately collected by the sigmoid sinuses drains through the jugular foramina to the internal jugular veins below.*

Cavernous Sinus (Paired). The cavernous sinus lies on the side of the sella turcica and occupies the broad expanded base of the diaphragma sellae. It receives blood

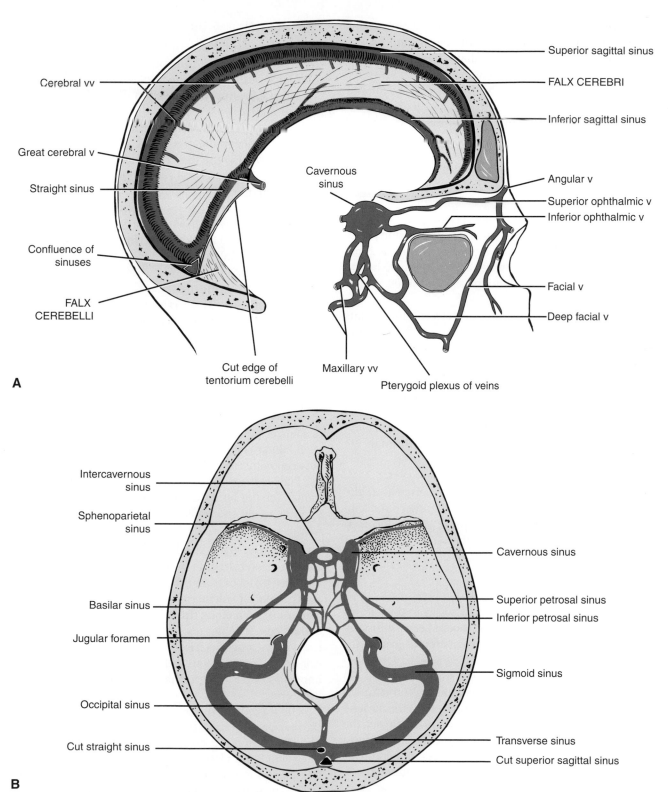

Figure 7-19 Internal aspect of the head with brain removed to show the cranial venous sinuses. **A,** Sagittal section. **B,** Horizontal section with the tentorium cerebelli removed.

from (1) the superior and inferior ophthalmic veins of the orbit, (2) cerebral veins draining the brain, and (3) the sphenoparietal sinus running medially under the shelter of the lesser wings of the sphenoid to the cavernous sinus. The cavernous sinus is drained by the superior and inferior petrosal sinuses.

Anterior and posterior **intercavernous sinuses** connect the right and left cavernous sinuses. A number of structures run through the cavernous sinus en route to the orbit. These are discussed under features of the middle cranial fossa (see pages 255 and 256).

Superior Petrosal Sinus. The superior petrosal sinus drains the cavernous sinus and travels laterally and posteriorly along the crest of the petrous ridge within the superior petrosal sulcus. As the sinus approaches the lateral limit of the ridge, it empties into the sigmoid sinus.

Inferior Petrosal Sinus. The inferior petrosal sinus drains the cavernous sinus, but drains downward and posteriorly within the dura-covered inferior petrosal sulcus to empty directly to the internal jugular foramen and vein.

Basilar Sinus. The basilar sinus lies below the dura of the clivus, scattered in a plexiform fashion. It receives blood from the cavernous sinus and inferior petrosal sinus and then drains to the vertebral plexus of veins through the foramen magnum.

Occipital Sinus. The occipital sinus travels within the base of the falx cerebelli down along the internal occipital crest. It skirts the posterior margin of the foramen magnum and communicates with the vertebral plexus of veins.

Emissary Veins

A small amount of venous blood passes from the venous sinuses directly through small skull openings via emissary veins. The emissary veins, in turn, communicate with extracranial veins of the scalp (see *Figure 7-16*).

The foramina that transmit emissary veins are (1) the **foramen cecum**—from the superior sagittal sinus to veins of the nasal cavity (in the fetus only), (2) the **parietal foramina**—from the superior sagittal sinus to veins of the scalp, (3) the **mastoid foramina**—from the sigmoid sinus to the posterior auricular vein, and (4) the **posterior condylar canal**—from the sigmoid sinus to the suboccipital veins.

Diploic Veins

The diploë is the spongy bone between the outer and inner tables of skull bones. Arterial supply to the bone is from meningeal arteries from within and scalp vessels from without. Venous drainage of the diploë is via diploic veins directly inward to intracranial venous sinuses.

THE BRAIN

The following brief description of the brain is intended solely to demonstrate the continuity of incoming blood supply and outgoing cranial nerves. More detailed descriptions of the brain are provided in textbooks dealing with neuroanatomy.

The brain (encephalon) consists of five components: (1) the **telencephalon** (cerebral hemispheres), (2) the **diencephalon,** (3) the **mesencephalon** (midbrain), (4) the **metencephalon** (pons and cerebellum), and (5) the **myelencephalon** (medulla oblongata).

Each portion of the brain consists of areas of **gray matter** (*cell bodies*), areas of **white matter** (*myelinated cell processes* commonly called *fibers*), and **hollow spaces** filled with cerebrospinal fluid (*ventricles*).

Cerebral Hemispheres

Surface Features. The cerebral hemispheres are the largest portion of the brain, occupying most of the cranial cavity (*Figure 7-20*). They are two bilaterally symmetrical hemispheres joined across the midline by a thick band of communicating fibers called the *corpus callosum*. The **cerebral cortex** is the surface layer (1 to 2 cm in thickness) that covers the cerebral hemispheres. The surface area of the hemispheres is increased significantly by a number of folds or convolutions. The grooves or spaces between each fold are called *sulci* (sing. *sulcus*); the ridges or folds between adjacent sulci are termed *gyri* (sing. *gyrus*). Key sulci divide the cerebrum into several lobes. The lobes are named for the bones of the skull under which they are found, namely, the *frontal, parietal, temporal,* and *occipital lobes.*

Key Sulci and Gyri. The **lateral sulcus** slashes obliquely across the lateral aspect of the brain separating the frontal and parietal lobes from the temporal lobe below.

The **central sulcus** runs from the superior pole of the cerebrum down along the lateral surface almost to the lateral sulcus. It separates the frontal lobe anteriorly from the parietal lobe posteriorly. The gyrus immediately anterior to the central sulcus is the **precentral gyrus;** the gyrus immediately posterior to the central sulcus is the **postcentral gyrus.**

The **precentral sulcus** delineates the anterior limit of the **precentral gyrus.** The **postcentral sulcus** delineates the posterior limit of the **postcentral gyrus.** The **parieto-occipital sulcus** is found mainly on the medial aspect separating the parietal lobe anteriorly from the occipital lobe posteriorly. The calcarine sulcus runs anteriorly on the medial aspect from the occipital pole of the cerebral hemisphere.

Lobes. The lateral, central, and parieto-occipital sulci are used to divide the cerebral hemispheres into four lobes: (1) **frontal lobe** anterior to the central sulcus and above the lateral sulcus, (2) **parietal lobe** posterior to the central sulcus and above the lateral sulcus, (3) **temporal lobe**

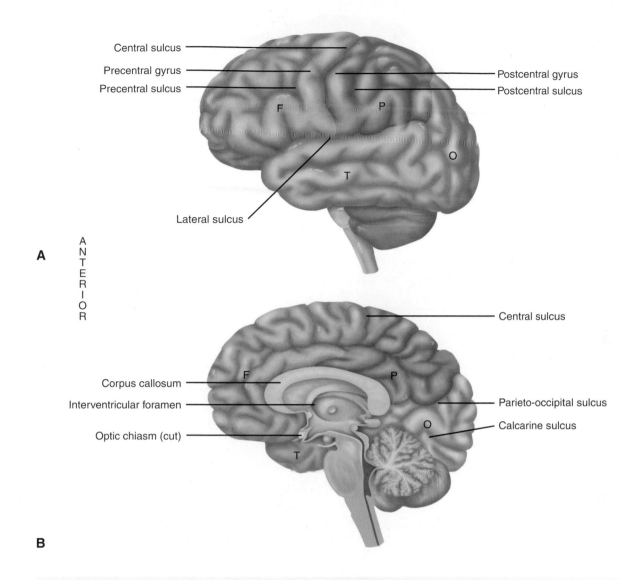

Figure 7-20 Gyri, sulci, and lobes of the brain. **A,** Lateral aspect of the left cerebral hemisphere. **B,** Left hemisphere removed to reveal the medial aspect of the right cerebral hemisphere. *F,* Frontal lobe; *P,* parietal lobe; *T,* temporal lobe; *O,* occipital lobe.

below the lateral sulcus, and (4) **occipital lobe** posterior to the parieto-occipital sulcus.

Functional Areas. The **primary motor area** lies within the *precentral gyrus* of the frontal lobe (*Figure 7-21*). It contains the cell bodies of upper motor neurons. Their axons descend through the *pyramidal tracts* and decussate to synapse with contralateral lower motor neuron in motor nuclei of the brainstem and ventral horns of the spinal cord. This is collectively termed the *pyramidal motor system,* and it is responsible for initiating voluntary movements.

The **general sensory (somesthetic) area** lies within the *postcentral gyrus* of the parietal lobe. It contains the cell bodies that ultimately receive impulses from the ascending sensory pathways conveying pain, temperature, touch,

and proprioception from the opposite side of the body. These sensory modalities are perceived within the postcentral gyrus.

The **primary visual area** lies on either side of the **calcarine sulcus** and receives visual impulses from the contralateral half of the visual field. The **taste area** lies at the most inferior portion of the postcentral gyrus in the parietal lobe.

The **areas of speech** for 95% of the population reside in the left cerebral hemisphere. This includes all right-handed people and most left-handed people. Speech and language are controlled by two separate but connected areas. The **motor speech (Broca's) area** is located just anterior to the inferior aspect of the precentral gyrus. Broca's area controls the ability to vocalize; damage results in

245

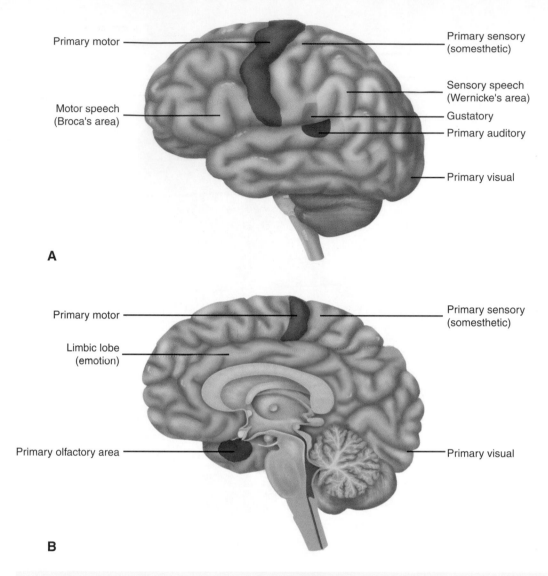

Figure 7-21 Functional areas of the brain. **A,** Lateral aspect of the left cerebral hemisphere. **B,** Left hemisphere removed to reveal medial aspect of the right cerebral hemisphere.

difficulty or an inability to articulate (motor aphasia). The **sensory speech (Wernicke's) area** lies within the junction of the parietal, occipital, and temporal lobes. It enables comprehension of the spoken language or language fluency. Damage to this area results in sensory aphasia.

The **auditory area** lies in the temporal lobe immediately anterior to the sensory speech area. The **olfactory area** is located on the anteroinferior aspect of the temporal lobe.

Association areas occupy the remainder of the cortical areas of the cerebral hemispheres. They control the integration of incoming stimuli and outgoing responses.

Internal Features. The internal aspect of the cerebral hemispheres consists primarily of white matter with isolated islands of gray matter (*Figure 7-22*).

White Matter. The white matter consists of myelinated nerve processes or nerve fibers that link the various areas of the brain and spinal cord. The fibers run in bundles or tracts. There are three types of fiber tracts.

Association tracts link cerebral centers within the same hemisphere. Short association fibers join adjacent, centers and long association fibers allow communication among lobes of the same hemisphere.

Commissural or **bridging fibers** join cerebral centers in one hemisphere with contralateral centers in the opposite hemisphere. Most commissural fibers travel in the corpus callosum; the remainder travel through the anterior commissure.

Projection fibers travel up or down linking higher and lower centers of the brain and spinal cord. Ascending (sensory) tracts eventually end in or project to the postcentral

246

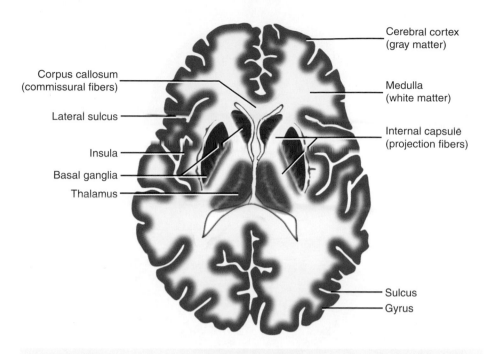

Figure 7-22 Horizontal stained section through the brain to demonstrate areas of gray and white matter.

gyrus. Descending (motor) tracts pass inferiorly to lower motor neurons located in cranial nerve motor nuclei of the brainstem or spinal nerve motor nuclei in the spinal cord (ventral horn).

Gray Matter: Basal Ganglia. Within the cerebrum are several nuclei collectively termed *basal ganglia*. These ganglia are really motor nuclei that belong to the *extrapyramidal motor system*. The pyramidal system described earlier initiates voluntary movement; the extrapyramidal motor system *adjusts and refines* the initial movements and provides *fine motor control*.

The Brainstem

Diencephalon. The diencephalon is a wedge-shaped area between the cerebral hemispheres (*Figure 7-23*); it is almost completely covered by the hemispheres. The lateral borders are difficult to demonstrate because they blend with the substance of each hemisphere. The diencephalon is seen to best advantage in a median section through the brain and brainstem (see *Figure 7-23, B*).

The diencephalon is divided into four functional areas.

Thalamus. The thalamus is the largest area and is basically a large sensory relay station containing tertiary neurons. All ascending sensory pathways (except olfaction) synapse in nuclei of the thalamus prior to projecting to the postcentral gyrus.

Epithalamus. The epithalamus sits above the thalamus and includes the pineal body and the habenular trigones. The function of both components of the epithalamus are not known at this point. Calcified deposits develop within the pineal body after the age of 16 years. This makes it a

useful landmark on radiographs of the head to determine whether trauma or disease has displaced the calcified pineal body from the midline.

Hypothalamus. The **hypothalamus,** including the **hypophysis cerebri,** is a small, yet important, area below and anterior to the thalamus that plays a major role in maintaining a *constant internal body environment (homeostasis)*. The hypothalamus plays a role in triggering responses to emotional changes and to needs signaled by hunger and thirst. It is the *integrating center for the autonomic nervous system*.

The Midbrain. The midbrain is immediately below the diencephalon and is about 2 cm in length. The **corpora quadrigemina** are a set of four bumps on the posterior surface of the midbrain. The **superior colliculi** ("small hills") are the upper set of bumps; the **inferior colliculi** are the lower set of bumps. The colliculi are *relay stations on the optic and auditory pathways* that initiate body responses to visual and auditory stimuli: for example, ducking a wild pitch or jumping at the unexpected sound of a loud noise.

The **cerebral peduncles (crura cerebri)** are two very large bundles of nerve fibers on the anterior aspect of the midbrain. The peduncles contain **descending motor fibers** of the **pyramidal pathway. Motor nuclei of cranial nerves III and IV** are found within the midbrain, surrounding the cerebral aqueduct. The **substantia nigra** and the **red nucleus** are motor nuclei involved with the **extrapyramidal motor system.**

The Pons. The pons is a relatively simple portion of the brainstem containing fibers running to and from its

247

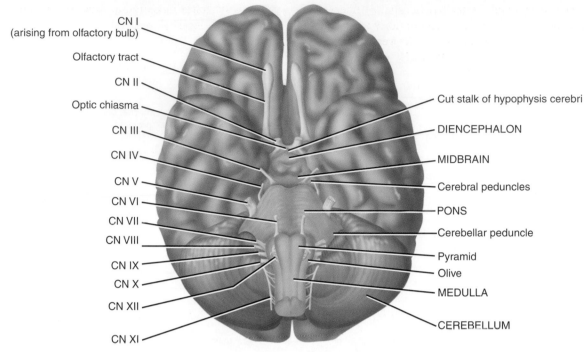

CN I
(arising from olfactory bulb)

Olfactory tract

CN II

Optic chiasma

CN III

CN IV

CN V

CN VI

CN VII

CN VIII

CN IX

CN X

CN XII

CN XI

Cut stalk of hypophysis cerebri

DIENCEPHALON

MIDBRAIN

Cerebral peduncles

PONS

Cerebellar peduncle

Pyramid

Olive

MEDULLA

CEREBELLUM

A

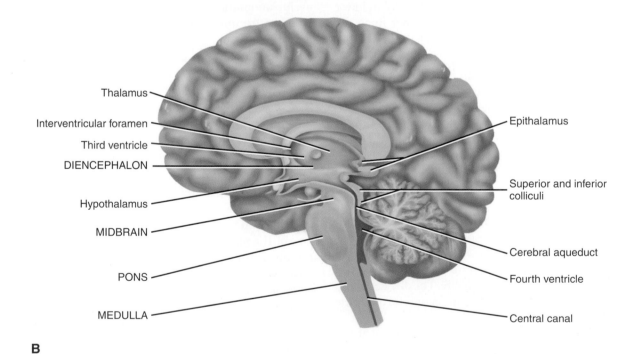

Thalamus

Interventricular foramen

Third ventricle

DIENCEPHALON

Hypothalamus

MIDBRAIN

PONS

MEDULLA

Epithalamus

Superior and inferior
colliculi

Cerebral aqueduct

Fourth ventricle

Central canal

B

Figure 7-23 **A** and **B**, Inferior view of brain to show the brainstem and cranial nerves.

posterior appendage, the cerebellum, and fibers in transit traveling up or down the brainstem. The **pontine nuclei** are relay stations for transversely crossing fibers.

Sensory and **motor nuclei associated with the trigeminal nerve (cranial nerve** V) are found within the pons.

Medulla Oblongata. The medulla oblongata is the transitional portion of the brainstem leading to the spinal cord below and extends between the pons above and the first cervical nerve below.

The **pyramids** are raised longitudinal fiber tracts on either side of the midline on the ventral aspect and contain the *descending pyramidal tract* (corticospinal) fibers. The **pyramidal decussation** can be seen inferiorly as pyramidal fibers crossing from left to right and vice versa.

The **nucleus gracilis** and the **nucleus cuneatus** are bilateral medial and lateral swellings of the dorsal aspect containing *second-order sensory neurons*, which synapse with proprioceptive fibers ascending from the spinal cord.

Cranial nerve nuclei of **cranial nerves VI, VII,** and **VIII** are found near the junction of the pons and medulla. **Cranial nerve nuclei of IX, X, XI,** and **XII** are found within the medulla.

The **reticular formation** consists of nuclei scattered loosely around the cranial nerve nuclei of the medulla, pons, and midbrain. The reticular formation is an *integrating center for complex reflexes* involving the cranial nerves. In addition, the reticular formation helps to *regulate visceral functions* and to *maintain arousal and consciousness.*

Cerebellum

The cerebellum sits atop the pons and a portion of the medulla and forms the roof of the fourth ventricle. It is somewhat similar to the cerebrum in that it consists of two hemispheres and has an external surface coated with gray matter that is thrown into folds. The folds, however, are arranged in a more orderly transverse fashion and are termed *folia.*

The cerebellum receives *vestibular information* from the semicircular canals of the inner ear and *proprioceptive information* from the muscles and joints of the body. It also receives collateral information from the descending pyramidal pathway. Armed with this information, the cerebellum then helps to *coordinate and synchronize* muscle movement initiated by the motor cortex. In addition, the cerebellum *maintains equilibrium and postural tone.*

Ventricular System

Formation of the brain begins with differentiation of the cephalic end of the hollow neural tube. Four hollow spaces, or **ventricles**, lined with ependymal cells evaginate into various areas of the brain. The ventricles interconnect and are filled with cerebrospinal fluid (CSF) produced by the **choroid plexus** (*Figure 7-24*).

The choroid plexus is formed by arterial capillaries covered with pia mater that have evaginated into the ventricular space. The plexus retains the ependymal lining of the ventricles. The CSF leaks across the choroid plexus membranes to fill and circulate within the ventricular system.

Lateral Ventricles within the Cerebral Hemispheres. The lateral ventricles (ventricles I and II) develop as C-shaped extensions of the lumen of the neural tube into the right and left *cerebral hemisphere.* The lateral ventricle has a **body** in the parietal lobe. An **anterior horn** extends anteriorly into the frontal lobe, a **posterior horn** extends posteriorly into the occipital lobe, and an **inferior horn** extends into the temporal lobe below.

Third Ventricle within the Diencephalon. The third ventricle is a midline cleft within the *diencephalon.* The **interventricular foramina** are two openings in the anterior aspect of the ventricle like two portholes on a ship's bow that communicate with the lateral ventricles.

Cerebral Aqueduct within the Midbrain. The cerebral aqueduct is a narrow canal that funnels downward from the floor of the third ventricle, passes through the *midbrain*, and opens into the fourth ventricle below.

Fourth Ventricle within the Pons and Medulla. As the cerebral aqueduct leaves the midbrain to enter the pons, it expands as the fourth ventricle, its roof and walls formed by the cerebellum and its floor formed by the dorsal aspect of the pons and medulla.

Two **lateral apertures** and a **midline median aperture** allow CSF to leave the ventricle and enter the subarachnoid space. Inferiorly, the ventricle narrows down to form the central canal of the medulla, which, in turn, becomes the **central canal** of the spinal cord.

BLOOD SUPPLY TO THE BRAIN: ARTERIAL CIRCLE (OF WILLIS)

Four large arteries enter the skull to form an arterial circle around the base of the brain (*Figure 7-25*). The circle of arterial flow ensures that blockage of arterial flow in one arterial branch to the brain is compensated for by flow from the other tributaries.

Four large arteries contribute to the formation of the arterial circle: the right and left internal carotid arteries and the right and left vertebral arteries.

Internal Carotid Artery

The right common carotid artery arises from the brachiocephalic artery; the left common carotid artery arises directly from the arch of the aorta. The common carotid artery ascends in the neck within the carotid sheath and, at the level of the hyoid bone, divides into two terminal branches. The external carotid artery continues on to supply the face. The internal carotid artery ascends to the carotid canal at the base of the skull and enters the petrous temporal bone; the artery passes obliquely through the carotid canal and turns upward at the junction of the carotid canal and the foramen lacerum to enter the skull. Within the skull, the internal carotid artery travels forward within the cavernous sinus lateral to the sella turcica and gives off branches to the wall of the cavernous sinus, pituitary gland, and trigeminal ganglion. Under the anterior clinoid process, the internal carotid artery curves upward, gives off the

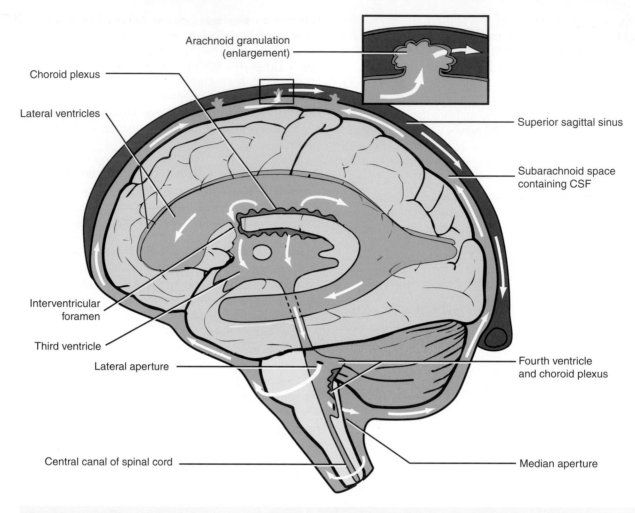

Choroid plexus

Lateral ventricles

Arachnoid granulation
(enlargement)

Superior sagittal sinus

Subarachnoid space
containing CSF

Interventricular
foramen

Third ventricle

Lateral aperture

Fourth ventricle
and choroid plexus

Central canal of spinal cord

Median aperture

Figure 7-24 Ventricles of the brain and a scheme of production, flow, and reabsorption of CSF. *CSF*, Cerebro spinal fluid.

ophthalmic artery to the orbit via the optic canal, and then curves anteriorly on itself. At this point the internal carotid artery gives off the posterior communicating artery, which travels posteriorly to join the posterior cerebral artery. The internal carotid artery ends by dividing into two terminal branches, the **anterior** and **middle cerebral arteries**.

The Vertebral Artery

The vertebral artery arises as the first branch from the subclavian artery in the root of the neck. The artery ascends toward the transverse process of vertebra C6 and enters its foramen transversarium. It then ascends through successively higher foramina transversaria, looping laterally, then medially, as it passes from C2 to C1. The arteries turn upward to enter the skull through the foramen magnum, along with the spinal cord.

Within the skull, two branches of the vertebral arteries join in the midline as the **anterior spinal artery**, which

descends back through the foramen magnum to supply the upper spinal cord. The two vertebral arteries converge toward the midline and give off the **posteroinferior cerebellar arteries**. The right and left vertebral arteries then unite as the single **basilar artery** on the grooved ventral surface of the pons. The basilar artery gives off the **anteroinferior cerebellar arteries**. At the superior border of the pons, the basilar artery divides as the right and left **posterior cerebral arteries**.

Communicating Arteries

Arterial communications complete the circle in the following manner: The **anterior communicating artery** joins the right and left anterior cerebral arteries; the **posterior communicating arteries** join the posterior cerebral artery to the internal carotid artery. Collateral branches of the vertebral and basilar arteries and communications between the basilar and internal carotid branches are shown in *Figure 7-25*.

Distribution of the Cerebral Arteries

The territories of the anterior, middle, and posterior cerebral arteries are shown in *Figure 7-25, B.*

THE CRANIAL NERVES

A general description of the central and peripheral nervous system is presented in Chapter 1 and should be reviewed at this point. The cranial nerves, in this chapter, are described in a physical sense, that is, the origin and course of each nerve from the brain, through the dura, and through its respective skull foramen to its ultimate destination (*Figure 7-26*). The functional components are discussed in Chapter 8.

Cranial Nerve I: Olfactory Nerve

The **olfactory tract** arises from the *olfactory trigone* on the inferior surface of the forebrain. The tract moves forward on the anterior cranial fossa floor and ends as two swellings, the **olfactory bulbs,** atop the *cribriform plate*. Tiny rootlets **(cranial I proper)** pass from the bulb through the dura and the perforations of the cribriform plate to the roof of the nasal cavity below.

Cranial Nerve II: Optic Nerve

The **optic tracts** originate from the *lateral geniculate bodies* at the base of the diencephalon. The tracts pass forward and converge at the midline to cross over at the **optic chiasma** (not all fibers cross). Passing forward from the chiasma are the right and left **optic nerves** (actually, they are still tracts). They pierce the dura to pass through the *optic foramen* to enter the orbit. Within the orbit, the optic nerve enters the posterior aspect of the eyeball to ultimately synapse with rod and cone cells within the retina.

Cranial Nerve III: Oculomotor Nerve

The oculomotor nerve emerges from the *interpeduncular fossa of the midbrain and travels forward to pierce the dura of the triangular fold* to enter the *cavernous sinus*. It passes through the sinus adherent to its lateral wall and leaves by passing through the *superior orbital fissure* to enter the orbit.

Cranial Nerve IV: Trochlear Nerve

The trochlear nerve is the only cranial nerve to arise from the dorsum of the brainstem. It arises as a slender thread *from below the inferior colliculus of the midbrain* and encircles the brainstem to pass anteriorly. It pierces the dura of the *triangular field* to enter the cavernous sinus, travels along the lateral sinus wall, and leaves through the *superior orbital fissure* to enter the orbit.

Cranial Nerve V: Trigeminal Nerve

The trigeminal nerve originates from the pons as a thick **sensory root** and a smaller but distinguishable **motor root**. It travels anteriorly over the petrous ridge and pushes the dura ahead of it to produce the *trigeminal (Meckel's) dural cave*. Within the cave, the stem dilates as the broad, flat **trigeminal ganglion**. Arising from the ganglion are the three divisions of the trigeminal nerve:

Cranial Nerve V-1: Ophthalmic Nerve. The ophthalmic nerve leaves the ganglion and the cave to enter the *cavernous sinus* anteriorly. It travels forward along the lateral wall of the sinus and exits via the *superior orbital fissure* to enter the orbit.

Cranial Nerve V-2: Maxillary Nerve. The maxillary division leaves the cave and passes anteriorly through the posteroinferior portion of the *cavernous sinus*. It leaves the sinus by passing through the *foramen rotundum* to enter the area of the pterygopalatine fossa.

Cranial Nerve V-3: Mandibular Nerve. The mandibular division leaves the cave and drops straight down through the *foramen ovale* to the infratemporal region. The *motor portion* of the trigeminal nerve travels only with the mandibular division.

Cranial Nerve VI: Abducens Nerve

The abducens nerve arises from the ventral aspect between the medulla and the pons, ascends on the clivus, pierces the dura to run below the dura, passes over the petrous temporal ridge, and enters the *cavernous sinus*. It passes through the sinus below the internal carotid artery and exits via the *superior orbital fissure* to enter the orbit.

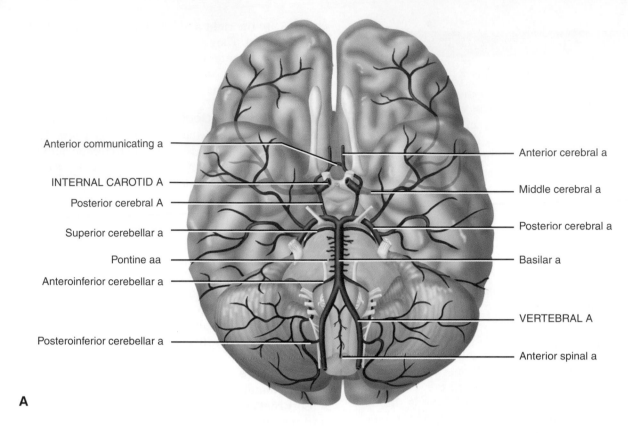

Anterior communicating a

INTERNAL CAROTID A

Posterior cerebral A

Superior cerebellar a

Pontine aa

Anteroinferior cerebellar a

Posteroinferior cerebellar a

Anterior cerebral a

Middle cerebral a

Posterior cerebral a

Basilar a

VERTEBRAL A

Anterior spinal a

A

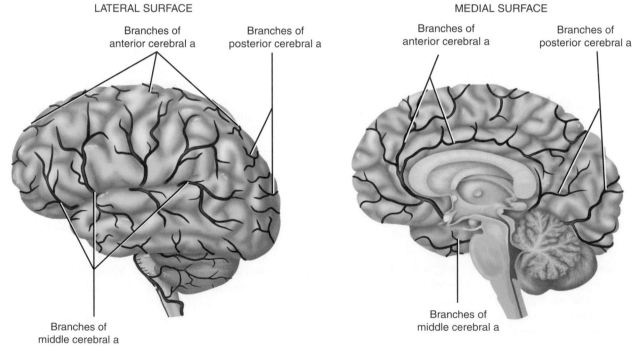

LATERAL SURFACE

Branches of anterior cerebral a

Branches of posterior cerebral a

MEDIAL SURFACE

Branches of anterior cerebral a

Branches of posterior cerebral a

Branches of middle cerebral a

Branches of middle cerebral a

B

Figure 7-25 Arterial blood supply to the brain. **A,** Inferior view to show arterial circle (of Willis). **B,** Distribution of cerebral arteries to lateral and medial surfaces of cerebral hemispheres.

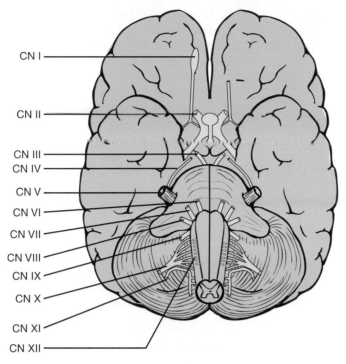

CN I

CN II

CN III
CN IV

CN V

CN VI

CN VII

CN VIII

CN IX

CN X

CN XI

CN XII

A

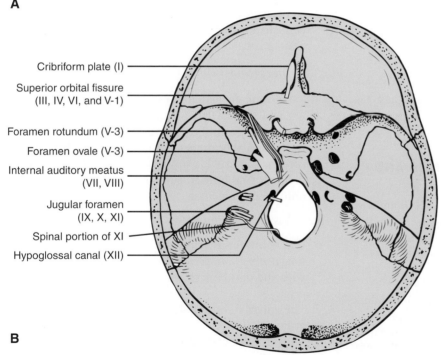

Cribriform plate (I)

Superior orbital fissure
(III, IV, VI, and V-1)

Foramen rotundum (V-3)

Foramen ovale (V-3)

Internal auditory meatus
(VII, VIII)

Jugular foramen
(IX, X, XI)

Spinal portion of XI

Hypoglossal canal (XII)

B

Figure 7-26 A, Inferior view showing cranial nerves arising from the brain. **B**, Internal aspect of base of skull showing foramina through which cranial nerves exit skull.

Cranial Nerve VII: Facial Nerve

The facial nerve leaves the lateral aspect of the brainstem between the pons and the medulla, passes laterally, pierces the dura, and exits through the *internal auditory meatus* to enter the petrous temporal bone. The facial nerve traverses the bone through the winding *facial canal* and ultimately exits inferiorly at the base of the skull through the *stylomastoid foramen.*

Cranial Nerve VIII: Vestibulocochlear Nerve

The vestibulocochlear nerve arises from the brainstem lateral to the facial nerve. It runs to the *internal auditory meatus* and enters the petrous temporal bone to supply the inner ear. Within the petrous temporal bone, it divides into a **cochlear portion** to the cochlea and a **vestibular portion** to the semicircular canals.

Cranial Nerve IX: Glossopharyngeal Nerve

The glossopharyngeal nerve arises as three or four rootlets from the lateral aspect of the medulla. The fibers converge as one bundle and pass to the *jugular foramen*. It pierces the dura and exits through the foramen to the external base of the skull.

Cranial Nerve X: Vagus Nerve

The vagus nerve arises as several rootlets from the medulla in line with and below the rootlets of the glossopharyngeal nerve. The rootlets combine and pass laterally to pierce the dura and exit through the *jugular foramen* to the neck below.

Cranial Nerve XI: Accessory Nerve

The accessory nerve arises from two sources: (1) the **cranial portion** arises as several converging rootlets below the vagus nerve, and (2) the **spinal portion** arises from motor spinal contributions of *spinal cord segments C1 to C6*. The filaments unite as they ascend, pass upward through the foramen magnum, and join the cranial portion. The accessory nerve pierces the dura and exits through the jugular foramen, and, at this point, the cranial portion splits off to join and be distributed along with the vagus nerve. The spinal portion exits alone through the *jugular foramen* to enter the neck.

Cranial Nerve XII: Hypoglossal Nerve

The hypoglossal nerve arises from the medulla in the cleft between the *olive* and the *pyramid* as several rootlets. The rootlets combine, pierce the dura, and exit through the *hypoglossal canal*.

REVIEW OF THE CAVERNOUS SINUS AND ITS CONTENTS

The cavernous sinus was described previously along with the other venous sinuses of the head (*Figure 7-27*). It is singled out here because several important structures pass through the blood-filled space en route to the orbital cavity.

Venous Communications

Emptying into the cavernous sinus are (1) the ophthalmic veins, (2) the sphenoparietal sinus, and (3) the pterygoid plexus via the foramen ovale. *Passing out of* the cavernous sinus are (1) the superior petrosal sinus and (2) the inferior petrosal sinus. The description of the facial vein should be reviewed at this point because of the vein's important indirect communications with the cavernous sinus.

Contents

In addition to venous blood, the cavernous sinus contains the (1) internal carotid artery, (2) sympathetic plexus, and (3) cranial nerves III, IV, VI, V-1, and V-2.

The Internal Carotid Artery. The internal carotid artery enters the skull through the foramen lacerum and passes anteriorly to enter the cavernous sinus. Within the sinus, it grooves the lateral aspect of the sella turcica and provides small branches to the **walls of the cavernous sinus, trigeminal ganglion**, and to the **pituitary gland**. Under the anterior clinoid process, it turns abruptly upward and leaves the cavernous sinus. Here it gives off the **ophthalmic artery**, a branch that passes anteriorly to the orbit through the optic canal. The internal carotid artery loops back upon itself and gives off the **posterior communicating artery**, which joins the posterior cerebral artery. The internal carotid artery ends as the **anterior cerebral** and **middle cerebral arteries**. In addition to the branches described previously, there are a number of smaller branches that arise from the internal carotid artery. The complete set of internal carotid branches are presented for reference purposes.

Eight collateral branches arise from the internal carotid artery before it ends by dividing into two terminal branches. *Within the carotid canal*:

1. The **caroticotympanic branch** passes to the middle ear to anastomose with the anterior tympanic branch of the maxillary artery.
2. A **pterygoid branch** passes through the pterygoid canal to anastomose with branches of the greater palatine artery.

Within the cavernous sinus:

3. Numerous **cavernous branches** arise to supply the walls of the cavernous and inferior petrosal sinuses and the trigeminal ganglion.
4. **Hypophyseal branches** arise to supply the hypophysis cerebri.
5. A **meningeal branch** supplies dura and bone of the anterior cranial fossa.

After the cavernous sinus:

6. The **ophthalmic artery** arises below the anterior clinoid process and passes through the optic canal along with the optic nerve. It supplies the contents of the orbit.
7. The **anterior choroidal artery** arises to help supply the brain.
8. The **posterior communicating artery** runs posteriorly to anastomose with the posterior cerebral branch of the basilar artery to help form the posterior segment of the circle of Willis.

Terminal branches:

9. The **anterior cerebral artery** passes forward to supply a large portion of the medial side of the cerebral hemisphere.
10. The **middle cerebral artery** passes laterally to supply the major portion of the lateral aspect of the cerebral hemisphere.

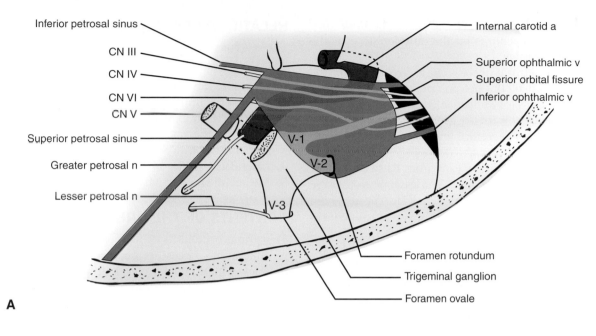

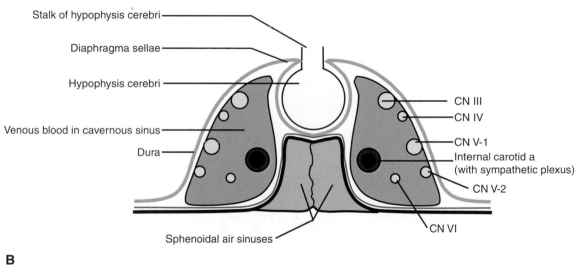

Figure 7-27 A, Superior view of the middle cranial fossa and its contents. The stem of the trigeminal nerve has been sectioned to show entry of internal carotid artery. **B,** Coronal section through cavernous sinuses to show their contents and relationships.

The Carotid Sympathetic Plexus. Postsynaptic sympathetic fibers arise from the superior cervical ganglion to pass to the internal carotid artery. The fibers surround the artery as a perivascular nerve plexus. The plexus hitchhikes with and is distributed by the internal carotid artery and its branches.

Cranial Nerves III, IV, VI, V-1, and V-2. Cranial nerves III, IV, and V-1 enter the sinus and pass through anteriorly, adherent to the lateral wall of the sinus. They leave the sinus by passing through the superior orbital fissure to enter the orbit.

Cranial nerve V-2 passes briefly through the posteroinferior portion of the sinus but leaves midway by dropping through the foramen rotundum.

Cranial nerve VI passes unattached through the blood-filled space and passes out anteriorly through the superior orbital fissure to enter the orbit.

THE PETROSAL NERVES

Two small, but important, nerves are encountered in the middle cranial fossa. They are described briefly here as contents of the neurocranium and as a prelude to fuller descriptions of the **otic** and **pterygopalatine ganglia.**

The nerves are called *petrosal nerves* because they appear from tiny openings on the anterior slope of the petrous temporal ridge.

The greater **petrosal nerve** is the more superior of the two. It passes out of the petrous ridge through a small opening called the *superior hiatus*. The nerve passes under the dura and heads toward the *foramen lacerum*. The nerve is a parasympathetic secretory branch of the facial nerve (cranial nerve VII).

The **lesser petrosal nerve** exits from its hiatus below that of the greater petrosal nerve. The lesser petrosal nerve passes under the dura to the foramen ovale. The nerve is a parasympathetic secretory branch of the glossopharyngeal nerve (cranial nerve IX).

3. The Orbital Cavity

SKELETON

The margins, walls, and various foramina of the orbit are described in Chapter 6 and are presented in *Figure 6-3*. These features should be reviewed. In addition, the features and relationships of the maxilla, sphenoid bone, and ethmoid bones should be reviewed.

RELATIONSHIPS

The relationships of the orbit and its contents are as follows (*Figure 7-28*):

1. Superior: the anterior cranial fossa and the frontal lobes of the brain
2. Inferior: the maxillary sinus
3. Posterior: the middle cranial fossa and the temporal lobes of the brain
4. Lateral: the temporal fossa
5. Medial: the nasal cavity

CONTENTS OF THE ORBIT

The prime occupants of the orbit are the eyeball and its optic nerve. Accessory occupants are (1) extraocular muscles, which move the eyeball into various positions; (2) nerves to the eyeball and muscles; (3) vessels to the muscles and eyeball; (4) the lacrimal gland; and (5) orbital fat, which acts as packing to prevent injury to the eyeball.

Muscles

All the muscles of the orbit, except one, have a common origin from a **tendinous ring**, or cuff (*Figure 7-29* and *Table 7-2*). The ring occupies the posterior pole of the orbit,

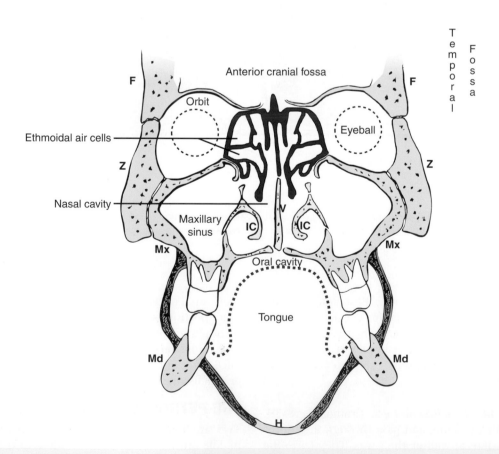

Figure 7-28 Coronal section through the skull to show relationships of orbits, nasal cavity, oral cavity, and paranasal air sinuses. Ethmoid is key to understanding these relationships.

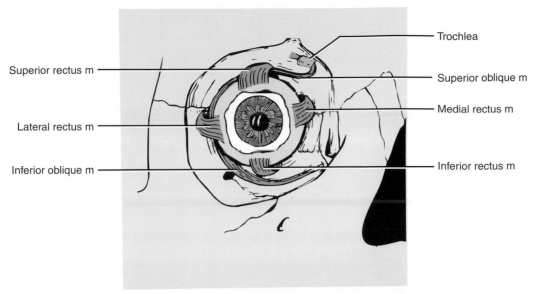

Superior rectus m

Trochlea

Superior oblique m

Medial rectus m

Lateral rectus m

Inferior oblique m

Inferior rectus m

A

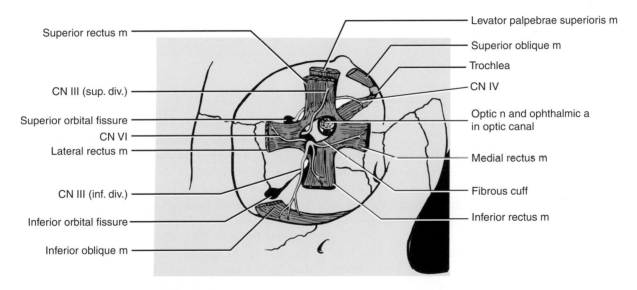

Superior rectus m

Levator palpebrae superioris m

Superior oblique m

Trochlea

CN III (sup. div.)

CN IV

Superior orbital fissure

Optic n and ophthalmic a in optic canal

CN VI

Lateral rectus m

Medial rectus m

CN III (inf. div.)

Fibrous cuff

Inferior orbital fissure

Inferior rectus m

Inferior oblique m

B

Figure 7-29 **A,** Right orbit with eyeball in place showing insertions of the extraocular muscles. **B,** Right orbit with eyeball removed showing origins of the extraocular muscles and their motor nerves.

attached to and surrounding the optic canal and the midportion of the superior orbital fissure. From this common origin, the muscles fan out anteriorly as a cone of muscles to attach to the eyeball. The most superior muscle of the cone is actually a muscle of the upper lid.

Levator Palpebrae Superioris. The levator palpebrae superioris originates from the superior position of the ring. It runs over and past the superior aspect of the eyeball and inserts into the skin of the upper lid. A few involuntary fibers insert into the tarsal plate (see *Figure 7-14*).

The muscle acts to open the palpebral fissure. The small involuntary portion is fired by *sympathetic innervation* and prevents drooping of the lid (ptosis). The remainder of the muscle is supplied by the *oculomotor nerve.*

Superior Rectus. The superior rectus also originates from the superior position of the tendinous ring and inserts anteriorly into the superior aspect of the eyeball behind the sclerocorneal junction. The superior rectus primarily turns the eyeball upward. It also turns the eyeball slightly

TABLE 7-2

Muscles of the Orbit

Extraocular Muscles	Origin	Insertion	Action	Cranial Nerve
Levator palpebrae superioris	Roof of orbit and superior position of tendinous ring	(a) Skin of upper eyelid (b) Tarsus of upper lid	(a) Elevates upper lid (voluntarily) (b) Elevates upper lid (involuntarily)	(a) III (b) Sympathetic
Superior rectus	Superior position of tendinous ring	Superior aspect of eyeball posterior to sclerocorneal junction	(a) Turns eye upward (b) Adducts eye	III
Medial rectus	Medial position of tendinous ring	Medial aspect of eyeball posterior to sclerocorneal junction	Adducts eye	III
Inferior rectus	Inferior position of tendinous ring	Inferior aspect of eyeball posterior to sclerocorneal junction	(a) Lowers eye (b) Adducts eye	III
Lateral rectus	Lateral position of tendinous ring	Lateral aspect of eyeball posterior to sclerocorneal junction	Abducts eye	VI
Superior oblique	Superomedial position of tendinous ring	Passes through trochlea and angles posteriorly and laterally to insert into superoposterolateral aspect of eyeball	Lowers eye and turns laterally	IV
Inferior oblique	Floor of orbit near posterior lacrimal crest	Posteroinferolateral aspect of eyeball	Turns eye up and laterally	III

medially or inward (adduction). It is supplied by a branch of the *oculomotor nerve*.

Medial Rectus. The medial rectus arises from the medial position of the tendinous ring and inserts into the medial aspect of the eyeball behind the sclerocorneal junction. The muscle acts to turn the eyeball inward (adduction) and is supplied by a branch of the *oculomotor nerve*.

Inferior Rectus. The inferior rectus arises from the inferior position of the tendinous ring, travels forward under the eyeball, and inserts into the inferior aspect of the eyeball behind the sclerocorneal junction. It turns the eye inferiorly and helps to turn the eye inward (adduction). The inferior rectus muscle is supplied by the *oculomotor nerve*.

Lateral Rectus. The lateral rectus arises from the lateral position on the tendinous ring, travels anteriorly, and inserts into the lateral aspect of the eyeball behind the sclerocorneal junction. It turns the eyeball outward (abduction) and is supplied by its very own cranial nerve, the *abducens nerve*, named after its action (abduction) on the eyeball.

Superior Oblique. The superior oblique muscle originates from the superomedial position on the tendinous ring and passes forward and medially toward the superomedial margin of the orbit. Here it narrows as an intermediate tendon and passes through an attached dense fibrous pulley, or **trochlea**. The tendon loops through the trochlea and changes direction. It resumes a fleshy belly and passes posteriorly and laterally to insert into the superior posterolateral aspect of the eyeball. The superior oblique muscle acts to turn the eye downward and laterally. It too possesses a private nerve supply, the *trochlear nerve*.

Inferior Oblique. The inferior oblique is the only muscle that does not originate from the tendinous ring but from the floor of the orbit near the posterior lacrimal crest. It passes obliquely backward and laterally to insert into the sclera of the posterior inferolateral aspect of the eyeball. It turns the eyeball superiorly and laterally and is supplied by a branch of the *oculomotor nerve*.

Movements of the Eyeball. A summary of the muscular actions of the eyeball is given in *Figure 7-30*.

Nerves
Motor Nerves to the Extraocular Muscles
Oculomotor Nerve (Cranial Nerve III). The oculomotor nerve enters the orbit through the superior orbital fissure within the cone of muscles. It divides into a superior and an inferior division that supply all of the extraocular muscles except the superior oblique and the lateral rectus muscles. The superior division supplies the superior rectus and levator palpebrae superioris muscles. The inferior division supplies the inferior rectus, medial rectus, and inferior oblique

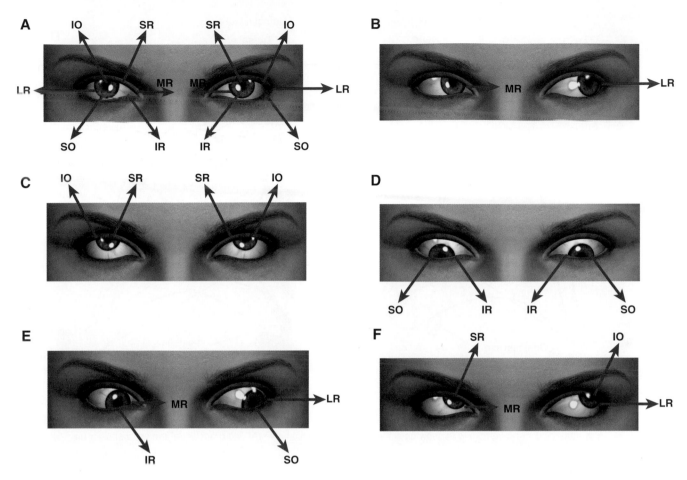

Figure 7-30 Actions of the extraocular muscles on the eyes. **A,** Eyes centered. **B,** Eyes turned to side. **C,** Eyes turned upward. **D,** Eyes turned downward to side. **F,** Eyes turned up and to the side.

muscles. In addition, the oculomotor nerve carries a parasympathetic component, and these fibers leave the nerve within the orbit to synapse within the ciliary ganglion.

Trochlear Nerve (Cranial Nerve IV). The trochlear nerve enters the orbit through the superior orbital fissure superior to and not within the cone of muscles; it supplies only the superior oblique muscle.

Abducens Nerve (Cranial Nerve VI). The abducens nerve enters the orbit through the superior orbital fissure within the cone of muscles. It passes to and supplies only the lateral rectus muscle.

Nerve Supply of Extraocular Muscles (a Mnemonic). By means of a mythical sulfate radical, the only two extraocular muscles not supplied by the oculomotor nerve (cranial nerve III) are easily remembered: LR_6SO_4 or lateral rectus, cranial nerve VI and superior oblique, cranial nerve IV. The remaining muscles, including the levator palpebrae superioris, are supplied by cranial nerve III.

Special Sensory Nerve, the Optic Nerve (Cranial Nerve II). The optic nerve passes through the optic

foramen from the middle cranial fossa and travels forward and slightly laterally toward the posterior aspect of the eyeball (*Figure 7-31*).

General Sensory Nerve, the Ophthalmic Nerve. The ophthalmic nerve leaves the middle cranial fossa through the superior orbital fissure and immediately breaks up into three terminal branches: (1) frontal nerve, (2) lacrimal nerve, and (3) nasociliary nerve (see *Figure 7-31, A*).

Frontal Nerve. The frontal nerve passes forward below the orbital roof. As it approaches the orbital margin, it divides into the **supraorbital** and **supratrochlear** nerves. These two nerves pass out of the orbit to the face to supply skin and conjunctiva of the upper lid and skin of the forehead and scalp.

Lacrimal Nerve. The **lacrimal nerve** passes to the lateral wall of the orbit toward the lacrimal gland. It picks up hitchhiking postsynaptic secretory fibers from the pterygopalatine ganglion and delivers them to the lacrimal gland and ends by passing to the face to supply sensation from the lateral aspect of the upper lid.

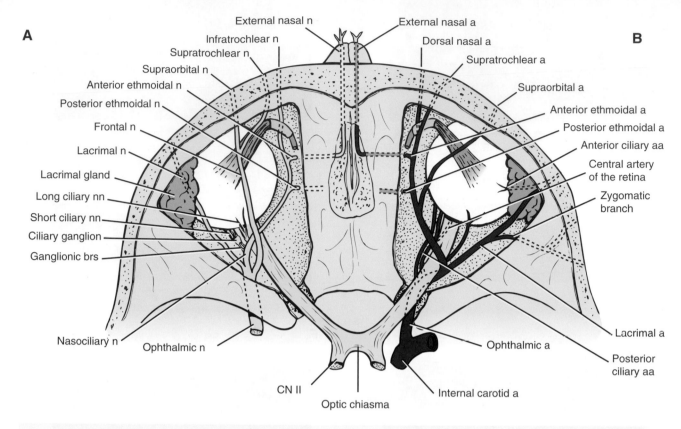

External nasal n
Infratrochlear n
Supratrochlear n
Supraorbital n
Anterior ethmoidal n
Posterior ethmoidal n
Frontal n
Lacrimal n
Lacrimal gland
Long ciliary nn
Short ciliary nn
Ciliary ganglion
Ganglionic brs
Nasociliary n
Ophthalmic n
CN II
Optic chiasma

External nasal a
Dorsal nasal a
Supratrochlear a
Supraorbital a
Anterior ethmoidal a
Posterior ethmoidal a
Anterior ciliary aa
Central artery of the retina
Zygomatic branch
Lacrimal a
Ophthalmic a
Posterior ciliary aa
Internal carotid a

Figure 7-31 Horizontal section through orbits to show branches of the ophthalmic nerve (**A**) and branches of the ophthalmic artery (**B**).

Nasociliary Nerve. The nasociliary nerve passes anteriorly and then swings medially behind the eyeball to parallel the medial orbital wall. The nasociliary nerve has three collateral and two terminal branches.

1. **Ganglionic branches** pass anteriorly to the **ciliary ganglion,** a small nerve swelling located between the optic nerve and the lateral rectus muscle. The branches of the ganglion are discussed shortly.
2. **Long ciliary branches** travel anteriorly to enter the posterior aspect of the eyeball. These are sensory to the eye and cornea.
3. The **posterior ethmoidal nerve** passes medially through the *posterior ethmoidal foramen* in the medial orbital wall to supply posterior ethmoidal air cells.
4. The **anterior ethmoidal nerve** is a terminal branch that passes medially through the *anterior ethmoidal foramen* in the medial orbital wall to supply anterior ethmoidal cells. The anterior ethmoidal nerve continues medially into the anterior cranial fossa and then leaves through the ethmoidal foramen anterior to the cribriform plate. This leads to the roof of the nasal cavity, and the nerve continues downward and forward along the internal aspect of the nasal bone. At the junction of the nasal bone and the lateral nasal cartilage, the nerve

emerges onto the nose as the **external nasal nerve**. It supplies a median strip of skin on the external nose.
5. The **infratrochlear nerve** is the second terminal branch. It passes deep to the trochlea and exits from the orbit to supply skin and conjunctiva of the medial angle of the upper lid.

Cranial Ganglia. Within the head are four parasympathetic synaptic relay stations, or ganglia. Each ganglion is associated with and attached to a branch of one of the divisions of the trigeminal nerve. Flowing into each ganglion are three types of nerve fibers:

1. **Sensory nerve fibers** from branches of the trigeminal nerve pass through the cranial ganglia *without synapsing.*
2. **Sympathetic nerve fibers** synapse in the superior cervical ganglion of the neck and hitchhike with the branches of the external and internal carotid arteries as a perivascular plexus. The closest arterial branch to the cranial ganglion supplies postsynaptic fibers to that ganglion. These pass through the ganglion *without synapsing.*
3. **Parasympathetic nerve fibers** arise from the brainstem and travel with cranial nerves III, VII, or IX. These fibers *do synapse* with secondary neurons within the cranial ganglia.

Flowing out of each of the four cranial ganglia are sensory, sympathetic, and parasympathetic mixed fibers.

The Ciliary Ganglion. The ciliary ganglion is a tiny swelling associated with the nasociliary nerve in the orbit (*Figure 7-32*). Like all cranial ganglia, it receives three roots: (1) *sensory fibers* come directly from the nasociliary nerve, (2) *sympathetic fibers* arise from the plexus of the internal carotid and ophthalmic arteries, and (3) *parasympathetic fibers* arise from the oculomotor nerve (cranial nerve III).

The outflow from the ciliary ganglion passes to the eyeball as the **short ciliary nerves** that provide (1) *general* *sensory* branches from the eyeball; (2) *sympathetic* branches that supply the **dilator pupillae muscle** of the eye; and (3) *parasympathetic fibers* that supply the **constrictor pupillae** and **ciliary muscles** of the eye. The actions of these muscles are described with the eyeball.

Blood Vessels

Ophthalmic Artery. The ophthalmic artery arises from the internal carotid artery within the middle cranial fossa (see *Figure 7-31, B*). It leaves the middle cranial fossa through the optic foramen, along with the optic nerve, to enter the orbit. Within the orbit, it gives off a number of branches that parallel the branches of the ophthalmic nerve.

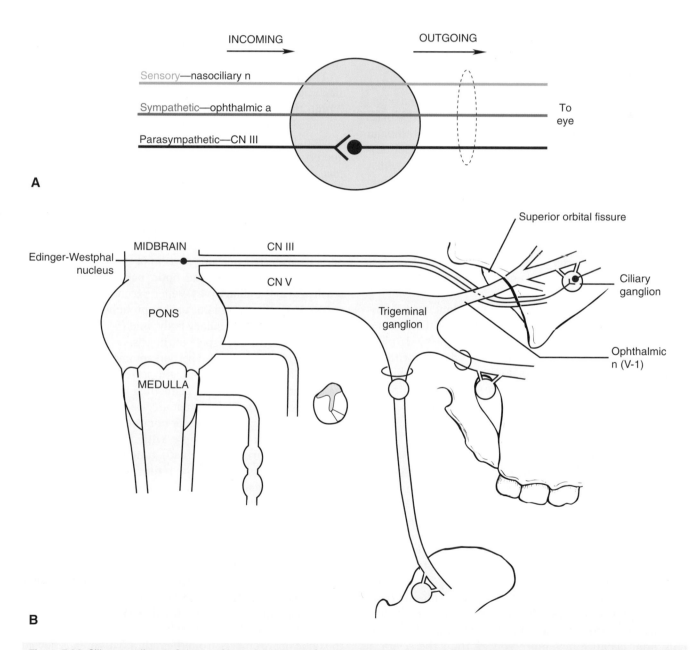

Figure 7-32 Ciliary ganglion. **A**, Scheme of incoming and outgoing nerve fibers. **B**, Origin of parasympathetic component from cranial nerve III.

1. **Muscular branches** arise to supply the muscles of the orbit.
2. **Posterior ciliary arteries** pass to the posterior aspect of the eyeball. One special ciliary branch pierces the optic nerve posterior to the eyeball. It enters the eye to supply the retina as the **central artery of the retina**. This artery is an end artery; that is, there are no additional anastomosing arterial flows to the retina. Blockage of the central artery results in blindness in that eye.
3. The **lacrimal artery** is a large branch that runs toward the lateral wall and the lacrimal gland. It gives off a **zygomatic branch** through the zygomatic canal, which ends up on the face as the **zygomaticofacial artery** and on the temple as the **zygomaticotemporal artery**. It also gives rise to **anterior ciliary branches** to the eyeball. The lacrimal artery ends on the face, supplying the lateral portion of the upper eyelid.
4. The **supraorbital artery** travels anteriorly over the eyeball and exits through the supraorbital notch, or foramen, onto the face. It supplies the upper lid, forehead, and scalp.
5. The **posterior** and **anterior ethmoidal arteries** pass medially through the posterior and anterior ethmoidal canals to supply ethmoidal air cells. The anterior ethmoidal artery ends as the external nasal nerve, which parallels the route of the **external nasal nerve** to supply the external nose. The ophthalmic artery ends as two terminal branches that pass to the face.
6. The **supratrochlear artery** passes over the trochlea to exit onto the face to supply the upper lid, forehead, and scalp.
7. The **dorsal nasal artery** (companion to the infratrochlear nerve) supplies the medial angle of the upper lid.

Ophthalmic Veins. The superior ophthalmic vein drains the orbital contents and passes back through the superior orbital fissure to the cavernous sinus (see *Figure 7-16*). The superior ophthalmic vein communicates directly with the facial vein anteriorly, and, because it contains no valves, blood flow from the facial vein can flow via the superior ophthalmic vein to the cavernous sinus (see later sections, "Cavernous Sinus (Paired)" and "The Facial Vein").

The Eyeball (Oculus Bulbi)
The eyeball is a hollow sphere, roughly 2 to 3 cm in diameter, and it is the organ for the special sense of sight (*Figure 7-33*). Part of the eyeball (the retina) forms as an outgrowth of the forebrain, and it remains connected to the brain by a tract. The eyeball consists of three concentric layers, or coats, and three refractive media.

Three Concentric Coats
Fibrous Coat. The **sclera** is a firm, smooth, fibrous outer covering of the posterior five sixths of the eyeball. The **transparent cornea** is the anterior one sixth of the eyeball, and, because it is more convex than the sclera, it sticks out anteriorly as a small lump. The cornea is over-

lapped slightly by the sclera at the corneoscleral junction. The cornea contains no blood vessels and gets its nutrients directly from peripheral blood vessels and its oxygen directly from the air. The transparent cornea allows light to pass through the pupil to enter the eyeball and provides a primary focus of light.

Vascular Coat. The vascular coat is immediately deep to the fibrous coat. It consists of the choroid, the ciliary body, and the iris. The **choroid** is a thin, vascular membrane covering the posterior two thirds of the eyeball. It consists of a dense network of venous and arterial capillaries.

The **ciliary body** surrounds the lens and suspends the lens around its entire periphery via the suspensory ligament. The ciliary body contains smooth muscle arranged in such a way that, upon contraction, the suspensory ligament loosens. The ciliary muscles are supplied by parasympathetic fibers of cranial nerve III.

The **iris** is a pigmented diaphragm. The aperture of the diaphragm is the pupil, which allows light to enter the eye. Within the iris are two sets of smooth muscles that control pupillary size. The **constrictor pupillae muscle** consists of circular smooth muscle fibers, which decrease pupil size upon contraction. It is supplied by *parasympathetic fibers of cranial nerve III via the ciliary ganglion*. The **dilator pupillae muscle** consists of radial fibers, which dilate the pupil upon contraction. It is controlled by *sympathetic fibers*.

Retina. The retina is the inner lining of the eyeball. It is composed of an external pigmented layer and an inner nervous layer. The nervous portion of the retina is divided into three regions: (1) the **optic part,** which is light-sensitive; (2) the **ciliary part,** which receives no light and is reduced to a thin, wavy line as it approaches and lines the internal aspect of the ciliary body; and (3) the **iridial part,** which lines the inner aspect of the iris.

The optic, light-sensitive portion contains a three-neuron pathway arranged in layers. Light passes through the nervous layer and stops at the pigmented layer. At this point, the light excites the light receptor cells: cone cells for acute vision and color and rod cells for nondiscriminative vision.

The receptor cells synapse with bipolar cells above, and these, in turn, synapse with ganglionic cells occupying the innermost layer of the retina (see *Figure 7-33, B*). Processes of the ganglionic cells stream toward the posterior pole of the eye to group and form the optic nerve.

The macula lutea is a small, yellowish area occupying the inner posterior pole of the retina (see *Figure 7-33, B*). Clustered in this area are proportionately more cone cells, and thus vision is most acute from this central point. Moving peripherally from the macula lutea, fewer and fewer cone cells in relation to rod cells are found, resulting in less discriminative vision from these areas.

The optic disc is the site where the outgoing fibers of the optic nerve emerge from the retina. This area is devoid of photoreceptor cells and is a blind spot.

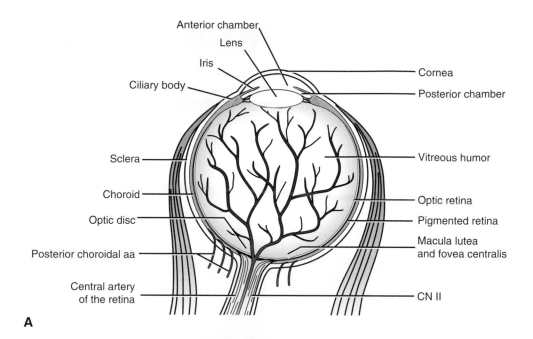

Anterior chamber
Lens
Iris
Ciliary body
Cornea
Posterior chamber
Sclera
Vitreous humor
Choroid
Optic retina
Optic disc
Pigmented retina
Posterior choroidal aa
Macula lutea and fovea centralis
Central artery of the retina
CN II

A

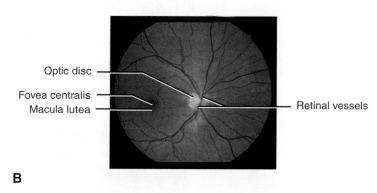

Optic disc
Fovea centralis
Macula lutea
Retinal vessels

B

Figure 7-33 A, Horizontal section through the right eyeball to demonstrate three concentric coats, three refractive media, and blood supply. **B,** The retina of the eye as revealed by ophthalmoscope. (Courtesy Dr. F. Feldman and Cynthia VandenHoven.)

Three Refractive Media. Light passing through the cornea travels through three refractive media before reaching the retina.

Aqueous Humor. The space between the posterior aspect of the cornea and the anterior aspect of the lens is filled with a clear fluid—the aqueous humor. The iris divides this confined space into an anterior and a posterior chamber connected by the pupillary aperture.

Vitreous Humor. The hollow space posterior to the lens and encapsulated by the retina is filled with a light-refractive gel called *vitreous humor.*

Lens. The lens is a transparent, biconvex disc that separates the aqueous and vitreous humors. It is composed of laminated clear fibers.

Lens Accommodation (Focusing)
Far Objects. When the eye is focused on distant objects, the elastic suspensory ligament holds the lens taut, thus

flattening the lens. This increases the focal length of the lens for distant vision.

Near Objects. As the eye is brought to focus on close objects, three phenomena occur, each controlled by the oculomotor nerve. Collectively the three phenomena are known as the ***accommodation reflex.***

1. The extraocular muscles turn the eyeballs inward.
2. The constrictor pupillae muscle cuts down on the light entering the eyeball (less light is needed for closer objects).
3. The ciliary muscles contract, thus loosening the suspensory ligament and allowing the lens to relax and assume its normal bulged shape; this decreases the focal length of the lens to accommodate for close vision.

Pupillary Light Reflex. A penlight shone into one eye constricts the pupil of that eye (direct pupillary reflex). It also constricts the pupil of the other eye (consensual

263

CLINICAL NOTES

Cataract

A cataract is a condition in which the lens becomes opaque, admits less light to the retina, and results in decreased vision. Removal of a cataract involves the actual removal of the opaque lens and replacement with an artificial lens.

Refractive Errors

Myopia, or nearsightedness, is caused by an elongated long axis of the eyeball. The focused image of distant objects falls short of the retina, and the resulting image is blurred. **Hyperopia**, or farsightedness, is the opposite situation. Focused images fall behind the retina, and blurred vision results when viewing close objects. **Astigmatism** is a condition that interferes with sharp vision and is caused by uneven curvature of the lens or the cornea, resulting in light rays that focus in different points on the retina.

Refractive Correction

Artificial lenses (glasses or contacts) are prescribed to focus the image properly on the retina and restore clear vision. **Refractive surgery** can be performed to alter the curvature of the cornea. This helps to focus the passing light rays closer to the retina and sharpen the image.

Glaucoma

Glaucoma is a common cause of blindness brought about by increased intraocular pressure that progressively and permanently destroys the exiting fibers of the optic nerve. The increased pressure is due to an obstructed outflow of aqueous humor. Pressures are measured with a tonometer, and it is extremely important that all adults have a baseline reading and regular checkups thereafter. Any elevation in subsequent readings should be suspect even if the pressure falls within normal limits.

pupillary reflex). Collateral branches of the optic tract pass into the midbrain, and project bilaterally to synapse near the superior colliculi. Bilateral postsynaptic fibers pass to the Edinger-Westphal nuclei and synapse, and these fibers join the oculomotor nerve as its parasympathetic component and are carried into the orbits. The parasympathetic fibers synapse in the ciliary ganglia, and the postsynaptic fibers pass to the dilator pupillae of both eyes.

Nerve Supply: A Review

Special Sensory. The optic nerve, tract, and optic radiation carry the stimuli received by the photoreceptor cells in the retina back to the visual cortex for appreciation of the special sensation of sight.

General Sensory. Sensory fibers to the eyeball arise from the ophthalmic nerve (cranial nerve V-1) as short and long ciliary nerves.

Parasympathetic. Parasympathetic fibers from cranial nerve III synapse in the ciliary ganglion and pass to the eyeball via short ciliary nerves. Postsynaptic fibers supply the constrictor pupillae and the ciliary muscle.

Sympathetic. Postsynaptic fibers of the superior cervical ganglion pass via the internal carotid plexus to the orbit. They supply the dilator pupillae muscle.

Blood Supply

Arteries. The arterial supply arises from the ophthalmic artery as posterior ciliary arteries and from the lacrimal branch of the ophthalmic artery as anterior ciliary arteries. The retina is supplied by the single, important end artery termed the *central artery of the retina*.

Veins. **Four choroidal veins** drain the eyeball and, in turn, drain to the superior and inferior ophthalmic veins.

The Lacrimal Apparatus

The lacrimal gland secretes tears, which moisten lubricate, and protect the eyeball (see *Figures 7-14* and *7-34*). Excess tears are removed by the nasolacrimal system.

CLINICAL NOTES

Dacryostenosis is a narrowing, or stricture, of the nasolacrimal duct that results in persistent tearing. **Dacryocystitis** is an infection of the lacrimal sac.

The Lacrimal Gland. The lacrimal gland is a serous gland situated just behind the superolateral margin of the orbit, deep to the superior conjunctival sac. The gland is wrapped around the free lateral border of the levator palpebrae superioris muscle, creating a *deep (orbital) lobe* and a *superficial (palpebral) lobe*. Approximately 10 to 12 tiny ducts open directly into the superior conjunctival sac.

Parasympathetic secretory fibers arise from the superior salivatory nucleus of the brainstem and leave the brain as a component of the *facial nerve (cranial nerve VII)*. The *greater petrosal nerve* arises from the *facial nerve* and synapses within the *pterygopalatine ganglion*. Postganglionic fibers enter the orbit through the inferior orbital fissure and hitchhike with the lacrimal nerve to the lacrimal gland.

Nasolacrimal System. At the junction of the ciliated and nonciliated margins of the lids are an **upper** and a **lower papilla**. The top of the papillae presents a tiny opening, or **punctum**, which sucks up excess tears. **Superior** and **infe-**

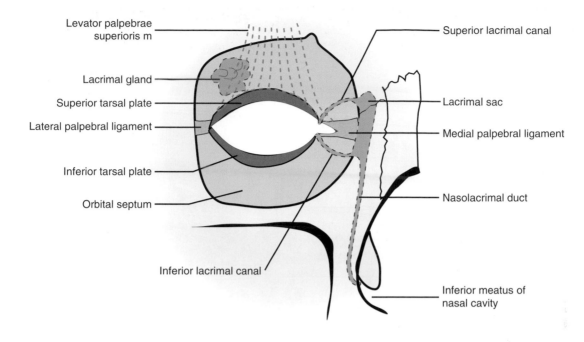

Levator palpebrae
superioris m

Lacrimal gland

Superior tarsal plate

Lateral palpebral ligament

Inferior tarsal plate

Orbital septum

Inferior lacrimal canal

Superior lacrimal canal

Lacrimal sac

Medial palpebral ligament

Nasolacrimal duct

Inferior meatus of
nasal cavity

Figure 7-34 The orbital septum and lacrimal apparatus.

rior lacrimal canals are fine tubes that convey the tears medially to a dilated lacrimal sac.

The **lacrimal sac** occupies the upper portion of the bony nasolacrimal canal.

The **nasolacrimal duct** is a membranous tube that drains the inferior aspect of the lacrimal sac. The duct opens below the inferior concha into the *inferior meatus of the nasal cavity*. This accounts for the nasal discharge during a good crying session.

4.   The Parotid Region

The parotid gland, the largest of the three salivary glands, occupies a rather complex area referred to as the *parotid bed*, or *region*.

SKELETON

The lateral view of the skull and all the features of the mandible should be reviewed (see Chapter 6).

BOUNDARIES

The region is roughly triangular in outline and has considerable depth.

1. Anterior: the posterior border of the ramus of the mandible and the posterior borders of the masseter and medial pterygoid muscles

2. Posterior: the anterior aspect of the mastoid process and the sternocleidomastoid muscle
3. Inferior: the posterior belly of the digastric and sty- lohyoid muscles
4. Medial: the styloid process of the skull and its attached musculature and ligaments

CONTENTS

Running through the parotid region are (1) the facial nerve and its branches; (2) the retromandibular vein and its tributaries; (3) the external carotid artery and its terminal two branches; and (4) the parotid gland, which surrounds and contains within its substance all the aforementioned structures (*Figure 7-35*).

Facial Nerve (Cranial Nerve VII)

The facial nerve exits through the stylomastoid foramen and passes directly into the parotid gland. Within the gland, it becomes plexiform and forms five sets of branches: *temporal, zygomatic, buccal, mandibular,* and *cervical*. These radiate from the anterior and inferior borders of the gland to spill onto the face and supply the superficial muscles of facial expression and the platysma muscle.

Retromandibular Vein

The retromandibular vein forms anterior and inferior to the ear through the union of the superficial temporal vein and the maxillary vein.

Tributaries. The **superficial temporal vein** drains the temple area, the anterior auricle, and the temporomandibular

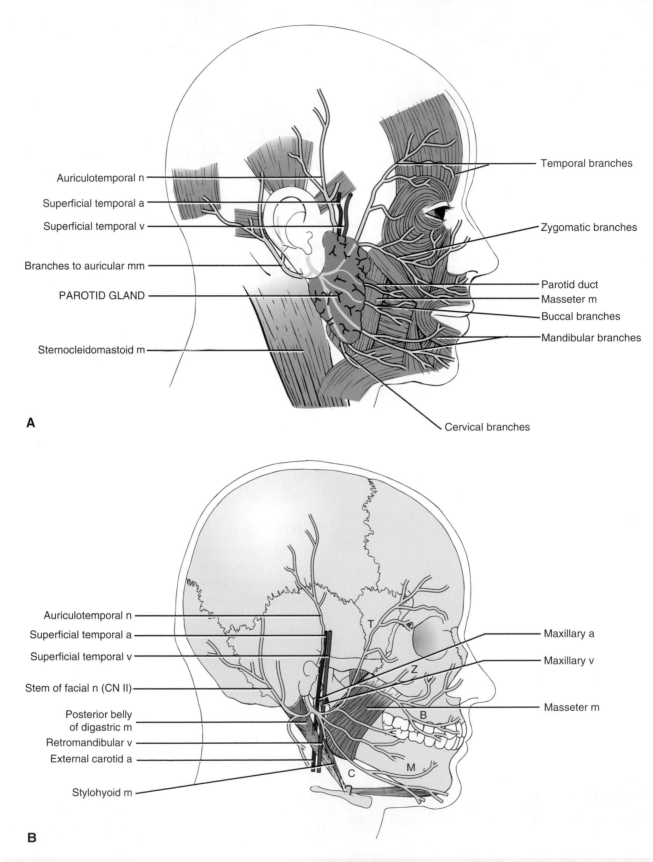

Auriculotemporal n

Superficial temporal a

Superficial temporal v

Branches to auricular mm

PAROTID GLAND

Sternocleidomastoid m

Temporal branches

Zygomatic branches

Parotid duct

Masseter m

Buccal branches

Mandibular branches

Cervical branches

A

Auriculotemporal n

Superficial temporal a

Superficial temporal v

Stem of facial n (CN II)

Posterior belly
of digastric m

Retromandibular v

External carotid a

Stylohyoid m

Maxillary a

Maxillary v

Masseter m

B

Figure 7-35 Parotid region. **A,** Parotid gland and branches of the facial nerve arising from its superior, anterior, and inferior borders. **B,** Parotid gland is removed to demonstrate structures of the parotid bed.

joint and passes inferiorly in front of the ear to enter the superior border of the parotid gland.

The **maxillary vein** drains the infratemporal region and pterygoid plexus of veins. It passes posteriorly deep to the neck of the mandibular condyle to enter the anterosuperior border of the gland and joins the superficial temporal vein within the gland.

Course and Branches. The retromandibular vein thus formed passes inferiorly through the parotid gland and, at its inferior border, enters the anterior triangle of the neck.

External Carotid Artery

The origin, course, and collateral branches of the external carotid artery are described as a feature of the anterior triangle of the neck. In the parotid region, the external carotid artery ascends within the parotid gland and provides some collateral glandular branches. Just below the ear, the external carotid artery ends as two terminal branches before it reaches the superior border of the gland.

The Maxillary Artery

This important branch passes anteriorly from the superior anterior border of the gland and passes deep to the neck of the mandibular condyle to enter the infratemporal region. The course and distribution of the maxillary artery are considered with the features of the infratemporal region.

The Superficial Temporal Artery

The superficial temporal artery leaves the superior aspect of the parotid gland and travels superiorly over the root of the zygoma anterior to the external auditory meatus. It then gives off several branches as it ascends on the side of the head.

1. The **transverse facial artery** arises within the parotid gland and passes anteriorly below the inferior border of the zygomatic arch. It supplies glandular branches to the parotid gland and duct, some muscular branches to masseter muscle, and cutaneous branches to overlying skin.
2. **Articular branches** supply the posterior portion of the temporomandibular joint.
3. **Anterior auricular branches** supply the external auditory meatus and the anterior portion of the auricle.
4. **Zygomatico-orbital** branches travel above the zygomatic arch toward the lateral angle of the eye to supply skin and the orbicularis oculi muscle. The side of the head is supplied by three terminal branches.
5. The **frontal branch** follows a tortuous course anteriorly and superiorly.
6. The **middle temporal branch** heads superiorly and passes deeply to supply a portion of temporalis muscle.
7. The **parietal branch** passes posteriorly and superiorly.

The Parotid Gland

The parotid gland is one of three major salivary glands that produce and secrete saliva for the oral cavity. It weighs about 25 g, is yellowish in the fresh state, and exhibits the typical lobulated appearance of exocrine glands. It consists entirely of serous secreting units.

Location. The name parotid is from *para* ("beyond") and *ous* ("ear"). It is actually anterior and inferior to the ear and occupies the aforementioned parotid space (see *Figures 7-35* and *7-36*).

The bed of the parotid gland is illustrated in *Figure 7-35, B.* Imagine taking a lump of plasticine and pushing it into this interval. It would surround the facial nerve, retromandibular vein, and external carotid artery. It would spill into the areas deep to the sternocleidomastoid muscle and the ramus of the mandible. Superficially, the excess would overflow the lateral surfaces of the sternocleidomastoid muscle and the masseter muscle overlying the ramus of the mandible. The plane of the facial nerve and its branches passing through the gland divides the gland into a superficial and a deep portion.

Capsule. The gland is wrapped in a fibrous capsule, which is continuous with the deep investing fascia of the neck. The *stylomandibular ligament* is an anterior thickening of the capsule, which runs from the styloid process to the angle of the mandible. It separates the parotid gland from the infratemporal region anteriorly and separates the parotid gland from the submandibular gland inferiorly and anteriorly.

The Parotid Duct. The ductules of the various lobules collect anteriorly and ultimately form a thick, wide duct. The duct is approximately 5 cm in length and 3 mm in internal diameter. Its walls are thick, consisting of an inner mucosal coat and an outer fibrous coat containing some smooth muscle cells.

The duct leaves the anterior (facial) process of the gland and may have about its origin small accessory lobules. The duct travels anteriorly about 1 fingerwidth below the zygomatic arch, over the lateral surface of the masseter muscle. At the anterior border of the masseter muscle and mandibular ramus, the duct turns abruptly deep to pierce the buccal fat pad and the buccinator muscle of the cheek and enters the oral cavity opposite the crown of the second maxillary molar.

Blood Supply. The parotid gland receives glandular branches from the external carotid and superficial temporal arteries.

Nerve Supply. The nerve supply to the parotid gland is extremely complicated. Although the facial nerve passes through the gland and is itself a carrier of parasympathetic fibers, the gland is actually supplied by parasympathetic components of the glossopharyngeal nerve (cranial nerve IX). The devious route by which these fibers reach the parotid gland is discussed with the otic ganglion in the infratemporal region.

CLINICAL NOTES

Infections (Parotitis)

Mumps is a viral infection that results in swelling of the parotid gland and occasional involvement of the gonads, meninges, or pancreas. Bacterial infection (noncontagious) is a localized infection and subsequent abscess in the gland. One possible cause is extremely poor oral hygiene and resultant tracking of infection back through the duct. The dentist must determine whether swellings of the cheek are caused by glandular involvement or abscesses of dental origin.

Facial Paralysis

The removal of a cancerous parotid gland would be a relatively simple procedure were it not for the facial nerve and its plexiform branches within the substance of the gland. The attending surgeon must laboriously pick away the gland piecemeal from around the facial nerve in a time-consuming and exacting operation. Injury to the nerve results in facial paralysis.

A temporary facial paralysis is occasionally caused by the dentist in attempting to secure anesthesia of the inferior alveolar nerve. *Figure 7-36* shows the relationship between the inferior alveolar nerve and the encapsulated parotid gland, immediately posterior to the nerve. If the needle tip is carried too far posteriorly, it could penetrate the capsule. Fluid injected into the capsule diffuses quickly through the gland and anesthetizes the facial nerve. The resulting facial paralysis is temporary; it wears off with the clearance of the anesthetic solution from the area. Assurance of the patient that it is only a passing phenomenon with no lasting effects is recommended.

Blocked Parotid Duct

Occasionally, a calcified deposit (sialolith) forms in the parotid duct and effectively blocks secretions. Pain and swelling result, and surgical removal of the sialolith is required.

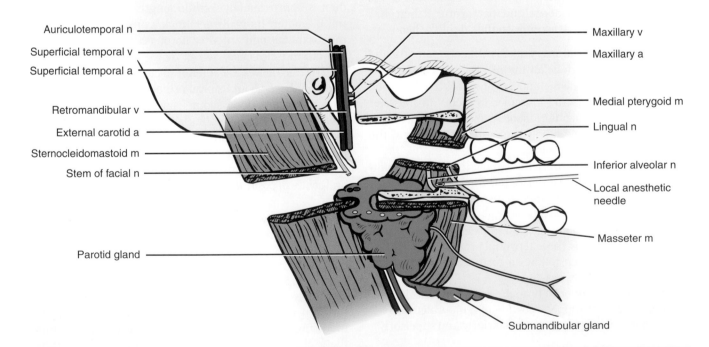

Figure 7-36 Horizontal section through the parotid and infratemporal regions to show relationships. Tip of the needle represents the injection site for inferior alveolar nerve. An injection delivered too far posteriorly can enter the parotid gland, anesthetize branches of the facial nerve, and produce temporary facial paralysis.

5.   The Masticator Region

Cervical fascia ascends to the head and splits at the lower border of the mandible to pass upward on either side of the ramus of the mandible. The resulting compartment is termed the *masticator space*, and its prime occupants are (1) the temporomandibular joint, (2) the muscles of mastication, (3) the mandibular nerve (cranial nerve V-3), (4) the maxillary artery, and (5) the pterygoid plexus of veins and the maxillary vein.

The masticator space includes (1) portions of the parotid region lateral to the ramus of the mandible, (2) the temporal fossa on the side of the head, and (3) the infratemporal fossa deep to the ramus of the mandible.

SKELETON

The lateral and basal aspects of the skull and all the features of the mandible should be reviewed (see Chapter 6).

BONY FOSSAE

Temporal Fossa

The temporal fossa is the shallow depression below the temporal lines of the skull. It funnels inferiorly to pass below the zygomatic arch and ends at the base of the skull. The infratemporal crest forms the inferior boundary of the temporal fossa and separates it from the infratemporal fossa below (*Figure 7-37*). The bed of the temporal fossa is made up of parts of the parietal, frontal, temporal, and sphenoid (greater wing) bones. The fossa contains and provides bony attachment for the temporalis muscle.

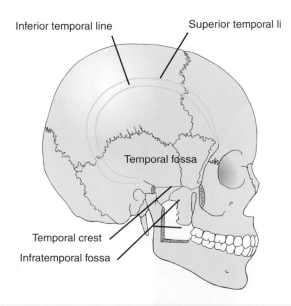

Figure 7-37 Temporal and infratemporal fossae of the skull.

Infratemporal Fossa

The **superior wall**, or roof, is formed by the inferior surface of the greater wing of the sphenoid and a small portion of squamous temporal bone. The infratemporal crest separates the roof from the temporal fossa above.

1. The **medial wall** is formed by the lateral surface of the lateral pterygoid plate.
2. The **lateral wall** is the medial aspect of the mandibular ramus.
3. The **anterior wall** is the posterior (infratemporal) surface of the maxilla.
4. The **inferior boundary** is imaginary and is marked by an inward extension of the mandibular plane of the mandible.
5. The **posterior wall** is not bony. The stylomandibular ligament separates the infratemporal region anteriorly from the parotid region behind.

TEMPOROMANDIBULAR JOINT*

The craniomandibular joint is a complex articulation of the movable mandible and the base of the skull. Articulation takes place in two areas: (1) between maxillary and mandibular teeth (interjaw dental occlusion) and (2) between the mandibular condyle and the temporal bone.

Occlusion is not discussed in this textbook but rather is left to books dealing specifically with dental anatomy and physiology. The temporomandibular joint (jaw joint) is a bilateral synovial joint. It permits a degree of freedom of movement of the mandible in three planes.

Bones Involved

The temporomandibular joint is named for the two bones that partake in the joint, namely, the temporal bone at the base of the skull and the moveable mandible (*Figure 7-38*).

Mandibular Process or Condyle of the Mandible. The mandibular condyle is roller-shaped and measures from 13 to 25 mm in mediolateral length (*Figure 7-39*). The long axis of the roller, when viewed superiorly, does not lie in a simple medial-lateral plane but angles slightly posteriorly from lateral to medial. The ends of the roller project medially and laterally as poles, with the **medial pole** projecting slightly more than the **lateral pole**. The superior surface is not completely rounded in an anteroposterior direction. A slight ridge runs from medial to lateral, resulting in a flattened superoanterior aspect and a convex posterosuperior aspect. The superior surface is convex in a medial-lateral direction.

The condyle varies in shape, ranging from a convex anterior profile to one that is rounded. Four main shapes have been described.

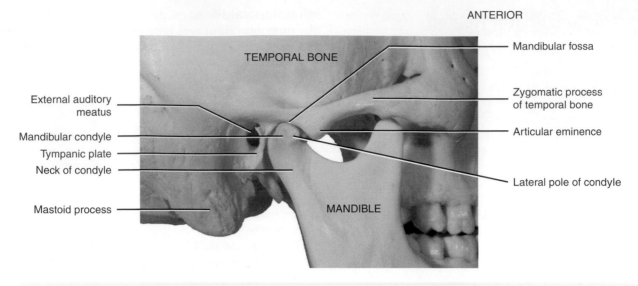

ANTERIOR

TEMPORAL BONE

Mandibular fossa

Zygomatic process of temporal bone

External auditory meatus

Mandibular condyle

Tympanic plate

Neck of condyle

Articular eminence

Lateral pole of condyle

Mastoid process

MANDIBLE

Figure 7-38 Lateral view of bones of the temporomandibular joint.

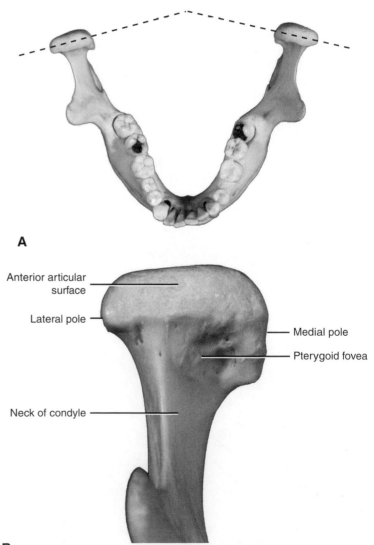

A

Anterior articular surface

Lateral pole

Medial pole

Pterygoid fovea

Neck of condyle

Figure 7-39 Condyles of the mandible. **A,** Superior view of condyles. Lines drawn through long axes extend posteriorly. **B,** Anterior view of the right condyle.

B

Temporal Bone.   The mandibular fossae are found on the base of the skull and are features of the right and left temporal bones (*Figure 7-40*). A number of features surround and limit the mandibular fossa.

Laterally, each fossa is limited by the root of the **zygomatic process of the temporal bone**. Medially, the fossa is limited by the **spine of the sphenoid bone**. Anteriorly, the fossa sweeps upward into a gently rounded bar of bone termed the *articular eminence*. Posteriorly, the **squamotympanic** and **petrotympanic fissures** separate the functional anterior portion of the mandibular fossa from the nonfunctional tympanic plate behind. Superiorly, the fossa is separated from the middle cranial fossa and the temporal lobes of the brain by a thin plate of bone at the apex of the fossa.

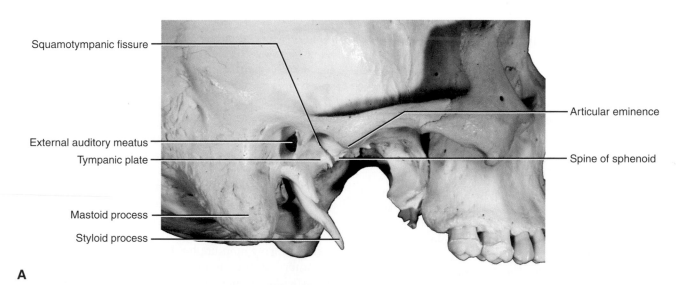

A

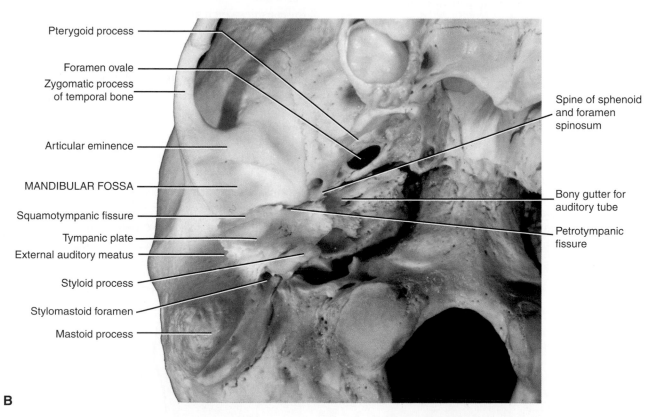

B

Figure 7-40   The mandibular fossae and articular eminence of temporal bone. **A,** Lateral aspect. **B,** Inferior aspect of base of the skull.

Articular Capsule, Temporomandibular Ligament, and Articular Disc

Review the features of a typical synovial joint with a disc in Chapter 1, section 4.

Articular Capsule and Temporomandibular Ligament.

The temporomandibular joint, like all synovial joints, possesses a fibrous capsule that encloses the joint surfaces like a sleeve that runs from the temporal bone superiorly to the condyle of the mandible inferiorly. The enclosed space between the articular surfaces is the **joint cavity**.

Superior Attachment. Superiorly the capsule attaches to the area surrounding the mandibular fossa and articular eminence of the temporal bone (see *Figures 7-40* and *7-41*). Note that the superior attachment extends as far anteriorly as the anterior slope of the articular eminence and as far posteriorly as the squamotympanic fissure.

Inferior Attachment. Inferiorly the joint capsule attaches to the periphery of the condylar neck below the medial and lateral poles of the condyle.

Temporomandibular (Lateral) Ligament. The temporomandibular ligament (see *Figure 7-41*) is a lateral thickening of the joint capsule and is similar to collateral ligaments of other joints. Because the temporomandibular joint is bilateral, the opposite temporomandibular ligament acts as a medial collateral ligament. The fibers of the temporomandibular ligament pass obliquely downward and posteriorly from the lateral aspect of the articular eminence (glenoid tubercle) to the posterior aspect of the neck of the mandibular. Deeper fibers run in a more horizontal plane from the glenoid tubercle to the lateral pole of the condyle. The temporomandibular ligament prevents posterior and inferior displacement of the condyle but allows limited anterior movements of the condyle.

Articular Disc

Features. An articular disc composed of dense fibrous tissue lies within the joint capsule, intervening between the condyle and the mandibular fossa (*Figure 7-42*). The disc features three zones of varying thickness. A prominent **posterior thickening** sits atop the condyle and fills the mandibular fossa above when the mandible is at rest.

A less prominent **anterior thickening** lies just below the posterior slope of the articular eminence, and a relatively thin **intermediate zone** lies between them. The resulting configuration is a biconcave disc that serves to provide reciprocal articular surfaces between its inferior aspect and the condyle and between its superior surface and the mandibular fossa and eminence. Only the peripheral attachments of the disc contain blood vessels; the disc itself is avascular, getting its nourishment by diffusion from the periphery and from synovial fluid.

Joint Cavities. The disc effectively divides the joint cavity into two distinct upper and lower compartments that allow two types of joint movement, a **hinge movement** in the *lower compartment* and a **translatory movement** in the *upper compartment*.

Attachments. The disc is attached to the inner periphery of the articular capsule by **superior** and **inferior sheets**, or **lamellae**, that continue superiorly and inferiorly to blend with the walls of the capsular ligament described earlier. The superior capsular attachments to the temporal bone above are *relatively loose*, allowing the condyle and the disc to translate forward on mandibular depression. Inferiorly, the attachments are *more tightly bound* to the capsule, causing the disc to translate forward with the condyle during mandibular depression.

Anteriorly, the superior lamella extends forward under the articular eminence and blends with the anterior wall of the capsule, which, in turn, fuses with the periosteum of the anterior slope of the articular eminence. The inferior lamella extends forward and then blends with the anterior capsule that loops posteriorly to blend with the periosteum of the condyle just below its articular surface.

Posteriorly, the superior and inferior lamellae diverge to enclose the **bilaminar** or **retrodiscal space** filled with loose, vascular connective tissue. The **superior lamella** of the posterior aspect of the disc contains *elastic fibers* that sweep upward to insert into the squamotympanic fissure. The **inferior lamella** contains only collagen fibers and passes inferiorly to fuse with the periosteum of the posterior condylar neck.

Relationship of Disc to Condyle During Opening Movements. *Figure 7-43* represents normal temporo-

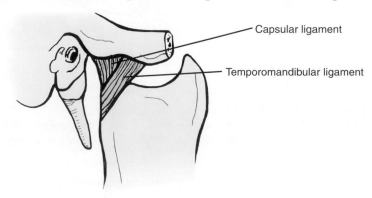

Capsular ligament

Temporomandibular ligament

Figure 7-41 Articular capsule and temporomandibular ligament of the right temporomandibular joint.

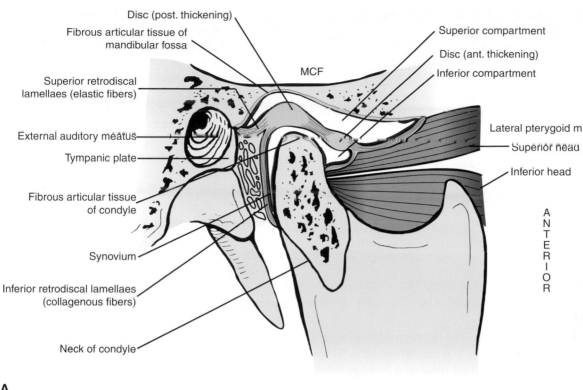

Disc (post. thickening)
Fibrous articular tissue of mandibular fossa
Superior retrodiscal lamellaes (elastic fibers)
External auditory meatus
Tympanic plate
Fibrous articular tissue of condyle
Synovium
Inferior retrodiscal lamellaes (collagenous fibers)
Neck of condyle

MCF

Superior compartment
Disc (ant. thickening)
Inferior compartment
Lateral pterygoid m
Superior head
Inferior head

ANTERIOR

A

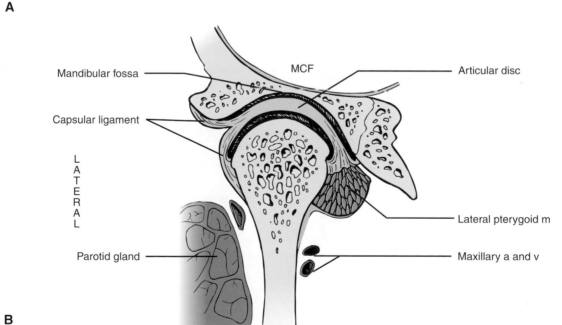

Mandibular fossa
Capsular ligament

LATERAL

Parotid gland

MCF

Articular disc

Lateral pterygoid m

Maxillary a and v

B

Figure 7-42 Internal features of the temporomandibular joint. **A,** Sagittal section. **B,** Coronal section. (MCF, middle cranial fossa.)

mandibular joint anatomy in the closed and open positions. Note how the relative sizes of the posterior and anterior recesses of the inferior joint space change in relative size. On opening, the posterior recess increases in size as the anterior recess decreases. Note that, upon opening, both the condyle and the disc translate forward to sit on the articular eminence. The disc lags slightly behind the condyle because the posterior thickening of the disc occupies a more posterior position in relation to the condylar head. This arrangement allows a nice reciprocal fit between the curvature of the articular eminence in the superior concavity of the disc and between the curvature of the condylar head and the inferior concavity of the disc.

CLINICAL NOTES

Discomalleolar (Pinto's) Ligament

The superior retrodiscal lamella that contains elastic fibers is thought to be a first arch remnant of the discomalleolar ligament. This ligament joins the medial posterosuperior aspect of the joint capsule and disc to the malleolus of the middle ear through Pinto's ligament that passes through the squamotympanic fissure. It is thought by some to play a role in tinnitus (ringing in the ear) secondary to inflammation of the temporomandibular joint. This ligament is seen through an arthroscope as the oblique protuberance.

Accessory Ligaments. Two accessory ligaments span the joint but probably do not significantly limit mandibular movements (*Figure 7-44*).

Sphenomandibular Ligament. The sphenomandibular ligament is another vestige of the first embryonic arch. It runs from the spine of the sphenoid bone as a band of thickened, fibrous tissue to the lingula of the mandible.

Stylomandibular Ligament. The stylomandibular ligament runs from the styloid process of the temporal bone to the angle of the mandible. It really serves as the thickened anterior portion of the parotid capsule, which separates the parotid region from the infratemporal region.

Articular Surfaces

The opposing articulating surfaces of most joints are covered with glass-smooth hyaline cartilage. This is true of joints between bones of endochondral ossification.

Synovial joints of bones that form from intramembranous ossification, however, are different in that their articular surfaces are coated with a yellowish, **dense fibrous tissue**. The clavicle and the mandible are both derived from intramembranous ossification. The sternoclavicular and acromioclavicular joints of the clavicle and the temporomandibular joints of the mandible contain dense fibrous articular tissue that, when dissected, feels and looks like hyaline cartilage. It is smooth, glossy, and perfectly suited for movement in a synovial joint.

The mandibular fossa of the temporal bone is lined with a thin layer of dense fibrous articular tissue (see *Figure 7-42*). Posteriorly, the articular tissue is limited by the squamotympanic fissure and does not cover the tympanic plate. Anteriorly, the articular tissue covers the articular eminence. The mandibular condyle is capped with the same dense fibrous articular tissue.

Synovial Membrane (Synovium)

A layer of synovium lines the inner aspects of the joint capsule. This relatively delicate membrane does not line the actual articular surfaces of joints because synovial joints are generally weight-bearing joints. Some investigators have reported synovium lining the mandibular fossa, and this would indicate that at least this part of the joint bears no pressure. The pressure, in fact, is borne by the occluded maxillary and mandibular teeth. The synovial membrane exhibits folding (**villi**), particularly in the fornices (reflections) of the joint cavity spaces. The degree of folding increases under pathological conditions and with age.

The synovial membrane consists of two layers: (1) an intimal cellular layer and (2) a vascular subintimal layer. The intimal layer contains two types of cells: type A cells appear to be phagocytic, and type B cells synthesize

NORMAL DISC POSITION

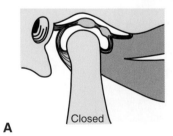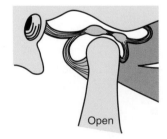

A

INTERNAL DISC DERANGEMENT

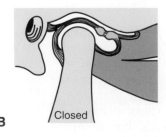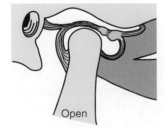

B

Figure 7-43 Relationships of condyle, disc, mandibular fossa, and articular eminence. **A,** Normal relationships in open and closed positions. **B,** Internal disc derangement in open and closed positions.

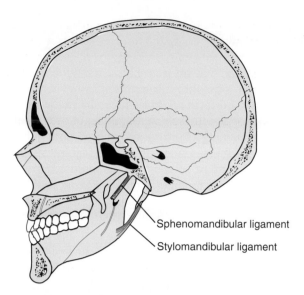

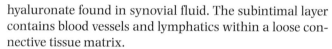

Figure 7-44 Medial view of the right temporomandibular joint to show accessory ligaments.

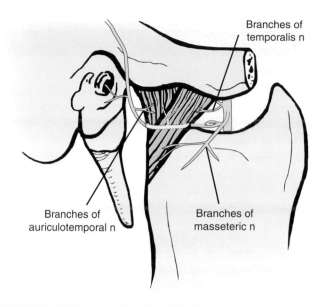

Figure 7-45 Sensory nerve supply of the temporomandibular joint.

hyaluronate found in synovial fluid. The subintimal layer contains blood vessels and lymphatics within a loose connective tissue matrix.

Synovium secretes synovial fluids for lubrication and possibly nourishment of the opposing articular surfaces. In addition, there is a constant turnover of synovial fluid to eliminate cellular debris within the joint cavity.

Nerve Supply

Most of the temporomandibular joint is supplied by sensory articular branches of the **auriculotemporal nerve** (*Figure 7-45*). A small anterior portion is supplied by sensory fibers arising from posterior temporal and masseteric branches of cranial nerve V-3.

The posterior and posterolateral regions of the joint capsule contain free nerve endings of C and A delta types of fibers that conduct **pain impulses** from the joint. This is part of a feedback mechanism that limits excessive mandibular movements.

The retrodiscal inferior lamella contains proprioceptive mechanoreceptors that detect condylar **movement** and **position**.

Blood Supply

Articular branches arise from the **superficial temporal artery** to supply most of the joint. In addition, there are small arterial "twigs" from muscular branches of the maxillary artery that supply the anterior aspect of the joint.

MASTICATION

The process of chewing food (mastication) involves a group of muscles that are capable of moving the mandible about the temporomandibular joint to grind and break up food between the occlusal surfaces of the maxillary and mandibular teeth.

In considering movements of the mandible, it is important to keep a few general points in mind: (1) muscles spanning the joint move the mandible; (2) muscles secure and then stabilize mandibular positions; (3) muscles determine the direction of mandibular movement; and (4) ligaments that also span the bones of the joint are arranged to limit the movements produced by the musculature.

Reference Positions of the Mandible

Rest Position. The mandible assumes a habitual rest position when not involved in some type of movement. Several millimeters separate the occlusal surfaces of the teeth (freeway space), and the condyles rest lightly on the posterior slope of the articular eminence.

The muscles of mastication act in harmony to maintain this postural position of rest against gravity.

Centric Occlusion. Centric occlusion is achieved on closing the freeway space and allowing the teeth to come into maximal contact in the midline. Malposed teeth may prevent individuals from acquiring a true centric relation, and they do the best they can by assuming an acquired habitual occlusion.

The condyles in centric occlusion sit within the mandibular fossae but exert little or no upward force. This is not a restful position (teeth clenched), because muscular effort is required to maintain centric occlusion.

Movements at the Temporomandibular Joint

The temporomandibular joint is a synovial joint with an intervening disc (*Figure 7-47*). The disc between the

275

CLINICAL NOTES

Arthritis

The temporomandibular joint, like all synovial joints, is susceptible to painful joint inflammation (arthritis) and changes in the apposing bones that are seen in medical imaging (osteoarthritis). The causes are varied, ranging from the ravages of time (primary degenerative arthritis) to abnormal function over a period of time (secondary degenerative arthritis). Abnormal function, in turn, may be the result of a structural problem such as dental malocclusion or a functional problem such as **bruxism** (clenching and grinding of the teeth). Manifestations of temporomandibular joint disorders are pain, which may radiate as facial pain to the muscles of mastication, restricted joint movements, and grinding noises from within the joint (crepitus).

Internal Disc Derangement (ID)

Internal disc derangement is a situation in which the disc is out of its normal position superior to the condyle. Instead it is located anterior and medial to the condyle brought about by weakened lateral and posterior disc attachments. On opening, in some cases, the disc snaps posteriorly with an audible "click" to assume its normal position (reduction) and, on closing, snaps anteriorly, sometimes with a reciprocal click. This is **disc derangement with reduction**. In other patients, the disc retains its abnormal position on opening. This is **disc derangement without reduction**.

Figure 7-43, B, illustrates an anteromedial meniscus displacement without reduction. In the closed position, the anterior recess of the inferior joint space is abnormally large and elongated with a concave superior border. In the open position, the condyle has translated only minimally forward and the anterior recess has changed little from its closed configuration. The disc changes from a biconcave to a biconvex configuration.

In later stages, the attaching tissues become thinner and the posterior attachment may perforate. Alternatively, perforation may occur in the intermediate zone or the attaching tissues anterior to the anterior thickening. Perforation allows communication between the superior and inferior joint spaces, allowing the condyle to rub directly against the anterior incline of the mandibular fossa. *Figure 7-46* illustrates a temporomandibular joint surgical procedure that has revealed a perforated disc and its subsequent removal.

Signs of internal derangement are: (1) locking with interincisal opening limited to 20 mm, (2) significant pain on attempted opening, (3) a history of clicking, and (4) crepitus on auscultation of the affected joint. Depending on the severity and the range of movement, treatment ranges from mild analgesics to fabrication of intraoral appliances and, in extreme cases, surgery.

Dislocation

Movement about a synovial joint is normally restricted by the joint ligaments. Loose or lax ligaments may result in painful joint dislocation or separation. Dislocation occurs in susceptible people following rigorous mastication, a forceful yawn, or a prolonged dental appointment with the mouth held open for a period of time. Dislocated condyles are carried anteriorly beyond the articular eminences to the infratemporal fossae. This is accompanied by painful spasms of the lateral pterygoid muscles. Reduction is effected by downward and backward pressure applied to the mandibular occlusal surfaces. Difficult cases are sometimes successfully treated with injection of a few drops of local anesthetic in the ipsilateral joint area.

---

articular surfaces divides the joint cavity in two and allows for more than one type of movement.

Hinge Movement. A hinge type of rotation takes place in the **lower compartment** between the inferior aspect of the stationary disc and the moving condyle. The axis of rotation is about a horizontal axis through the condyles.

Plane (Gliding) Movement. A gliding type of movement takes place in the **upper compartment** between the superior surface of the disc, which moves with the condyle, and the stationary mandibular fossa and eminence. The condyle and the disc move bodily forward.

The descriptions of the two basic movements are simplistic, to say the least, and the actual excursions through which the mandible moves involve a combination of gliding and hinge movements.

Mandibular Movements

The mandible is capable of six basic movements about the temporomandibular joint: (1) protrusion or protraction, (2) retrusion or retraction, (3) elevation or closing, (4) depression or opening, (5) right lateral excursion, and (6) left lateral excursion (see *Figure 7-47*).

The actual process of chewing involves combinations of the six basic movements. To demonstrate the

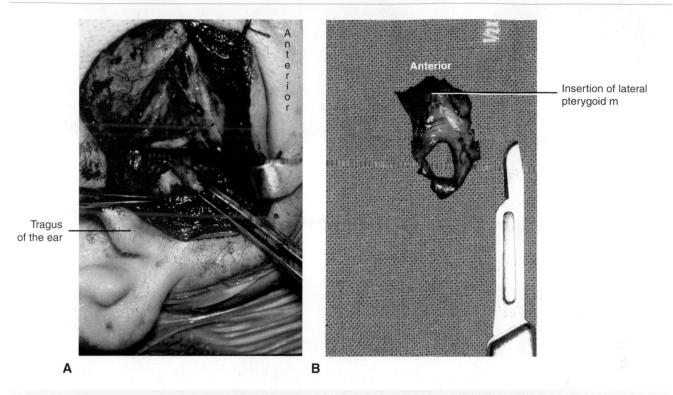

A

B

Tragus of the ear

Anterior

Anterior

Insertion of lateral pterygoid m

Figure 7-46 Perforated disc. **A,** Surgical exposure of the temporomandibular joint. **B,** Perforated disc removed. (Courtesy Dr. B. Kryshtalskyj.)

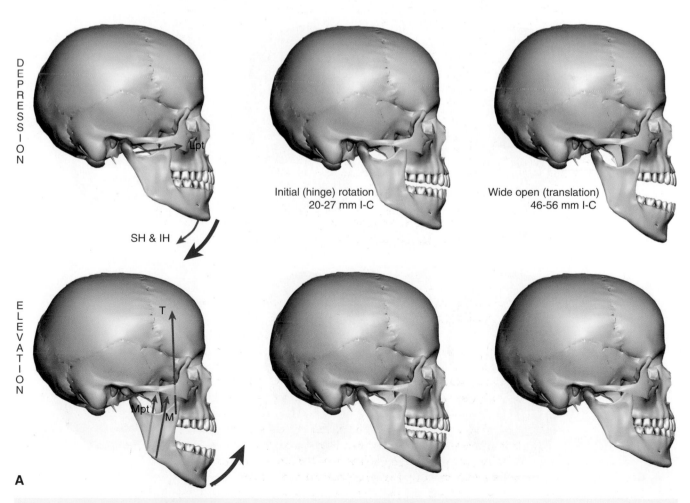

DEPRESSION

ELEVATION

Lpt

SH & IH

T

Mpt M

Initial (hinge) rotation 20-27 mm I-C

Wide open (translation) 46-56 mm I-C

A

Figure 7-47 Six basic movements of the mandible and the muscles that produce these movements.

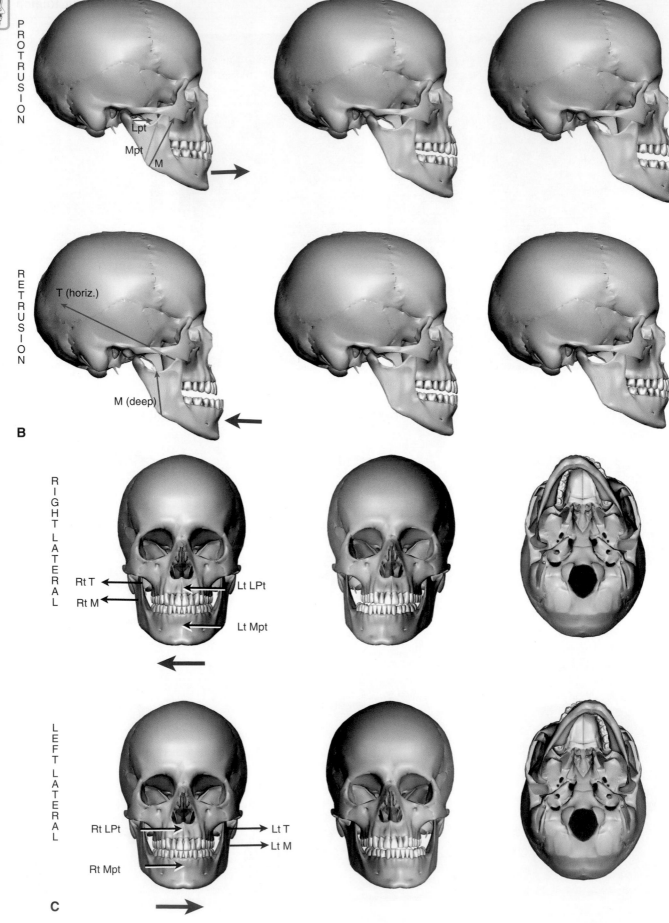

PROTRUSION

Lpt
Mpt
M

RETRUSION

T (horiz.)

M (deep)

B

RIGHT LATERAL

Rt T
Rt M
Lt LPt
Lt Mpt

LEFT LATERAL

Rt LPt
Rt Mpt
Lt T
Lt M

C

Figure 7-47 Cont'd.

movements, palpate your condyles immediately anterior to the tragus of the ear and go through the following movements.

Protrusion. With the teeth in centric occlusion, slide the mandible forward, maintaining dental contact until the incisors bite end-to-end. Maximal protrusion results in the lower incisors being a few **millimeters** anterior to the maxillary incisors.

The condyles move anteriorly and inferiorly along the posterior slope of the articular eminence. This movement takes place in the upper compartment; that is, the disc and the condyle together pass downward and forward along the slope of the eminence.

Retrusion. From the protruded position, slowly move the mandible posteriorly while maintaining dental contact until the teeth are once more in the centric position. The condyles and the discs move upward and backward on the articular eminence and reoccupy the mandibular fossae.

Depression. From the normal occluded position, slowly depress the mandible. The occlusal surfaces of the teeth diverge, and the chin swings downward. The condyles undergo a slight rotation in the lower compartment during the initial 20 to 27 mm of opening. Then the condyles and discs begin to move downward and forward along the eminence. When maximal opening is attained, the condyles rest atop the articular eminences. The axis of rotation is roughly through the mandibular foramina. A continuous hinge rotation through a condylar axis would send the mandible crashing into the pharynx behind.

Elevation. The opposite sequence of events takes place. As the chin swings upward and forward, the condyles move backward and upward along the articular eminence. As the occlusal surfaces approach each other, the mandible hinges upward about a condylar axis to once more attain centric occlusion.

Right and Left Lateral Excursions. From a centric occluded position, slide the teeth to the right while maintaining occlusal contact. Then slide back to centric and beyond to the left side. This is the basic side-to-side movement, which allows us to grind food.

In traveling to the right, the right condyle shifts slightly medially and then rotates through a vertical axis. The left condyle travels downward and forward along the articular eminence. Extreme lateral movements are physically impossible because the excursion is blocked by the ramus

of the contralateral side banging into the contralateral maxillary buccal segments.

MUSCLES OF MASTICATION

The muscles of mastication originate from the skull, span the temporomandibular joint, and insert into the mandible (*Table 7-3*). On contraction, they act to move the mandible during movements of mastication.

Masseter Muscle

The masseter muscle is a quadrilateral muscle that covers most of the lateral aspect of the ramus of the mandible (*Figure 7-48*). Lying superficial to the muscle is a portion of the parotid gland (facial process), the parotid duct, the transverse facial artery, and the various branches of the facial nerve (see *Figure 7-35, A*).

The muscle is clearly divided into a superficial and a deep portion, which blend as a single anterior border.

Origin. The superficial portion arises as a thick tendon from the zygomatic process of the maxilla and as fleshy fibers from the inferior border of the anterior two thirds of the zygomatic arch. The deep portion arises from the inner aspect of the zygomatic arch and the inferior border of the posterior third of the zygomatic arch.

Insertion. The superficial fibers sweep inferiorly and posteriorly to insert into the angle of the mandible and the lower portion of the lateral aspect of the ramus. They cover the deep portion.

The deep fibers pass vertically downward to insert into the upper portion of the lateral aspect of the ramus. They do not insert into the mandibular condyle, neck, nor the upper portion of the coronoid process.

Actions
1. **Elevation (bilateral):** The masseter muscle is a powerful elevator of the mandible and is very active during forceful (clenched) centric occlusion.
2. **Ipsilateral excursion (unilateral):** The origin of the masseter muscle is slightly lateral to its insertion, and, therefore, a single masseter muscle can move the mandible to the same side.
3. **Retrusion (bilateral):** When the mandible is in a protruded position, the deep fibers are in a position to help retrude the mandible.

Temporalis Muscle

To see the full extent of the temporalis muscle, it is necessary to remove the zygomatic arch (*Figure 7-49*).

TABLE 7-3

Muscles of Mastication

Muscle	Origin	Insertion	Action	Cranial Nerve
Masseter				
Superficial head	Zygomatic process of maxilla and inferior border of anterior two thirds of zygomatic arch	Angle of mandible and lower portion of lateral aspect of ramus	Elevation (bilateral)	V-3
			Ipsilateral excursion (unilateral) Protrusion (bilateral—superficial head)	
Deep head	Inner aspect of zygomatic arch and posterior third	Upper portion of lateral aspect of ramus	Retrusion (bilateral—deep head)	
Temporalis	Lower temporal line of skull	Coronoid process of mandible	Maintain resting tonus Elevation (bilateral)	V-3
	Temporal fossa Overlying temporal fascia	Anterior border of ramus of mandible	Ipsilateral excursion (unilateral) Retrusion (bilateral—posterior, horizontal fibers)	
Medial pterygoid	Medial aspect of lateral pterygoid plate	Medial aspect of mandibular ramus and angle of mandible	Elevation (bilateral)	V-3
			Protrusion (bilateral) Contralateral excursion (unilateral)	
Lateral pterygoid	Lateral aspect of lateral pterygoid plate	Pterygoid fovea of condylar neck	Protrusion (bilateral)	V3
Inferior head			Depression (bilateral) Contralateral excursion (unilateral)	
Lateral pterygoid	Roof of infratemporal fossa (greater wing of sphenoid)	Pterygoid fovea of condylar nec with interior head	Elevation—particularly during power stroke	V3
Superior head		Capsule and disc of TMJ		

TMJ, Temporomandibular joint.

The temporalis muscle is fan shaped, with the periphery of the fan attached to the side of the skull and the handle of the fan attached to the coronoid process of the mandible. The muscle is covered by a strong membranous sheet of fascia, which attaches superiorly to the superior temporal line. Below, the fascia splits to attach to the medial and lateral aspects of the zygomatic arch. Lying within the split portion above the arch is a variable amount of fat, some small vessels, and nerves.

Origins. The temporalis muscle originates as fleshy fibers from (1) the curvilinear lower temporal line, (2) the temporal fossa below the temporal line, and (3) the overlying temporal fascia. The fibers, arranged as a fan, can be divided on the basis of function into vertical anterior and middle vertical fibers and almost horizontal posterior fibers.

Insertion. The anterior, middle, and posterior fibers converge and pass downward deep to the zygomatic arch as a thick tendon, to insert into the medial aspect of the coronoid process and the anteromedial border of the ramus of the mandible.

Actions
1. **Resting tonus (bilateral):** The temporalis muscle maintains normal mandibular rest position when the subject is in the upright position.
2. **Elevation (bilateral):** The fibers of temporalis are active during end-to-end and centric occlusal biting positions; the muscle is most active, however, in centric occlusion.
3. **Retrusion (bilateral):** The posterior fibers of temporalis lie in an almost horizontal plane and, therefore, are in

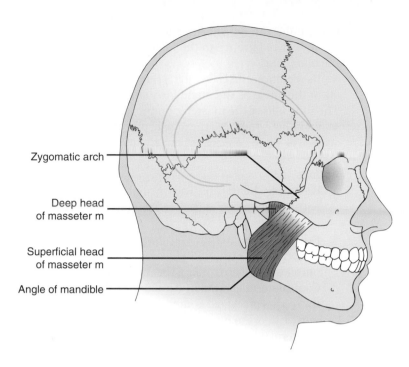

Zygomatic arch

Deep head
of masseter m

Superficial head
of masseter m

Angle of mandible

Figure 7-48 Right masseter muscle.

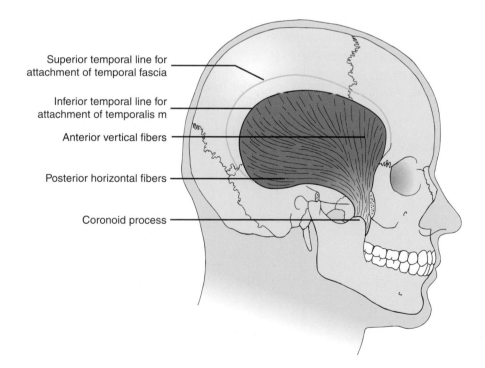

Superior temporal line for
attachment of temporal fascia

Inferior temporal line for
attachment of temporalis m

Anterior vertical fibers

Posterior horizontal fibers

Coronoid process

Figure 7-49 Right temporalis muscle.
The zygomatic arch has been removed
to reveal insertion into coronoid process.

a good position to pull the protruded mandible back to
a centric position.

4. **Ipsilateral excursion (unilateral):** The insertion of
temporalis is medial to the origin, and, therefore the
temporalis muscle acting singly is capable of pulling
the mandible to the same, or ipsilateral, side.

Medial Pterygoid Muscle

The medial and lateral pterygoid muscles are occupants of
the infratemporal fossa. To see them, it is necessary to remove
a portion of the ramus of the mandible (*Figure 7-50*).

The medial pterygoid muscle is almost a mirror
image of the masseter muscle. It is rhomboidal and runs

practically in the same direction on the inner surface of the mandibular ramus.

Origin. The origin is fleshy from the medial aspect of the lateral pterygoid plate. A few fibers arise from the maxillary tuberosity.

Insertion. The fibers run downward, backward, and slightly medially to insert into the medial aspect of the mandibular ramus. The insertion extends from just below the mylohyoid groove to the inferior border and angle of the mandible.

Its tendinous insertion joins that of the masseter muscle at the angle of the mandible to form a common sling. The sling allows the masseter on the lateral surface of the mandibular ramus and the medial pterygoid on the medial surface to act in concert as powerful elevators of the jaw.

Actions

1. **Elevation (bilateral):** The medial pterygoids, acting with the masseter muscles, are powerful elevators of the mandible.
2. **Protrusion (bilateral):** The insertion of the muscle is posterior to its origin and, therefore the right and left muscles aid in protruding the mandible.
3. **Contralateral excursion (unilateral):** The insertion of the medial pterygoid is lateral to its origin, allowing the muscle fibers to move the mandible to the opposite side in lateral movements.

Lateral Pterygoid Muscle

The lateral pterygoid is almost triangular in shape with two distinct heads, inferior and superior, each with contrasting functions. It is the only muscle of the four muscles of mastication to occupy primarily a horizontal position (*Figure 7-51*).

Origins. The **inferior head** arises as fleshy fibers from the lateral aspect of the lateral pterygoid plate of the sphenoid bone.

CLINICAL NOTES

Myofascial Pain Syndrome (Fibromyalgia)

Myofascial pain syndrome involves pain emanating from fibrous muscle sheaths, muscle, tendons, and ligaments. Curiously there is no evidence of inflammation in these tissues. Common target areas are the occipital region, neck, low back and thighs, and pain in the masticator region that involves the muscles of mastication and their fascial coverings. Myofascial pain in the masticator region occurs more frequently in women, particularly women in their early twenties and those near menopause. The immediate cause is usually nocturnal bruxism (clenching or grinding the teeth during sleep). Treatment consists of mild analgesics and fabrication of an acrylic night guard or splint with occlusal bite pads that is worn intraorally at night to prevent bruxism.

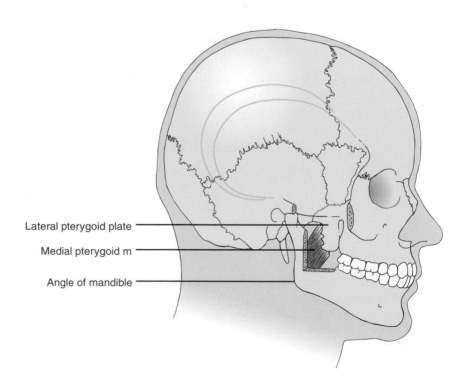

Lateral pterygoid plate

Medial pterygoid m

Angle of mandible

Figure 7-50 Right medial pterygoid muscle. Portion of ramus has been removed.

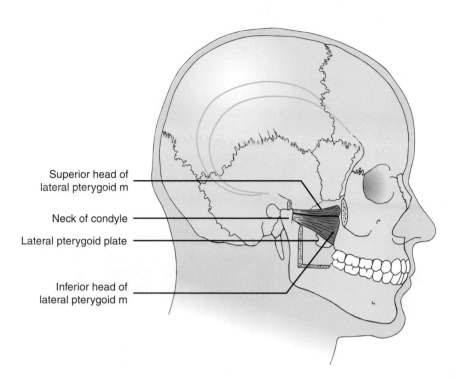

Superior head of
lateral pterygoid m

Neck of condyle

Lateral pterygoid plate

Inferior head of
lateral pterygoid m

Figure 7-51 Right lateral pterygoid muscle.

The **superior head** originates as fleshy fibers from the inferior aspect of the greater wing of sphenoid, which forms the roof of the infratemporal fossa.

Insertions. The **inferior head** passes backward, upward, and slightly laterally to insert into the pterygoid fovea on the anterior aspect of the condylar neck.

The **superior head** passes posteriorly and somewhat laterally to insert into the articular capsule and the articular disc and anterior aspect of the condylar neck. Most of the inserting fibers blend with the tendon of the inferior head to insert into the pterygoid fovea of the condylar neck. A smaller number of deeper or more medial fibers insert into the medial aspect of the capsule and disc. The discal insertion is somewhat contentious among investigators but tugging on the superior head in cadavers invariably produces movement of the disc indicating direct or at least indirect attachment.

Actions of the Inferior Head
1. **Protrusion (bilateral):** The inferior lateral pterygoids acting together are the prime protractors of the mandible. The fibers are in a perfect position to haul the condyles and articular disc forward in moving the mandible into a protrusive position.
2. **Depression (bilateral):** To understand this action, one must remember that the prime axis of rotation during mandibular depression is through the mandibular foramen. Thus, contractions of both lateral pterygoids not only pull the condyles forward but also, along with the suprahyoid and infrahyoid muscles, help in depressing the mandible.

3. **Contralateral excursion (unilateral):** The insertion of the lateral pterygoid is lateral to its origin, and thus the lateral pterygoid muscle acting singly moves the mandible to the opposite side.

Actions of the Superior Head. The superior lateral pterygoids are inactive during opening. They are active, however, during mandibular elevation or closing along with the temporalis, masseter, and medial pterygoid muscles. The superior heads are particularly active when the teeth, upon closure, encounter resistance such as a bolus of food. *Closure on resistance* is termed the *power stroke*, and the superior lateral pterygoids play an active role in the power stroke.

Accessory Muscles of Mastication
Other muscles that are active in mastication include the suprahyoid and infrahyoid muscles of the neck described in Chapter 5. Both groups of muscles are active in helping to depress the mandible.

Summary of Muscles of Mastication
Elevation (Closing). The muscles that elevate the mandible during closing are (1) the right and left temporalis, (2) the right and left masseter, and (3) the right and left medial pterygoid muscles (see *Figures 7-47* and *7-52*).

Depression (Opening). The muscles responsible for depression of the mandible during opening are (1) the inferior heads of the right and left lateral pterygoid muscles, (2) the right and left suprahyoid muscles of the neck, and (3) the right and left infrahyoid muscles of the neck.

283

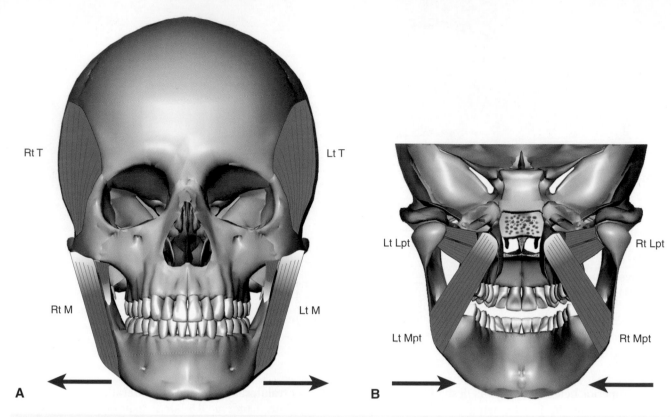

Figure 7-52 A, Anterior view of masseter and temporalis muscles to demonstrate their ability to draw the mandible to the same (ipsilateral) side. **B,** Posterior view of medial and lateral pterygoid muscles to demonstrate their ability to perform contralateral movements. *T,* Temporalis muscle; *M,* masseter muscle; *Mpt,* medial pterygoid muscle; *Lpt,* lateral pterygoid muscle.

Protrusion. The muscles that protrude or protract the mandible are (1) the right and left lateral pterygoid, (2) the right and left medial pterygoid muscles, and (3) the right and left superficial heads of the masseter muscles.

Retrusion. The muscles that retrude or retract the mandible include: (1) the posterior fibers of the right and left temporalis and (2) the deep heads of the right and left masseter muscles.

Right Lateral Excursion. The muscles that swing the mandible to the right are (1) the right masseter, (2) the right temporalis, (3) the left medial pterygoid, and (4) the left lateral pterygoid muscles.

Left Lateral Excursion. The muscles that swing the mandible to the left are (1) the left masseter, (2) the left temporalis, (3) the right medial pterygoid, and (4) the right lateral pterygoid muscles.

Nerve Supply

All four muscles are supplied by motor branches arising from the mandibular nerve (cranial nerve V-3). The distribution of the mandibular nerve is described fully in the following section.

Arterial Supply

The four muscles of mastication receive arterial branches from the second part of the maxillary artery described in the next section.

THE MANDIBULAR NERVE (CRANIAL NERVE V-3)

The mandibular nerve is the nerve of the mandibular process of the first branchial arch, and consequently it supplies all the structures that arise from the mandibular process.

Origin

The mandibular nerve arises within the middle cranial fossa from the trigeminal ganglion. It consists of a large sensory component and a smaller motor component, which merge as a single trunk after leaving the ganglion. The sensory component arises directly from the trigeminal ganglion. The motor portion arises from the pons, passes deep to the ganglion, and joins the sensory portion as a single trunk or stem. The nerve drops through the foramen ovale to enter the infratemporal region. Here it lies deep to the lateral pterygoid muscle and almost immediately divides into an anterior and a posterior branch.

Branches arise from the stem, anterior division, and posterior division (*Figure 7-53*).

Branches of the Stem

The stem lies deep to the lateral pterygoid muscle. The stem gives off three motor branches and one sensory branch.

Attached to the medial aspect of the stem is the otic ganglion, which is discussed shortly.

Nerve to Medial Pterygoid (Motor). The medial pterygoid nerve arises from the mandibular stem and travels inferiorly to supply the medial pterygoid muscle.

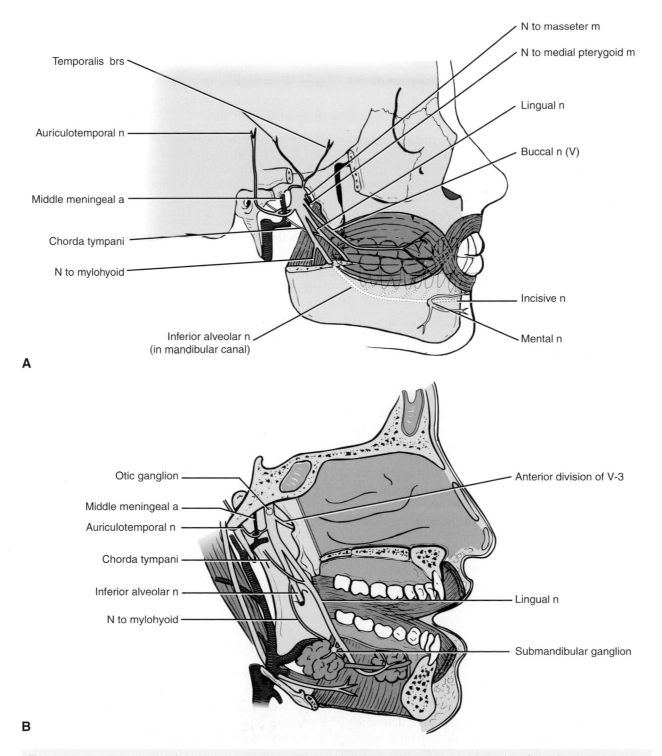

Figure 7-53 Mandibular nerve (V-3) and its branches. **A,** Lateral view of the right mandibular nerve. **B,** Medial view of the left mandibular nerve.

Nerve to Tensor Tympani (Motor). The tensor tympani nerve arises from the stem, traverses the otic ganglion, and passes backward to enter the origin of the tensor tympani muscle from the cartilaginous portion of the auditory canal. The tensor tympani muscle is discussed with the middle ear.

Nerve to Tensor Veli Palatini (Motor). The tensor palate nerve arises from the stem and passes medially to enter and supply the tensor veli palatini muscle of the soft palate.

Nervus Spinosus (Sensory). The nervus spinosus arises from the stem and heads superiorly to enter the skull through the foramen spinosum. It supplies dura of the middle cranial fossa.

Branches of the Anterior Division

Three motor branches and one sensory branch arise from the anterior division of the mandibular nerve.

Nerve to Masseter (Motor). The masseter nerve is generally the first to arise from the anterior division and passes between the roof and the superior head of the lateral pterygoid muscle. It then passes through the mandibular notch to enter the deep surface of the masseter muscle. The nerve to the masseter muscle also carries a few sensory fibers, which it supplies to the anterior portion of the temporomandibular joint.

Nerve to Temporalis (Motor). Three branches, anterior, middle, and posterior temporal nerves, pass between the superior head of the lateral pterygoid muscle and the roof of the infratemporal fossa. The branches sweep upward under the overlying temporalis muscle, enter it, and supply it.

Nerve to Lateral Pterygoid (Motor). Deep to the lateral pterygoid muscle, two branches are given off. One goes to the superior head; the other branch passes to the inferior head.

Buccal Branch (Long Buccal Nerve) (Sensory). The buccal branch of cranial nerve V-3 passes forward and laterally, emerging between the two heads of the lateral pterygoid muscle. The nerve continues inferiorly and anteriorly, pierces the tendon of the temporalis muscle, passes through the buccal fat pad, and emerges onto the buccinator muscle of the cheek from under cover of the ramus of the mandible. The buccal branch is sensory to the mucosa and skin of the cheek and sensory to the mandibular buccal gingiva of the molar region.

Branches of the Posterior Division

Two sensory branches and one mixed (sensory and motor) branch arise from the posterior division of the mandibular nerve.

Auriculotemporal Nerve (Sensory). The auriculotemporal nerve is mainly sensory but carries hitchhiking postsynaptic parasympathetic and sympathetic outflow from the otic ganglion. The auriculotemporal nerve passes posteri-

orly and then splits to pass around the middle meningeal artery. The nerve passes lateral to the spine of the spheroid and medial to the mandibular condyle. It then passes laterally behind the capsule of the temporomandibular joint and emerges superficially between the jaw joint and the external auditory meatus. The nerve passes upward over the root of the zygoma and ascends on the side of the head. During its course it gives off several branches.

Auricular Branches. Auricular branches are sensory to the external auditory meatus and the lateral aspect of the tympanic membrane.

Articular Branches. The articular branches supply the sensory nerves that convey most sensation from the temporomandibular joint.

Secretory Fibers. Postsynaptic parasympathetic secretory fibers from the otic ganglion pass to the facial nerve, which, in turn, distributes the secretory fibers to the parotid gland. The secretory fibers are described under the otic ganglion.

Temporal Branches. Temporal branches continue superiorly on the temples to supply overlying skin and the lateral aspect of the scalp.

Lingual Nerve (Sensory). The lingual nerve is a large branch that passes downward, forward, and slightly laterally. It appears from under the inferior border of the lateral pterygoid muscle and continues downward and forward over the lateral aspect of the medial pterygoid muscle. From here, it heads toward the lingual aspect of the third molar alveolar area and enters the area of the floor of the mouth.

Chorda Tympani Nerve (Parasympathetic and Special Sense: Taste). The chorda tympani nerve is a branch of the facial nerve (**cranial nerve VII**) that carries special sensory taste and parasympathetic secretory fibers. It leaves the facial nerve within the facial canal of the petrous temporal bone and enters the middle ear. It passes anteriorly across the medial aspect of the tympanic membrane and exits from the skull through the petrotympanic fissure. The chorda tympani passes anteriorly and inferiorly, medial to the spine of the spheroid, and joins the posterior aspect of the lingual nerve deep to the inferior border of the lateral pterygoid muscle. The chorda tympani continues as part of the lingual nerve and is carried to the floor of the mouth.

Distribution of the Lingual Nerve. The course of the lingual nerve is presented in the section dealing with the floor of the mouth. Its distribution there is the following:

1. **General sensory afferent**: This component supplies (1) mucosa of the anterior two thirds of the tongue, (2) mucosa of the floor of the mouth, and (3) mandibular lingual gingiva.
2. **Parasympathetic efferent**: The parasympathetic fibers contained within the chorda tympani are carried with the lingual nerve to the floor of the mouth, where they

synapse within the submandibular ganglion. From the ganglion, postsynaptic fibers pass to (1) the submandibular gland, (2) the sublingual gland, and (3) minor glands of the floor of the mouth.

3. **Special sensory taste:** Special sensory fibers of taste within the chorda tympani are distributed by the lingual nerve to the mucosa of the anterior two thirds of the tongue.

Inferior Alveolar Nerve (Sensory and Motor). The inferior alveolar nerve passes downward behind the lateral pterygoid muscle, along with the lingual nerve. As they both appear from under the inferior border of the lateral pterygoid muscle, the lingual nerve pursues a deeper and more anterior course on its way to the floor of the mouth. The inferior alveolar nerve continues downward and slightly laterally as it heads toward the mandibular foramen. At this point it lies between the medial pterygoid muscle medially and the ramus of the mandible laterally.

The mandibular foramen lies roughly at the center point of the internal aspect of the ramus, about 1.5 to 2 cm below the mandibular notch. It is just about at the same level as a posterior extension of the mandibular occlusal plane. The inferior alveolar nerve makes contact with the ramus just above the mandibular foramen and, at this point, gives off the nerve to the mylohyoid.

Nerve to Mylohyoid (Motor). The mylohyoid nerve is a slender motor branch that runs downward in a shallow groove on the medial aspect of the ramus just below the mandibular foramen. The nerve passes to the submandibular region to supply the mylohyoid muscle and the anterior belly of the digastric muscle.

Intramandibular Portion of the Inferior Alveolar Nerve. The inferior alveolar nerve enters the mandibular foramen and passes downward and anteriorly through the mandibular canal. As it passes below the root apices of the mandibular molars, premolars, and anterior teeth, it sends small branches to supply the pulps of the teeth. Innervation is one-sided and generally stops at the midline with no crossover of nerve fibers. If there is crossover, it is slight and does not go beyond the opposite central incisor.

The Mental Nerve. The mental nerve branches from the inferior alveolar nerve and passes to the face through the mental foramen. The mental foramen is generally in the region of the second premolar, at the midpoint between the alveolar crest and the inferior mandibular border. The mental nerve sends branches to supply the (1) skin and mucous membrane of the lower lip, (2) skin of the chin, and (3) vestibular gingiva of the mandibular incisors.

Some authors describe the inferior alveolar nerve as having two terminal branches: the mental nerve, as just described, and the incisive nerve, which continues within the mandibular canal to supply the mandibular anterior teeth.

The Otic Ganglion. The otic ganglion is a small swelling about 3 mm in diameter (see *Figure 7-53, B*). It is attached

to the medial aspect of the stem of the mandibular nerve as it passes through the foramen ovale. The otic ganglion, like other cranial ganglia, receives fibers from three sources (*Figure 7-54*).

Incoming Fibers

1. **Sensory fibers** arise from the stem of the mandibular nerve and pass through the ganglion without synapsing.
2. **Sympathetic fibers** arise from the perivascular plexus of the middle meningeal artery. They too, pass through the ganglion without synapsing.
3. **Parasympathetic fibers** arrive in a bizarre, roundabout route and originate from the glossopharyngeal nerve (cranial nerve IX); as cranial nerve IX exits from the skull through the jugular foramen, it gives off a tympanic branch that reenters the base of the skull through the tympanic canal. The tympanic canal leads to the middle ear cavity, and here the tympanic branch forms a plexus that supplies the mucosa of the middle ear. The *lesser petrosal nerve* arises from the tympanic plexus, passes through a canal in the petrous temporal bone, and emerges in the middle cranial fossa through the hiatus for the lesser petrosal nerve. The nerve then heads toward the foramen ovale and passes through to join the otic ganglion on the medial aspect of the stem of the mandibular nerve. These parasympathetic fibers synapse within the otic ganglion.

CLINICAL NOTES

Local Anesthesia

The various branches of the mandibular nerve that supply oral and dental structures can be anesthetized. The anatomy of local anesthesia is covered in Chapter 8.

Outgoing Fibers. Postsynaptic sympathetic and parasympathetic fibers hitchhike with the auriculotemporal nerve to continue their odyssey toward the parotid gland. Postsynaptic parasympathetic fibers are motor secretory, but it is not entirely clear as to the function of the sympathetic fibers.

THE MAXILLARY ARTERY

The external carotid artery is described in the anterior triangle of the neck and in the parotid region of the head. At the level of the neck of the mandibular condyle, the external carotid artery divides as two terminal branches. The superficial temporal artery was traced onto the side of the head, and its branches were noted in discussion of the parotid region.

The maxillary artery passes anteriorly deep to the neck of the mandibular condyle and traverses the infratemporal fossa (*Figure 7-55*). It passes over the lateral pterygoid

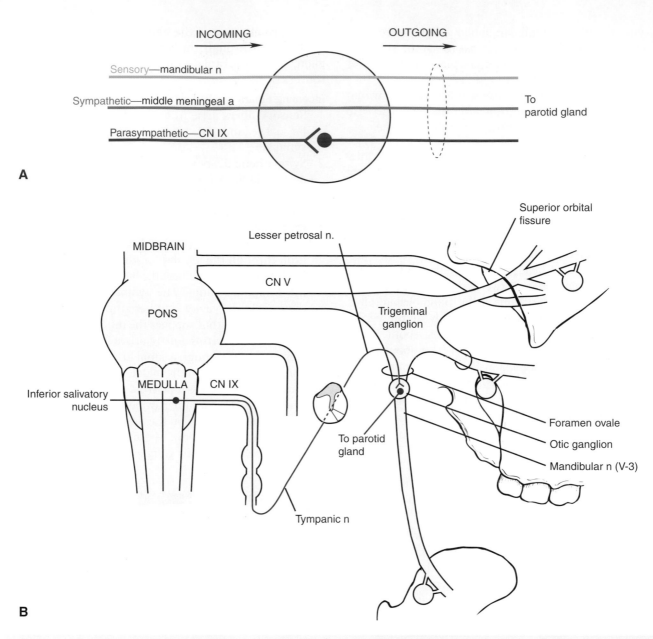

Figure 7-54 Otic ganglion. **A,** Scheme of incoming and outgoing nerve fibers. **B,** Origins of parasympathetic component form cranial nerve IX.

muscle and then disappears in the pterygopalatinine fossa. (In some individuals, the maxillary artery passes deep to the inferior head of the lateral pterygoid muscle.)

The lateral pterygoid muscle is used as a landmark to conveniently divide the maxillary artery into three parts: part 1 is the portion before the muscle, part 2 is the portion passing over the muscle, and part 3 is the part after crossing the muscle.

Parts 1 and 2 provide companion arterial branches for each branch of the mandibular nerve (cranial nerve V-3). Part 3 provides companion arterial branches for branches of the maxillary nerve (cranial nerve V-2) and is discussed with the maxillary nerve.

Branches of Part 1

There are four branches of part 1; these pass through four openings of the skull.

Deep Auricular Artery. The deep auricular artery passes upward and backward to travel with the auricular branches of the auriculotemporal nerve. It supplies skin of the external auditory meatus and the lateral aspect of the tympanic membrane.

Anterior Tympanic Artery. The anterior tympanic artery is the companion artery to the chorda tympani nerve. It ascends behind the temporomandibular joint and passes

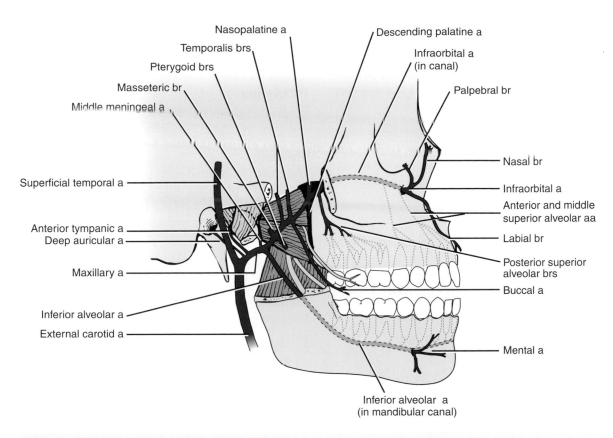

Figure 7-55 Branches of the maxillary artery.

through the petrotympanic fissure to enter the middle ear cavity and supply its lining.

Middle Meningeal Artery. The middle meningeal artery is the companion artery to the nervus spinosus, and it ascends to pass through the foramen spinosum to enter the middle cranial fossa. It ascends on the internal aspect of the lateral wall of the skull and divides into an anterior (frontal) branch and a posterior (parietal) branch. These anastomose with anterior and posterior meningeal arteries. The middle meningeal artery supplies the dura mater, the inner table of bone, and the diploë of the cranial vault. It also supplies small branches to the trigeminal nerve roots and ganglion.

CLINICAL NOTES

Trauma

The relatively thin bone of the temporal fossa is easily fractured, and laceration of the underlying middle meningeal artery is possible. Subsequent extradural hemorrhage compresses the motor cortex of the brain and produces paralysis of the opposite side.

The accessory meningeal artery, when present, supplements the supply of the middle meningeal artery. It passes upward through the foramen ovale into the cranial cavity to help supply the trigeminal ganglion, bone, and dura.

Inferior Alveolar Artery. The inferior alveolar artery descends toward the mandibular foramen, pursuing a parallel course to the inferior alveolar nerve. It gives off a companion artery to the nerve to the mylohyoid and then enters the mandibular foramen and canal to supply the mandible. As it passes below the roots of the mandibular teeth, it gives off small branches to the root apices. At the level of the second premolar, the artery gives off the mental branch, which exits through the mental foramen along with the mental nerve. It supplies the lower lip, the vestibular gingiva of the mandibular incisors, and the chin.

Branches of Part 2

All the branches of part 2 go to supply the four muscles of mastication and the buccinator muscle.

Deep Temporal Arteries. Anterior and posterior deep temporal branches arise from the maxillary artery and ascend deep to the temporalis muscle to supply it.

Pterygoid Arteries. Pterygoid arteries arise to supply the medial and the lateral pterygoid muscles.

Masseteric Arteries. Small masseteric branches pass laterally through the mandibular notch to enter the deep surface of the masseter muscle.

Buccal Artery. A small buccal branch travels downward and anteriorly along with the buccal branch of cranial nerve V-3. It pierces the tendon of the temporalis muscle and passes through the buccal fat pad to end up on the lateral surface of the buccinator muscle.

Branches of Part 3

The branches of part 3 of the maxillary artery run as companion arteries with the various branches of the maxillary nerve (cranial nerve V-2). The branches of part 3 are considered following the description of the maxillary nerve in the next section.

THE PTERYGOID PLEXUS OF VEINS AND THE MAXILLARY VEIN

The venous flow from areas supplied by the maxillary artery does not return in a nice neat fashion to the maxillary vein (*Figure 7-56*). Instead the tributaries form a complex configuration termed the pterygoid plexus of veins. The venous plexus is of considerable size and occupies areolar spaces between the temporalis and lateral pterygoid muscles and between the medial and lateral pterygoid muscles, and surrounds the maxillary artery.

Tributaries

The pterygoid plexus receives veins that correspond to the various branches of the maxillary artery.

Drainage

The plexus is drained posteriorly by the short maxillary vein, which parallels the course of part 1 of the maxillary artery. The maxillary vein passes backward deep to the neck of the mandibular condyle, enters the substance of the parotid gland, and unites here with the superficial temporal vein to form the retromandibular vein.

Communications

The pterygoid plexus communicates with the following:

1. The **cavernous sinus** via small veins passing through the foramen ovale.
2. The **inferior ophthalmic vein** via veins passing through the inferior orbital fissure.
3. The **pharyngeal plexus** of veins via communicating veins.
4. The **facial vein** via the deep facial vein.

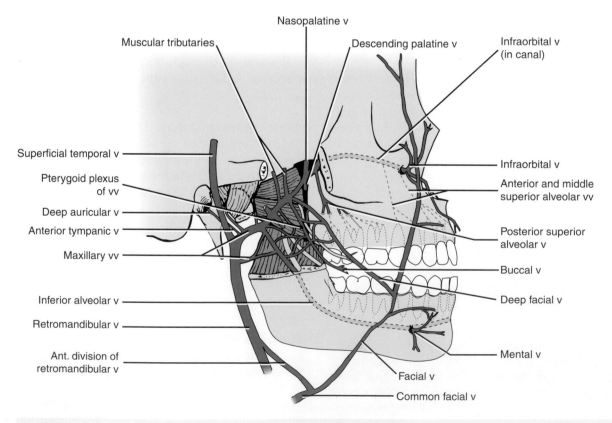

Figure 7-56 The pterygoid plexus of veins and its tributaries and communications.

Vascular Accidents

Local anesthetic injections are routinely administered in the infratemporal fossa and, on occasion, the needle can puncture one of the many vessels in the area.

Facial Hematoma

Puncture of a blood vessel in the infratemporal region can cause a hemorrhage into the space. Puncture of a venous tributary of the pterygoid plexus of veins leaks slowly into the space. Puncture of an arterial branch of the maxillary artery leaks quickly into the space. The hemorrhaging bulges into the superficial fascia of the face in the cheek region and produces a swelling or **hematoma**. There is generally nothing one can do to prevent its occasional unfortunate occurrence. Like bruises anywhere else in the body, the hematoma undergoes several color changes over time before it resolves.

Inadvertent Intravascular Local Anesthetic Injections

A cardinal rule when administering a local anesthetic injection is to determine whether the tip of the needle has entered a blood vessel. If blood is aspirated into the syringe, the needle must be repositioned to ensure that the anesthetic fluid is not injected into the bloodstream. The reagents, particularly the epinephrine commonly packaged with the anesthetic, can produce mild to severe reactions in the patient.

6. The Pterygopalatine Fossa

SKELETAL REVIEW

The skeletal features of the middle cranial fossa and the maxilla, sphenoid, and palatine bones should be reviewed (see Chapter 6).

LOCATION AND TERMINOLOGY

The pterygopalatine fossa is located on the lateral aspect of the skull and is best seen with the zygomatic arch removed (*Figure 7-57*). The fossa is seen through a narrow cleft, the **pterygomaxillary fissure**, between the pterygoid process of the sphenoid bone and the posterior wall of the maxilla. The medial wall of the fossa is the vertical plate of the palatine bone.

There are seven exits and entrances of the pterygopalatine fossa; these communicate with other regions of the head.

1. The **foramen rotundum**, because it has length, is really a canal. It leaves the middle cranial fossa at the junction of the greater wing and body of sphenoid bone and enters the superoposterior aspect of the pterygopalatine fossa.
2. The **pterygoid canal** is located by finding the foramen lacerum at the external aspect of the skull; it arises from a small opening in the anterior border of the foramen lacerum and passes through the base of the medial pterygoid plate to enter the pterygopalatine fossa inferior and medial to the foramen rotundum.
3. The **sphenopalatine foramen** is situated on the superior aspect of the medial wall of the fossa. It is so named because it is formed by the sphenopalatine notch of the palatine bone and the body of the sphenoid bone above. The foramen opens medially into the lateral wall of the nasal cavity.
4. The **inferior orbital fissure** is the cleft between the lesser wing of the sphenoid and the maxilla. The fissure communicates with the bony orbit.
5. On the inferior aspect of the inferior orbital fissure is a small notch leading to the uncovered **infraorbital groove**. The groove continues anteriorly and laterally across half the length of the floor of the orbit; acquires a thin, bony roof; and becomes the **infraorbital canal**. The canal exits onto the face just below the orbital margin.
6. The **greater and lesser palatine canals** leave the pterygopalatine fossa at its V-shaped base and appear again as the greater and lesser palatine foramina on the posterior aspect of the hard palate.
7. The posterior **superior alveolar foramina** are located in the infratemporal surface of the maxilla. They appear as small perforations on the posterior convex surface of the maxilla and lead to the interior of the maxillary sinus.

CONTENTS

The pterygopalatine fossa contains portions of the maxillary nerve (cranial nerve V-2) and the maxillary artery (part 3).

The Maxillary Nerve (Cranial Nerve V-2)

The maxillary nerve is the sensory supply to all the eventual derivatives of the maxillary process. It is the second of three large divisions to arise from the trigeminal ganglion within the middle cranial fossa. The maxillary nerve follows a somewhat complicated course through four regions of the head and gives rise to sensory branches as it passes through each region.

291

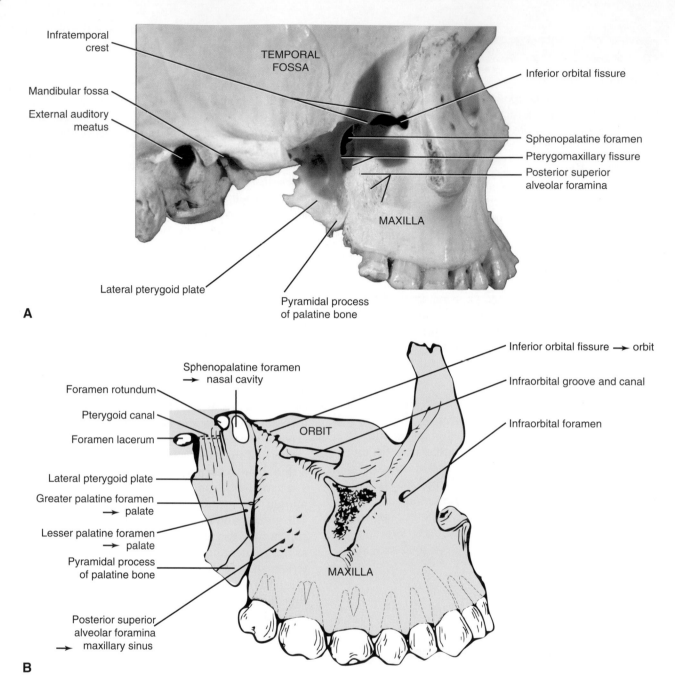

Figure 7-57 **A,** Right lateral view of the skull with the zygomatic arch removed to show pterygopalatine fossa. **B,** Scheme of pterygopalatine fossa to show its entrances and exits.

Intracranial. Within the middle cranial fossa, the maxillary nerve runs anteriorly in the lateral wall of the cavernous sinus and then leaves the sinus and the middle cranial fossa by dropping through the foramen rotundum (see *Figure 7-27*).

Meningeal branches arise to supply the dura mater of the middle cranial fossa.

Pterygopalatine Fossa. After passing through the foramen rotundum, the maxillary nerve enters the pterygopalatine fossa (*Figure 7-58*). The nerve runs across the upper portion of the fossa, turns laterally, and heads for the infraorbital groove in the posterior aspect of the maxilla. Three branches are given off within the pterygopalatine fossa.

Ganglionic Branches. Communicating branches suspend the pterygopalatine ganglion from the maxillary nerve. These branches supply sensory fibers to the ganglion and convey mixed sensory, parasympathetic, and sympathetic fibers back to the maxillary nerve.

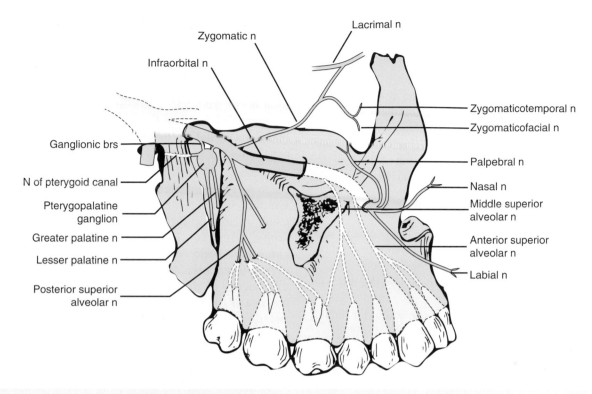

Zygomatic n
Infraorbital n
Lacrimal n
Zygomaticotemporal n
Zygomaticofacial n
Ganglionic brs
Palpebral n
N of pterygoid canal
Nasal n
Middle superior alveolar n
Pterygopalatine ganglion
Greater palatine n
Anterior superior alveolar n
Lesser palatine n
Labial n
Posterior superior alveolar n

Figure 7-58 The maxillary nerve and its branches.

Zygomatic Nerve. The zygomatic nerve leaves the fossa through the inferior orbital fissure to enter the orbit. It runs anteriorly along the lateral wall of the orbit and communicates with the lacrimal branch of cranial nerve V-1. Postganglionic fibers from the pterygopalatine ganglion travel with the lacrimal nerve to supply the lacrimal gland with parasympathetic secretory fibers. The zygomatic nerve leaves the orbit through a tiny zygomatic canal in the lateral wall. The canal is Y-shaped and diverges within the bone. The zygomatic nerve divides as two terminal branches within the canal: (1) the **zygomaticofacial nerve** travels along one limb of the canal and exits onto the face at the prominence of the cheek to supply overlying skin; (2) the **zygomaticotemporal nerve** travels along the other limb of the Y and exits from the zygomatic bone into the temporal fossa. There it ascends deep to the temporalis muscle, pierces the muscle above the zygomatic arch, and surfaces as cutaneous branches to the skin of the temple.

Posterior Superior Alveolar Nerve. The last branch to arise from the maxillary nerve within the pterygopalatine fossa is the posterior superior alveolar nerve. The nerve descends along the infratemporal surface of the maxilla and enters the perforated area of the infratemporal surface as several branches. The nerves pass through the posterior superior alveolar foramina and enter the maxillary sinus. Here they descend toward the roots of the maxillary molar teeth in small grooves deep to the mucosal lining of the sinus. As they approach the molar teeth, the nerves become plexiform and form the posterior portion of the **superior alveolar plexus.**

1. **Dental branches** arise from the plexus to supply the pulps of the maxillary molar teeth.
2. **Maxillary sinus branches** supply the mucosal lining of the maxillary sinus.
3. **Gingival branches** do not enter the posterior superior alveolar foramina but rather continue downward and forward, external to the maxilla, to supply the vestibular (buccal) gingiva of the maxillary molars and a small superior portion of the cheek.

Infraorbital Portion. As the maxillary nerve enters the infraorbital groove, it becomes the **infraorbital nerve.** Two sensory branches arise from the infraorbital nerve.

Middle Superior Alveolar Nerve. This nerve leaves the infraorbital nerve and passes inferiorly through the floor of the orbit to enter the maxillary sinus. It runs downward in a small, bony groove in the lateral wall of the maxillary sinus deep to the mucosal lining and forms the intermediate portion of the superior alveolar plexus. The middle superior alveolar nerve supplies the following branches:

1. **Dental branches** arise from the plexus to supply the pulps of the premolar teeth and, allegedly, the mesiobuccal root of the first molar (the middle superior alveolar nerve may not always be present, and in these cases, the premolar teeth are supplied by the anterior superior alveolar nerve and the posterior superior alveolar nerve).

293

2. **Maxillary sinus branches** supply the mucosal lining of the maxillary sinus.
3. **Gingival branches** supply the vestibular gingiva of the maxillary premolars.

Anterior Superior Alveolar Nerve. Before the exit of the infraorbital nerve onto the face, the anterior superior alveolar nerve is given off. It enters the *sinuous canal* on the anterior wall of the maxillary sinus, turns medially, and then descends to form the anterior portion of the superior alveolar plexus over the roots of the maxillary anterior teeth. Branches of the anterior superior alveolar nerve are the following:

1. **Dental branches,** which arise from the plexus to supply the pulps of the central and lateral incisors and the canine teeth.
2. **Maxillary sinus branches,** which supply the mucosal lining of the maxillary sinus.
3. **Gingival branches,** which supply the vestibular (labial) gingiva of the incisors and canine teeth.
4. **Nasal branches,** which pass medially to supply small portions of the nasal septum, lateral wall, and floor of the nasal cavity.

Facial Portion. The infraorbital nerve exits onto the face through the infraorbital foramen and immediately breaks up into three terminal groups of branches, deep to the levator labii superioris muscle.

Inferior Palpebral Branches. These ascend to the orbit deep to the orbicularis oculi muscle, pierce the muscle, and supply skin and conjunctiva of the lower eyelid.

Lateral Nasal Branches. These branches travel toward the lateral aspect of the external nose to supply the skin of the lateral aspect of the nose and mucous membrane of the movable cartilaginous portion of the nasal septum.

Superior Labial Branches. The superior labial branches descend deep to the levator labii superioris and supply the skin and mucous membrane of the upper lip.

The Pterygopalatine Ganglion. The pterygopalatine ganglion is a small swelling that hangs from the maxillary nerve as it traverses the pterygopalatine fossa (*Figure 7-59*). The ganglion receives three types of nerve fibers—only the parasympathetic synapses in the ganglion.

Incoming Fibers
1. **Sensory branches** arise directly from the maxillary nerve.
2. **Sympathetic branches** arise from the postganglionic plexus surrounding the internal carotid artery as the deep petrosal nerve; these fibers have already synapsed in the sympathetic superior cervical ganglion.
3. **Parasympathetic preganglionic fibers** leave the genu of the facial nerve (cranial nerve VII) within the facial canal of the petrous temporal bone as the **greater petrosal nerve**.

The greater petrosal nerve leaves the petrous bone through the superior hiatus to enter the middle cranial fossa (see *Figure 7-27, A*). It then heads toward the foramen lacerum, drops partially through it, and enters the mouth of the pterygoid canal, along with the sympathetic **deep petrosal nerve**. The two nerves unite as the single **nerve of the pterygoid canal** and pass through the canal and into the pterygopalatine fossa to enter the pterygopalatine ganglion. Only the parasympathetic fibers synapse in the ganglion.

Outgoing Fibers. Mixed sensory, sympathetic, and parasympathetic fibers arise from the pterygopalatine ganglion, including the palatal, nasal, pharyngeal, and orbital branches (*Figure 7-60*). The sympathetic and parasympathetic components travel with each of the nerves listed hereafter to supply the minor glands of the mucosa of the hard and soft palate, nasal mucosa, mucosa of the paranasal air sinuses, and mucosa of the superior portion of the pharynx. In addition, sympathetic and parasympathetic fibers travel to the orbit to supply the lacrimal gland.

1. The **greater palatine nerve** passes inferiorly in the pterygopalatine fossa and exits via the *greater palatine canal* onto the hard palate. It travels anteriorly along the hard palate to supply the mucous membrane of the hard palate, including the palatal glands and the lingual or palatal gingiva. The greater palatine nerve supplies the mucosa of the hard palate as far anteriorly as the maxillary canines.
2. The **lesser palatine nerve** travels posterior to the greater palatine nerve, drops through the *lesser palatine canal*, and emerges through the palatal opening. It travels posteriorly to supply mucous membrane and glands of the soft palate.

CLINICAL NOTES

Allergies
Sometimes the pterygopalatine ganglion is referred to as the *hay fever ganglion* because it controls everything that one associates with hay fever and allergies, such as stuffy, runny nose and watery eyes.

3. The **nasopalatine nerve** (long sphenopalatine nerve) exits medially through the *sphenopalatine foramen* to enter the nasal cavity. It travels medially across the roof of the nasal cavity and deflects downward and forward along the nasal septum. It descends to the *incisive canal*, passes through, and emerges onto the hard palate. Its branches are (1) nasal to the nasal septum and (2) palatal to the palatal mucosa anterior to the maxillary canines.

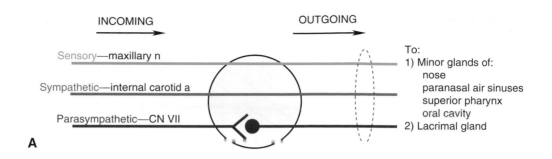

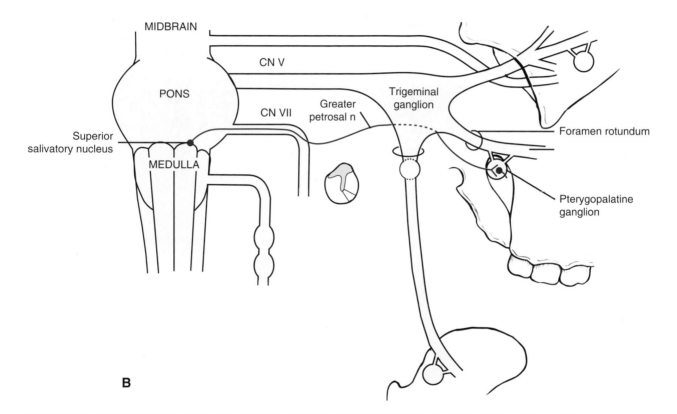

Figure 7-59 Pterygopalatine ganglion. **A,** Scheme of incoming and outgoing nerve fibers. **B,** Origins of parasympathetic component form cranial nerve VII.

4. **Posterolateral nasal branches** (short sphenopalatine nerves) exit through the *sphenopalatine foramen* to enter the nasal cavity. They supply mucous membrane of the lateral wall of the nasal cavity.

5. **Pharyngeal branches** arise from the ganglion, exit through the *sphenopalatine foramen,* and turn immediately posteriorly to enter the *palatinovaginal (pharyngeal) canal* between the vaginal process of the palatine bone and the body of the sphenoid bone. The nerve supplies mucous membranes of the sphenoidal air sinus and the roof of the pharynx.

6. Two or more tiny **orbital branches** leave the ganglion and pass through the *inferior orbital fissure* to enter the orbit. They supply (1) sensory fibers to periosteum of the orbit, (2) sympathetic fibers to orbitalis muscle (smooth muscle that bridges the inferior orbital fissure,

the function of which is unknown), and (3) secretory parasympathetic fibers to the lacrimal gland.

Maxillary sinus branches pass back up to the maxillary nerve to be distributed with the posterior, middle, and anterior superior alveolar nerves to the maxillary sinus.

CLINICAL NOTES

Local Anesthesia

The various branches of the maxillary nerve that supply oral and dental structures can be anesthetized. The anatomy of local anesthesia is covered in Chapter 8.

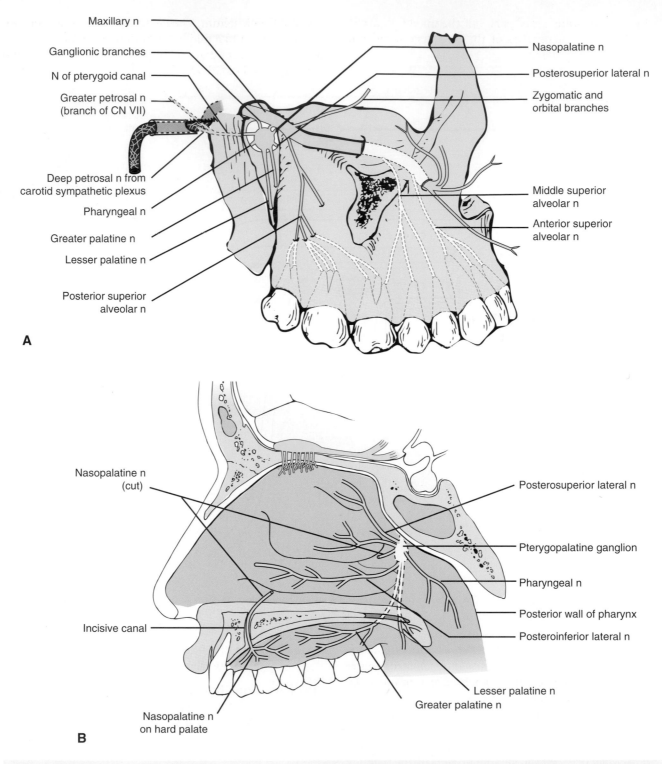

Figure 7-60 Branches of the right pterygopalatine ganglion. **A,** Lateral view. **B,** Medial view showing branches passing to the nasal cavity and pharynx.

Maxillary Artery (Part 3)

Parts 1 and 2 of the maxillary artery were studied along with the mandibular nerve in the infratemporal region (see *Figure 7-55*). Part 3 leaves the infratemporal region through the pterygomaxillary fissure to enter the pterygopalatine fossa. Here it parallels the course of the maxillary nerve through the fossa and leaves the fossa with the nerve through the infraorbital groove. At this point, it becomes the infraorbital artery.

In general, branches of part 3 of the maxillary artery follow the various branches of the maxillary nerve and pterygopalatine ganglion.

Branches

Posterior Superior Alveolar Artery. This artery leaves the maxillary artery and descends toward the posterior wall of the maxilla. Here it divides into several branches that pass through the posterior superior alveolar foramina to enter the maxillary sinus. They supply (1) the pulps of the molar and premolar teeth, (2) the mucosal lining of the maxillary sinus, and (3) the vestibular gingiva of the molar and premolar regions.

Descending Palatine Artery. This branch drops inferiorly and divides as two further branches. The greater palatine artery passes to the palate through the greater palatine canal and then passes forward to supply the mucosa of the hard palate posterior to the maxillary canine. The lesser palatine artery descends to the palate through the lesser palatine canal and passes posteriorly to supply the soft palate. There may be more than one branch and canal.

Artery of the Pterygoid Canal. A small branch travels posteriorly through the pterygoid canal to supply portions of the superior pharynx, auditory tube, and middle ear.

Sphenopalatine Artery. This artery passes medially through the sphenopalatine foramen and breaks into two branches. **Posterolateral branches** supply the lateral wall of the nasal cavity and portions of the maxillary, ethmoidal, and sphenoidal air sinuses. The **posterior septal artery** deflects off the nasal septum and descends anteriorly with the nasopalatine nerve. The artery passes through the incisive foramen and anastomoses with the greater palatine artery.

Infraorbital Artery. The infraorbital artery passes anteriorly in the infraorbital groove and canal. Within the canal, it gives off the anterior superior alveolar artery. The anterior superior alveolar artery supplies the pulps of the maxillary incisors and canines and the mucosa of the anterior wall of the maxilla.

The infraorbital artery exits onto the face through the infraorbital foramen and sends branches to the lower eyelid, the lateral aspect of the external nose, and the upper lip.

7. The Nasal Cavity and Paranasal Air Sinuses

The nose is the upper portion of the respiratory tract. The external nose is described as a feature of the face in section 1 of this chapter. The nostrils, or nares, on the inferior aspect of the external nose lead to the nasal cavity within.

The nasal cavity is a chamber consisting of bony walls covered with respiratory pseudostratified, ciliated, columnar epithelium. The cavity has a floor, a roof, two lateral walls, and a midline partition, or septum, of bone and cartilage that divides the nasal cavity into right and left portions. Posteriorly, the nasal cavity communicates with the nasopharynx through the posterior nasal apertures or choanae.

The nasal cavity is about 6 to 7 cm in length (anteroposteriorly) and 2 cm wide inferiorly and tapers to a narrowed width of 0.5 cm superiorly. The functions of the nose and nasal cavity are (1) respiration, (2) olfaction, (3) filtration of particulate matter, (4) humidification of inspired air, and (5) reception of secretions from communicating paranasal air sinuses and from the nasolacrimal duct of the orbit.

SKELETON

The features of the nasal bones, frontal bone, maxillae, ethmoid bone, sphenoid bone, palatine bones, and vomer should be reviewed.

RELATIONSHIPS

Figure 7-61 represents a coronal section through the skull to demonstrate various important relationships of the nasal cavity. *Figure 7-62* is a sagittal section through the nasal cavity to demonstrate the continuity of the nasal cavity with the nasopharynx posteriorly.

Superior

The nasal cavity is separated from the anterior cranial fossa above by the perforated cribriform plate. Lying atop the cribriform plates are the olfactory bulbs, which, in turn, receive filaments of the olfactory nerve (cranial nerve I) from mucosa of the roof of the nasal cavity.

Lateral

Lateral to the upper half of the lateral wall of the nasal cavity is the ethmoidal air sinus, and lateral to the ethmoid sinus is the medial wall of the orbit. Lateral to the lower half of the lateral nasal wall is the maxillary air sinus.

Inferior

Below the floor of the nasal cavity is the oral cavity. The hard palate forms a common partition separating the oral cavity below from the nasal cavity above.

Posterior

Behind the nasal cavity and beyond the choanae is the nasopharynx.

Anterior

The nares lead inward to a slightly dilated area that is termed the *vestibule*. The vestibule is lined with skin and contains coarse hairs, which occasionally can develop infections or furuncles. The vestibule constricts posteriorly

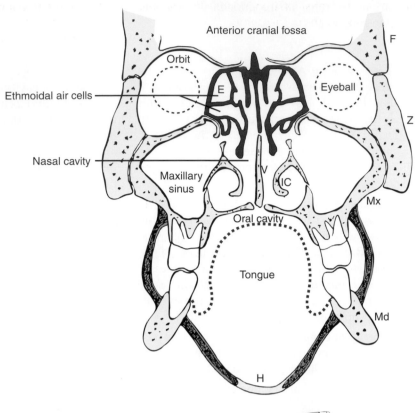

Temporal Fossa

Anterior cranial fossa

Orbit

Ethmoidal air cells

Eyeball

F

Nasal cavity

E

Z

Maxillary sinus

V

IC

Mx

Oral cavity

Tongue

Md

H

Figure 7-61 Coronal section through the skull to demonstrate the relationship of the nasal cavity to orbits, anterior cranial fossa, and oral cavity.

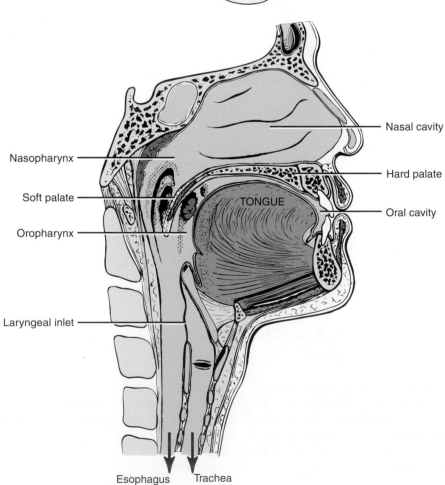

Nasopharynx

Soft palate

Oropharynx

Laryngeal inlet

Nasal cavity

Hard palate

TONGUE

Oral cavity

Esophagus

Trachea

Figure 7-62 Sagittal section through the head to illustrate the relationships of the nasal cavity, oral cavity, and the three divisions of pharynx.

as it leads to the respiratory portion of the nasal cavity. This constriction marks the transition from skin of the vestibule to respiratory mucosa of the nasal cavity.

BOUNDARIES

Floor

The floor of the nasal cavity is the hard palate. The palatal processes of the maxillae contribute to the anterior two thirds and the palatal processes of the palatine bone contribute to the posterior third. The floor of the nasal cavity is convex in a mediolateral direction.

Roof

From anterior to posterior, the roof is formed by the lateral nasal cartilages, the nasal bones, the nasal spine of the frontal bone, the cribriform plate of the ethmoid bone, and the anterior and inferior aspects of the body of the sphenoid bone.

Lateral Wall

The bony composition of the lateral wall is complicated, with many bones contributing in part (*Figure 7-64*). These include the nasal bone, maxilla, ethmoid bone, palatine bone, sphenoid bone, and inferior concha.

Three Conchae. Three elevations arise from the lateral wall as fragile scrolls of bone covered by mucous membrane. The **superior** and **middle conchae** are medial extensions of the ethmoid bone. The larger **inferior concha** is

a separate bone attached to the lateral wall. The superior border of the inferior concha articulates with the lacrimal bone, maxilla, ethmoid bone, and palatine bone. The inferior edge of the inferior concha is free.

Four Spaces. The space below each concha is termed a *meatus.* Below the inferior concha is the **inferior meatus,** below the middle concha is the **middle meatus,** and below the superior concha is the **superior meatus.** The space above and behind the superior concha is the **sphenoethmoidal recess.**

Nasal Septum

The septum of the nose divides the nasal cavity into right and left portions (*Figure 7-63*). These portions are generally unequal, because the septum deviates to one side or the other. The septum is formed by the following elements that in turn are covered with nasal mucosa: (1) the **septal cartilage** represents the movable portion of the septum and is not seen in the dried skull; (2) the **vertical plate of the ethmoid bone** contributes to the anterosuperior portion of the bony septum; and (3) the **vomer** contributes to the posteroinferior portion of the bony septum.

In addition, various bones contribute in a small way to the septum with midline projections or crests. These include **nasal crests** of the frontal bone, nasal bones, and sphenoid bones above; and **nasal crests** of the maxillae and palatine bones below.

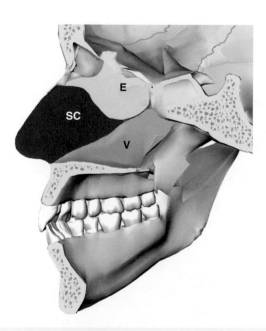

Figure 7-63 Components of the nasal septum. *SC,* Septal cartilage; *E,* vertical plate of ethmoid bone; *V,* vomer.

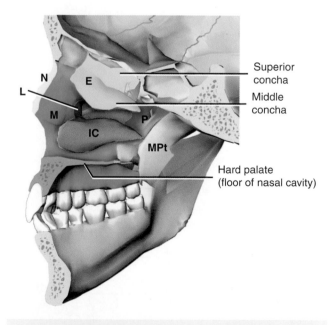

Figure 7-64 The skeletal components of the lateral wall of the nasal cavity. *M,* Maxilla; *N,* nasal bone; *L,* lacrimal bone; *E,* ethmoid bone; *P,* palatine bone; *MPt,* medial pterygoid plate of sphenoid bone; *IC,* inferior concha.

BLOOD AND NERVE SUPPLY

Nerves (*Figure 7-65*)

General Sensation. The general sensory nerves are branches of either the ophthalmic nerve (cranial nerve V-1) or the maxillary nerve (cranial nerve V-2).

Anterior Ethmoidal Nerve (Cranial Nerve V-1). The anterior ethmoidal nerve arises from the nasociliary branch of the ophthalmic nerve within the orbit. The anterior ethmoidal branch passes medially through the *anterior ethmoidal*

canal of the orbital wall to supply anterior ethmoidal air cells. The nerve continues medially to enter the anterior cranial fossa briefly and then exits through the *ethmoidal canal* anterior to the cribriform plate. The canal leads to the roof of the nasal cavity, and here the anterior ethmoidal nerve divides. Internal branches pass to the lateral nasal wall and septum. External nasal branches continue downward on the internal aspect of the nasal bone to exit onto the external nose as the *external nasal nerve*.

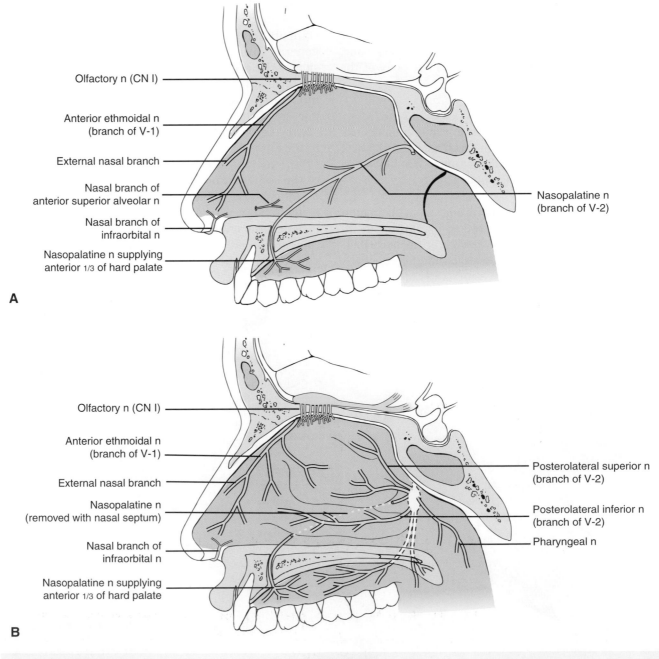

Figure 7-65 Nerve supply to the nasal cavity. **A,** Nasal septum. **B,** Lateral wall.

Nasal Branches of Infraorbital Nerve (Cranial Nerve V-2). The nasal branch of the infraorbital nerve supplies skin of the ala of the nose. An internal branch penetrates to the vestibule to supply skin of the vestibule and the movable portion of the nasal septum.

Nasal Branch of Anterior Superior Alveolar Nerve (Cranial Nerve V-2). As the anterior superior alveolar nerve descends in its canal in the anterior wall of the maxillary sinus, it gives off an internal nasal branch that passes to the nasal cavity just below the inferior concha. It supplies mucosa of the anterior portion of the inferior meatus.

Posterosuperior Lateral Nasal Nerves (Short Sphenopalatine Nerves; Cranial Nerve V-2). These arise from the pterygopalatine ganglion and pass medially through the sphenopalatine foramen to supply the posterior two thirds of the lateral nasal wall. Posteroinferior lateral nasal branches arise from the greater palatine branch of the pterygopalatine ganglion as it descends in its canal. The branches leave the canal to supply the inferoposterior lateral aspect of the nasal wall.

Nasopalatine Nerve (Long Sphenopalatine Nerve; Cranial Nerve V-2). This nerve arises from the pterygopalatine ganglion and passes medially through the sphenopalatine foramen to the nasal cavity. It continues medially and is deflected downward and anteriorly along the nasal septum, supplying it as it goes. It ends by passing through the incisive canal to the oral cavity below, where it is sensory to the oral mucosa of the anterior aspect of the hard palate.

Special Sensation: Smell. The mucosa of the superior concha and upper third of the nasal septum is the olfactory region of the nose. It is yellowish in the fresh state in contrast to the pink respiratory mucosa below. The olfactory mucosa contains bipolar olfactory cells. Peripheral processes pass to the mucosal surface as hairlike smell receptor endings. Central processes pass upward as approximately 20 bundles of filaments (olfactory nerve proper). These filament bundles pass through the cribriform plate and end by synapsing in the olfactory bulbs with ganglionic cells. Central processes of the ganglionic cells pass back to the brain through the olfactory tracts.

Autonomic Nerve Supply. Parasympathetic and sympathetic nerve supplies to the glands of the nasal mucosa arise from postganglionic fibers of the ciliary ganglion traveling with the anterior ethmoidal nerve and from postganglionic fibers of the pterygopalatine ganglion traveling with the posterolateral nasal and nasopalatine nerves.

Arteries
The mucosa of the nasal cavity receives a rich blood supply from several sources that anastomose freely (*Figure 7-66*). The important and largest arteries are the **anterior ethmoidal branch** of the *ophthalmic artery* and the **sphenopalatine branch** of the *maxillary artery* (see *Figure 7-66*).

In addition, *small nasal branches* arise from the *facial* and *infraorbital arteries*.

Veins
The venous return collects as a plexus from which veins drain to ophthalmic veins, pterygoid plexus, facial vein, and infraorbital veins.

NASAL BREATHING AND SMELLING
Most individuals are capable of nasal breathing, that is, inspiration and expiration through the nasal passages with the lips closed. Air inspired through the nose is warmed and humidified by the warm, moist mucosa of the nasal cavities. Most of the inspired air is directed back through the inferior meatus, whereas most expired air leaves along the middle meatus. Cilia of the mucosa filter particulate matter from the inspired air and then pass it back toward the nasopharynx. The pattern of the waving cilia moves particles posteriorly.

Small currents of inspired air find their way to the roof of the nose so that strong or pungent odors are detected during quiet nasal breathing. Subtler odors, however, are discerned by sniffing air, which tends to direct more air upward to the olfactory mucosa.

PARANASAL AIR SINUSES
Development
During the fetal period, the nasal mucosa invades various surrounding bones, eroding solid bones and producing hollow, air-filled spaces lined with nasal mucosa. The bones thus hollowed (*pneumatic bones*) are (1) the frontal bone, (2) the ethmoid bone, (3) the sphenoid bone, and (4) the right and left maxillae. The original route of the evaginations into the surrounding bones persist in the adult as openings. Thus the nasal mucosa is continuous with the mucous lining of each of the sinuses. Secretions from the mucosa of the air sinuses eventually drain to the nasal cavity through their respective openings, or **ostia**.

At birth, the sinuses are small and rudimentary but grow to maximum size in the adult. They follow a general growth pattern: that is, slow continuous growth during childhood and rapid growth during adolescence.

Drainage
All paranasal air sinuses drain to the nasal cavity through openings, or ostia, in the lateral nasal wall (*Figure 7-67*). These openings are obscured by the nasal conchae and are seen only in the cadaver when the conchae are *snipped away* from the lateral wall.

The **hiatus semilunaris** is a curved depression found in the middle meatus. Its superior and inferior aspects are open and lead to the paranasal air sinuses. The superior opening leads to a channel that drains the frontal sinus; the inferior opening leads directly to the maxillary sinus.

301

CLINICAL NOTES

Nasal Obstruction

Obstruction of the nasal air passages may occur for a variety of reasons. **Chronic obstruction** may be caused by a deviated nasal septum. Usually the conchae of the opposite side tend to grow toward the midline, causing partial blockage of the good side.

Chronically infected **palatine and pharyngeal tonsils** may enlarge and block the posterior passages, or choanae. The pharyngeal tonsils are commonly referred to as *adenoids* and when enlarged cause a characteristic nasal twang in the speech through the blockage.

Chronic nasal obstruction forces the patient to breathe through the mouth, and this may result in excessively dried and inflamed anterior labial gingiva. In addition, holding the mandible in a constant open position is unnatural; this causes the cheeks to press against the buccal segments of the teeth and eventually collapse them lingually. Collapsed narrow dental arches may be treated orthodontically once the primary cause of the malocclusion (nasal obstruction) is removed.

Occasional obstruction is caused by temporary inflammation of the nasal mucosa (**rhinitis**) brought on by (1) viruses (common cold), (2) bacteria (secondary bacterial infection), and (3) allergens (allergies).

Rhinorrhea refers to a drippy nose that accompanies rhinitis. Secretions of the swollen mucosa pass anteriorly as a drippy nose or pass posteriorly to the pharynx, where they are swallowed or coughed up as phlegm (postnasal drip).

Cerebrospinal Fluid Rhinorrhea

This is a spontaneous discharge of clear CSF that leaks into the nose following a fracture of the cribriform plate and tearing of the meninges.

Epistaxis (Nosebleed)

Several anastomosing arteries contribute to the blood supply of the nasal cavity. In addition, there is an extensive venous plexus. Nosebleed is a common problem resulting from trauma or sometimes occurring spontaneously. Kieselbach's area on the anterior aspect of the nasal septum is the site of several converging arteries and is particularly susceptible to bleeding (see *Figure 7-66, A*). Applying pressure by squeezing the external nose usually stems the flow. Recurring and troublesome cases may require cautery or, occasionally, ligation of the external carotid artery.

The **bulla ethmoidalis** is a swelling on the superior border of the hiatus semilunaris caused by ballooning underlying anterior ethmoidal air cells. Several openings on the bulla and the lateral surface of the middle meatus drain the anterior ethmoidal air cells to the nasal cavity.

Posterior ethmoidal air cells drain through several small openings in the lateral wall of the superior meatus. The sphenoidal air sinuses drain to the sphenoethmoidal recess through its two ostia.

Secretions of another kind also find their way to the nasal cavity for discharge. Tears produced by the lacrimal glands are removed from the conjunctival sacs by the nasolacrimal apparatus. The nasolacrimal duct ultimately drains to the inferior meatus of the nose through an oblique, inconspicuous opening.

Locations

The Maxillary Sinus (Antrum). The paired maxillary sinuses are the largest and clinically, perhaps, the most troublesome of the paranasal air sinuses (*Figures 7-68 to 7-72*). They lie within the bodies of the right and left maxillae and are variable in size (age and individual variation). Each sinus is pyramidal in shape, the base being the lateral wall of the nose and the apex extending into the zygomatic process of the maxilla. The walls of the maxilla are thin and translucent in areas.

Walls. The **posterior wall** of the maxillary sinus is the thin infratemporal surface of the maxilla. In a bony specimen, the small posterior superior alveolar foramina are seen entering the posterior wall of the maxilla. Small channels in the bone lead from the foramina downward toward the floor of the sinus overlying the maxillary molar root apices. These channels carry branches of the posterior superior alveolar nerves and vessels to and from the maxillary molars.

The **roof** of the maxillary sinus is the thin orbital plate of the maxilla. The plate separates the sinus below from the orbit and its contents above. Running along the orbital roof and then spilling onto the anterior wall is the infraorbital nerve within a bony ridge. The canal carries the infraorbital nerve and vessels from the inferior orbital fissure to the infraorbital foramen on the face. In a bony specimen, small canals may be seen leaving the infraorbital canal and leading to the floor of the sinus overlying the premolar root apices. The canals carry branches of the middle superior alveolar nerves and vessels to the premolar teeth.

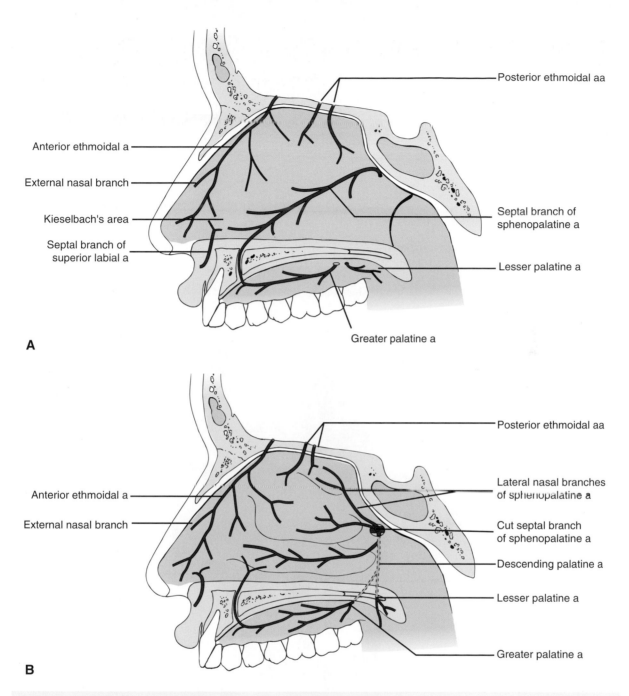

Figure 7-66 Arterial supply to the nasal cavity. **A,** Nasal septum. **B,** Lateral wall.

The **anterior wall** is formed by the facial surface of the maxilla. The infraorbital canal deflects from the roof of the sinus onto the anterior wall, descends slightly, and then exits onto the face with its contents. Just before it exits, a small, sinuous canal leaves the infraorbital canal, carrying anterior superior alveolar nerves and vessels. These pass to the apical areas of the maxillary incisors and canines.

The **medial** or **nasal wall** (*Figure 7-69*) is the common partition separating the nasal cavity and maxillary sinus.

This wall is formed primarily by the maxilla, which has a large deficiency termed the *maxillary hiatus*. Obliterating portions of this hiatus are parts of the vertical plate of the palatine bone, a bit of lacrimal bone, and a portion of the inferior concha. The remaining opening to the nasal cavity is thus considerably smaller and is rendered even smaller by covering nasal mucosa. The ostium, therefore, is relatively small leading to the hiatus semilunaris of the middle meatus of the nose.

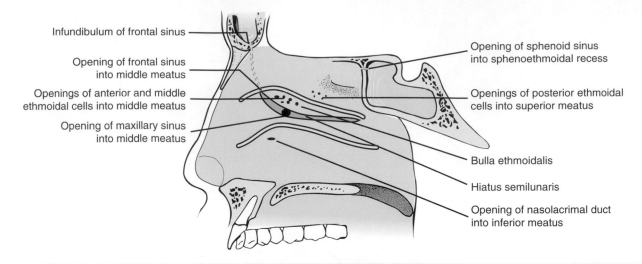

Infundibulum of frontal sinus

Opening of frontal sinus
into middle meatus

Openings of anterior and middle
ethmoidal cells into middle meatus

Opening of maxillary sinus
into middle meatus

Opening of sphenoid sinus
into sphenoethmoidal recess

Openings of posterior ethmoidal
cells into superior meatus

Bulla ethmoidalis

Hiatus semilunaris

Opening of nasolacrimal duct
into inferior meatus

Figure 7-67 Lateral wall of the nasal cavity with conchae removed to illustrate opening of paranasal sinuses into the nasal cavity.

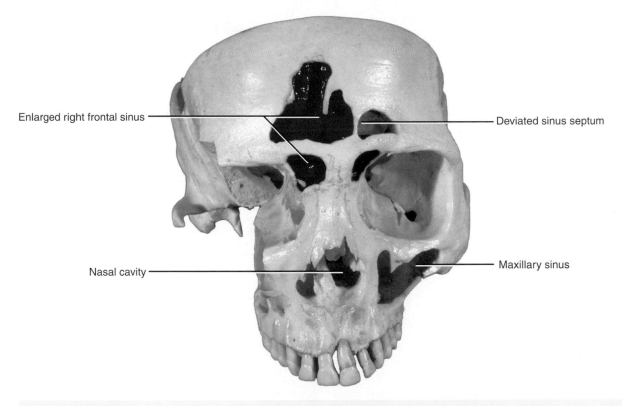

Enlarged right frontal sinus

Nasal cavity

Deviated sinus septum

Maxillary sinus

Figure 7-68 Frontal view of the maxillary and frontal air sinuses. Note extreme asymmetry of the frontal air sinuses.

The **lateral wall** is actually the blunted apex of the pyramid, which extends into the zygomatic process of the maxilla.

The **floor** of the maxillary sinus dips down below the level of the nasal cavity into the alveolar process. The roots of the first and second molars may be in close proximity to the floor of the sinus and also, variably, *the roots of the third molar*, *the premolars*, and *even the canines*. Occasionally, the roots of the maxillary molars protrude

into the sinus and are separated from the sinus only by the thin antral mucosa (*Figure 7-70*).

Relationships. *Figure 7-61* demonstrates quite nicely the important relationships of the maxillary sinus.

1. **Superior:** The orbits and their contents lie immediately above the maxillary sinuses and are separated from them by only a thin plate of bone.

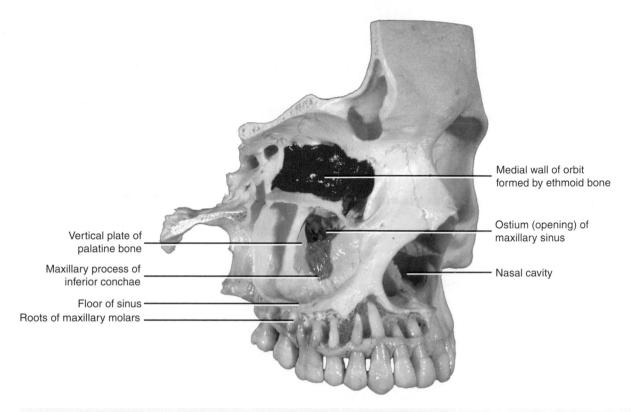

Medial wall of orbit formed by ethmoid bone

Ostium (opening) of maxillary sinus

Nasal cavity

Vertical plate of palatine bone

Maxillary process of inferior conchae

Floor of sinus

Roots of maxillary molars

Figure 7-69 The right maxillary sinus with its lateral wall removed. Note relationship of the sinus to the orbit and relationship of the sinus to the maxillary teeth.

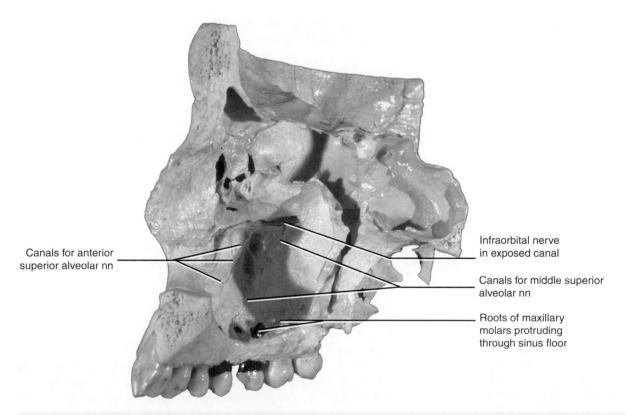

Canals for anterior superior alveolar nn

Infraorbital nerve in exposed canal

Canals for middle superior alveolar nn

Roots of maxillary molars protruding through sinus floor

Figure 7-70 The right maxillary sinus with its medial (nasal) wall removed to reveal internal features. Note root apices of the maxillary molars, in this case, protruding through the floor of the sinus.

2. **Medial**: The nasal cavity lies medial to the maxillary sinuses, which drain medially via small openings, or ostia, into the middle meatus.
3. **Inferior**: The alveolar process and maxillary tooth roots lie immediately below the maxillary sinuses; moving from distal to mesial in the maxillary dental arch, the molar tooth roots are in proximity to the sinus, the premolar teeth less so, and the anterior roots are generally far removed from the maxillary sinus.

Nerve and Blood Supply. The superior alveolar (anterior, middle, and posterior) nerves, branches of the maxillary nerve, supply the maxillary sinus. The blood supply arises as superior alveolar branches of the maxillary artery (part 3). In addition, branches of the greater palatine artery contribute somewhat to the floor of the sinus. Venous drainage is to the pterygoid plexus of veins.

Drainage of Secretions. The maxillary sinus drains to the middle meatus of the nose through its ostium, which passes medially to the inferior aspect of the hiatus semilunaris. The opening may be large or small and is sometimes chronically blocked. The opening is also placed rather high on the medial wall. Occasionally, an accessory opening is found inferiorly and posteriorly to the main opening. Normal amounts of secretion are moved from the sinus by a spiral pattern of beating cilia centered around the ostium.

Variations in Size and Shape. The maxillary sinus in the adult can vary greatly in size and shape. *Figure 7-71* illustrates a small maxillary sinus in which the molar roots are

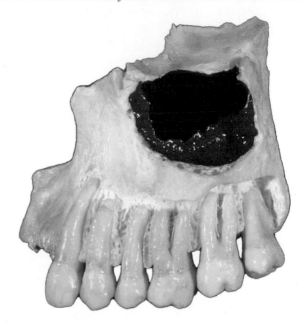

Figure 7-71 Small left maxillary sinus viewed from lateral aspect. Roots of the molars are remote from the sinus floor. Compare with Figure 7-70.

CLINICAL NOTES

Maxillary Sinusitis

Abnormal amounts of secretion fill the lumen of the sinus to the high level of the ostium before mechanical drainage is affected. Obstructed openings can lead to secondary infections and a painful inflammation of the mucosal lining (sinusitis). The condition is treatable with antibiotics, but chronic obstruction may require creating an artificial opening through the lateral wall of the inferior meatus.

The maxillary sinuses can be transilluminated in a dark room. A penlight is placed under the palate under the sinuses. If one side is infected, it does not transilluminate as well as the noninfected side.

Referred Pain

Toothache in the maxillary arch is occasionally caused by referred pain from an infected sinus. Because the maxillary teeth roots lie in proximity to the sinus floor, and because the teeth and the maxillary sinus share a common nerve supply, sinusitis may manifest as a generalized ache arising from the teeth. The sensitivity of the teeth is in direct relationship to the distances of the roots from the sinus floor. Therefore, on percussion (tapping with an instrument), the posterior teeth are more sensitive and the anterior teeth are less sensitive.

Oral Surgery

The proximity of the maxillary molar teeth to the sinus floor may pose a number of problems to the dentist. Surgical removal of maxillary molar teeth can, occasionally, result in fracture of one of the three diverging roots, usually the most divergent—the palatal root. Improper retrieval attempts can drive the pointed, bullet-shaped root fragment upward into the maxillary sinus. This may create two problems: (1) creation of a communication between the oral cavity and the maxillary sinus (**oral-antral fistula**) that hampers normal attempts to create a nasal-oral seal during blowing and sucking functions; and (2) introduction of oral bacteria to the maxillary sinus, creating an infection of the sinus (sinusitis).

The root fragment may be removed by making a window in the floor of the sinus, but the deficiency must be properly sealed and allowed to heal. Antibiotics are generally prescribed to prevent infection, and patients are instructed not to blow their noses or suck through straws following such a procedure until healing occurs.

far removed from the floor of the sinus. *Figure 7-72* shows an edentulous maxilla in which the sinus is large, extending well down into the alveolar ridge.

The Ethmoidal Sinuses. The ethmoidal sinuses lie within the labyrinths of the ethmoid bone (*Figures 7-73* and *7-74*). Extremely thin septa of bone covered with mucosa form a variable number of incomplete interconnecting compartments that ultimately drain medially to the lateral wall of the nose. The number of compartments varies from about 18 small ones to 3 or so large ones.

The ethmoid cells encroach on the frontal sinus anteriorly and the sphenoidal sinus posteriorly. Laterally, only a thin plate of bone separates the ethmoid sinuses and the orbits.

Nerve and Blood Supply. The anterior and posterior ethmoidal branches of the nasociliary nerve supply the ethmoidal sinuses. The nasociliary nerve, in turn, is a branch of the ophthalmic nerve (cranial nerve V-1). The anterior and posterior ethmoidal branches of the ophthalmic artery provide the blood supply to the ethmoidal sinuses.

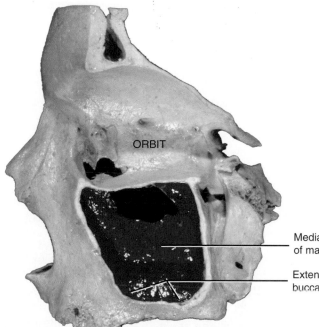

ORBIT

Medial wall of maxillary sinus

Extension of sinus into buccal alveolar ridge

Figure 7-72 Left, edentulous maxilla viewed from the lateral aspect. Sinus floor extends down into the alveolar ridges.

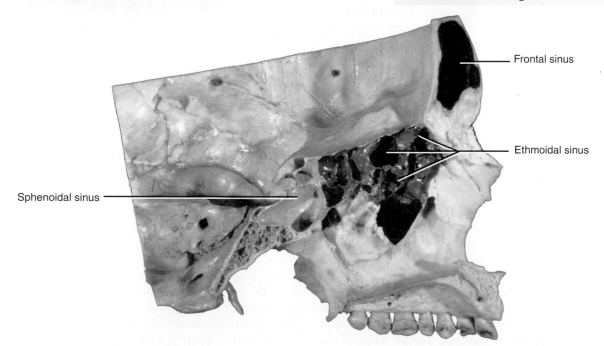

Frontal sinus

Ethmoidal sinus

Sphenoidal sinus

Figure 7-73 Sagittal section through the skull to show frontal, ethmoidal, and sphenoidal air sinuses.

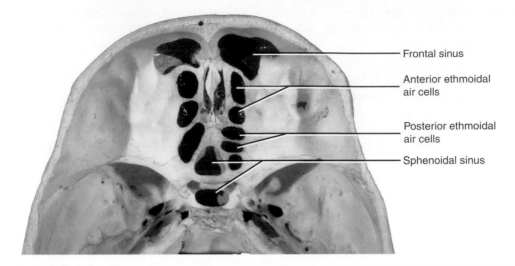

Frontal sinus

Anterior ethmoidal
air cells

Posterior ethmoidal
air cells

Sphenoidal sinus

Figure 7-74 Portions of the anterior and middle cranial fossae have been dissected away to display a superior view of the frontal, ethmoidal, and sphenoidal air sinuses.

Drainage. The anterior ethmoidal air cells open directly to the middle meatus or indirectly via the frontal infundibulum. The posterior ethmoidal air cells open directly to the superior meatus.

The Frontal Sinuses. The frontal sinuses lie behind the superciliary arches of the frontal bone, fanning up into the squama and posteriorly into the orbital plates (see *Figures 7-68, 7-69,* and *7-74*). They are relatively large in the male, smaller in the female, and rudimentary in the child. A septum divides the sinuses into right and left, usually asymmetrical portions. Smaller, incomplete septa may divide each chamber into smaller but interconnecting subchambers.

Nerve and Blood Supply. The nerve supply is from branches of the supraorbital nerve, itself a branch of the ophthalmic nerve (cranial nerve V-1).

Drainage. Each frontal sinus drains downward through a funnel-like infundibulum that eventually opens into the upper end of the hiatus semilunaris of the middle meatus of the nose.

The Sphenoidal Air Sinuses. The sphenoidal sinuses lie within the body of the sphenoid bone (see *Figures 7-73* and *7-74*). They are variable in size, extending from the ethmoidal air sinuses anteriorly to almost the occipital bone posteriorly. The body of the sphenoid bone is actually a fragile, hollow cube. Only thin plates of bone separate the sinuses within from vital structures: (1) anteriorly lies the optic chiasma; (2) superiorly is the hypophyseal fossa containing the hypophysis cerebri; and (3) laterally lie the internal carotid arteries within the cavernous venous sinuses (see *Figure 7-27*).

CLINICAL NOTES

Orbital Infection

If the nasal drainage is blocked, infections of the ethmoidal cells may break through the fragile medial orbital wall to the orbital contents, producing an orbital cellulitis. Severe infections of this nature may lead to blindness. Some posterior cells lie in proximity to the optic nerve canal, and spread of infection may involve the optic nerve.

Nerve and Blood Supply. The posterior ethmoidal nerve and artery and superior pharyngeal nerve and artery supply the sphenoidal air sinuses.

Drainage. The sphenoidal sinuses drain through their respective ostia in the anterior wall of the body of sphenoid to the sphenoethmoidal recess of the nasal cavity.

8. The Oral Cavity

The mouth, or oral cavity, is associated with many pleasurable functions, but the most basic are eating and drinking. The mouth is the gateway to the gastrointestinal system, and it is in the mouth that food and drink are initially tasted and savored. Food is mixed with saliva, masticated, and, if deemed palatable, voluntarily swallowed. Subsequent processing and movement of food through the remainder of the gut are automatic.

The tissues of the oral cavity are, unfortunately, subject to various disease conditions, and so widespread are these diseases that a separate health profession, dentistry, has evolved, which is devoted primarily to the care and preservation of the oral tissues.

SKELETON

Review the features of the maxillae, palatine bones, mandible, and hyoid bone.

BOUNDARIES AND RELATIONSHIPS

The oral cavity consists of two areas (see *Figures 7-61* and *7-62*). The **vestibule** is the space between the teeth and the inner mucosal lining of the lips and cheeks. The **oral cavity proper** is the space contained within the upper and lower dental arches.

Anterior and Lateral. The anterior and lateral boundaries of the vestibule are the intraoral surfaces of the lips and cheeks. The mouth aperture is controlled by the circumoral facial muscles.

The anterior and lateral boundaries of the oral cavity proper are the lingual surfaces of the teeth and corresponding alveolar processes. The opening to the oral cavity proper is guarded by the teeth, and this opening is controlled by the muscles of mastication.

With the teeth clenched, the only communication between the vestibule and the oral cavity proper is a common open area posteriorly between the last molars and the anterior border of the ramus of the mandible.

Posterior. Posteriorly, the oral cavity communicates with the pharynx through the oropharyngeal isthmus. The isthmus may be opened or sealed by the musculature of

---

CLINICAL NOTES

Oral Infections and Cancer (Oral Medicine and Pathology)

Various systemic diseases may manifest as some lesion of the oral cavity. A physical examination by the physician always includes an inspection of the oral cavity to spot any telltale sign of a systemic disease in the mouth. The dentist, in addition, performs a detailed intraoral visual and radiographic inspection, and patients with suspected systemic disorders are referred to the medical practitioner. Localized sores and infections are treated in the dental office.

Oral cancer is largely screened during routine dental examinations. Cancerous or precancerous conditions are suspected when lesions do not heal within 2 weeks, and subsequent diagnosis is based on examination of a tissue smear or biopsy specimen.

Dental Caries (Restorative Dentistry)

Decay of the dental hard tissues is an almost universal affliction. Treatment consists of removal of the decay, followed by restoration of the anatomy of the tooth with a suitable material.

Pulpitis and Tooth Abscess (Endodontics)

Neglected caries, over time, invades and inflames the pulpal tissues. An infective process is set up that spreads through the root canals to the supporting alveolar bone, producing an abscess. The condition may be treated by gaining access to the pulpal cavity and root canals, cleansing and enlarging them, then filling them to seal the root apex foramina to prevent further infection.

Tooth Removal (Oral Surgery)

Occasionally it is not practical to perform endodontics because of economic circumstances or extreme tooth destruction. The only alternative is removal of the infected tooth.

Unerupted third molars pose another fairly common problem. They are the last teeth to erupt in the dental arches, and often there is not enough room for them. They become lodged (impacted) under the distal aspect of the second molar and should be removed.

Periodontal Disease (Periodontics)

Improper oral hygiene and neglect result in gingivitis or inflammation of the gums. If left unchecked, the disease spreads to the other supporting structures and alveolar bone, causing *periodontitis* (inflammation and destruction of the periodontal ligament and alveolar bone). Total neglect over a variable period results in increasing mobility and eventual loss of the teeth.

Treatment involves thorough scaling and polishing of the teeth, possible surgery and removal of diseased tissues, and instructions in proper home care.

Restoration of Missing Teeth (Prosthodontics)

Missing teeth may be replaced by removable or fixed bridgework. Loss of the entire dentition is treated by fabrication of a full denture. Dental implants may be inserted to replace individual teeth or to serve as abutments for fixed or removable bridgework.

Malocclusion (Orthodontics)

Malocclusion, or improper bite, may manifest itself in the developing child for a variety of reasons: (1) the unfortunate inheritance of large teeth from one parent and small jaws from the other; (2) retained infantile oral habits, such as thumb sucking and tongue thrusting during swallowing; (3) chronic mouth breathing caused by nasal obstruction; and (4) premature loss of deciduous molars, which hold the space for succeeding premolar teeth. Malposed teeth can be treated by applying orthodontic forces to move the teeth through alveolar bone to new positions.

Improper Jaw Relationships (Orthodontics/Oral Surgery)

Some malocclusions are a result of improper jaw relationships, for example, a large upper jaw in relation to the lower jaw (weak chin) or large lower jaw in relation to the upper jaw (prominent chin). Mild cases are treated orthodontically. Severe adult cases are treated with a combination of maxillofacial surgery to realign the jaws and postsurgical orthodontic treatment to effect a fine realignment of the teeth.

---

the tongue and the soft palate. The posterior limit of the oral cavity is the palatoglossal arch.

Superior. The roof of the oral cavity is the hard palate, which partitions the oral cavity from the nasal cavity above.

Inferior. Inferiorly, the mylohyoid muscle forms a muscular diaphragm that supports the tongue and structures of the floor of the mouth.

VISUAL INSPECTION OF THE ORAL CAVITY

The topography of the oral cavity is obviously important to the dental student (*Figure 7-75*). Because the oral cavity is so readily accessible, it is advantageous, at this point, to examine it in the living person prior to embarking on the standard anatomical descriptions. This is accomplished by examining one's own mouth in a mirror or, better still, by examining the mouth of a partner. The clinic is the ideal place to do this; however, a flashlight and a tongue depressor in the laboratory setting are adequate for intraoral inspection.

The Lips and Cheeks

Examine the lips and cheeks and review their structures in section 1 of this chapter. Note the skin of the external aspect of the **lip** and the **vermilion border** that marks the abrupt beginning of the transition zone. Here the skin is so thin that it imparts the underlying color of the blood vessels. The transition zone gives way intraorally to mucous membrane. Look for and feel the mucous labial and molar glands, which lie below the thin mucosa. Grasp the upper or lower lip between the thumb and forefinger to feel the pulsations of the labial branches of the facial artery.

The Vestibule and Gingivae

Vestibular Fold. The mucous membrane of the lip reflects back onto the alveolar bone as alveolar mucosa (*Figure 7-76*). This reflection is termed the *vestibular fold.*

Anteriorly, it is generally referred to as the *mucolabial fold;* posteriorly, it is referred to as the *mucobuccal fold.*

Alveolar Mucosa. Note the color and texture of the alveolar mucosa. It is thin, red, and loosely bound to the underlying alveolar bone.

Gingivae. As the alveolar mucosa approaches the necks of the teeth, it changes in color and texture to become true, attached gingivae, or gums. In the healthy individual, gingivae are pink and stippled in contrast to the red, shiny alveolar mucosa. They are also firmly attached to the necks of the teeth and the alveolar crests. Interdentally, the gingivae appear as firm, pointed projections.

Labial Frenula. Look for the frenula of the upper and lower lips. These are free-edged folds of mucous membrane, which run in the median plane from the inner aspect of the lip to the vestibular gingiva between the central incisors. Overly large frenula can cause a space between the central incisors. Large lower frenula may tug on the labial gingiva and cause eventual gingival recession. Occasionally, smaller frenula appear in the premolar vestibular regions.

Other Vestibular Features. In the lower vestibule, palpate the **external oblique ridge** of the mandible deep to the vestibular mucous membrane. Follow the ridge back and up as it becomes the anterior border of the ramus. Your finger is now in the **coronoid notch**. Slide the finger slightly medially to engage the **internal oblique crest,** or **temporal crest**. Your finger now resides in the **retromolar fossa** and marks the injection site for local anesthesia of the inferior alveolar nerve. The soft tissue overlying this fossa is the retromolar pad.

In the upper vestibule, palpate the inferior border of the zygomatic arch. By alternately clenching and unclenching the teeth, the anterior border of masseter muscle becomes

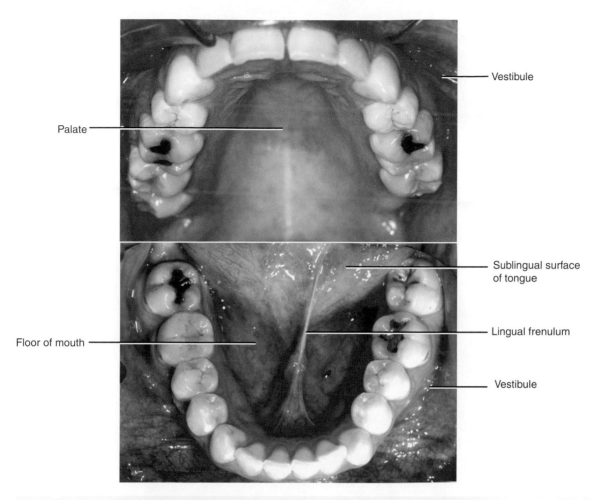

Palate

Vestibule

Sublingual surface
of tongue

Lingual frenulum

Floor of mouth

Vestibule

Figure 7-75 Features of the oral cavity.

apparent. With the subject's mouth half open, palpate the **zygomatic process of the maxilla**. This marks the injection landmark for anesthesia of the posterior superior alveolar nerve. Note that when the subject is asked to open wide, the palpating finger is displaced by the coronoid process of the mandible and the attached temporalis tendon.

On the buccal mucosa of the cheek, look for a papilla opposite the crown of the second maxillary molar. Opening from the papilla into the vestibule is the **orifice of the parotid duct** (*Figure 7-77*).

The Oral Cavity Proper and the Teeth

Examine the teeth of the maxillary and mandibular arches. The complete human adult dentition contains 32 *teeth*; the child's dentition contains 20 *deciduous teeth*. By convention, the teeth are divided into four quadrants, and each quadrant is assigned a number (*Figure 7-78*): The upper right quadrant; upper left quadrant; lower left quadrant; and lower right quadrant are assigned numbers 1, 2, 3, and 4, respectively.

CLINICAL NOTES

Teeth may be missing for a variety of reasons.

Failure to Develop

Commonly, upper or lower or both sets of third molars fail to develop; less commonly, lateral incisors, canines, or premolars fail to develop. Adult retention of a deciduous tooth is generally a clue.

Impaction

The tooth may have developed but failed to erupt for lack of space. This occurs commonly with third molars and less commonly with premolars and canines.

Previous Extractions

More often than not, missing teeth are due to extractions at a previous visit.

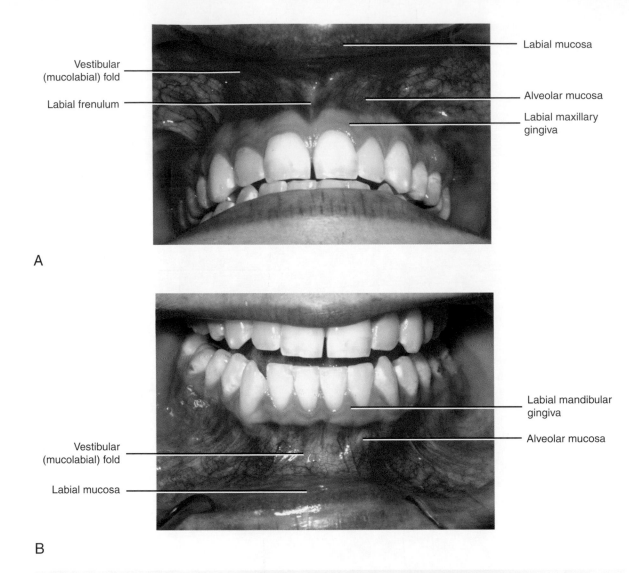

Labial mucosa

Vestibular (mucolabial) fold

Labial frenulum

Alveolar mucosa

Labial maxillary gingiva

A

Labial mandibular gingiva

Alveolar mucosa

Vestibular (mucolabial) fold

Labial mucosa

B

Figure 7-76 Vestibule and vestibular gingivae of the oral the cavity. **A,** Maxilla. **B,** Mandible.

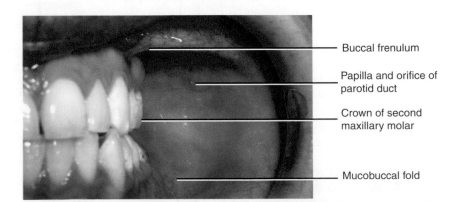

Buccal frenulum

Papilla and orifice of parotid duct

Crown of second maxillary molar

Mucobuccal fold

Figure 7-77 Buccal vestibule and mucosa of the cheek. Opening of the parotid duct is seen opposite the second maxillary molar.

The teeth in each quadrant are numbered from 1 to 8: 1—central incisor; 2—lateral incisor; 3—canine; 4—first premolar; 5—second premolar; 6—first molar; 7—second molar; and 8—third molar. Thus, the symbol for the lower right first molar is 4.6 (4 for lower right quadrant, 6 for first molar).

In the deciduous arch, the quadrants are numbered from 5 to 8: 5—upper right quadrant; 6—upper left quadrant; 7—lower left quadrant; and 8—lower right quadrant. The deciduous teeth are numbered from 1 to 5: 1—central incisor; 2—lateral incisor; 3—canine; 4—first molar;

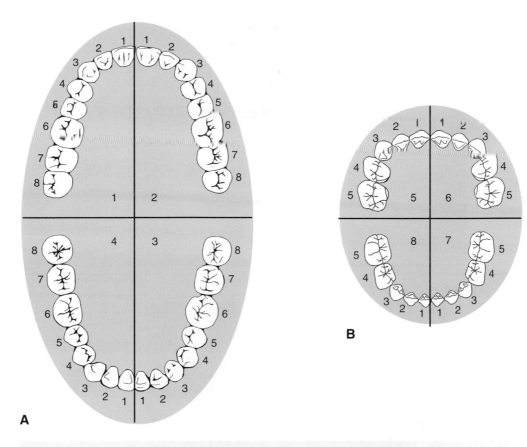

Figure 7-78 Numerical symbols for the dentition and quadrants. **A,** Adult. **B,** Child.

and 5—second molar. The symbol for the lower right first deciduous molar is 8.4 (the 8 represents the lower right deciduous quadrant, and the 4 indicates the first deciduous molar).

Count the number of teeth present, and note any missing teeth.

The Hard and Soft Palates

Note the mucosa of the hard palate. It is tightly bound to the underlying bone, and, therefore, submucous injections into the palatal area are extremely painful. The lingual or palatal gingiva of the maxillary arch is continuous with the mucosa of the palate (*Figure 7-79*).

Behind the maxillary central incisors, look for the **incisive papilla,** an elevation directly anterior to the underlying incisive foramen. This marks the site of injection for anesthesia of the nasopalatine nerve. Radiating laterally from the incisive papilla are six or so parallel transverse ridges, or **palatal rugae.** These aid in manipulating food during mastication. Running posteriorly from the incisive papilla is the midline **palatal raphé.** Numerous minor glands open onto the palatal mucosa as small pits.

The soft palate is the movable posterior third of the palate. It possesses no bony skeleton and hangs like a limp trap door into the pharynx behind. It ends posteriorly as a free edge with a midline pendulous projection, the **uvula.**

The soft palate is supported posteriorly by two arches (the fauces). The **anterior arch** runs from the soft palate down to the lateral aspects of the tongue as the *palatoglossal arch*. The **posterior arch** is the free posterior border of the soft palate, which continues laterally to blend with the lateral wall of the pharynx as the *palatopharyngeal arch*.

The **palatine tonsils** are rounded masses of lymphoid tissue occupying the triangular intervals between the anterior and posterior pillars. The oral surface of the tonsil is pitted with blind-ended *tonsillar crypts*. The palatine tonsils are large during childhood and begin to atrophy greatly with the onset of puberty. Inflammation of the tonsils (tonsillitis) causes hypertrophy, and extremely large tonsils may meet in the midline. Chronic inflammation generally calls for removal of the tonsils (tonsillectomy).

Palpate the maxillary tubercle behind the last molar tooth, and then slide the finger medially onto the palate to engage the hamulus of the medial pterygoid plate. Just anterior to the anterior arch, feel for the anterior border of the medial pterygoid muscle.

The Tongue. Inspect the pinkish upper surface (dorsum) of the tongue, and note that it is covered with small papillae of various shapes and colors (*Figure 7-80*). The *anterior two thirds* of the tongue resides in the oral cavity; the *posterior third* is vertical and extends down into the

313

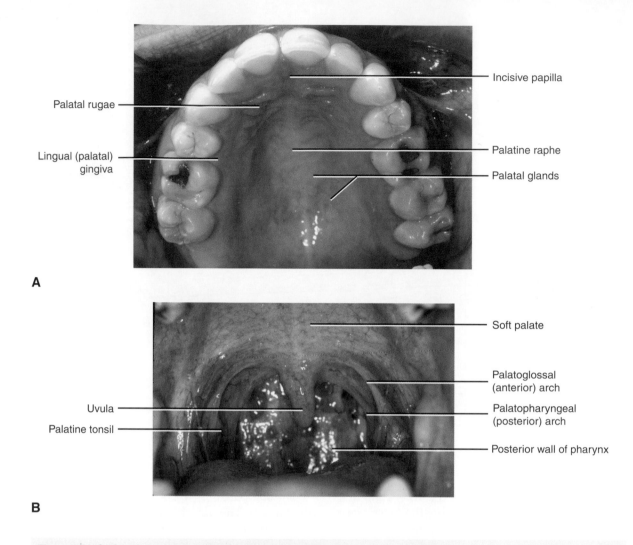

Palatal rugae

Lingual (palatal) gingiva

Incisive papilla

Palatine raphe

Palatal glands

A

Soft palate

Palatoglossal (anterior) arch

Uvula

Palatine tonsil

Palatopharyngeal (posterior) arch

Posterior wall of pharynx

B

Figure 7-79 Surface features of the hard (**A**) and soft (**B**) palates.

pharynx. Note the *median sulcus* of the tongue running posteriorly from the tip.

Have your subject raise the tongue while you inspect its inferior (sublingual) surface. The mucosa here is thin, smooth, shiny, and transparent, disclosing hundreds of small blood vessels. The **lingual frenulum** is a midline fold of mucous membrane running from the lingual gingiva behind the mandibular central incisors posteriorly to the undersurface of the tongue.

Look for two small **papillae** on either side of the lingual frenulum just behind the central incisors. Opening through the papillae into the mouth are the **openings of the submandibular ducts**. Two smaller, rudimentary *fimbriated folds* parallel the midline lingual frenulum on either side.

Examine now the thin mucosa overlying the floor of the mouth below the tongue. Running posteriorly and laterally in a horseshoe shape from the submandibular

papillae is the **sublingual ridge** produced by the underlying sublingual salivary glands.

Finally, palpate the lingual mucosa overlying the root of the mandibular third molar and try to roll the lingual nerve below the mucosa.

9. Structures and Areas of the Oral Cavity

HARD PALATE

The palate, or roof of the mouth, separates the nasal cavity above from the oral cavity below. The superior (nasal) surface, therefore, is covered with *respiratory mucosa*, and the inferior (oral) surface is covered with *oral mucosa*. The superficial features of the palate were discussed under inspection of the oral cavity.

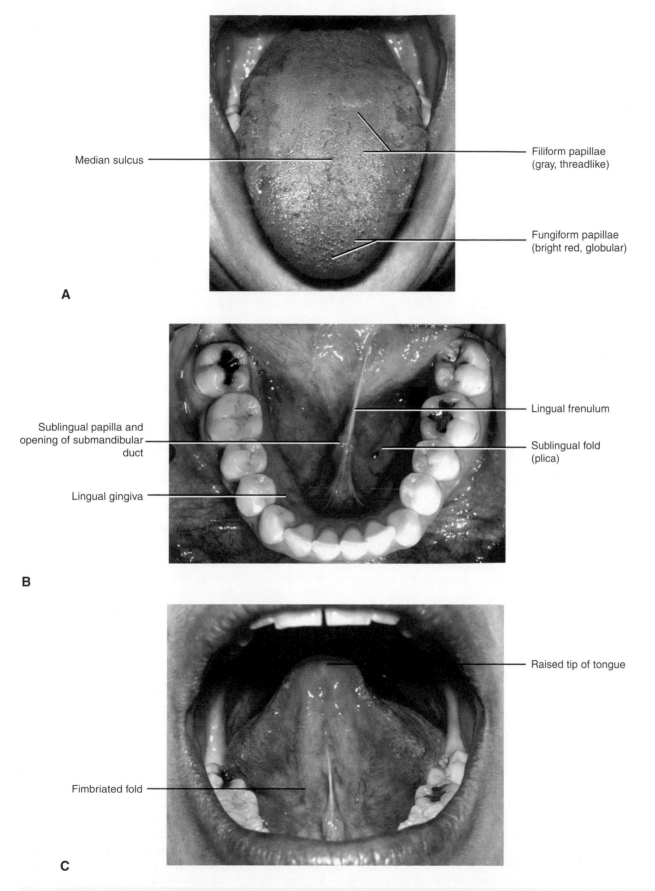

Median sulcus

Filiform papillae
(gray, threadlike)

Fungiform papillae
(bright red, globular)

A

Sublingual papilla and
opening of submandibular
duct

Lingual gingiva

Lingual frenulum

Sublingual fold
(plica)

B

Raised tip of tongue

Fimbriated fold

C

Figure 7-80 Surface features of the tongue. **A,** Dorsum of tongue. Note roughened appearance due to papillae. **B,** Floor of the mouth. Note thin mucosa and numerous underlying blood vessels. **C,** Sublingual aspect of the tongue.

Skeleton

The **palatal processes of the right and left maxillae** form the anterior two thirds of the skeleton of the hard palate; the **palatal processes of the right and left palatine bones** form the posterior third of the skeleton of the hard palate (see *Figure 6-8*).

Three foramina open onto the oral aspect of the hard palate: (1) the **incisive foramen** opens distally to the maxillary central incisors in the midline and transmits the nasopalatine vessels and nerves; (2) the **greater palatine foramen** opens medially to the roots of the third molar and transmits the greater palatine vessels and nerve; (3) the **lesser palatine foramen** opens posteriorly to the greater palatine foramen and medially to the maxillary tuberosity and transmits the lesser palatine vessels and nerve.

The hard palate is concave, or vaulted, and this space is normally filled by the dorsum of the tongue at rest.

Palatal Gingiva and Mucosa

The mucous membrane and submucosa of the hard palate line the concavity or vault of the hard palate. A thin strip of peripheral mucosa adjacent to the lingual aspects of the maxillary teeth is closely and firmly applied to the underlying alveolar bone. This strip is the **palatal gingiva,** and it is continuous with the vestibular gingiva through interdental papillae that pass between the teeth. In the healthy individual, the lingual gingiva, interdental papillae, and the vestibular gingiva form a tight cuff around the teeth.

The palatal gingiva is continuous with the mucosa of the palate, but the palatal mucosa is thicker and spongier. Unlike the gingival area, there is a distinct differentiation between the lamina propria of the mucosal layer, submucosa, and the periosteum. Strong bands of connective tissue bind the palatine mucosa to the periosteum of the hard palate. Packed among the anchoring strands of connective tissue are **palatal mucous glands** and fat globules. The glands are larger and more numerous in the posterior parts of the palate. The mucosa of the hard palate is continuous with the mucosa of the soft palate posteriorly.

SOFT PALATE

The soft palate contains no bony framework but instead contains a membranous aponeurosis. At rest, it hangs from the posterior aspect of the hard palate into the cavity of the pharynx. It separates the nasopharynx above from the oropharynx below and is actually a component of the pharynx.

The structures of the soft palate are (1) a mucosal lining (nasal mucosa superiorly, oral mucosa inferiorly); (2) palatal mucous glands below the mucosa; (3) a membranous palatine aponeurosis; and (4) five paired skeletal muscles, which attach to the aponeurosis.

Muscles

Palatopharyngeus. This muscle originates from the palatine aponeurosis and runs posteriorly and downward to insert into the lateral wall of the pharynx (*Figure 7-81* and *Table 7-4*). It is covered by a layer of mucous membrane and thus forms the posterior pillar, or palatopharyngeal arch.

The muscle fibers contract to help approximate the tongue and soft palate, and this action *seals the oropharyngeal isthmus* or closes the oral cavity from the oropharynx.

Palatoglossus. The palatoglossus muscle originates from the palatine aponeurosis and passes laterally and downward to insert into the side of the tongue. It, too, is covered with mucous membrane and outwardly forms the anterior pillar, or palatoglossal arch. The muscle acts in concert with the palatopharyngeus muscle to *close the oropharyngeal isthmus* by approximating the tongue and soft palate.

Levator Veli Palatini. The levator veli palatini muscle originates from the medial aspect and floor of the auditory tube at the base of the skull. It passes downward, forward, and medially as a thick band of fibers to insert directly to the palatine aponeurosis. It acts to elevate the soft palate to *seal the nasopharynx from the oropharynx.*

Tensor Veli Palatini. The tensor veli palatini muscle originates from the lateral aspect of the auditory tube (from the bony gutter and membrane of the tube) and the scaphoid fossa. The fibers form as a fan-shaped belly and pass downward along the medial aspect of the medial pterygoid plate. The fibers converge as a tendon as they approach the hamulus, and the tendon hooks over the hamulus. The tendon spreads out into the broad membranous palatine aponeurosis, blending with the aponeurosis of the opposite muscle.

Using the hamulus as a pulley, the muscle fibers contract to *tense the soft palate.* At the same time, they pull open the membranous portion of the normally collapsed auditory tube at the origin of the muscle.

Uvular Muscle. The uvular muscle is a paired muscle that arises from the posterior nasal spine and travels posteriorly on either side of the midline to insert into the submucosa of the uvula. Contraction of the muscle fibers *shortens the uvula and pulls it upward* to help seal the nasopharynx.

Nerve Supply of the Palatal Muscles. All the palatal muscles except for the tensor veli palatini muscle receive a motor supply from the **cranial accessory nerve (cranial nerve XI)** traveling with the **vagus nerve (cranial nerve X).** The tensor veli palatini muscle is supplied by motor branches of the mandibular nerve (cranial nerve V-3).

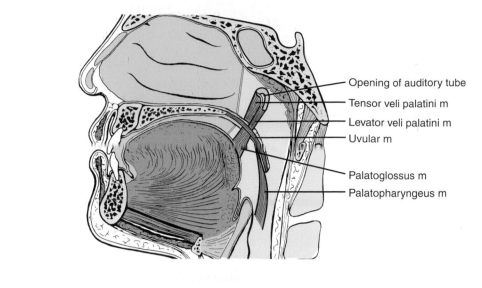

A

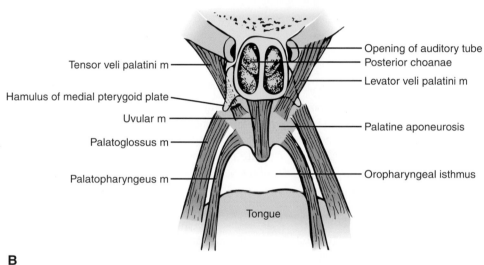

B

Figure 7-81 Muscles of the soft palate. **A,** Lateral aspect. **B,** Posterior aspect. The left veli palatini muscle has been cut to reveal tensor veli palatini muscle.

Functions. The soft palate performs two functions:

1. **Closure of the oropharyngeal isthmus:** The palatopharyngeus and palatoglossal muscles approximate the dorsum of the tongue and the soft palate, thus sealing the oral cavity from the oropharynx behind. This occurs automatically during the act of **sucking.** Sealing of the oropharyngeal isthmus still allows the infant to breathe through the nose while suckling. Test this by placing a finger in the mouth, sucking on it, and breathing through the nose.

2. **Closure of the oropharynx from the nasopharynx:** The levator veli palatini, tensor veli palatini, and uvular muscles contract to raise the soft palate and seal it like a trap door against the posterior pharyngeal wall. This occurs during the act of **swallowing,** thus preventing food from being pushed up to the nasopharynx and nasal cavity. Laughing during the swallowing of a liquid relaxes the soft palate at the wrong time, allowing liquids to be forced upward through the nasal cavity and out the external nares.

Sensory Nerve and Blood Supply to the Entire Palate

Sensory Nerves. The nerve supply is basically from the pterygopalatine ganglion associated with the maxillary nerve (cranial nerve V-2), and these structures should be reviewed.

Nasopalatine Nerve. The nasopalatine nerve arises from the pterygopalatine ganglion and passes to the nasal cavity, which it helps supply. It travels downward and forward along

317

TABLE 7-4

Muscles of the Soft Palate

Muscle	Origin	Insertion	Action	Cranial Nerve
Palatopharyngeus	Palatal aponeurosis	Lateral wall of pharynx and posterior border of thyroid cartilage	Elevates pharynx and larynx Closes oropharyngeal isthmus	XI via X
Palatoglossus	Palatal aponeurosis	Dorsum and lateral aspect of tongue	Closes oropharyngeal isthmus	XI via X
Levator veli palatini	Medial aspect of auditory tube Medial aspect of bony gutter on inferior aspect of petrous temporal bone	Directly into palatine aponeurosis	Elevates palate during swallowing, yawning	XI via X
Tensor veli palatini	Lateral aspect of membranous portion of auditory tube, scaphoid fossa sphenoid bone	Tendon hooks under hamulus and inserts into palatine aponeurosis	Tenses palate and opens mouth of auditory tube during swallowing and yawning	V-3
Uvular	Posterior nasal spine	Uvula	Raises uvula to help seal oral from nasal pharynx	XI via X

the vomer and leaves the nasal cavity by dropping through the incisive foramen. It appears on the oral surface and travels through the submucosa to supply lingual gingiva and palatal mucosa anterior to the maxillary canines (*Figure 7-82*).

Greater Palatine Nerve. This nerve arises from the pterygopalatine ganglion and drops inferiorly through the greater palatine canal to surface on the oral aspect of the palate medial to the second molar tooth. The nerve passes anteriorly through the submucosa to supply lingual gingiva and palatal mucosa from the maxillary canines posteriorly.

Lesser Palatine Nerve. The lesser palatine nerve arises from the pterygopalatine ganglion and drops inferiorly through the lesser palatine canal to emerge on the oral aspect of the palate posterior to the greater foramen. The nerve turns posteriorly through the submucosa to supply the soft palate mucosa.

Arteries. The arterial supply arises from part 3 of the maxillary artery and closely parallels the nerve supply (see *Figure 7-55*).

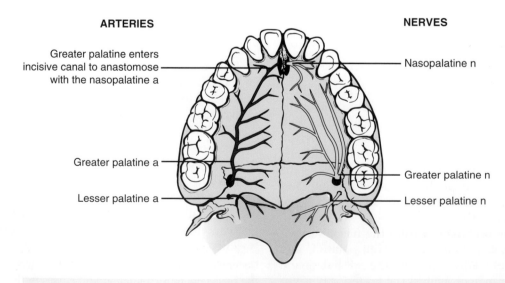

ARTERIES

Greater palatine enters incisive canal to anastomose with the nasopalatine a

Greater palatine a

Lesser palatine a

NERVES

Nasopalatine n

Greater palatine n

Lesser palatine n

Figure 7-82 Blood and sensory nerve supply to the hard and soft palates.

Greater Palatine Artery. The **descending palatine artery** arises from part 3 of the maxillary artery and descends in the pterygopalatine fossa. The artery divides into two branches that enter the greater and lesser palatine canals. The **greater palatine artery** enters the greater palatine canal and descends through it to pass on to the palate through the greater palatine foramen. The artery passes anteriorly and anastomoses with the septal branch of the sphenopalatine artery.

CLINICAL NOTES

Cleft Lip and Palate

A cleft palate results in a communication between the oral cavity below and the nasal cavity above; cleft palate interferes with sucking and swallowing in the newborn. A removable palatal appliance (obturator) is fitted to seal the cleft. Corrective surgery can permanently close the defect. There are two types of clefts.

Clefts of the anterior or **primary palate** occur when the maxillary prominence fails to unite with the merged medial nasal prominences during development. The severity of the cleft can range from a hardly noticeable notching of the vermilion border of the lip to a complete cleft through the lip and alveolar process. The cleft may be unilateral or bilateral.

Cleft of the posterior or **secondary palate** occurs when the lateral palatine processes fail to fuse together in the midline and fail to fuse with the nasal septum above. The defect may range from a mild bifid uvula to a wide separation between the palatal shelves.

Torus Palatinus

A torus is a benign lump of bone, or exostosis, that can develop below the mucosa on the roof of the mouth or palate. Tori are generally not a problem unless they are very large. They sometimes interfere with the fabrication of a full upper or removable partial denture.

Lesser Palatine Artery. The **descending palatine artery** also gives rise to the **lesser palatine artery**, which descends through the lesser palatine canal and exits onto the palate through the lesser palatine foramen. The artery passes posteriorly to supply the soft palate.

Ascending Palatine Artery. The soft palate also receives some supply from the ascending palatine branch of the **facial artery**.

THE TONGUE

The tongue can be likened to a mucous membrane bag stuffed with muscles (see *Figure 7-80*). It has a fixed base, or root, and a mobile body and tip that can take on a variety of shapes and positions. At rest, the tongue occupies most of the oral cavity.

The tongue is an important organ, responsible for a number of functions: (1) speech, (2) manipulation and positioning of food (the antagonist of the orbicularis oris and buccinator muscles), (3) tasting, (4) swallowing, and (5) cleansing of the oral cavity. (Following a meal, the tongue darts from crevice to crevice, seeking out and retrieving bits of retained food in the oral cavity.)

Parts and Surfaces of the Tongue (*Figure 7-83*)

1. The **body** of the tongue is the anterior two thirds of the tongue, found in the oral cavity.
2. The **root** of the tongue is the posterior third that turns vertically downward to reside in the pharynx.
3. The **sulcus terminalis** is a V-shaped groove, the apex of which points posteriorly in the midline; it divides the tongue into the anterior two thirds and posterior third.
4. The **foramen cecum** is a small pit at the apex of the sulcus terminalis and is a vestige of the proximal end of the thyroglossal duct (see *Figure 5-23*).
5. The **dorsum** is the superior and posterior roughened aspects of the tongue.
6. The **sublingual surface** of the tongue is covered with thin, transparent mucosa through which one can see many underlying vessels.
7. The **lingual frenulum** is a thin fold of mucous membrane that extends from the floor of the mouth, immediately posterior to the mandibular central incisors in the midline, to the inferior surface of the tongue.

Mucosa of the Dorsum of the Tongue

Anterior Two Thirds. The anterior two thirds of the tongue is covered superiorly with velvety papillae. There are four varieties of papillae.

1. **Filiform papillae** are the most numerous. They are pinkish gray in color and project as tapering, threadlike points. They are arranged in V-shaped rows paralleling the sulcus terminalis. The filiform papillae impart a rough texture to the dorsum of the tongue, which aids in handling foods. In addition, they contain sensory nerve endings—touch corpuscles that are highly sensitive. Because of its mobility and high degree of sensitivity, the tongue can efficiently seek out foreign particles in the mouth.
2. **Fungiform papillae** are scattered among the filiform papillae like rubies in the sand. They are globular and bright red in color. They are found mainly at the tip and lateral margins of the tongue.

3. **Vallate papillae** are circular and large (about 2 mm in diameter). About 12 of them are placed in a V-shaped row anterior and parallel to the sulcus terminalis. Each is surrounded by a circular trough, or moat.

4. **Foliate papillae** are found on the lateral margins of the tongue as three to four short vertical folds. These are rudimentary in human beings.

Taste buds are receptor organs for the special sensation of taste. They are pale, oval bodies about 70 μm in length. Most are located in the troughs surrounding the vallate papillae; a few are found on the fungiform and foliate papillae. In addition, a few taste buds are found scattered through the epithelium of the oral surface of the soft palate, the posterior wall of the pharynx, and the epiglottis.

Posterior Third. The mucosa of the posterior third of the tongue is devoid of small papillae. Instead, its surface is thrown into many larger, rounded elevations, or nodules, composed of lymphoid tissue beneath a thin layer of epithelium. Collectively, the lymphoid nodules are called the ***lingual tonsil***.

Muscles of the Tongue

The bulk of the tongue (filling the mucous membrane bag) is composed of voluntary striated skeletal muscle. A thin median fibrous septum divides the tongue into equal right and left halves, so the musculature of the tongue is paired.

Two types of muscle are found within the tongue. **Extrinsic muscles** originate from remote structures and insert into the tongue. They act to move the tongue bodily. **Intrinsic muscles** originate from the tongue and insert into the tongue. They act to change the tongue's shape. Three paired extrinsic muscles and three paired intrinsic muscles are present.

The *infrahyoid* and *suprahyoid muscles*, which were considered with the neck, are **accessory muscles** of the tongue. They act to move the hyoid bone up and down and with it the base of the tongue.

Extrinsic Muscles

Genioglossus Muscle. The genioglossus muscle originates from the superior mental spine (genial tubercle) of the mandible as a narrow tendon (*Table 7-5*). The muscle fans out into the tongue posteriorly, and its fibers insert into the entire extent of the dorsum. The lowest fibers insert straight into the hyoid bone.

The inferior and middle fibers act to pull the dorsum of the tongue forward; that is, they protrude the tongue. The superior fibers act to retract the tip of the tongue and pull it inferiorly.

Hyoglossus Muscle. The hyoglossus muscle originates from the upper surface of the greater horn and the lesser horn of the hyoid bone. It is a flat, parallelogram-shaped sheet of muscle that angles upward and anteriorly to insert into the lateral aspect of the tongue.

Its fibers act to pull the sides of the tongue downward and depress the dorsum of the tongue. The muscle also aids in retrusion of the tongue.

Styloglossus Muscle. The styloglossus muscle originates from the anterior aspect of the styloid process, passes downward and forward, and inserts into the lateral aspect of the tongue. The muscles act to draw up the sides of the tongue to create a trough for swallowing. They also aid in retracting the tongue.

Intrinsic Muscles. These are named according to the three spatial planes in which they run. The intrinsic fibers intermingle with the extrinsic fibers.

Longitudinal Fibers. The longitudinal fibers run in an anteroposterior direction and are distributed *as superior* and *inferior* bundles. The *superior bundle* runs just below the mucosa of the dorsum; the *inferior bundle* runs between

---

TABLE 7-5

Extrinsic Muscles of the Tongue

Muscle	Origin	Insertion	Action	Cranial Nerve
Genioglossus	Superior mental spine	Superior fibers: tip of tongue	Superior fibers: retract tip of tongue	XII
		Middle fibers: dorsum of tongue	Middle fibers: depress dorsum of tongue	
		Inferior fibers: into body of hyoid bone	Inferior fibers: advance hyoid bone	
Hyoglossus	Upper surface of greater horn and lesser horn of hyoid bone	Lateral aspect of tongue	Helps retrude tongue, draws sides of tongue downward	XII
Styloglossus	Anterior aspect of styloid process	Lateral aspect of tongue	Helps retrude tongue, draws sides of tongue upward	XII

the genioglossus and hyoglossus muscles at the base of the tongue. The fibers contract to shorten the length of the tongue and to curl the tip of the tongue up and back.

Transverse Fibers. These muscle fibers run horizontally at right angles just below the superior longitudinal bundle. The transverse fibers act to narrow the tongue and help to form a longitudinal trough on the dorsum of the tongue.

Vertical Fibers. The vertical fibers run from the dorsum of the tongue down to the inferior surface. They act to flatten and broaden the tongue.

Actions of the Tongue: A Summary

1. **Protrusion**: genioglossi muscles, inferior and middle fibers
2. **Retrusion**: hyoglossi muscles, styloglossi muscles, superior fibers of genioglossi muscles
3. **Depression**: genioglossi and hyoglossi muscles
4. **Elevation**: styloglossi muscles with help from the palatoglossi muscles
5. **Shortening**: longitudinal intrinsic fibers
6. **Narrowing**: transverse intrinsic fibers
7. **Flattening**: vertical intrinsic fibers

In addition, the tongue may take a variety of shapes and positions through combined actions of the various muscles.

Motor Nerve Supply. The three pairs of extrinsic and three pairs of intrinsic muscles are supplied by the **hypoglossal nerve (cranial nerve XII)**.

CLINICAL NOTES

Paralyzed Tongue

A fractured mandible may damage the hypoglossal nerve, causing the nonaffected tongue muscles to pull the tongue to the same side. General anesthesia results in a looseness, or flaccidity, of muscles. A paralyzed or flaccid tongue tends to fall back into the airway, causing suffocation, unless a patent airway is maintained (see Figure 7-100 later in this chapter).

Tongue Tie

A large lingual frenulum can limit the mobility of the tongue and interfere with speech. The condition is easily repaired by cutting the frenulum (**lingual frenectomy**).

Sensory Nerve Supply. The mucosa of the tongue is supplied with general sensation nerves and special sensation (taste) nerves (see *Figure 7-83, B*).

General Sensation. The **lingual nerve** (a branch of the anterior division of **cranial nerve V-3**) carries general sensation from the anterior two thirds of the tongue. The **glossopharyngeal nerve (cranial nerve IX)** carries general sensation from the posterior third of the tongue. The **vagus nerve (cranial nerve X)** carries general sensation from the area surrounding the epiglottis.

Special Sensation: Taste. The **facial nerve (cranial nerve VII)** (via the chorda tympani) conveys taste sensation from the anterior two thirds of the tongue. The **glossopharyngeal nerve (cranial nerve IX)** carries taste sensation from the posterior third of the tongue. The **vagus nerve (cranial nerve X)** carries taste sensation from the area surrounding the epiglottis.

THE FLOOR OF THE MOUTH

The floor of the mouth is the space between the medial aspect of the mandibular body above the mylohyoid line and the base of the tongue (*Figures 7-84 and 7-85*). Inferiorly, the flat mylohyoid muscles limit the floor of the mouth and act as a muscular diaphragm. Superiorly, the contents of the floor of the mouth are covered with a thin layer of mucosa.

The mucous membrane of the tongue is continuous with the mucous membrane of the floor of the mouth. In turn, the floor mucosa reflects upward on the inner aspect of the mandible to end superiorly as the lingual gingiva.

Found within the floor of the mouth are a number of important structures: (1) three nerves and a ganglion, (2) two major salivary glands and their ducts, and (3) an artery.

The Lingual Nerve

The lingual nerve was described previously as a content of the infratemporal region (see *Figures 7-53, 7-84, and 7-85, and Chapter 7, section 5*).

Course. The lingual nerve arises as a branch of the posterior division of the mandibular nerve (cranial nerve V-3) within the infratemporal fossa. The lingual nerve curves downward, slightly laterally, and forward to emerge between the medial and lateral pterygoid muscles; it is joined at this point by the slender chorda tympani branch of cranial nerve VII. The lingual nerve continues anteriorly and downward, entering the floor of the mouth just medial to the root of the mandibular third molar.

In the floor of the mouth, the lingual nerve curves downward and then loops upward on the lateral surface of the hyoglossus muscle. The nerve ends superiorly by supplying branches to the dorsum of the anterior two thirds of the tongue.

Branches. Two or more short ganglionic branches suspend the submandibular ganglion from the lingual nerve

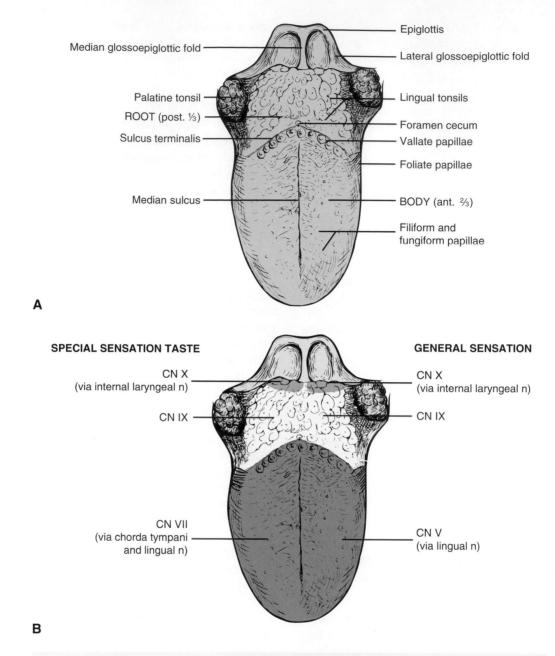

Figure 7-83 **A,** Surface features of the tongue. **B,** General and special sensory (taste) nerve supply.

as it loops on the surface of the hyoglossus muscle. The branches carry sensory and parasympathetic fibers to the ganglion.

General sensory branches pass to the mucosa of the anterior two thirds of the tongue, sublingual mucosa, and the mandibular lingual gingiva. **Special sensory taste fibers** from the accompanying fibers of the chorda tympani pass to the mucosa of the anterior two thirds of the tongue, along with the general sensory branches. Sensory branches also supply all of the mandibular lingual gingiva.

Submandibular Ganglion. The submandibular ganglion is a flattened small swelling that hangs by ganglionic branches from the lingual nerve (see *Figures 7-84* and *7-86*). Like all parasympathetic cranial ganglia, the ganglion receives sensory and sympathetic fibers in addition to incoming parasympathetic fibers.

Incoming Fibers

1. **Sensory fibers** pass to the ganglion from the lingual branch of cranial nerve V-3. They do not synapse in the ganglion.

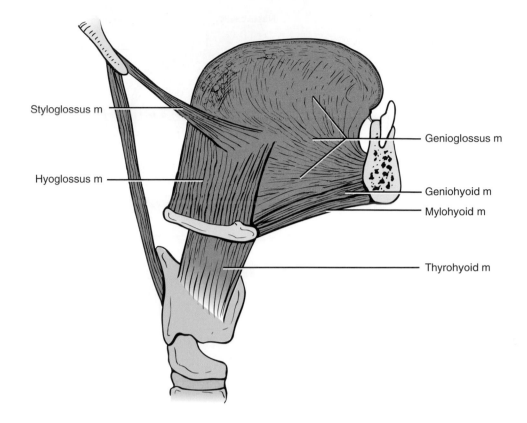

Styloglossus m

Hyoglossus m

Genioglossus m

Geniohyoid m

Mylohyoid m

Thyrohyoid m

A

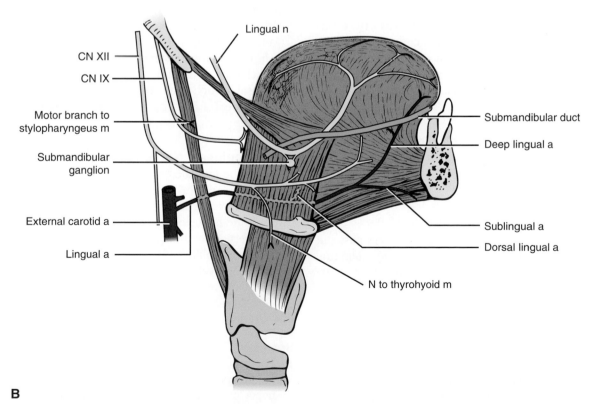

CN XII

CN IX

Motor branch to
stylopharyngeus m

Submandibular
ganglion

External carotid a

Lingual a

Lingual n

Submandibular duct

Deep lingual a

Sublingual a

Dorsal lingual a

N to thyrohyoid m

B

Figure 7-84 Lateral aspect of the tongue to show extrinsic and accessory muscles of the tongue (**A**) and vessels and nerves associated with the tongue (**B**).

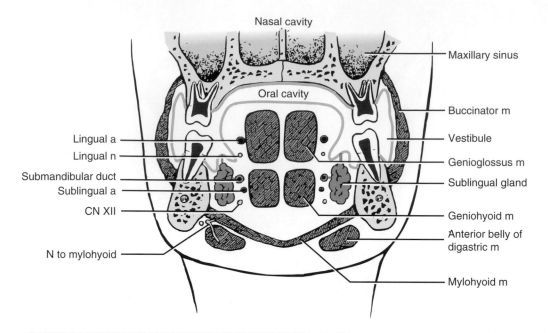

Nasal cavity

Maxillary sinus

Oral cavity

Buccinator m

Lingual a

Vestibule

Lingual n

Genioglossus m

Submandibular duct

Sublingual gland

Sublingual a

CN XII

Geniohyoid m

Anterior belly of
digastric m

N to mylohyoid

Mylohyoid m

Figure 7-85 Coronal section through the oral cavity and floor of the mouth.

2. **Sympathetic fibers** arise from the postsynaptic perivascular nerve plexus surrounding branches of the external carotid artery. The arteries that convey these fibers to the submandibular ganglion are the lingual and perhaps the facial arteries. The fibers do not synapse in the ganglion; they merely pass through. (They have already synapsed in the superior cervical ganglion of the sympathetic trunk.)

3. **Parasympathetic fibers of cranial nerve VII** are carried to the submandibular ganglion via the chorda tympani nerve travelling with the lingual nerve. Parasympathetic fibers pass to the submandibular ganglion via the ganglionic branches of the lingual nerve and synapse within the ganglion with secondary neurons.

Outgoing Fibers. Postganglionic outgoing fibers pass out to supply (1) the submandibular gland, (2) the sublingual gland, and (3) minor mucous glands of the floor of the mouth.

The Glossopharyngeal Nerve (Cranial Nerve IX)

Course. The glossopharyngeal nerve arises from the medulla and passes through the jugular foramen to the external base of the skull (see *Figure 7-84*). Here it passes to the pharynx between the borders of the superior and middle constrictors and continues forward deep to the tonsillar bed. It ends by plunging into the posterior third of the tongue.

Branches

1. **Pharyngeal branches** are general sensory to the mucosal lining of the pharynx.
2. The **nerve to the stylopharyngeus** is a single motor branch, which supplies this longitudinal muscle of the pharynx.
3. **Glossal branches** spread out to the mucosa of the posterior third of the tongue and convey general sensation and the special sensation of taste.

The Hypoglossal Nerve (Cranial Nerve XII)

Course. The hypoglossal nerve was described previously as a content of the submandibular region (see *Figures 5-16* and *7-84*). The nerve arises from the medulla, exits through the hypoglossal canal, and then descends in the neck superficial to the carotid sheath and its contents. It picks up hitchhiking spinal nerve contributions from APR of C1. At the level of the tip of the greater horn of the hyoid bone, the nerve curves anteriorly and disappears deep to the mylohyoid muscle to enter the floor of the mouth. It then branches to supply the musculature of the tongue.

Branches

1. The **superior limb of the ansa cervicalis** contains most of the spinal nerve contribution of C1; it leaves the hypoglossal nerve as the nerve loops anteriorly. It continues downward in the neck to help form the ansa cervicalis, which, in turn, supplies the infrahyoid strap muscles of the neck.

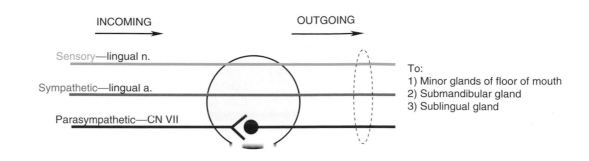

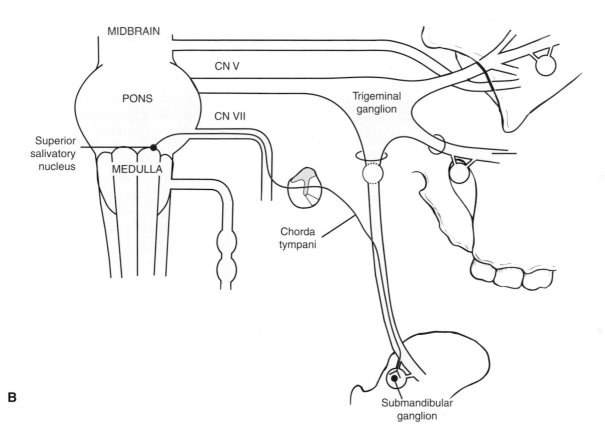

Figure 7-86 Submandibular ganglion. **A,** Scheme of incoming and outgoing nerve fibers. **B,** Origins of parasympathetic component from cranial nerve VII.

2. The **nerve to the thyrohyoid and geniohyoid muscles** is given off, and it represents the remaining fibers of the spinal nerve contribution C1.
3. **Glossal motor branches** pass to each of the extrinsic and intrinsic muscles of the tongue.

Lingual Artery

Origin and Course. The lingual artery arises as a collateral branch of the external carotid artery just above the tip of the greater horn of the hyoid bone (see *Figures 7-84* and *7-85*). It passes through the submandibular region and leaves by passing forward between the deeper genioglossus and the more superficial hyoglossus muscle into the floor of the mouth. The artery follows a somewhat tortuous route and divides into three sets of branches.

Branches
1. **Dorsal lingual branches** arise to supply the posterior third of the tongue.
2. A **sublingual branch** tracks deeply to supply the sublingual gland and the floor of the mouth.
3. The **terminal portion** of the lingual artery loops upward to supply the anterior two thirds of the tongue.

The Submandibular Gland

The submandibular gland is one of three major salivary glands. It is a *mixed serous* and *mucus-secreting gland*, and it is found partly in the submandibular region and partly in the floor of the mouth.

Location. The superficial portion of the gland was described as part of the submandibular region of the neck (see *Figure 5-19*). The gland wraps itself around the posterior free border of the mylohyoid muscle and becomes the deep portion within the floor of the mouth (*Figure 7-87*). The deep portion extends anteriorly between the body of the mandible and the base of the tongue as far as the second molar tooth. At this point, it continues forward as the submandibular duct.

The Submandibular Duct. The submandibular duct continues forward between the sublingual gland laterally and the body of the tongue medially (see *Figures 7-85* and *7-87*). The duct ends anteriorly by opening into the oral cavity through the sublingual papilla just lateral to the midline lingual frenulum.

Nerve and Blood Supply. The submandibular gland is supplied by *postganglionic autonomic fibers* of the **submandibular ganglion**. These fibers include a parasympathetic component (cranial nerve VII) and a sympathetic component. Glandular branches of the facial artery supply the submandibular gland.

The Sublingual Gland

The sublingual gland is primarily a *mucus-secreting* salivary gland.

Location. The sublingual gland is found entirely in the floor of the mouth (see *Figures 7-85* and *7-87*). Laterally, it nestles against the sublingual fossa of the mandible and medially lies along the base of the tongue. The gland is elongated, and its long axis lies in an anteroposterior direction. The right and left glands meet anteriorly, forming a horseshoe that surrounds the base of the tongue. Superiorly, only a thin lining of mucosa separates the gland from the oral cavity above. The sublingual fold within the oral cavity betrays the location of the gland (see *Figure 7-80*).

Sublingual Ducts. Approximately 12 tiny ducts empty directly upward through the sublingual fold to the oral cavity. A few of the more anterior ducts may drain medially to the closely adherent submandibular duct to mix with submandibular gland secretions.

Nerve and Blood Supply. The sublingual gland, like the submandibular gland, receives *postganglionic autonomic fibers* from the **submandibular ganglion**. These fibers include a parasympathetic component (cranial nerve VII) and a sympathetic component. The blood supply is from glandular branches of the **sublingual artery**.

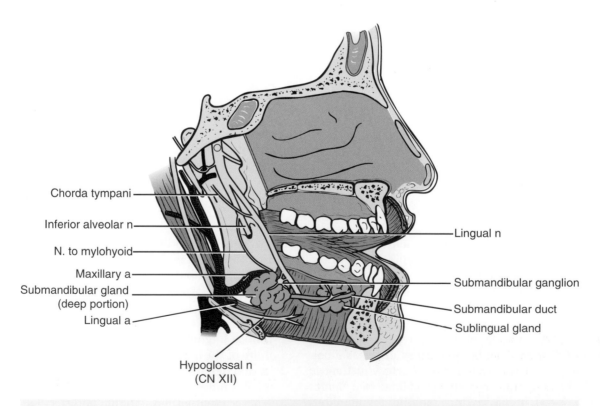

Chorda tympani
Inferior alveolar n
N. to mylohyoid
Maxillary a
Submandibular gland (deep portion)
Lingual a
Hypoglossal n (CN XII)

Lingual n
Submandibular ganglion
Submandibular duct
Sublingual gland

Figure 7-87 Medial view of the floor of the mouth with tongue removed to show structures of floor of the mouth.

TABLE 7-6

The Major Salivary Glands

Gland	Location	Secretion	Duct	Cranial Nerve Supply
Parotid	Parotid region: interval between posterior border of ramus and upper anterior border of sternomastoid m	Serous	Parotid duct travels anteriorly along lateral border of masseter m, rolls over anterior border of masseter to pierce cheek, and empties into oral cavity at occlusal level 2nd max. molar	Preganglionic: lesser petrosal nerve, a branch of IX Synapse: otic ganglion Postganglionic: fibers leave otic ganglion and travel with auriculotemporal branch of V-3 to parotid region
Submandibular	Superficial portion: submandibular region between lateral aspect of mylohyoid m and submandibular fossa of mandible Deep portion: in floor of mouth between base of tongue and sublingual gland	Serous and mucous	Submandibular duct continues forward from deep portion of gland and empties into oral cavity behind lower central incisors	Preganglionic: chorda tympani nerve, a branch of VII Synapse: submandibular ganglion Postganglionic: fibers leave ganglion and pass to gland
Sublingual	Floor of mouth, medial to sublingual fossa of mandible; above the mylohyoid muscle	Mucous	Sublingual ducts open directly into oral cavity through openings in sublingual fold Anterior ducts open medially into submandibular duct	Preganglionic: chorda tympani nerve, a branch of VII Synapse: submandibular ganglion Postganglionic: fibers leave ganglion and pass to gland

Summary of the Salivary Glands

A summary of the three salivary glands is presented in *Table 7-6.* Details of the parotid gland are discussed in section 4 of this chapter.

Accessory Salivary Glands. Small mucous glands throughout the oral mucosa empty their secretions directly to the mouth through individual tiny ducts.

Glandular Nerve Supply. Although the parasympathetic division of the autonomic nervous system is traditionally described as controlling salivation, it is becoming increasingly evident that the sympathetic division also plays a role in salivation. Parasympathetic stimulation regulates the water and electrolyte release; sympathetic stimulation induces protein secretion. Anxiety, such as in a nervous patient, results in a depression of parasympathetic stimulation and an increase in sympathetic stimulation. The saliva continues to flow but assumes a thicker, ropier consistency.

THE TEETH

On the surface, it may seem ludicrous that a textbook written for students of dentistry contains less information about teeth than do some medical anatomy texts. The fact is, however, that dental anatomy is traditionally taught as a separate course and several excellent texts devoted solely to dental anatomy are available.

For our purposes, a simple description of teeth and their supporting structures is offered as a prelude to reviewing the nerve supply to the teeth and supporting structures.

CLINICAL NOTES

Saliva

Saliva is important in mastication and the initial stages of the processing of food. Saliva also plays a critical role in the maintenance of the dentition, particularly during the first 2 years following tooth eruption, playing a role in posteruption maturation of the enamel. Saliva is also capable of remineralizing early carious lesions.

The salivary glands continually produce saliva, which flows through their respective ducts to the oral cavity. Stimulation by the sight or smell of food brings about an initial, rapid expulsion of saliva (watering of the mouth) by contraction of the myoepithelial cells surrounding the acini and intercalated ducts. During the course of a day, some 640 to 1200 mL of saliva are secreted. Production during the night drops dramatically to about 10 mL. Occasionally, strong, almost painful, contractions of the mylohyoid muscles rapidly squeeze the deep portion of the submandibular gland, producing squirts of saliva through the submandibular orifices.

CLINICAL NOTES

Calculus

Saliva contains high levels of calcium phosphate, which can precipitate spontaneously as a chalky material on the teeth as *supragingival calculus*. Saliva from the submandibular gland seems to be particularly at fault because calculus forms most readily on the lingual surfaces of the mandibular anterior teeth, directly anterior to the orifices of the submandibular ducts. Some patients are more susceptible to this formation and form abundant depositions of calculus, which must be periodically scaled to prevent gingival inflammation.

Blocked Submandibular Duct

Occasionally, a calcified deposit (sialolith) obstructs the duct and causes a backup and swelling of the submandibular gland. An attempt may be made to milk the sialolith forward through the duct and out the orifice but it is generally too large to pass through the duct orifice unless it can be palpated and crushed. Occasionally, it must be surgically removed.

Sialography (*Figure 7-88*)

The course and degree of patency of the parotid and submandibular ducts may be examined radiographically. A small cannula is introduced into the duct orifice, and a radiopaque substance is injected. The procedure is followed radiographically, and any blockage of the duct becomes immediately apparent.

Xerostomia (Dry Mouth)

Xerostomia is caused by reduced production of saliva as seen in elderly patients and in patients undergoing radiation therapy. This condition results in a drying of the tissues, with pain upon swallowing. It also results in increased dental caries and caries on tooth surfaces that are not normally affected. To date, the treatment of choice is the regular and frequent use of oral rinses or artificial saliva.

External Features (*Figure 7-89*)

Teeth are either **single-rooted** or **multirooted,** and sit in bony sockets, or **alveoli,** within the alveolar processes of the maxilla and mandible. The root supports a short **neck,** which is tightly surrounded by a cuff of gingival tissue. Above the neck and visible in the oral cavity is the **crown** of the tooth.

Dental Tissues

Pulp Chamber. This is a hollow space within the crown and neck of the tooth (*Figures 7-90* and *7-91*). It contains the pulpal soft tissues: (1) *odontoblasts* on the periphery, which produce dentine; (2) ordinary *connective tissue* cells; and (3) *blood vessels* and *nerves*. The pulp cavity funnels down to a narrow root canal in a single-rooted tooth or to one canal per root in a multirooted tooth. The canal opens at the root apex as a tiny *apical foramen*. It is through this foramen that vessels and nerves enter or leave the pulp chamber.

Dentine. Dentine forms the walls of the pulpal cavity and the root canal. It also forms the bulk of the structure of the crown and root. *Dentinal tubules* maintain continuity with the odontoblasts of the pulpal chamber. By some mechanism not yet understood, stimulation of cut dentine in a vital tooth is transmitted via the tubules to the nerves of the pulp. These stimuli are transported by the peripheral nervous system to the brain, where they are ultimately perceived as pain.

Cementum. This is a thin layer of bonelike material that coats the root surface externally. It is this material that anchors and supports the collagenous fibers of the periodontal ligament.

Enamel. Enamel is the extremely hard yet brittle (if not supported) material that caps and overlies the dentine of the crown of the tooth. It is composed of tightly packed calcified prisms, or rods.

Dental Surfaces and Terminology

The crown of each tooth as it appears in the oral cavity presents five named surfaces:

1. The **occlusal surface** is the masticating, or biting, surface.
2. The **vestibular surface** faces the vestibule. Older terminology describes a buccal surface of posterior teeth (facing the cheek) and a labial surface of anterior teeth (facing the lip).
3. The **lingual surface** is the side facing the tongue.
4. The **mesial surface** is the side closest to the midline of the dental arch.
5. The **distal surface** is the side farthest from the midline of the dental arch.

Mesial and distal surfaces approximate in all teeth except for the mesial approximations of the central incisors and the lone distal surface of the last tooth in the dental arch.

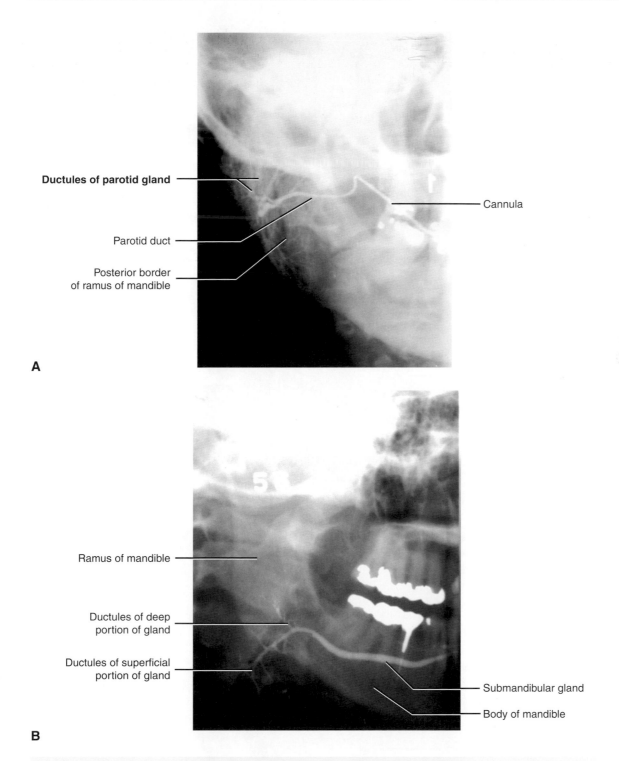

Ductules of parotid gland ⎯⎯⎯

Cannula

Parotid duct ⎯⎯⎯

Posterior border
of ramus of mandible ⎯⎯⎯

A

Ramus of mandible ⎯⎯⎯

Ductules of deep
portion of gland ⎯⎯⎯

Ductules of superficial
portion of gland ⎯⎯⎯

Submandibular gland

Body of mandible

B

Figure 7-88 Sialographs. **A,** Parotid gland. **B,** Submandibular gland. (Courtesy Dr. N. Marcus.)

DECIDUOUS TEETH   PERMANENT TEETH

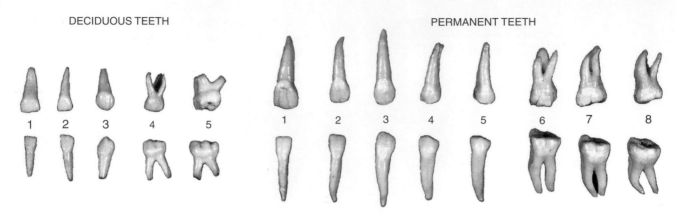

ADULT MAXILLARY DENTITION

Central incisor
Lateral incisor
Canine
First premolar (bicuspid)
Second premolar (bicuspid)
First molar
Second molar
Third molar

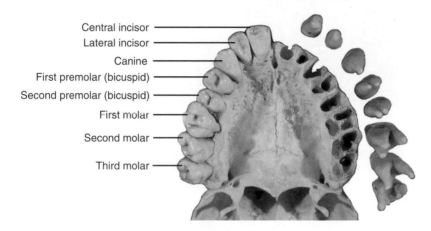

ADULT MANDIBULAR DENTITION

Third molar
Second molar
First molar
Second premolar (bicuspid)
First premolar (bicuspid)
Canine
Lateral incisor
Central incisor

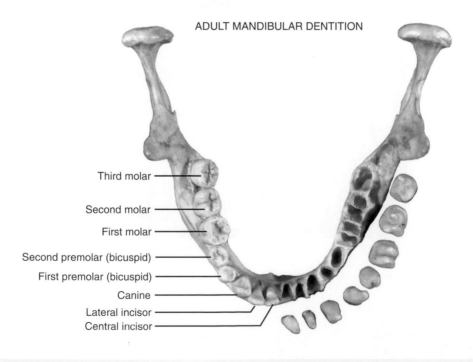

Figure 7-89 Deciduous and adult dentitions.

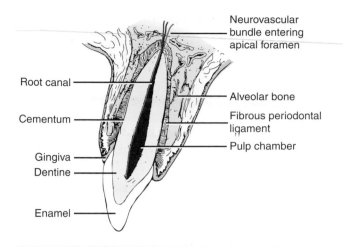

Neurovascular bundle entering apical foramen

Root canal

Cementum

Gingiva

Dentine

Enamel

Alveolar bone

Fibrous periodontal ligament

Pulp chamber

Figure 7-90 Sagittal section through the maxillary incisor to show its features.

Dental Nerve Supply. In general, all stimuli to the tooth (temperature, touch, pressure) are perceived as discomfort (see *Figures 7-53* and *7-58*). Extreme stimuli are translated as brilliant, flashing pain. The cutting of dentine in cavity preparation elicits pain, and for most patients the only way to prepare a cavity is to block the sensory nerve pathway somewhere and prevent transmission of pain perception impulses.

Sensation is carried from the maxillary dentition by the maxillary nerve (cranial nerve V-2) and from the mandibular dentition by the mandibular nerve (cranial nerve V-3). Specifically, the nerve supply to the upper and lower dentition is the following.

Maxillary Teeth

1. The central incisor, lateral incisor, and canine teeth are supplied by terminal branches of the **anterior superior alveolar nerve** (see *Figure 7-58*).

2. The first and second premolars and the mesiobuccal root of the first molar are supplied by the **middle superior alveolar nerve**.

3. The first molar (excluding the mesiobuccal root), second molar, and third molar are supplied by terminal branches of the **posterior superior alveolar nerve**.

In the primary dentition, the central incisor, lateral incisor, and canine are supplied by the **anterior superior alveolar nerve**; the first and second molars are supplied by the **middle superior alveolar nerve**.

Mandibular Teeth. All the mandibular teeth on the right side are supplied by the **right inferior alveolar nerve**; those on the left side are supplied by the **left inferior alveolar nerve**. In the primary dentition, all the primary teeth are supplied by the inferior alveolar nerves (see *Figure 7-53*).

Dental Blood Supply

Each tooth must have a blood supply. Small arterial "twigs" enter the apical foramen to pass through the root canal to the pulp chamber. Here they pass through a capillary bed to supply pulpal tissues (see *Figure 7-90*). Venules and lymphatics collect the tissue fluids from the capillary beds and leave through the apical foramen.

Arterial Supply. Both dental arches are supplied by branches of the maxillary artery (see *Figure 7-55*). Maxillary teeth are supplied by part 3 of the maxillary artery, which parallels the superior alveolar nerves as the **posterior, middle,** and **anterior superior alveolar arteries**. Mandibular teeth are supplied by the **inferior dental branch** of the first part of the maxillary artery. It parallels the course and distribution of the inferior alveolar nerve.

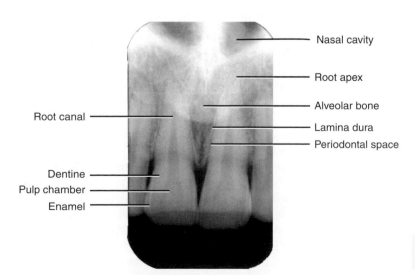

Nasal cavity

Root apex

Alveolar bone

Lamina dura

Periodontal space

Root canal

Dentine

Pulp chamber

Enamel

Figure 7-91 Periapical radiograph of the maxillary central incisors to show its internal features.

CLINICAL NOTES

Dentoalveolar Abscess

One problem in dental practice is the treatment of the nonvital tooth, that is, a tooth that loses its blood supply. In such a case, the pulpal tissues die and the remaining necrotic debris inevitably becomes infected.

A tooth may lose its blood supply following a blow to the tooth that disrupts the flimsy vessels at the root apex. More commonly, loss of blood supply is due to the invasion of the pulp chamber by a deep carious lesion. This infects and irritates the pulpal tissues and sets up a defensive inflammatory process (pulpitis). Elsewhere in the body, local inflammation does not pose a serious problem and is generally resolved. The pulp cavity, however, is a rigid, enclosed space, and the swelling pulpal tissues cause considerable pain. The small vessels in the narrow root canal are strangled by the pressure of the swollen inflamed tissues. The tissues die, and, ultimately, built-up pressure of the dead infected tissues forces the material out through the apical foramen to secondarily infect the alveolar bone and produce a dentoalveolar abscess.

Venous Return. The venous return of both dental arches is to the **pterygoid plexus of veins** (see *Figure 7-56*). The plexus eventually forms posteriorly as the **maxillary vein,** which, in turn, unites with the **superficial temporal vein** to form the **retromandibular vein.**

The Supporting Dental Structures

The Periodontal Ligament. The junction of tooth root and alveolar bone was described in Chapter 1 as a gomphosis type of joint in which many short collagenous fibers suspend the tooth root in the bony alveolar socket. The fibers are embedded in the thin cementurn overlying the root and run across a short periodontal space (about 0.2 mm) to embed in the alveolar bone.

The periodontal ligament contains many *sensory pressure receptors*, which probably monitor occlusal biting forces. This information is relayed to the brain to help modify mandibular movements during mastication.

The collagenous fibers are arranged in groups: (1) **Oblique fibers** prevent masticatory forces from driving the tooth into the socket. (2) **Horizontal groups** help maintain the tooth in an upright position and prevent tilting. (3) **Circular fibers** encircle the neck of the tooth as a tight cuff within the gingiva. (4) **Gingival fibers** arise from the cementurn of the neck and the alveolar bony crest and pass to the gingiva, anchoring the gingiva to the tooth and alveolar bone.

The alveolar nerves and vessels that supply the teeth also supply the corresponding periodontal ligaments.

The Gingivae (Gums)

Alveolar Mucosa. In the mandibular arch, oral mucosa sweeps upward from the vestibular fold and from the floor of the mouth on the lingual side. This mucosa is shiny, red, and nonkeratinizing. It is thin and, therefore, imparts the underlying color of the blood vessels below (see *Figure 7-76*). The alveolar mucosa is not firmly attached to the underlying bone.

In the maxillary arch, the vestibular mucosa sweeps from the vestibular fold down onto the alveolar base as loose alveolar mucosa. The lingual or palatal mucosa is firmly anchored to the bones of the hard palate and sweeps downward onto the alveolar process. Unlike the vestibular alveolar mucosa, it is firmly attached to alveolar bone and is keratinizing.

Gingiva Proper. As the alveolar mucosa approaches the neck of the tooth, it changes abruptly in nature and color. It becomes pink, stippled, and keratinizing. It is firmly anchored to the underlying alveolar bone. The vestibular and the lingual gingiva are connected through interdental papillae that pass between the crowns of the teeth. The buccal, lingual, and interdental papillae surround the neck of the tooth as a tight cuff.

Nerve and Blood Supply to the Gingivae

Maxillary Vestibular Gingivae (Labial and Buccal)

1. The gingivae overlying the central incisors, lateral incisors, and canines are supplied by gingival branches of the anterior superior alveolar nerves and vessels. Labial branches of the infraorbital nerve and vessels help supply the area.
2. The gingivae overlying the premolars are supplied by gingival branches of the middle superior alveolar nerve and vessels.
3. The gingivae overlying the first, second, and third molars are supplied by gingival branches of the posterior superior alveolar nerve and vessels.

Maxillary Lingual (Palatal) Gingivae. The lingual gingivae of the maxillary incisors and canines are supplied by gingival branches of the *nasopalatine nerve and vessels*. The lingual gingivae of the maxillary premolars and molars are supplied by gingival branches of the *greater palatine nerve and vessels*.

Mandibular Vestibular Gingivae (Labial and Buccal)

1. The vestibular gingivae of the mandibular incisors, canines, and premolars are supplied by gingival branches of the *inferior alveolar nerve* and vessels (the incisive branches); labial and gingival branches of the *mental nerve and vessels* help to supply the area.
2. The vestibular gingivae of the mandibular molars are supplied by gingival branches of the *buccal nerve* (a branch of cranial nerve V-3) and gingival branches of the *buccal artery* (a branch of the maxillary artery—part 3).

Gingivitis

Neglect and improper oral hygiene leave food deposits in tooth and gingival crevices. This results in irritation and inflammation of the gingivae. The gingivae lose the pink stippled appearance. They swell and turn red, creating a pocket, or sulcus, around the tooth, which leads to further entrapment of food particles.

Periodontitis

Chronic neglect of oral hygiene leads to an eventual breakdown of the gingival cuff surrounding the neck of tooth, forming a pocket. If untreated, the pocket progressively increases in depth. Breakdown of the periodontal ligament and alveolar bone progresses in an apical direction, and, if unchecked, the teeth are eventually lost.

Mandibular Lingual Gingivae. The lingual gingivae of all the mandibular teeth are supplied by gingival branches of the *lingual nerve and vessels*.

Summary of Nerve Supply to Jaws, Teeth, and Surrounding Soft Tissues

Figure 7-92 is presented as a review and summary of the innervation to the soft and hard tissues of the maxillary and mandibular arches.

10. The Pharynx

After food is swallowed, it passes from the oral cavity posteriorly to the pharynx, a funnel-shaped fibromuscular tube that is a common area for air and food passages. Both the nasal cavity and the oral cavity communicate posteriorly with the pharynx. Inferiorly, air passes through the more anteriorly

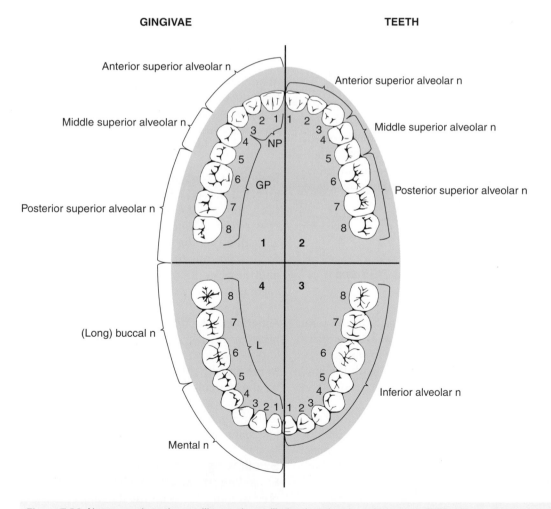

GINGIVAE   **TEETH**

Figure 7-92 Nerve supply to the maxillary and mandibular dental arches. Arches are divided by convention into four quadrants starting with upper right. The right side shows nerve supply gingiva and surrounding oral mucosa; the left side shows nerve supply to teeth. *NP*, Nasopalatine nerve; *GP*, greater palatine nerve; *L*, lingual nerve.

placed larynx on its way to the trachea and the bronchial tree. Food passes behind the larynx to enter the esophagus.

SKELETON

Review the features of the base of the skull (see Chapter 6), and the skeleton of the larynx (see *Figure 7-96*).

WALLS OF THE PHARYNX

Although air passes through the pharynx, the area structurally belongs to the gastrointestinal system. The pharyngeal walls contain the same four basic layers as the rest of the gut.

1. An **areolar coat** covers the exterior of the pharynx. It is continuous with the areolar fascia overlying the buccinator muscle, so it is termed *buccopharyngeal fascia.* Like all fascial layers, it acts as a neurovascular transport medium. Running through the fascia is a pharyngeal plexus of veins and nerves.
2. A **muscular coat** consists of five paired muscles, which form an outer semicircular layer, and two inner longitudinal muscles.
3. The **submucosa,** or **pharyngobasilar fascia,** is a tough, fibrous coat. It anchors the pharynx to the base of the skull at a U-shaped attachment. The area of attachment to the base of the skull is as follows: trace a line posteriorly from the medial pterygoid plate to the anterior border of the carotid canal—this marks the lateral limit. A line joining the anterior aspects of the right and left carotid canals marks the posterior border. This line passes through the pharyngeal tubercle. The pharynx opens anteriorly to the nasal cavity above and the oral cavity below.
4. The **mucosa** coats the internal aspect of the pharynx, and the internal features are discussed shortly.

MUSCLES OF THE PHARYNX (*Figure 7-93* and *Table 7-7*)
Semicircular Constrictor Muscles
Superior Constrictor Muscle. This muscle arises from the length of the pterygomandibular raphé, a ligament that runs from the hamulus above to the retromolar area of the mandible below. It is a shared origin with the buccinator muscle, which sweeps anteriorly from the raphé. A few fibers arise from the tongue.

The superior constrictor fibers fan out posteriorly and turn medially to meet their opposite muscle in a midline posterior, or pharyngeal, raphé. Superiorly, the pharyngeal raphé is anchored to the pharyngeal tubercule at the base of the skull.

Middle Constrictor Muscle. This muscle *arises from the bony interval between the greater and lesser horns of the hyoid bone* and a small inferior portion of the stylohyoid

ligament. The fibers sweep posteriorly and medially to join their opposite muscle at the midline pharyngeal raphé. The fibers of the middle constrictor partially overlap the superior constrictor muscle above.

Inferior Constrictor Muscle. The inferior constrictor muscle originates from the lateral aspects of the thyroid and cricoid cartilages. The muscle fibers fan out posteriorly and medially to meet fibers of the opposite muscle in the midline pharyngeal raphé. The lower portion of the inferior constrictor muscle is usually termed the *cricopharyngeus muscle.*

Functions. The functions of the constrictor muscles are discussed under swallowing.

Nerve Supply. The constrictor muscles are supplied by pharyngeal branches of the vagus nerve (**cranial nerve X**). The motor fibers originate from the cranial accessory nerve (cranial nerve XI), which travel with cranial nerve X.

Longitudinal Muscles
Palatopharyngeus Muscle. This muscle was described previously as a muscle of the soft palate. It originates mainly from the palatal aponeurosis but a few slips arise from the mouth of the auditory tube as the salpingopharyngeus muscle. The fibers pass inferiorly to insert into the posterolateral aspect of the pharynx and the posterior aspect of the hyoid bone and thyroid cartilage.

Stylopharyngeus Muscle. It originates from the medial aspect of the styloid process and passes medially and inferiorly through the gap between the superior and inferior constrictors to enter the pharynx. Here, its fibers mingle with those of the palatopharyngeus muscle and insert with them into the posterolateral wall of the pharynx and the posterior aspects of the hyoid bone and thyroid cartilage.

Functions. The two longitudinal muscles act to raise the pharynx and larynx during the act of swallowing.

Nerve Supply. The palatopharyngeus muscle is supplied by the **cranial accessory nerve (cranial nerve XI)** travelling with the **vagus nerve (cranial nerve X).** The stylopharyngeus muscle is supplied by a motor branch of the glossopharyngeal nerve (cranial nerve IX).

Swallowing or Deglutition
Stage One (Voluntary). Following mastication, the food is pressed into a bolus on the dorsum of the tongue against the hard palate (*Figure 7-94*). The swallow is initiated by pushing the food posteriorly into the oropharynx by the tongue.

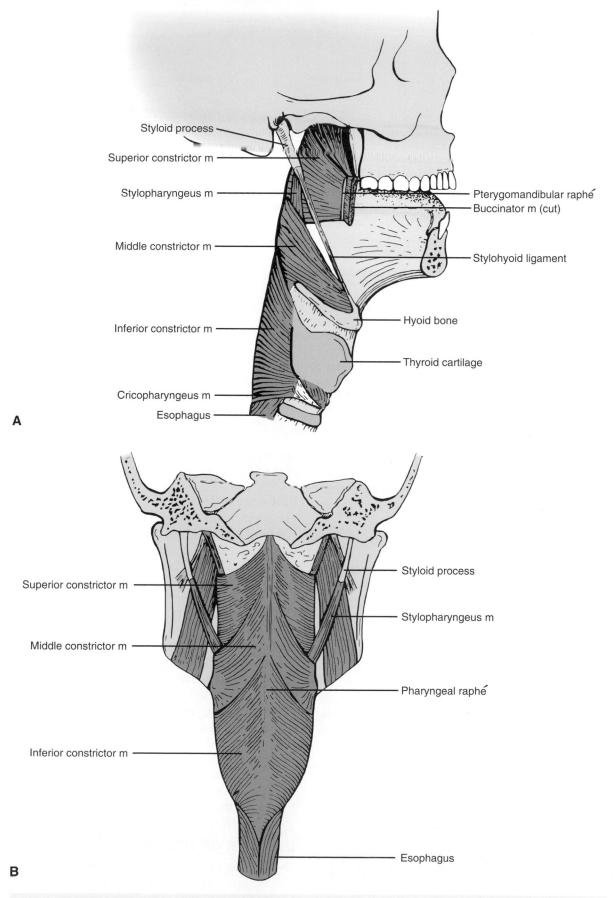

Styloid process

Superior constrictor m

Stylopharyngeus m

Middle constrictor m

Inferior constrictor m

Cricopharyngeus m

Esophagus

Pterygomandibular raphé

Buccinator m (cut)

Stylohyoid ligament

Hyoid bone

Thyroid cartilage

A

Superior constrictor m

Middle constrictor m

Inferior constrictor m

Styloid process

Stylopharyngeus m

Pharyngeal raphé

Esophagus

B

Figure 7-93 Muscles of the pharynx. **A,** Lateral view. **B,** Posterior view.

TABLE 7-7

Muscles of the Pharynx

Muscle	Origin	Insertion	Action	Cranial Nerve
Semicircular				
Superior constrictor	Pterygomandibular raphé, hamulus of medial pterygoid plate, lateral aspect of tongue, posterior aspect of mylohyoid ridge of mandible	Pharyngeal tubercle on base of skull, median pharyngeal raphé	All constrictors constrict pharynx in sequence from superior to inferior during swallowing	XI via X
Middle constrictor	Interval between greater and lesser horns of hyoid bone, stylohyoid ligament	Median pharyngeal raphé		XI via X
Inferior constrictor	Oblique line of thyroid cartilage, lateral aspect of cricoid cartilage	Median pharyngeal raphé		XI via X
Longitudinal				
Stylopharyngeus	Styloid process	Posterolateral wall of pharynx, posterior aspect of thyroid cartilage and hyoid bone	Elevate the pharynx and larynx during swallowing and speech	IX
Palatopharyngeus		Posterolateral wall of pharynx, posterior aspect of thyroid cartilage and hyoid bone	Elevate the pharynx and larynx during swallowing and speech	XI via X

Stage Two (Involuntary). The soft palate elevates to seal the oropharynx from the nasopharynx and prevents regurgitation of food into the nasal cavity. The stylopharyngeus and palatopharyngeus muscles and the suprahyoid muscles contract to raise the larynx.

Stage Three (Involuntary). The three constrictor muscles contract in a sequential fashion as peristaltic waves. From superior to inferior, each pair of muscles contracts for approximately 0.33 second. Just as the muscles physically overlap, so do their contractions overlap from superior to inferior.

Stage Four (Involuntary). The bolus enters the esophagus and is propelled downward by peristaltic action.

The cricopharyngeus muscle (lower fibers of the inferior constrictor muscle) is in a constant state of contraction and prevents passage of air to the esophagus below. During the act of swallowing, the cricopharyngeus relaxes to allow passage of the bolus into the esophagus below.

CLINICAL NOTES

Pharyngeal Dysphagia
Dysphagia is difficulty in swallowing and passing the bolus from the pharynx to the esophagus. It is generally caused by neurological or muscular disorders.

The bolus is propelled to the stomach by peristaltic waves of the esophagus.

Pharyngeal Gaps
The superior and inferior borders of the constrictor muscles form four gaps through which pass several key structures (*Figure 7-95*).

Gap 1 is located between the base of the skull and the superior border of the superior constrictor muscle. Passing through are the auditory tube, the levator veli palatini muscle, and the ascending palatine branch of the facial artery.

Gap 2 is between the superior and middle constrictors; passing through the gap are the stylopharyngeus muscle and the glossopharyngeal nerve (cranial nerve IX).

Gap 3 is between the middle and inferior constrictor muscles, and it transmits the internal laryngeal branch of cranial nerve X and the superior laryngeal branch of the superior thyroid artery.

Gap 4 is between the inferior constrictor and the esophagus; passing through this gap are the recurrent laryngeal nerve and the inferior laryngeal branch of the inferior thyroid artery.

INTERIOR OF THE PHARYNX

The interior of the pharynx is lined by mucosa and is divided into three functional areas: (1) nasopharynx, (2) oropharynx, and (3) laryngeal pharynx (*Figure 7-96*).

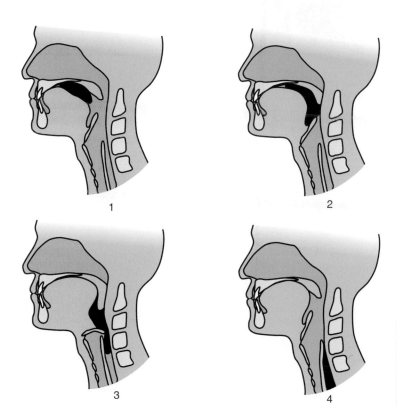

Figure 7-94 Four stages of swallowing. *1,* Tongue pushes bolus of food to back of oral cavity. *2,* Soft palate is raised to prevent bolus from entering nasopharynx. *3,* Tongue elevates and epiglottis seals laryngeal inlet, preventing bolus from entering airway. *4,* Pharyngeal constrictors have propelled food into esophagus.

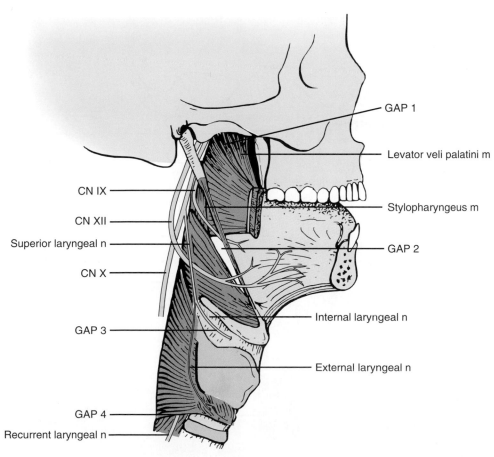

Figure 7-95 Pharyngeal gaps and the structures that traverse them.

337

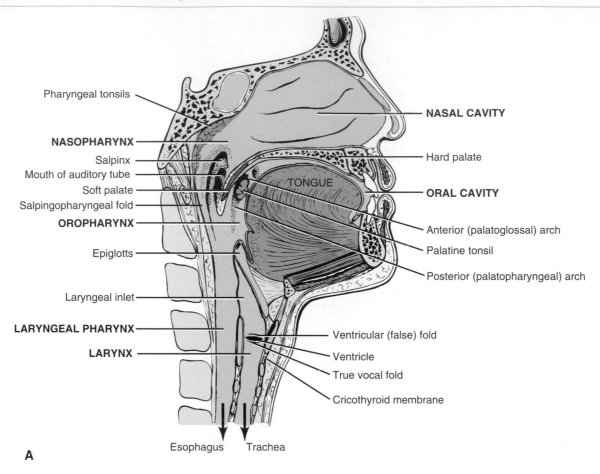

Pharyngeal tonsils

NASOPHARYNX

Salpinx

Mouth of auditory tube

Soft palate

Salpingopharyngeal fold

OROPHARYNX

Epiglotts

Laryngeal inlet

LARYNGEAL PHARYNX

LARYNX

NASAL CAVITY

Hard palate

TONGUE

ORAL CAVITY

Anterior (palatoglossal) arch

Palatine tonsil

Posterior (palatopharyngeal) arch

Ventricular (false) fold

Ventricle

True vocal fold

Cricothyroid membrane

Esophagus   Trachea

A

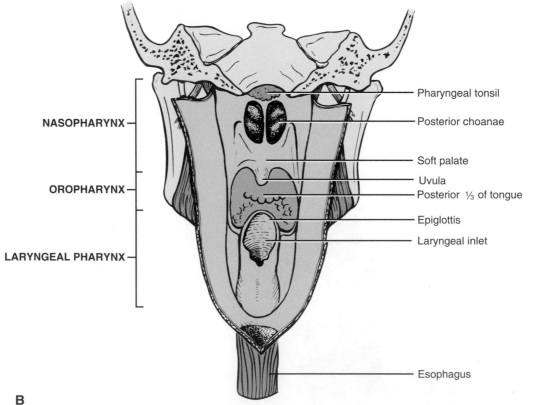

NASOPHARYNX

OROPHARYNX

LARYNGEAL PHARYNX

Pharyngeal tonsil

Posterior choanae

Soft palate

Uvula

Posterior ⅓ of tongue

Epiglottis

Laryngeal inlet

Esophagus

B

Figure 7-96 Subdivisions of the pharynx and their relationships to oral and nasal cavities. **A,** Sagittal section. **B,** Posterior view of pharynx with posterior wall cut and spread laterally to reveal internal features.

Nasopharynx

The nasopharynx is the superior portion of the pharynx lying above the soft palate and communicates with the nasal cavity anteriorly through the choanae. The walls of the nasopharynx are lined with respiratory ciliated columnar pseudostratified epithelium. The following features are found within the nasopharynx:

1. The **mouth of the auditory (pharyngotympanic)** tube bulges out into the lateral wall of the nasopharynx about 1.25 cm behind the inferior concha. The raised mouth is mucous membrane-covered cartilage called the *salpinx* (*trumpet*), and the middle of the salpinx presents a vertical slit, the auditory tube orifice.
2. The **salpingopharyngeal fold** consists of a small muscle covered with mucous membrane. The fold continues inferiorly from the posterior aspect of the salpinx and blends with the lateral wall of the nasopharynx. The salpingopharyngeus muscle is a small portion of the palatopharyngeus muscle.
3. The **pharyngeal recess** is a vertical cleft between the salpingopharyngeal fold and the posterior wall of the pharynx.
4. The **pharyngeal tonsils**, or **adenoids**, are a collection of nodular lymphoid tissue found on the superoposterior wall of the nasopharynx. It also extends laterally into the pharyngeal recess.

Oropharynx

The oropharynx lies below the soft palate and communicates anteriorly with the oral cavity. When the soft palate is at rest, the nasopharynx communicates with the oropharynx. When the soft palate is raised, it hinges upward to form a seal against the posterior wall of the pharynx. This occurs during the act of swallowing.

The oropharynx may be sealed from the oral cavity by approximation of the soft palate and the dorsum of the tongue. This occurs during the act of sucking. The following features are found within the oropharynx:

1. The **anterior** and **posterior pillars** are two folds of mucous membrane extending laterally and inferiorly from the soft palate. The more anterior fold is the **palatoglossal arch** running down to the lateral aspect of the tongue. Below the fold is the palatoglossus muscle.

   The posterior fold runs from the soft palate to the lateral wall of the pharynx as the **palatopharyngeal arch**. Below the mucous membrane of the arch is the palatopharyngeus muscle.
2. The **palatine tonsil** is a rounded elevation of lymphoid tissue covered by mucous membrane. It sits in the triangular interval between the anterior and posterior pillars. Its size is variable, but it is generally relatively large during childhood and begins to atrophy after the onset of puberty.

The tonsillar bed between the two arches consists of a number of important structures. Immediately deep to the palatine tonsil is the pharyngobasilar fascia. The fascia, in turn, lies on the superior constrictor, palatopharyngeus, and styloglossus muscles and the glossopharyngeal nerve.

The blood supply to the palatine tonsil is from tonsillar branches of the ascending palatine artery and facial artery. Other tonsillar branches arise from the dorsal lingual artery, ascending pharyngeal artery, and lesser palatine artery.

Venous drainage passes medially and is collected by the external palatine vein descending from the soft palate above and draining to the pharyngeal plexus of veins. Drainage is also to the facial vein.

Laryngeal Pharynx

The larynx projects upward into the pharynx, and that part of the pharynx adjacent to the larynx is called the *laryngeal pharynx*. The laryngeal pharynx ends inferiorly at vertebral level C6 by funnelling downward into the esophagus. The following features are found within the laryngeal pharynx:

1. The **epiglottis** is a leaflike, elastic cartilage structure that guards the oval opening into the larynx. The epiglottis is fully discussed as a feature of the larynx.
2. The **glossoepiglottic folds** are three folds of mucous membrane that run anteriorly from the epiglottis to the base of the posterior third of the tongue; there is a median fold and two lateral folds on either side (see *Figure 7-83*).
3. The **valleculae** are two small depressions created by the three folds; they lie on either side of the median glossoepiglottic fold.
4. The **piriform recess** is a vertical gutter on the lateral wall of the laryngeal pharynx; it lies between the lateral glossoepiglottic fold and the side wall of the pharynx and continues downward on either side of the larynx like two troughs to the esophagus below.

NERVE AND BLOOD SUPPLY TO THE PHARYNX

Nerves

Motor Nerves. All the muscles of the pharynx (except for the stylopharyngeus muscle) are supplied by **pharyngeal branches** of the **vagus nerve** (*fibers of cranial nerve XI travelling with cranial nerve X*). The stylopharyngeus muscle is supplied by a muscular branch of the **glossopharyngeal nerve (cranial nerve IX)**.

Sensory Nerves
1. The **glossopharyngeal nerve (cranial nerve IX)** is the main sensory supply from the pharynx.
2. The **maxillary nerve (cranial nerve V-2)** supplies the soft palate and pharyngeal roof via its lesser palatine and pharyngeal branches, respectively.
3. The **vagus nerve (cranial nerve X)** is sensory from the area surrounding the laryngeal inlet.

Blood Supply

Arteries. The pharynx receives a very rich anastomosing blood supply from various sources: (1) **ascending pharyngeal branch** of the external carotid artery, (2) **superior thyroid branch** of the external carotid artery, and (3) **inferior thyroid branch** from the thyrocervical trunk. In addition, the soft palate and tonsillar area are supplied by the **facial artery** (tonsillar and ascending palatine branches) and the **maxillary artery** (lesser palatine branch).

Veins. The veins draining the pharyngeal wall and the soft palate form a plexus within the buccopharyngeal fascia. The plexus ultimately regroups as a pharyngeal vein, which joins the internal jugular vein deep to the angle of the mandible. The **pharyngeal plexus** also communicates anteriorly with the pterygoid plexus of veins.

RETROPHARYNGEAL SPACE

The pharynx cannot be fixed to the underlying prevertebral fascia; it must be free to move up and down during the act of swallowing. To accommodate this movement, an areolar space exists between the posterior wall of the pharynx and the vertebral unit behind. This areolar space extends from the base of the skull above to the superior mediastinum below. Its significance is further discussed in Chapter 8, dealing with the section on spreads of infection in the head and neck.

11.   The Larynx

Inspired air passes posteriorly through the nasal or oral cavity to the pharynx behind, which is a common air and food chamber. The larynx protrudes up into the pharynx and extends from the base of the tongue (vertebral level C3) down to the trachea (vertebral level C6). The inlet to the larynx lies immediately behind the posterior third of the tongue and is guarded by the flaplike epiglottis. Thus, inspired air passes through the laryngeal inlet and down through the larynx to the trachea. Food and drink continue inferiorly behind the larynx to the esophagus below.

FUNCTIONS

The larynx performs three basic functions. It acts as (1) an **air passage** linking the pharynx above to the trachea below, (2) a **sphincter** preventing food in the pharynx from entering the air passage, and (3) an organ of **phonation**.

SKELETON

The skeleton of the larynx consists of three large unpaired cartilages (thyroid, epiglottis, and cricoid cartilages) and three smaller paired cartilages (arytenoid, cuneiform, and corniculate cartilages) (*Figure 7-97*). In addition, the hyoid bone is closely related functionally to the skeleton of the larynx.

Thyroid Cartilage

This is the largest of the laryngeal cartilages and consists of two four-sided plates, or laminae, joined anteriorly in the midline. The cartilage is open posteriorly, and, viewed from above, the thyroid cartilage is V-shaped, the apex of the V facing anteriorly. The following features are characteristic of the thyroid cartilage:

1. The **thyroid prominence** is the upper, prominent portion of the angular union of the laminae; it is felt subcutaneously as the Adam's apple and is very prominent in adult men.
2. The **thyroid notch** is located in the midline directly above the prominence.

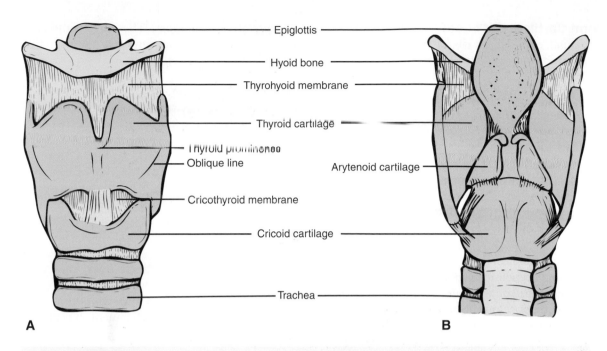

Figure 7-97 Skeleton of the larynx. **A,** Frontal view. **B,** Posterior view.

3. The **superior horns,** or **cornua,** sweep upward and backward as slender processes from the free posterior borders of the laminae.
4. The **inferior horns,** or **cornua,** project downward and anteriorly from the free posterior border as two smaller processes.
5. The **oblique line** is a raised ridge that slopes inferiorly and anteriorly on the lateral aspect of each lamina. It runs from the base of the greater horn to the inferior border of the lamina.

Cricoid Cartilage

The cricoid cartilage sits immediately below the thyroid cartilage at vertebral level C6. It is shaped and sized somewhat like a signet ring, with the signet portion facing posteriorly. The following features are characteristic of the cricoid cartilage:

1. The **lamina** is the signet portion, which faces posteriorly. The lower border of the lamina is horizontally straight; the upper border dips obliquely downward and laterally from the midline.
2. The **arch** of the cricoid is the anterior narrow ring portion. It may be palpated below the thyroid prominence.
3. The **cricoid lumen** is round and is approximately the diameter of an index finger.

Epiglottis

The epiglottis is a fibroelastic cartilage in the shape of a leaf. Its stem, or stalk, is anchored to the internal aspect of the angle of the thyroid laminae. The broad leaf portion

angles upward and backward and ends as a curved border above the level of the hyoid bone, just behind the posterior third of the tongue.

The epiglottis presents an anterior and a posterior surface, both covered with mucous membrane. A median and two **lateral glossoepiglottic folds** sweep from the anterior surface to the posterior third of the tongue. Below the mucous membrane of the anterior surface, the **hyoepiglottic ligament** runs from the epiglottis to the body of the hyoid bone. The posterior surface below the mucous membrane is pockmarked to accommodate large mucous glands.

Arytenoid Cartilages (Paired)

These are two pyramid-shaped cartilages perched like caps on the lateral aspects of the superior border of the lamina. Each possesses three surfaces and a base and three angular processes. The posterior surface is smooth and concave; the medial surface is flat; the anterolateral surface is convex and rough; and the base is smooth and concave for articulation with the lamina of the cricoid cartilage.

The **apex** is the slender superior process that curves backward and medially; the **vocal process** points anteriorly and provides attachment for the vocal cord; the **muscular process** projects laterally and is the site of insertion for various intrinsic laryngeal muscles.

Corniculate Cartilages (Paired)

These are tiny elastic cartilages sitting atop the apices of the arytenoid cartilages. They function merely to extend the lengths of the apical processes and may be fused to them.

341

Cuneiform Cartilages (Paired)

These are small, club-shaped islands of elastic fibrocartilage stranded in the aryepiglottic folds.

JOINTS OF THE LARYNX

Two sets of synovial joints are found in the larynx.

Thyrocricoid Joint

The inferior horns of the thyroid cartilage articulate with two facets on the lateral aspects of the cricoid cartilage. The joint is surrounded by a capsular ligament. The bilateral joint allows the thyroid cartilage to tilt forward and backward on the stationary cricoid cartilage.

Cricoarytenoid Joint

The base of each arytenoid cartilage articulates with the superior border of the cricoid lamina. These synovial joints allow two basic types of movements: (1) rotation about a roughly vertical axis and (2) translation medially and laterally along the sloping superior laminar border of the cricoid cartilage.

LIGAMENTS OF THE LARYNX

External Ligaments

Thyrohyoid Membrane. This is a fibroelastic sheet joining the inferior surface of the hyoid bone to the superior aspect of the thyroid cartilage. The posterior borders of the ligament are free and thickened and are called the *lateral thyrohyoid ligaments.*

Occasionally, a nodule of cartilage develops in the lateral thyrohyoid ligament.

Median Cricothyroid Ligament. This is a triangular median ligament running from the anterosuperior aspect of the cricoid cartilage to the anteroinferior border of the thyroid cartilage.

Internal Ligaments

Just below the internal mucous membrane lining of the larynx are a number of elastic and fibroelastic ligaments (*Figure 7-98, A*).

Vocal Ligaments. These are thick bands of elastic fibers running from the vocal processes of the arytenoid cartilages forward to converge as a V on the internal laminar angle of the thyroid cartilage. They are covered by mucous membrane to form the vocal folds, or **true vocal folds**.

Ventricular Ligaments. These ligaments are two bands of fibers that run from the lateral borders of the arytenoid cartilages to the internal angle of the thyroid lamina. These ligaments run above the vocal folds and are covered with mucous membrane to form the ventricular folds, or **false vocal folds**.

Aryepiglottic Ligaments. These ligaments pass upward from the apices of the arytenoid cartilages to the superior lateral borders of the epiglottis.

Quadrangular Membrane. The area between the aryepiglottic ligament above and the ventricular ligament below is filled with a thin, fibroelastic sheet that is called the *quadrangular ligament* because of its shape. It is a bilateral structure.

Cricothyroid Membrane. The triangular area between the vocal folds above and the superior border of the cricoid cartilage below is filled with a fibroelastic sheet. It is a single structure sweeping in U-shaped fashion from the vocal process of one arytenoid cartilage around to that of the opposite arytenoid cartilage. Inferiorly, it attaches as a semicircle to the superior border of the lamina of the cricoid cartilage. Anteriorly, it fuses with the more externally placed median cricothyroid ligament. It is also referred to as the *conus elasticus.*

INTERIOR OF THE LARYNX

The internal aspect of the larynx is lined with respiratory mucosa (*Figure 7-98, B*).

Features

The Laryngeal Inlet, or Aditus. The laryngeal inlet allows air to pass from the pharynx above to the lumen of the larynx below. It is formed anteriorly by the curved superior border of the epiglottis, laterally by the aryepiglottic folds, and posteriorly by the interarytenoid fold of mucous membrane. The plane of the opening is oblique, with the anterior border being higher than the posterior border.

The Lumen of the Larynx. The lumen extends from the inlet above to the lumen of the trachea below. Two sets of mucous membrane-covered folds project from the lateral walls into the lumen: the **ventricular folds** are the superior set; the **vocal folds** are the inferior set. These impinge farther into the lumen than do the ventricular folds and, thus, the vocal folds may be seen from above in a superior view of the laryngeal lumen.

The two vocal folds seen from above are together termed the *glottis*. The opening between the vocal folds is termed the *rima glottidis*. The **rima glottidis** may be opened or closed.

The true vocal folds and the ventricular (false) folds divide the lumen into three areas.

1. The **vestibule** is the portion of the lumen above the ventricular folds. It is wide above and constricted below.
2. The **ventricle** is the small midportion between the ventricular folds and the vocal folds; it extends laterally.

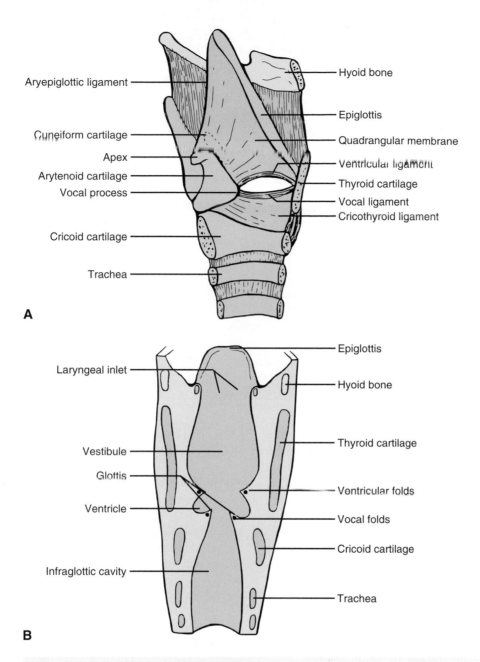

Figure 7-98 **A,** Midsagittal cut through the larynx to reveal laryngeal ligaments and membranes. **B,** Coronal section to show features of the lumen.

From the ventricle, a blind pouch extends upward for about 1 cm as the **laryngeal saccule**.

3. The **infraglottic cavity** is the portion of the lumen inferior to the vocal folds.

MUSCLES OF THE LARYNX
Extrinsic Muscles
These muscles have a remote origin but insert into the larynx or the hyoid bone (*Table 7-8*). Because of this remote anchorage, the extrinsic muscles are able to move the larynx bodily up or down. These include the suprahyoid muscles and the longitudinal pharyngeal muscles that pull the hyoid bone and larynx upward, as well as the infrahyoid strap muscles that pull the hyoid bone and larynx downward.

Intrinsic Muscles
Intrinsic muscles originate from the larynx and insert into the larynx (*Figure 7-99*). They are, therefore, able to move one laryngeal cartilage in relation to another. There are eight paired intrinsic muscles of the larynx.

TABLE 7-8

Muscles of the Larynx

Muscle	Origin	Insertion	Action	Cranial Nerve
Cricothyroid	Anterior aspect of cricoid cartilage	Posteroinferior border of thyroid cartilage	Stretch the vocal cords	XI via X—external laryngeal branch
Transverse arytenoid	Muscular process of arytenoid cartilage	Muscular process of opposite arytenoid cartilage	Draw arytenoids toward each other	XI via X—recurrent laryngeal branch
Posterior cricoarytenoid	Posterior aspect of the cricoid lamina	Muscular process of arytenoid cartilage	Abduct or open vocal cords	
Lateral cricoarytenoid	Lateral aspect of cricoid cartilage	Muscular process of arytenoid cartilage	Adduct or close vocal cords	
Aryepiglottic	Muscular process of arytenoid cartilage	Apex of opposite arytenoid, epiglottis	Approximate epiglottis and arytenoids to help close airway during swallowing	XI via X—recurrent laryngeal branch
Thyroarytenoid	Internal aspect of thyroid lamina	Lateral border of arytenoid cartilage	Help to close the vestibule	XI via X—recurrent laryngeal branch
Thyroepiglottic	Thyroid cartilage	Epiglottis	Help to close the vestibule	XI via X—recurrent laryngeal branch
Vocalis	Internal aspect of thyroid lamina (inferior fibers of thyroarytenoid m)	Vocal process of arytenoid cartilage	Shorten the vocal cords	XI via X—recurrent laryngeal branch

Cricothyroid Muscle. This muscle arises from the anterior aspect of the cricoid cartilage just off the midline. The fibers fan upward to insert into the posteroinferior border of the thyroid cartilage. The muscles act to tilt the thyroid cartilage forward over the cricoid cartilage at the cricothyroid joints. In doing so, they stretch the vocal folds.

The remaining intrinsic muscles originate from or insert into the arytenoid cartilage.

Transverse Arytenoid Muscle. This muscle arises from the muscular process and lateral aspect of the arytenoid cartilage and passes across the midline to insert into the same area of the opposite arytenoid cartilage. The fibers contract to approximate the right and left arytenoid cartilages.

Posterior Cricoarytenoid Muscle. The posterior cricoarytenoid has a broad origin from the posterior aspect of the cricoid lamina. The fibers taper upward and laterally to insert into the muscular process of the arytenoid cartilage. The right and left muscles contract to spin the arytenoid cartilages about vertical axes at the cricothyroid joints. This causes the vocal processes and attached vocal folds to diverge (abduct), thus opening the rima glottidis.

Lateral Cricoarytenoid Muscle. This muscle arises from the lateral aspect of the cricoid cartilage and passes upward and medially to insert into the muscular process of the arytenoid cartilage. The muscles contract bilaterally to turn the arytenoids about vertical axes at the cricoarytenoid

joints. This causes the vocal processes and attached vocal folds to converge (adduct) to close the rima glottidis.

Aryepiglottic Muscle. The fibers of this muscle arise from the muscular process of the arytenoid cartilage and sweep upward and medially to cross the midline. Some fibers insert into the apex of the opposite arytenoid cartilage; the rest continue upward to insert into the lateral aspect of the epiglottis. Fibers of the right and left muscles decussate in the midline. The muscles help close the vestibule by approximating the epiglottis and the arytenoids.

Thyroarytenoid Muscle. This muscle lies just above the lateral cricoarytenoid muscle. It arises from the internal aspect of the thyroid lamina and inserts into the entire lateral border of the arytenoid cartilage. The muscles act to help close the vestibule.

Thyroepiglotticus Muscle. These are wispy fibers lying atop the quadrangular membrane. They run from the thyroid cartilage to the epiglottis and help close the vestibule.

Vocalis Muscle. The lower medial fibers of the thyroarytenoid muscle pass as a distinct band of muscle fibers to insert on the vocal process of the arytenoid cartilage. The muscle fibers run below and lateral to the vocal ligament. The fibers contract to approximate the thyroid cartilage and arytenoid cartilages, thus shortening the vocal ligaments. This muscle is the antagonist of the cricothyroid muscle.

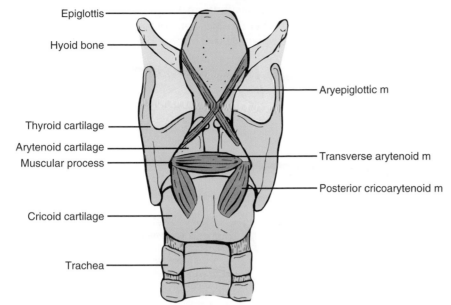

Epiglottis

Hyoid bone

Thyroid cartilage

Arytenoid cartilage

Muscular process

Cricoid cartilage

Trachea

Aryepiglottic m

Transverse arytenoid m

Posterior cricoarytenoid m

A

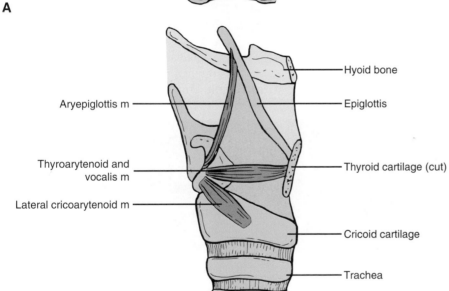

Aryepiglottis m

Thyroarytenoid and vocalis m

Lateral cricoarytenoid m

Hyoid bone

Epiglottis

Thyroid cartilage (cut)

Cricoid cartilage

Trachea

B

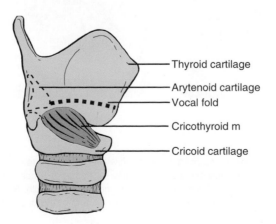

Thyroid cartilage

Arytenoid cartilage

Vocal fold

Cricothyroid m

Cricoid cartilage

C

Figure 7-99 Intrinsic muscles of the larynx. **A,** Posterior view. **B,** Lateral view with the right thyroid lamina removed. **C,** Right lateral view to show the cricothyroid muscle.

Actions of Intrinsic Muscles of the Larynx: A Review

The intrinsic muscles perform three separate functions: (1) some open the rima glottidis to allow passage of air in and out; (2) some close the vestibule and rima glottidis during swallowing to prevent aspiration of food; and (3) other muscles control the rima glottidis and tension of the vocal folds for phonation (*Figure 7-100*).

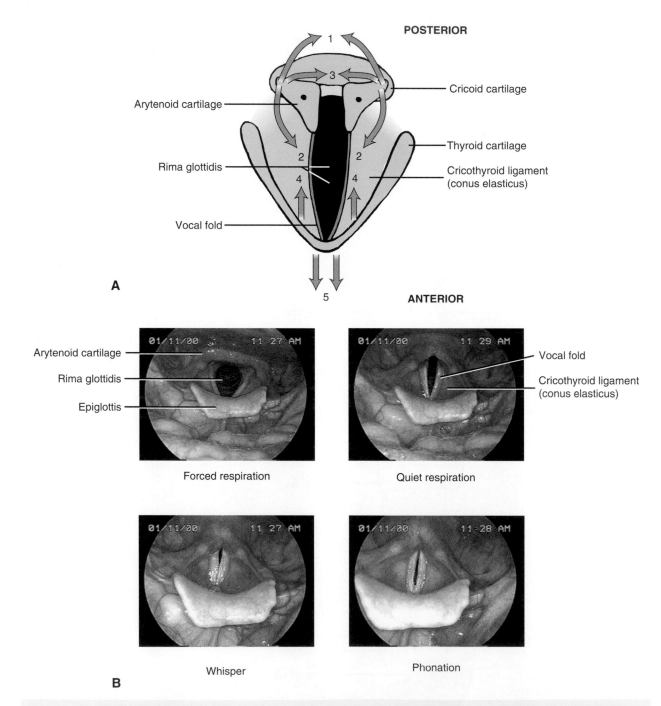

Figure 7-100 Movements of the intrinsic laryngeal muscles. **A,** Superior view of the vocal folds and arytenoid cartilages. Muscle actions are represented by arrows, and muscles are represented by numbers. *1,* Posterior cricoarytenoid muscle; *2,* lateral cricoarytenoid muscle; *3,* transverse arytenoid muscle; *4,* vocalis muscle; *5,* cricothyroid muscle. **B,** Laryngoscopic views of the glottis. Note that the pictures are oriented with the anterior aspect toward the bottom of the page and the posterior aspect toward the top. (Courtesy Dr. J.A. Anderson.)

Muscles that Control the Vestibular Opening. During swallowing, the vestibule is closed by the sphincteric action of (1) aryepiglotticus muscles, (2) thyroepiglotticus muscles, and (3) thyroarytenoid muscles.

Muscles that Open (Abduct) the Vocal Folds. The right and left posterior cricoarytenoid muscles are the only abductors of the vocal folds.

Muscles that Close (Adduct) the Vocal Folds. The lateral cricoarytenoids, aided by the thyroarytenoids, approximate the vocal folds. The transverse arytenoids approximate the vocal folds posteriorly by drawing the arytenoids together.

Muscles that Control Tension of the Vocal Folds. The cricothyroid muscles pull the thyroid cartilage down and forward at the cricothyroid joint. This stretches the vocal folds (the tighter the stretch, the higher the pitch in voice). The posterior cricoarytenoids contract as fixators to prevent forward tilting of the arytenoid cartilages. The vocalis muscles act to shorten the vocal folds and provide fine adjustment to the degree of cord tension.

NERVE AND BLOOD SUPPLY

Nerves

Motor Nerves. All the intrinsic muscles. of the larynx are supplied by **laryngeal branches of the vagus nerves** (*fibers of cranial nerve XI—cranial portion, traveling with cranial nerve X*). All of the laryngeal muscles, except one, are supplied by the **recurrent laryngeal branch**. The sole exception is the cricothyroid muscle, which is supplied by the **external laryngeal branch**.

Sensory Nerves. The **vagus nerve** is the sensory nerve of the larynx via two laryngeal branches. The **internal laryngeal branch** is sensory from the mucous membrane above the vocal folds. The **recurrent laryngeal nerve** is sensory from the mucous membrane below the vocal folds.

Vessels

Arteries. The larynx receives its blood supply from two arteries. (1) The **superior thyroid artery** arises from the external carotid artery and loops downward to supply the thyroid gland. It also gives off an internal laryngeal branch, which accompanies the internal laryngeal nerve through the thyrohyoid membrane. (2) The **inferior thyroid artery** arises from the thyrocervical trunk. It gives off an inferior laryngeal branch, which accompanies the recurrent laryngeal nerve to the larynx.

Veins. Laryngeal veins drain to the superior thyroid veins, and these, in turn, drain to the internal jugular veins. The inferior portion of the gland is drained by inferior laryngeal veins, which drain to the inferior thyroid veins. These then drain to the left brachiocephalic vein.

CLINICAL NOTES

Upper Airway Obstruction

Most of us have experienced the phenomenon of food or drink "going down the wrong way." This means that the food or drink enters the laryngeal inlet rather than proceeding posteriorly and inferiorly to the esophagus. This phenomenon is usually coincidental with talking or laughing during the act of swallowing. Happily, a good coughing session expels the material, and, aside from an irritated throat, all is fine.

Food Obstruction

Occasionally, not all goes well. A large mass of food stuck in the vestibule or the rima glottidis mechanically obstructs the airway and causes suffocation. Even a small amount of material may irritate the laryngeal mucosa and trigger a reflex spasm of the vocal folds, with a resultant closing of the airway. Surveys of such accidents reveal that many such victims are older people who are partially edentulous and cannot chew their food (particularly meat) into a manageable bolus. Incomplete chewing, ingestion of alcohol, and laughter may result in obstruction.

Foreign Bodies and Dental Accidents

Small objects, such as crowns, amalgam scraps, extracted teeth, and small instruments, are sometimes lost down the patient's throat. Fortunately, the patient usually coughs and produces the truant object. Sometimes it is swallowed and passed to the gut. Trouble arises, however, if the object is aspirated, that is, passed to the larynx. The object could obstruct the larynx or produce laryngospasm. If the object passes through the vocal cords to the trachea and beyond, the patient is not in immediate danger, but the object must be located and removed as quickly as possible.

Allergic Reactions

One of several ways in which an allergic reaction to drugs, foods, insect bites, and so on may manifest is a massive swelling, or edema, of subcutaneous and mucous membrane tissues (angioedema). Edema of the vestibule can obstruct the airway.

Clearing an Airway Obstruction

Qualification in **cardiopulmonary resuscitation (CPR)** is required in most dental schools prior to the student's first encounter with patients. Clinicians must have a plan of action and have access to an emergency kit should emergency problems such as airway obstruction arise.

Artificially Opening the Airway: Cricothyrotomy

If all initial attempts to initiate breathing fail, the obstructed vocal folds may be bypassed by surgically creating an airway. Extend the victim's head and palpate under the chin, in succession, the hyoid bone, the laryngeal prominence, a dip, and then the cricoid bone. The dip is the cricothyroid space, and below the skin is the median cricothyroid ligament.

An incision is made through the skin and cricothyroid ligament in the midline and continued deeply and angled inferiorly, to puncture the airway below the vocal cords. The incision is kept open by inserting a length of tubing (an empty ballpoint pen barrel would do nicely if a proper emergency kit is not available). This opening bypasses the obstructed vocal folds and allows the victim to breathe directly through the opening. Oxygen, if available, can be flowed over the open tube. The cadaver in the dissecting laboratory provides an ideal opportunity to simulate this emergency procedure.

In a hospital environment, under controlled conditions, the entry is usually made inferiorly into the trachea (tracheostomy). Care is taken to avoid structures that cover the trachea anteriorly, such as the thyroid gland isthmus and the inferior thyroid veins.

In an emergency, however, the safer but more disfiguring cricothyrotomy is preferred because there are no important structures between the cricothyroid membrane and the skin.

Endotracheal Intubation

Endotracheal intubation is the passing of a flexible tube through the mouth or nose, past the vocal folds, and into the trachea (*Figure 7-101*). This procedure is commonly performed to administer a general anesthetic agent and oxygen through the tube directly to the trachea and the lungs. It provides, if necessary, a direct airway in patients with acute laryngeal obstruction.

The laryngoscope is really a metal tongue depressor with a light and is used to visualize the epiglottis and glottis behind the posterior third of the tongue. A lubricated tube is then passed through the oral cavity, down into the oropharynx, and through the glottis between the vocal folds and left in the trachea.

In dental operations, a tube passed through the oral cavity would be in the way. In these cases, the tube is inserted through the external nares, along the floor of the nose, and back to the nasopharynx. The tube then deflects inferiorly along the posterior pharyngeal wall and drops below the soft palate into the oropharynx. At this point, the tube is visualized and directed through the vocal folds into the trachea. Great care is taken to ensure that the tube passes through the glottis rather than through the esophageal opening posteriorly.

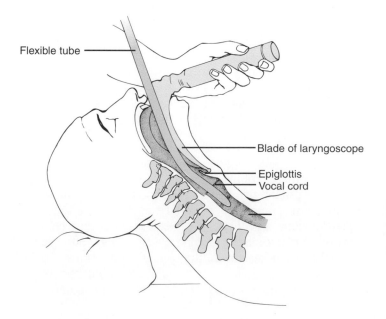

Flexible tube

Blade of laryngoscope

Epiglottis

Vocal cord

Figure 7-101 Endotracheal intubation. With the laryngoscope as a guide, a flexible tube is passed through vocal folds to the trachea below to carry controlled mixtures of anesthetic gases and oxygen for general anesthesia.

12. The Ear

SKELETON
Review the features of the temporal bone.

PARTS
The ear can be functionally and regionally divided into five distinct portions (*Figure 7-102*). (1) The **outer ear** consists of the auricle and the external auditory meatus, or canal, which funnel air vibrations inward to the tympanic membrane, or eardrum. (2) The **tympanic membrane** stretches across the medial end of the external auditory meatus, and it vibrates in sympathy with the incoming sound waves. (3) The **middle ear** is a chamber within the temporal bone that contains air and bony ossicles that conduct vibrations from the tympanic membrane to the inner ear. (4) The **inner ear** consists of the *cochlea*, which contains sound receptors, and the *semicircular canals*, which contain balance receptors. (5) The **auditory (pharyngotympanic) tube** joins the middle ear cavity to the nasopharynx and serves as an air pressure compensatory mechanism.

External Ear
Auricle. The features of the auricle were noted previously, along with the superficial structures of the face.

External Auditory Meatus. The external auditory meatus, or canal, is approximately 2.5 cm in length, and it func-

tions as the stem of a funnel carrying air vibrations from the concha of the external ear to the tympanic membrane that limits the medial end of the meatus.

The cartilage of the auricle is continued as a tube into the bony meatus for about one third of its length. This lateral third of the meatus is lined with skin that contains hair follicles, sebaceous glands, and modified sweat glands. These produce a hard, waxy exudate called *cerumen* (ear wax), which, when it accumulates, can cause pain and partial deafness in the affected ear. The medial two thirds of the meatus is bone lined with a thin layer of stratified squamous epithelium, a continuation of the skin.

Arteries and Nerves
Arteries. The arterial supply is from three branches of the external carotid artery: (1) auricular branches, which arise from the superficial temporal artery; (2) deep auricular branches, which arise from the first part of the maxillary artery; and (3) the posterior auricular artery.

Nerves. The sensory nerve supply is derived from three cranial nerves: (1) the auricular branch of the auriculotemporal nerve, a branch of V-3, supplies most of the external auditory meatus; (2) the auricular branch of the vagus nerve (cranial nerve X); and (3) the auricular sensory branches from the facial nerve (cranial nerve VII) supply only a small portion of the meatus.

Tympanic Membrane (Eardrum)
Features. The external auditory meatus ends medially at a somewhat circular membrane (8 to 9 mm in diameter).

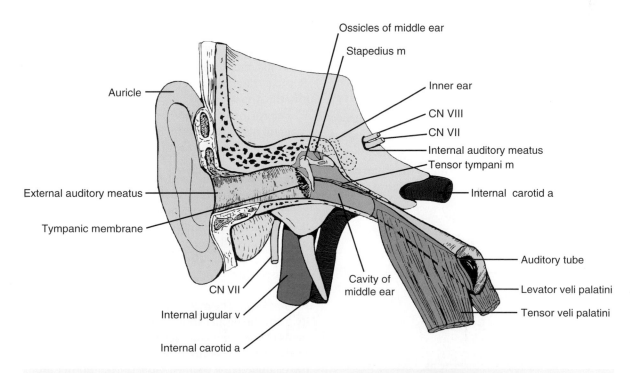

Figure 7-102 Coronal section through the skull to show the external, middle, and internal ear.

It sits obliquely at the end of the canal, facing laterally but tipped downward and slightly forward when viewed through the canal. Its surface domes inward.

CLINICAL NOTES

Inspection Using an Otoscope

The **handle of the malleus,** one of the ear ossicles, is adherent to the medial aspect of the membrane, and the radial fibers seem to radiate out from the handle (*Figure 7-103*). Superiorly, the fibers do not radiate from the handle, and this portion is loose and is called the **pars flaccida.** The lowest part of the handle draws the membrane inward as the **umbo.** When the membrane is viewed from the external auditory meatus with an ear speculum, a cone of light is seen radiating downward and forward from the umbo.

The membrane itself consists of circular and radial fibers. The lateral, or superficial, aspect is layered with stratified squamous epithelium that is continuous with the skin lining the external auditory meatus. The medial, or deep, aspect is covered with mucous membrane that is continuous with the lining of the middle ear cavity.

The chorda tympani nerve passes across the medial aspect of the upper portion of the membrane. It is attached to the mucous membrane by a pair of malleolar mucosal folds.

Nerve and Blood Supply. The tympanic membrane presents two surfaces: an outer surface lined by epidermis and an inner surface lined by mucous membrane. Each surface has a separate nerve and blood supply.

Outer (Lateral) Aspect. This surface shares the same nerve and blood supply as the external auditory meatus noted previously.

Inner (Medial) Aspect. This surface shares the same blood and nerve supply as the middle ear mucosal lining.

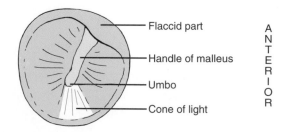

Figure 7-103 The right tympanic membrane as viewed by an otoscope through the external auditory meatus.

Middle Ear Cavity (Tympanic Cavity)

Deep to the tympanic membrane is the cavity of the middle ear. The cavity is likened to a small chamber with four walls, a roof, and a floor within the petrous temporal bone. It is roughly 15 mm high and 4 to 6 mm wide, with its lateral wall compressed inward. The cavity is lined with mucous membrane, and it contains air, three ossicles, a nerve, and two tiny muscles. The cavity presents six surfaces, or walls: (1) a lateral wall, (2) a roof, (3) a floor, (4) a posterior wall, (5) an anterior wall, and (6) a medial wall.

Lateral Wall. This wall is largely filled by the tympanic membrane, described previously. A small portion of the middle ear extends upward beyond the tympanic membrane as the **epitympanic recess** (*Figure 7-104*). The **chorda tympani,** a small branch of the facial nerve (cranial nerve VII), emerges from a small canal in the posterior wall and crosses the medial surface of the tympanic membrane.

Roof. The roof is a thin plate of bone termed the ***tegmen tympani.*** It separates the middle ear below from the middle cranial fossa above.

Floor. The floor is also a thin plate of bone that separates the middle ear above from the jugular bulb below.

Posterior Wall. The posterior wall contains an opening on its upper aspect termed the *aditus.* The aditus is a short canal that leads posteriorly to the mastoid antrum. The mastoid antrum communicates further with the air cells that honeycomb the interior of the mastoid process.

Lower on the posterior wall is a short conical projection, the **pyramid.** The pyramid houses the tiny belly of the stapedius muscle, and its tendon passes through the apex of the pyramid to enter the middle ear cavity and insert into the stapes.

Lateral to the pyramid is the tiny opening for the chorda tympani nerve. The canal extends posteriorly to the facial canal containing the facial nerve.

Anterior Wall. This wall is narrow and consists of two openings separated by a thin wedge of bone. The larger, lower opening is the medial opening of the **auditory tube.** It leads anteriorly and medially to the nasopharynx and will be discussed shortly. The smaller, upper opening transmits the tendon of the **tensor tympani muscle,** and it too is discussed shortly.

Medial Wall. The medial wall separates the middle ear cavity from the deeper inner ear (*Figure 7-105*). Two components of the inner ear encroach as bony projections on the medial wall. The **promontory** is a rounded projection formed by the underlying cochlea. Superiorly, another prominence is formed by the underlying lateral semicircular canal.

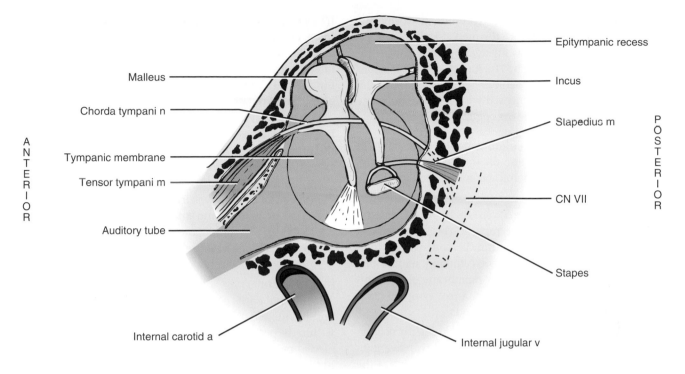

Epitympanic recess

Malleus

Incus

Chorda tympani n

Stapedius m

Tympanic membrane

Tensor tympani m

CN VII

Auditory tube

Stapes

Internal carotid a

Internal jugular v

ANTERIOR

POSTERIOR

Figure 7-104 Lateral wall of the right middle ear and middle ear ossicles.

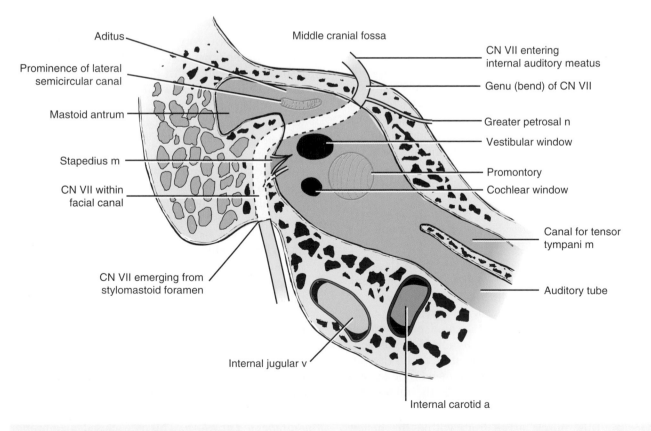

Aditus

Middle cranial fossa

CN VII entering internal auditory meatus

Prominence of lateral semicircular canal

Genu (bend) of CN VII

Mastoid antrum

Greater petrosal n

Vestibular window

Stapedius m

Promontory

CN VII within facial canal

Cochlear window

Canal for tensor tympani m

CN VII emerging from stylomastoid foramen

Auditory tube

Internal jugular v

Internal carotid a

Figure 7-105 Medial wall of the right middle ear.

Between these two features is a third prominence formed by the facial canal bulging out into the medial wall.

The **vestibular window** is an oval opening that communicates with the inner ear. The foot plate of the stapes covers this opening. The **cochlear window** is a smaller, inferior, rounded window covered with a thin membrane that communicates with the inner ear.

Ossicles. Three small articulating bones form a chain from the tympanic membrane on the lateral wall across the cavity to the vestibular window on the medial wall (see *Figure 7-104*).

Malleus (Hammer). This bone consists of a round head that projects upward into the epitympanic recess, two short processes, and a long process, or handle, that extends inferiorly onto the medial aspect of the tympanic membrane. The handle is fixed to the mucous membrane of the tympanic membrane. The tendon of the tensor tympani muscle inserts into the handle of the malleus.

Incus (Anvil). The incus is actually shaped like a tiny deciduous molar tooth with a crown, or body, and two diverging roots, or processes, one long and one short. The head of the malleus articulates with the body of the incus through a synovial joint. The long process of the incus projects medially.

Stapes (Stirrup). The stapes consist of a small head that articulates with the incus, a short neck that leads to an arch, and a flat, oval foot plate forming the base of the arch that covers the vestibular window. The tendon of the stapedius muscle inserts into the neck of the stapes.

Movements. Sound, in the form of waves, is funneled by the auricle and external auditory meatus to the tympanic membrane. Inward movements of the membrane move the attached handle of the malleus and, in turn, the chain of articulating ossicles. Ultimately, the foot plate of the stapes pushes into the vestibular window, and the fluid of the inner ear reacts by bulging out the membrane of the cochlear window below. The opposite sequence of events occurs when the tympanic membrane is moved outward.

Muscles. The movements of the ossicles are modified or dampened by the protective action of two tiny muscles, the tensory tympani and the stapedius muscles.

Tensor Tympani. This muscle originates from the cartilaginous and bony roof of the auditory tube. The muscle passes posteriorly and laterally in a tiny, bony canal that finally opens into the anterior wall of the tympanic cavity. The tendon of the muscle leaves the canal, passes around a bony pulley, and inserts into the handle of the malleus. By pulling on the handle of the malleus, it tenses the tympanic membrane; that is, it pulls the membrane inward. The muscle is supplied by a branch of the mandibular nerve (cranial nerve V-3).

Stapedius. This muscle arises from within the hollow, bony pyramid on the posterior wall of the middle ear cavity. Its tiny tendon passes through the pyramidal apex and inserts into the neck of the stapes. Upon contraction, the stapedius muscle pulls the anterior aspect of the foot plate laterally, thus dampen its action to counteract loud, low-tone sound. The stapedius muscle is supplied by a branch of the facial nerve (cranial nerve VII).

Nerve and Blood Supply. The sensory nerve supply to the mucosa of the tympanic cavity (including the medial aspect of the tympanic membrane) arises from the tympanic branch of the glossopharyngeal nerve (cranial nerve IX). The arterial supply is from tympanic branches of the posterior auricular and maxillary arteries, plus small "twigs" from the middle meningeal artery, the ascending pharyngeal artery, and the artery of the pterygoid canal.

Internal Ear

The internal ear is concerned with the reception of sound and balance. It is found medial to the middle ear cavity within the petrous temporal bone. The internal ear consists of two parts: (1) The **bony labyrinth** is an interconnecting system of twisted canals and is filled with a plasmalike fluid called *perilymph*. (2) The **membranous labyrinth** is suspended within the perilymph of the bony labyrinth, and it too is filled with fluid called the *endolymph*.

Bony Labyrinth. The bony labyrinth is itself divisible into three parts (*Figure 7-106*).

1. The **vestibule** is a centrally located area that communicates with the other two areas of the internal ear and also communicates with the middle ear through the vestibular and cochlear windows.
2. The **cochlea** is the **hearing organ**. It communicates with the anterior aspect of the vestibule. The cochlea is shaped like the shell of a snail and consists of a bony core, or modiolus, around which is wrapped the cochlear canal (two and three-fourths turns). Radiating screwlike from the central core is a bony shelf, or lamina, which is further continued outward by a basilar membrane. These effectively divide the cochlear canal into two halves, or scalae, which communicate at the apex of the cochlea. The upper half (vestibular scala) communicates with the vestibule. The lower half (scala tympani) communicates with the middle ear through the membrane-covered cochlear window. The base of the cochlea is the end of the internal auditory meatus, which transmits the vestibulocochlear nerve.
3. The **semicircular canals** are the receptor organs of **balance**. There are three canals that occupy three planes in space: superior, lateral, and posterior canals. Each canal communicates with the vestibule.

Membranous Labyrinth. This is a closed membranous system of tubes suspended within the bony labyrinth. The

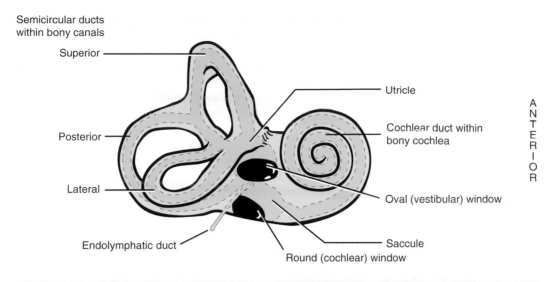

Semicircular ducts
within bony canals

Superior

Posterior

Lateral

Endolymphatic duct

Utricle

Cochlear duct within
bony cochlea

Oval (vestibular) window

Saccule

Round (cochlear) window

ANTERIOR

Figure 7-106 Structures of the inner ear.

membranous labyrinth occupies the bony canals as membranous ducts, that is, the cochlear duct and the semicircular ducts. There are two membranous expansions within the vestibule: the utricle and the saccule.

Vestibulocochlear Nerve (Cranial Nerve VIII). The vestibulocochlear nerve leaves the brainstem and passes laterally into the internal auditory meatus to enter the petrous temporal bone. At the lateral limit of the meatus, the nerve divides into a cochlear portion, which passes anteriorly to the cochlea, and a vestibular portion, which passes posteriorly to the vestibule and the semicircular canals.

Cochlear Nerve (Hearing). The cochlear nerve enters the base of the modiolus through the spiral canal, and within the canal the nerve dilates as the **spiral ganglion.** The ganglion contains the cochlear nerve cell bodies, and these, in turn, give rise to short, peripheral fibers that end on receptor organs within the cochlear duct (**spiral organ of Corti**). Central nerve processes pass back through the internal auditory meatus as the cochlear component of cranial nerve VIII to the brainstem. Ascending pathways within the brainstem pass the stimulus up to the auditory cortex of the temporal lobe where sound is perceived.

Vestibular Nerve (Balance). The cell bodies of the vestibular nerve are found within the vestibular ganglion in the internal auditory meatus. Peripheral fibers pass to the saccule, utricle, and semicircular canals, where they end on receptor cells. Movements of the head produce corresponding movements in the endolymph, which stimulates the receptor cells. These, in turn, stimulate the peripheral nerve endings of the vestibular ganglion. Central processes of the ganglion convey the stimulus to the brainstem and ascending pathways. The pathways within the

central nervous system are complex, and the nerve fibers communicate with the cerebellum and motor nuclei, which activate muscles of the body in response to incoming vestibular stimuli.

The Auditory (Pharyngotympanic) Tube

The auditory air tube runs from the lateral aspect of the nasopharynx to the anterior wall of the tympanic cavity (see *Figures 7-81, 7-102, 7-104,* and *7-105*). The tube passes backward, laterally, and slightly upward.

Components. The lateral 1.2 cm comprise a **bony canal** lined with mucosa. The medial 2.5 cm consists of a **cartilaginous** and **membranous tube** that occupies a bony gutter on the base of the skull. The cartilage in cross section is J-shaped, and it forms the roof of the tube and the medial wall. The floor and the lateral wall of the tube consists of membrane.

Functions. The auditory tube serves to equalize air pressure on both sides of the tympanic membrane. Normally, the membranous walls of the tube lie collapsed against the rigid cartilaginous walls, thus closing the lumen of the tube. The tensor veli palatini muscle originates from the membrane of the tube. When the muscle contracts, as in swallowing and yawning, the membrane is pulled away from the cartilage and the lumen of the tube is opened.

Sudden changes in atmospheric pressure (as in ascension in an elevator or airplane) can painfully stretch the tympanic membrane. Swallowing contracts the tensor veli palatini muscle. This in turn drags the lumen of the auditory tube open and allows the atmospheric and middle-ear pressures to equalize.

Nerve and Blood Supply. The mucosa of the auditory tube is supplied by sensory branches of the tympanic and pharyngeal branches of the glossopharyngeal nerve (cranial nerve IX). The arterial supply is from "twigs" of the ascending pharyngeal and middle meningeal arteries and the artery of the pterygoid canal.

The Facial Nerve (Cranial Nerve VII)

The facial nerve is studied here because it is so closely related to the middle and inner ear structures (see *Figures 7-104* and *7-105*). The facial nerve arises from the brainstem as a large motor root and a mixed special sensory taste and parasympathetic secretory nerve called the *nervus intermedius.* The two roots enter the internal auditory meatus collectively as the facial nerve. At the lateral limit of the meatus, the facial nerve enters the facial canal, which carries the nerve laterally above the vestibule to the medial wall of the middle ear. Here the canal and nerve turn abruptly as a sharp bend (genu) and pass posteriorly deep to the medial wall. On reaching the posterior wall of the middle ear, the canal dives inferiorly and exits from the skull through the stylomastoid foramen. At this point the facial nerve leaves the skull, enters the parotid gland, and breaks up into five sets of branches, which supply the muscles of facial expression. The cell bodies of the special sensation taste component lie in the geniculate ganglion located within the genu (bend) of the facial nerve within the facial canal.

Branches of the Facial Nerve

Greater Petrosal Nerve. This slender branch arises from the genu of the facial nerve. It passes medially and anteriorly through a small canal in the petrous temporal bone. The nerve emerges through a hiatus on the anterior petrosal slope within the middle cranial fossa of the skull (see *Figure 7-27*). Here it tracks to the foramen lacerum, drops through, and then turns anteriorly through the pterygoid canal to synapse within the pterygopalatine ganglion (see *Figure 7-60, A*). The greater petrosal nerve carries (1) parasympathetic motor fibers to the **lacrimal gland** and **minor glands** of the oral and nasal cavities and (2) special sensory taste fibers from the palate.

Nerve to Stapedius. This nerve branches from the descending portion of the facial canal and passes anteriorly to the stapedius muscle within the pyramid.

Chorda Tympani Nerve. This, too, arises from the descending part of the facial nerve and passes forward to enter the middle ear. Here it continues anteriorly,

---

CLINICAL NOTES

Otitis Externa

This translates as an inflammation of the external ear, which can develop in the skin of the external auditory meatus. It can be caused by obsessive poking of the ear canal with a finger, which may cause a skin furuncle. It can also be caused by retained water in the ear after swimming. Water is trapped within the external auditory meatus. Normally the water drains spontaneously or after a vigorous hop on one foot. Retained water in the canal and attempts to clear it can result in an inflamed canal or "swimmer's ear."

Otitis Media

This is an infection and inflammation of the middle ear. The resulting fluid, or exudate, from the inflamed mucosal lining of the middle ear cavity place outward painful pressure on the tympanic membrane. Migrating infection from the nasopharynx passes through the auditory tube to infect the middle ear. This is especially true of children, who demonstrate a higher incidence of otitis media because their auditory tubes are relatively shorter in comparison to those of adults. Chronic, untreated otitis media can lead to impaired hearing because of scarring and more limited movements of the ossicles within the middle ear.

Ruptured Tympanic Membrane

Otitis media and fluid pressure can rupture or tear the tympanic membrane. Small tears generally heal without a loss of hearing. Occasionally, pressure is relieved surgically with a small incision to release the buildup of fluid and exudate in the middle ear. The incision is made in the posteroinferior aspect of the eardrum to avoid the more vascular pars flaccida above and to avoid the handle of the malleus and chorda tympani nerve.

Mastoiditis

The middle ear communicates posteriorly with the mastoid air cells via a short canal termed the *aditus*. Infection within the labyrinth of mastoid air cells is difficult to eradicate. Before antibiotics were available, an infected mastoid had to be surgically opened and drained.

Internal Ear Infections

Infections from the middle ear can track to the inner ear through the oval and round windows and can result in tinnitus (a buzzing or ringing sound), loss of hearing, and vertigo.

crossing the medial aspect of the tympanic membrane and passing over the medial aspect of the handle of the malleus. The nerve then leaves the middle ear through the petrotympanic fissure to enter the infratemporal region below the skull, where it joins the lingual nerve (see *Figure 7-53*).

The component fibers of the chorda tympani nerve are (1) parasympathetic secretory to the submandibular and sublingual glands and to the minor glands of the floor of the mouth and (2) special sensory taste fibers from the anterior two thirds of the tongue.

External Motor Branches. The facial nerve goes on to supply the muscles of facial expression, including the platysma muscle, the stylohyoid muscle, and the posterior belly of the digastric muscle.

Review Questions

1. The buccal artery is a branch of the
   _____.
   a. facial artery
   b. inferior alveolar artery
   c. superficial temporal artery
   d. transverse facial artery
   e. maxillary artery

2. All of the following are direct or eventual branches
   of the ophthalmic nerve (V-1) EXCEPT the
   _____.
   a. zygomatic nerve
   b. dorsal nasal nerve
   c. external nasal nerve
   d. posterior ethmoidal nerve
   e. lacrimal nerve

3. All of the following bones contribute to the bony
   orbit EXCEPT the _____.
   a. zygomatic bone
   b. temporal bone
   c. lacrimal bone
   d. sphenoid bone
   e. ethmoid bone

4. The three divisions of the trigeminal nerve pass
   through openings in the _____.
   a. sphenoid bone
   b. maxilla
   c. temporal bone
   d. frontal bone
   e. ethmoid bone

5. The common facial vein is formed by a union of
   the facial vein and the _____.
   a. anterior jugular vein
   b. anterior division of the retromandibular vein
   c. posterior auricular vein
   d. posterior division of the retromandibular vein
   e. external jugular vein

6. Numbness at the tip of the nose could indicate a
   problem with the _____.
   a. anterior ethmoidal nerve
   b. long buccal nerve
   c. infratrochlear nerve
   d. zygomaticofacial nerve
   e. nasopalatine nerve

7. Damage to the oculomotor nerve (cranial nerve
   III) would affect all of the following EXCEPT the
   _____.
   a. ability to turn the eye upward
   b. ability to turn the eye downward

   c. ability to turn the eye medially
   d. ability to focus on distant objects
   e. ability to constrict the pupil

8. As a result of an inadvertent injection of local
   anesthetic into the parotid gland, a patient
   exhibits a transient facial paralysis. On the
   affected side, the patient is unable to perform
   all of the following movements EXCEPT
   _____.
   a. opening the eyelids
   b. closing the eyelids
   c. opening the lips
   d. closing the lips
   e. pushing food lingually onto the occlusal
      surfaces

9. Branches of the maxillary artery supply all of the
   following EXCEPT the _____.
   a. soft palate
   b. middle ear
   c. mandibular teeth
   d. maxillary sinus
   e. anterior nasal septum

10. The parotid gland is separated from the
    infratemporal fossa and submandibular gland by
    the _____.
    a. stylohyoid ligament
    b. sphenomandibular ligament
    c. stylomandibular ligament
    d. pterygomandibular ligament
    e. temporomandibular ligament

11. Depression of the mandible is accomplished by
    bilateral contractions of the _____.
    a. posterior fibers of the temporalis muscles
    b. deep fibers of the masseter muscles
    c. medial pterygoid muscles
    d. inferior heads of the lateral pterygoid
       muscles
    e. superior heads of the lateral pterygoid
       muscles

12. A patient is requested to say "Ah," and the uvula
    is pulled to the left. The cranial nerve that may be
    damaged is the _____.
    a. right mandibular division of the trigeminal
       nerve
    b. left hypoglossal nerve
    c. right cranial accessory nerve traveling with the
       right vagus nerve
    d. right glossopharyngeal nerve
    e. left facial nerve

13. All of the following muscles are active during the act of sucking EXCEPT the _____.
a. orbicularis oris muscle
b. levator veli palatini muscle
c. palatoglossus muscle
d. palatopharyngeus muscle
e. buccinator muscle

14. The lingual vein usually drains into the _____.
a. retromandibular vein
b. common facial vein
c. pterygoid plexus of veins
d. facial vein
e. internal jugular vein

15. Which of the following statements concerning the lacrimal apparatus is TRUE?
a. Tears are released by small ducts into the medial side of the superior fornix of the conjunctival sac.
b. The maxillary artery supplies the lacrimal gland.
c. The lacrimal gland is supplied by postsynaptic parasympathetic branches of the pterygopalatine ganglion.
d. Tears are carried to the middle meatus of the nose by the nasolacrimal duct.
e. The lacrimal gland is wrapped around the medial free border of the levator palpebrae superioris muscle.

16. The narrowest portion of the larynx is the _____.
a. piriform recess
b. vestibule
c. rima glottidis
d. laryngeal inlet
e. infraglottic cavity

17. Choose one correct alternative. The tympanic membrane _____.
a. is convex laterally
b. separates the middle ear from the internal ear
c. is tensed by a muscle supplied by cranial nerve V-3
d. is supplied on its lateral wall by sensory branches of cranial nerve IX
e. is supplied on its medial wall by sensory branches of cranial nerve V-3

18. The tensor veli palatini muscles are supplied by motor branches of cranial nerve _____.
a. V-3
b. VII
c. IX
d. XI via X
e. XII

19. The pterygoid plexus of veins receives tributaries from all the following EXCEPT the _____.
a. mandibular teeth
b. maxillary teeth
c. muscles of mastication
d. tongue
e. cavernous sinus

20. Posterior ethmoidal air cells normally drain to the _____.
a. medial wall of the orbit
b. superior meatus of the nose
c. middle meatus of the nose
d. inferior meatus of the nose
e. sphenoethmoidal recess

21. The glossopharyngeal nerve supplies all of the following structures or areas EXCEPT the _____.
a. mucosa of the middle ear
b. parotid gland
c. carotid sinus
d. taste buds of the posterior third of the tongue
e. palatopharyngeus muscle

22. Which of the following statements concerning the auditory tube is FALSE?
a. It opens into the nasopharynx.
b. It can transmit infection to the middle ear and mastoid antrum.
c. Its lateral component resides within a bony canal.
d. Its opening to the pharynx is normally closed.
e. The palatopharyngeus muscles contract to open the auditory tube.

23. Sensitivity to loud, low-tone sounds indicates possible damage to _____.
a. the great auricular nerve
b. a branch of the facial nerve
c. a branch of the mandibular nerve
d. a branch of the glossopharyngeal nerve
e. a branch of the vagus nerve

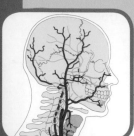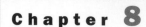

Chapter 8

Systemic Anatomy of the Head and Neck

1. Arteries 358

2. Veins.. 358

3. Lymphatics and Lymph Nodes 358

4. Cranial Nerves and Cranial Autonomics 368

1. Arteries

The arteries that ultimately supply the head and neck originate from the **subclavian and common carotid arteries.** On the right side, the common carotid and subclavian arteries originate from the **brachiocephalic artery** just posterior to the right sternoclavicular joint in the root of the neck. On the left side, the common carotid and subclavian arteries originate separately from the **arch of the aorta** within the superior mediastinum.

The arteries of the head and neck are illustrated in *Figure 8-1* and listed in *Table 8-1*. Regional detailed descriptions of the arteries are found in Chapter 7.

2. Veins

The venous drainage of the head and neck may be conveniently grouped into a set of *external* or *superficial veins* and a set of *deep* or *intracranial veins*. The superficial veins drain to either the external jugular vein or the internal jugular vein; the deep veins drain to the internal jugular vein.

The **external jugular vein** picks up tributaries from posterior superficial structures of the head and face and descends along the sternocleidomastoid muscle.

Inferiorly, it enters the posterior triangle and joins the **subclavian vein.**

The **internal jugular vein** drains intracranial structures, leaves the skull through the jugular foramen, and descends in the neck within the carotid sheath. At the root of the neck, it joins the **subclavian vein** to form the large **brachiocephalic vein.** In the superior mediastinum the right and left brachiocephalic veins unite to form the **superior vena cava,** which, in turn, drains to the **right atrium** of the heart.

The veins of the head and neck are illustrated in *Figures 8-2* and *8-3* and listed in *Table 8-2*. Regional detailed descriptions of the veins are found in Chapter 7.

3. Lymphatics and Lymph Nodes

Knowledge of the routes by which lymph flows from the head and neck back to the venous system is essential to understand lymphatic spread of infections and cancer (*Table 8-3*). For a general discussion of the lymphatic system, see Chapter 1, Section 6.

The lymphatics of the head and neck, as in other areas of the body, drain toward groups of lymph nodes. The nodes act as *filters* and add *lymphocytes* to the lymph fluid. In the head and neck, the lymph nodes may be conveniently grouped into (1) a horizontal ring of superficial nodes, (2) a horizontal ring of deep nodes, and (3) two vertical chains of deep cervical nodes. Both horizontal rings drain to the two deep vertical chains (*Figure 8-4*).

SUPERFICIAL RING OF NODES

The superficial ring surrounds the transition area of neck to head and is arranged into five main groups (*Figure 8-5*; see *Table 8-3*). These nodes are palpable when infected.

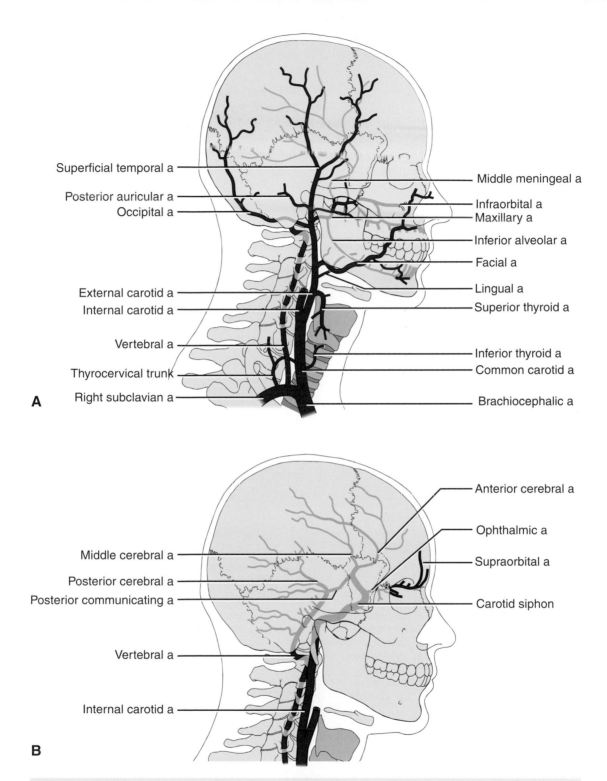

Figure 8-1 Arteries of the head and neck. **A,** Right external carotid artery and its branches. **B,** Right internal carotid and vertebral arteries and their branches within the skull.

Submental Nodes

The submental lymph nodes are located under the chin within the submental triangle and on the surface of the mylohyoid muscle.

Afferent Vessels. The submental nodes receive lymphatics, which drain (1) the lower lip, (2) the chin, (3) the tip of the tongue, and (4) the anterior floor of the mouth.

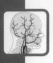

Efferent Vessels. The submental nodes drain either (1) to the submandibular nodes or (2) directly to the jugulo-omohyoid node of the deep cervical chain.

Submandibular Nodes

The submandibular nodes lie within the submandibular region, scattered over the surface of the submandibular salivary gland and in the interval between the salivary gland and the medial surface of the mandible. An exten-sion of the submandibular group overlies the cheek supe-riorly as the *buccal group of nodes.*

Afferent Vessels. The submandibular nodes receive afferent vessels from the (1) submental nodes; (2) cheek, nose, and upper lip of the face; (3) maxillary teeth; (4) vestibular gingivae; (5) mucosa and gingivae of the hard palate; (6) posterior floor of the mouth; and (7) tongue.

TABLE 8-1

Arteries of the Head and Neck

Artery	Origin	Branches	Structures Supplied
I. Vertebral	Subclavian a	1. Spinal 2. Muscular 3. Meningeal 4. Anterior and posterior spinal 5. Basilar (union of right and left vertebral)	Cervical spinal cord via intervertebral foramina Suboccipital mm Dura and bone of posterior cranial fossa Cervical spinal cord via foramen magnum Brain

II. Thyrocervical trunk	Subclavian a	1. Suprascapular
		2. Transverse cervical
		3. Inferior thyroid
		    (a) Muscular
		    (b) Ascending cervical
		    (c) Inferior laryngeal
		    (d) Pharyngeal
		    (e) Tracheal
		    (f) Glandular
			Neck and back mm
			Neck mm
			
			Infrahyoid strap mm of the neck
			Deep mm of neck and spinal cord
			Larynx
			Pharynx
			Upper trachea
			Lower portion of thyroid gland

III. Costocervical trunk	Subclavian a	1. Costal 2. Cervical	 First and second intercostal spaces
IV. Common carotid	Brachiocephalic (right side) a Arch of aorta (left side) a	1. Internal carotid 2. External carotid	Deep cervical structures and spinal cord Brain and orbit Face and jaws

A. Internal carotid	Common carotid a	1. Caroticotympanic
		2. Pterygoid
		3. Cavernous branches
		4. Hypophyseal
		5. Meningeal
		6. Ophthalmic
		    (a) Lacrimal
		
		    (b) Posterior ciliary
		    (c) Central artery of retina
		    (d) Supraorbital
		    (e) Posterior ethmoidal
		    (f) Anterior ethmoidal
		    (g) Supratrochlear
		    (h) Dorsal nasal
		7. Anterior choroidal
		8. Posterior communicating
		9. Anterior cerebral
		10. Middle cerebral
			Middle ear
			Pterygopalatine fossa via pterygoid canal
			Trigeminal ganglion, walls of cavernous sinus
			Hypophysis cerebri (pituitary gland)
			Bone and dura of anterior cranial fossa
			
			Zygomatic to face and temple, anterior ciliary to eye, glandular to lacrimal gland, palpebral branches to upper eyelid
			Eye
			Retina of eye (end a)
			Upper lid, forehead, and scalp
			Posterior ethmoidal air cells
			Anterior ethmoidal air cells and external nose
			Upper lid, forehead, and scalp
			Lacrimal sac, medial aspect of eyelids
			Brain
			Brain
			Terminal branch to brain
			Terminal branch to brain

mm, Muscles; *m,* muscle; *a,* artery.

TABLE 8-1

Arteries of the Head and Neck—cont'd

Artery	Origin	Branches	Structures Supplied
B. External carotid	Common carotid a	1. Superior thyroid	
		(a) Muscular	Sternomastoid mm
		(b) Superior laryngeal	Larynx
		(c) Glandular	Superior portion of thyroid gland
		2. Ascending pharyngeal	Pharynx, middle ear
		3. Lingual	
		(a) Dorsal lingual	Dorsum of posterior third of tongue
		(b) Sublingual	Floor of mouth, mm of tongue, sublingual gland
		4. Facial	
		(a) Ascending palatine	Soft palate, palatine tonsils, auditory tube
		(b) Tonsillar	Palatine tonsil and bed
		(c) Glandular	Submandibular gland
		(d) Submental	Structures of submental triangle
		(e) Inferior labial	Lower lip
		(f) Superior labial	Upper lip
		(g) Angular	Medial angle of eye
		5. Occipital	
		(a) Muscular	Sternocleidomastoid, posterior belly of digastric and stylohyoid mm
		(b) Mastoid	Mastoid air cells via mastoid foramen
		(c) Auricular	Posterior of auricle
		(d) Meningeal	Dura and bone of posterior cranial fossa via jugular foramen
		(e) Scalp	Occipital portion of scalp
		6. Posterior auricular	
		(a) Muscular	Sternocleidomastoid, posterior belly of digastric and stylohyoid mm
		(b) Glandular	Parotid gland
		7. Superficial temporal	(Terminal branch)
		(a) Transverse facial	Parotid gland and duct
		(b) Auricular	Auricle
		(c) Temporal	Lateral aspect of temple and scalp
		8. Maxillary	(Terminal branch)
		Part 1	
		(a) Deep auricular	EAM and lateral aspect of tympanic membrane
		(b) Anterior tympanic	Middle ear via petrotympanic fissure
		(c) Middle meningeal	Dura and bone of middle cranial fossa via foramen spinosum
		(d) Accessory meningeal	Dura and bone of middle cranial fossa and trigeminal ganglion via foramen ovale
		(e) Inferior alveolar	Mandibular teeth and mandible via mandibular canal
		(1) Mental	Lower lip, chin, and mandibular labial gingiva via mental foramen
		Part 2	
		(f) Temporal	Temporalis m
		(g) Pterygoid	Lateral and medial pterygoid mm
		(h) Masseteric	Masseter m via mandibular notch
		(i) Buccal	Buccinator m and cheek
		Part 3	
		(j) Palatine	
		(1) Greater palatine	Posterior of hard palate via greater palatine foramen
		(2) Lesser palatine	Soft palate via lesser palatine foramen
		(k) Pharyngeal	Roof of nasopharynx, sphenoidal sinus, and auditory tube via pharyngeal canal
		(l) Artery of pterygoid canal	Superior aspect of pharynx, auditory tube, and middle ear via pterygoid canal
		(m) Sphenopalatine	
		(1) Posterolateral nasal	Posterolateral wall of nasal cavity
		(2) Posterior septal	Nasal septum

EAM, External auditory meatus.

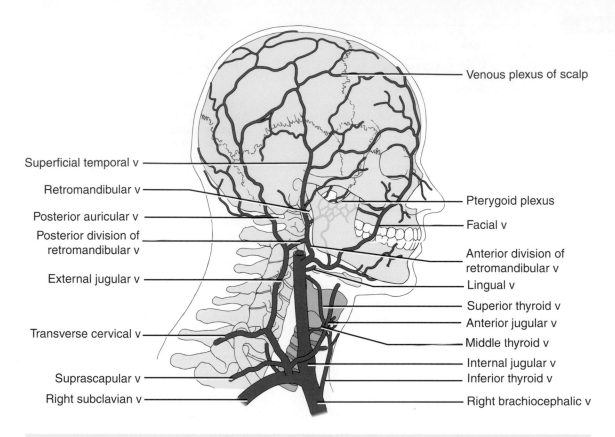

Venous plexus of scalp

Superficial temporal v

Retromandibular v

Posterior auricular v

Posterior division of
retromandibular v

External jugular v

Transverse cervical v

Suprascapular v

Right subclavian v

Pterygoid plexus

Facial v

Anterior division of
retromandibular v

Lingual v

Superior thyroid v

Anterior jugular v

Middle thyroid v

Internal jugular v

Inferior thyroid v

Right brachiocephalic v

Figure 8-2 Superficial veins of the head and neck.

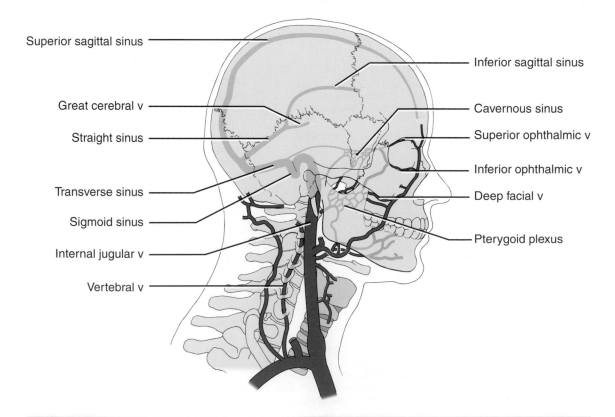

Superior sagittal sinus

Great cerebral v

Straight sinus

Transverse sinus

Sigmoid sinus

Internal jugular v

Vertebral v

Inferior sagittal sinus

Cavernous sinus

Superior ophthalmic v

Inferior ophthalmic v

Deep facial v

Pterygoid plexus

Figure 8-3 Deep veins of the head and neck and communications with facial vein.

TABLE 8-2

Veins of the Head and Neck

Artery	Termination	Tributaries	Areas Drained
I. Superficial Veins			
A. Facial	Common facial	1. Supratrochlear	Scalp, forehead, upper eyelid
		2. Supraorbital	Scalp, forehead, upper eyelid
		3. Nasal	Scalp, forehead, upper eyelid
		4. Superior labial	Upper lip
		5. Inferior labial	Lower lip
		6. Muscular	Masseter and buccinator mm
		7. Submental	Submental structures
		8. Tonsillar	Palatine tonsil and tonsillar bed
		9. Submandibular	Submandibular gland
B. Superficial temporal	Retromandibular	1. Scalp	Anterior and posterior regions of scalp
		2. Glandular	Parotid gland
		3. Auricular	External ear
		4. Articular	Temporomandibular joint
		5. Transverse facial	Side of face and cheek
C. Pterygoid plexus of veins	Maxillary veins and small contribution to cavernous sinus	1. Infraorbital	Lower eyelid, external nose, upper lip, maxillary teeth
		2. Sphenopalatine	Nasal cavity, anterior of hard palate
		3. Muscular	Muscles of mastication
		4. Buccal	Cheek and buccal mandibular gingivae
		5. Palatine	
		(a) Greater palatine	Posterior two thirds of hard palate
		(b) Lesser palatine	Soft palate
		6. Inferior alveolar	Mandibular teeth
		(a) Mental	Lower lip, chin, mandibular labial gingivae
		7. Deep facial	A direct communication with the facial
D. Maxillary	Retromandibular	Pterygoid plexus	See above
E. Retro-mandibular	Anterior and posterior divisions	1. Superficial temporal	See above
		2. Maxillary	See above
F. Common facial	Internal jugular	1. Facial	See above
		2. Retromandibular (anterior division)	See above
G. External jugular	Subclavian	1. Retromandibular (posterior division)	See above
		2. Posterior auricular	Scalp posterior to ear, external ear
		3. Transverse cervical	Neck
		4. Suprascapular	Neck and upper back
		5. Anterior jugular	Structures of anterior triangle of neck
II. Deep Veins			
A. External cerebral	Intracranial venous sinuses	1. External cerebral v	Brain
		2. Arachnoid granulations	Brain
B. Internal cerebral	Great cerebral	External cerebral v	See above
C. Superior sagittal sinus	Right transverse sinus	1. Great cerebral v	CSF of subarachnoid space
		2. Inferior sagittal sinus	See above
D. Inferior sagittal sinus	Straight sinus	External cerebral vv	See above
E. Straight sinus	Left transverse sinus	1. Great cerebral v	See above
		2. Inferior sagittal sinus	See above

mm, Muscles; *CSF,* cerebrospinal fluid; *v,* vein; *vv,* veins

Continued

TABLE 8-2

Veins of the Head and Neck—cont'd

Artery	Termination	Tributaries	Areas Drained
F. Lateral sinus (paired)	Sigmoid sinus	1. Right-superior sagittal sinus 2. Left-straight sinus 3. Cerebral and cerebellar	See previous entry
G. Sigmoid sinuses (paired)	Internal jugular	1. Lateral sinuses 2. Superior petrosal sinus	See previous entry Cavernous sinus
H. Cavernous sinus (paired)	Superior petrosal sinus Inferior petrosal sinus	1. Ophthalmic 2. Sphenoparietal sinuses 3. External cerebral v 4. Pterygoid plexuses (small portion) 5. Intercavernous sinus	Eyeball and orbital contents Dura and meningeal v of middle cranial fossa Brain Infratemporal structures Joins right and left cavernous sinuses
I. Superior petrosal sinus (paired)	Sigmoid sinus	Cavernous sinus	See above
J. Inferior petrosal sinus (paired)	Internal jugular	Cavernous sinus	See above
K. Occipital sinus	Sigmoid sinus	Cerebral veins	Cerebellum
L. Basilar sinus	Vertebral plexus	—	Joins right and left inferior petrosal sinuses
M. Middle meningeal	Variable pterygoid plexus via foramen spinosus, foramen ovale; sphenoparietal sinus; cavernous sinus	1. Meningeal 2. Cerebral	Meninges of brain Brain
N. Emissary v	External v of skull via emissary foramina	—	Venous sinuses
O. Diploic v	Intracranial venous sinuses	—	Diplöe of skull bones
III. Internal Jugular	Brachiocephalic	1. Intracranial venous sinuses 2. Lingual 3. Pharyngeal v 4. Occipital 5. Common facial 6. Superior thyroid 7. Middle thyroid	See above Tongue Pharynx Posterior scalp See above Thyroid gland and larynx Thyroid gland and larynx
IV. Vertebral	Brachiocephalic	Basilar sinus	See above
V. Inferior Thyroid	Brachiocephalic		Thyroid gland and larynx

v, Vein.

Efferent Vessels. The submandibular nodes, in turn, drain to the nodes of the deep cervical chain.

Superficial Parotid Nodes
The superficial parotid nodes lie superficial to the capsule of the parotid gland, clustered about the superficial temporal and transverse facial arteries.

Afferent Vessels. The superficial parotid nodes receive afferent vessels from (1) the eyelids, (2) the temples, (3) the prominence of the cheek, and (4) the auricle.

Efferent Vessels. Efferent channels drain to (1) deep parotid nodes or (2) deep cervical nodes.

Deep Parotid Nodes
The deep parotid nodes lie within the parotid gland.

TABLE 8-3

Lymph Nodes of the Head and Neck

Lymph Node	Structures Drained (Afferents)	Efferents
Superficial Horizontal Ring		
Submental	Lower lip, chin, tip of tongue, anterior floor of mouth	Submandibular nodes, jugulo-omohyoid nodes
Submandibular	Submental nodes, cheek, nose, upper lip, maxillary teeth, vestibular gingivae, mucosa and gingivae of the hard palate, posterior floor of mouth, lateral aspects of anterior two thirds of tongue	Nodes of deep cervical chain
Parotid (Preauricular)		
Superficial	Eyelids, temples, prominence of the cheek, auricle	Deep parotid nodes, deep cervical nodes
Deep	Middle ear, external auditory meatus, soft palate, posterior aspect of nasal cavity, superficial parotid nodes	Deep cervical nodes
Mastoid (retroauricular)	Scalp, auricle	Deep cervical nodes
Occipital	Posterior scalp	Deep cervical nodes
Deep Horizontal Ring		
Retropharyngeal	Posterior nasal cavity, nasopharynx, soft palate, middle ear, external auditory meatus	Deep cervical nodes
Paratracheal, pretracheal, prelaryngeal, and infrahyoid	Larynx, trachea, pharynx, esophagus	Deep cervical nodes
Deep Cervical Vertical Chain		
Jugulodigastric, Jugulo-omohyoid, and other nodes of the cervical chain	Entire chain receives afferents from the superficial horizontal ring of nodes and the deep horizontal ring of nodes	Left side: joins thoracic duct at junction of left subclavian and internal jugular veins Right side: joins right subclavian and right bronchomediastinal lymph trunks to enter junction of right subclavian and right internal jugular veins

Afferent Vessels. The deep parotid nodes receive lymph drainage from (1) the middle ear and external auditory meatus, (2) the soft palate, (3) the posterior aspect of the nasal cavity, and (4) the superficial parotid nodes.

Efferent Vessels. Efferent vessels drain to the deep cervical lymph nodes.

Retroauricular (Mastoid) Nodes

The retroauricular nodes lie over the mastoid process in proximity to the posterior auricular artery.

Afferent Vessels. The retroauricular nodes receive drainage from (1) the scalp and (2) the auricle.

Efferent Vessels. The nodes, in turn, drain to the deep cervical nodes.

Occipital Nodes

The occipital nodes lie just below the superior nuchal line atop the trapezius muscle and in proximity to the occipital artery.

Afferent Vessels. The occipital nodes receive lymphatics from the scalp.

Efferent Vessels. The efferent vessels drain to the deep cervical nodes.

DEEP RING OF LYMPH NODES

A deeper horizontal group of lymph nodes surrounds and drains the visceral structures of the neck. The deep ring, in turn, drains outwardly to the vertical chain of deep cervical nodes.

Retropharyngeal Nodes

The retropharyngeal nodes lie within the retropharyngeal space, that is, the fascial space between the posterior wall of the pharynx and the prevertebral fascia of the vertebral unit.

Afferent Vessels. The retropharyngeal nodes receive afferents from (1) the posterior nasal cavity and nasopharynx,

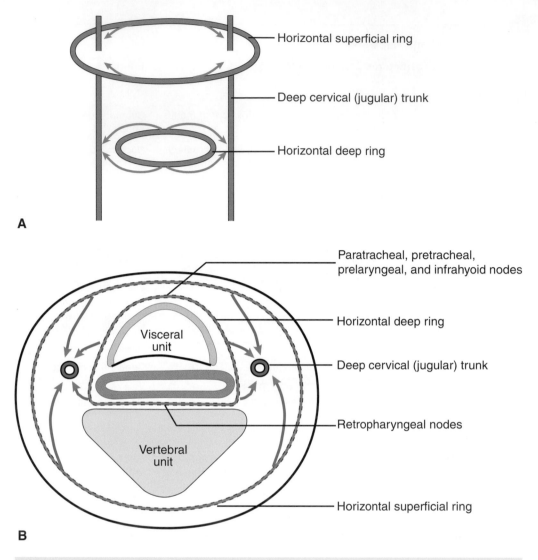

Figure 8-4 A, Scheme of lymphatic drainage of head and neck. **B,** Coronal section through the upper neck to show scheme of lymphatic drainage to deep cervical trunk.

(2) the soft palate, and (3) the middle ear and external auditory meatus.

Efferent Vessels. The efferent vessels drain to the upper group of deep cervical nodes.

Paratracheal, Pretracheal, Prelaryngeal, and Infrahyoid Nodes

The paratracheal, pretracheal, prelaryngeal, and infrahyoid nodes lie lateral and anterior to the visceral structures of the neck.

Afferent Vessels. The paratracheal, pretracheal, prelaryngeal, and infrahyoid nodes receive afferents from (1) the larynx and trachea and (2) the pharynx and esophagus.

Efferent Vessels. The efferent vessels drain to the deep cervical nodes.

DEEP CERVICAL (JUGULAR) VERTICAL CHAIN

The deep cervical chains descend from the base of the skull down to the root of the neck, and they parallel the courses of the right and left internal jugular veins. The deep cervical chain receives afferent drainage from the nodes of the superficial ring and the deeper visceral ring of lymph nodes. As the deep cervical chains approach their terminations, they form the right and left jugular lymph trunks.

On the left side, the jugular trunk joins the thoracic duct or enters the junction of the subclavian vein and internal jugular vein independently. *On the right side*, the

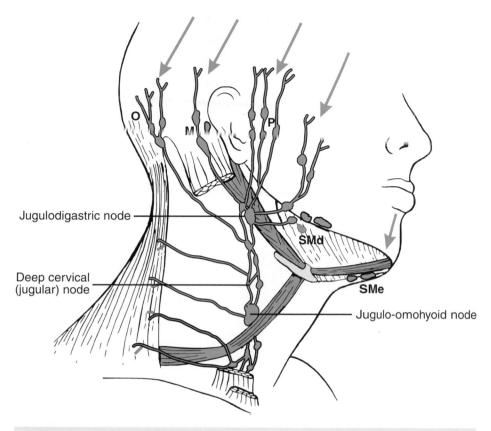

Figure 8-5 Lymphatic drainage of the face. *SMe*, Submental nodes; *SMd*, submandibular nodes; *P*, parotid (preauricular) nodes; *M*, mastoid (postauricular) nodes; *O*, occipital nodes.

right jugular, subclavian, and bronchomediastinal lymph trunks may join to form a common right lymphatic duct, which, in turn, empties to the confluence of the right subclavian and internal jugular veins. Alternatively, the right jugular trunk may independently enter the venous system at the same point.

Two large nodes are singled out in the deep cervical chain: (1) the jugulodigastric and (2) jugulo-omohyoid nodes.

DRAINAGE OF SPECIFIC STRUCTURES AND AREAS

Teeth
The maxillary teeth drain to vessels that pass to the face via the infraorbital canal and then pass inferiorly to enter the submandibular nodes.

The mandibular dental lymphatics drain backward through the mandibular canal and end in the deep cervical nodes.

Gingivae
The vestibular gingivae of the mandibular and maxillary arches drain to the submandibular nodes.

Mandibular lingual gingivae and the mucosa of the floor of the mouth drain to the submandibular nodes or directly to the deep cervical chain. The anterior segment drains initially to the submental nodes.

The maxillary palatal gingivae and the palatal mucosa drain to the submandibular or to the retropharyngeal nodes.

Lips
The upper lip drains to the submandibular nodes; the lower lip drains to the submental nodes.

Tongue
The tip of the tongue drains to the submental lymph nodes, the lateral aspects of the anterior two thirds drain to the submandibular nodes, and the medial portion of the anterior two thirds drain directly to the deep cervical nodes (*Figure 8-6*).

The posterior third of the tongue drains posteriorly to the retropharyngeal group of lymph nodes.

There is some crossing over the midline of lymphatic drainage of the tongue. Thus a lesion on one side of the tongue may spread to the opposite side via crossing lymphatics.

367

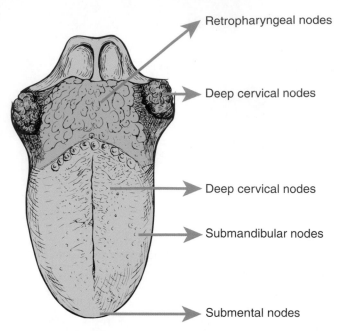

Retropharyngeal nodes

Deep cervical nodes

Deep cervical nodes

Submandibular nodes

Submental nodes

Figure 8-6 Drainage of lymph from various areas of the tongue and palatine tonsils.

Palatine Tonsils

The palatine tonsils drain to the jugulodigastric node of the deep cervical chain.

Nasal Cavity, Paranasal Air Sinuses, and Nasopharynx

The anterior portion of the nasal cavity drains to the submandibular nodes. The posterior nasal cavity, sinuses, and nasopharynx drain directly to the deep cervical chain or indirectly via the deep parotid nodes or the retropharyngeal nodes.

Ear

Drainage of the auricle and external auditory meatus may be to the retroauricular or deep parotid nodes or directly to the deep cervical chain. The middle ear drains to the deep cervical chain.

Larynx and Trachea

The lymphatics of the larynx above the vocal cords drain initially to the infrahyoid nodes or directly to the deep cervical chain. The laryngeal lymphatic vessels below the vocal cords drain to the prelaryngeal and pretracheal nodes or directly to the deep cervical chain.

Lymphatic vessels of the trachea pass to the pretracheal and paratracheal nodes or pass directly to the deep cervical chain.

Pharynx and Esophagus

The lymphatic vessels of the pharynx and esophagus drain to the retropharyngeal or paratracheal nodes or may pass directly to the deep cervical nodes.

4. Cranial Nerves and Cranial Autonomics

CRANIAL NERVES

A general description of the nervous system is found in Chapter 1, Section 7, and a description of the brain and attached cranial nerves is presented in Chapter 7, Section 2. In addition, a description of each cranial nerve is given as it appears in the various regions of the head. A summary of the cranial nerves is presented in *Table 8-4*.

Twelve pairs of cranial nerves arise from the brain. The first two nerves are remote from the brain and communicate with the brain via long extensions, or **tracts.** The remaining ten nerves arise directly from the brainstem.

Cranial nerves may perform one or more functions; possible functional components include (1) *somatic afferent* (general sensory from body structures), (2) *visceral afferent* (visceroceptive from glands and viscera), (3) *special afferent* (special sensory smell, sight, taste, hearing, and balance), (4) *somatic efferent* (motor to muscles derived from somites), (5) *branchial efferent* (motor to muscles derived from branchial arches), and (6) *visceral efferent* (autonomic motor to smooth muscle and glands).

Cranial Nerve I: Olfactory Nerve

Functional Component. The **special sensation of smell** is the only functional component of the olfactory nerve (*Figure 8-7*). The olfactory nerve originates from bipolar olfactory cells within the nasal mucosa, where peripheral processes end as specialized smell receptors in the mucosa covering the superior concha and upper nasal septum. Central processes collect as 18 to 20 branches of the olfactory nerve proper. These pass upward through the *cribriform plate* to the anterior cranial fossa and enter the overlying *olfactory bulbs*. Here they synapse with *mitral cells*, and their central processes pass back along the *olfactory tract* to the olfactory area of the forebrain.

Cranial Nerve Test. Each nostril, in turn, is challenged with various common odors. The patient is blindfolded and asked to correctly identify the odor. Lesions of the olfactory system result in loss of smell (anosmia).

Cranial Nerve II: Optic Nerve

Functional Component. The **special sensation of sight** is the sole functional component of this cranial nerve (*Figure 8-8*). Classically (but incorrectly) the optic nerve is described as the section that passes posteriorly from the eyeball to the optic chiasma. Actually, the optic nerve proper is contained within the retina of the eye and originates from *rod cells* (nondiscriminating sight) and *cone cells* (discriminating sight and color). These receptor cells occupy the most external portion of the retina and receive incoming light. Central processes pass inward to synapse

TABLE 8-4

Cranial Nerves

Cranial Nerve	Skull Foramen	Brainstem Nucleus	Functional Components and Distribution
Olfactory I	Cribriform plate	Mitral cells in olfactory bulb	Special sensory smell
Optic II	Optic canal	Ganglion cells of retina	Special sensory vision
Oculomotor III	Superior orbital fissure	Oculomotor	Somatic motor to all extraocular mm except superior oblique and lateral rectus mm
		Edinger-Westphal	Visceral motor (parasympathetic) to sphincter pupillae and ciliary mm of eye
Trochlear IV	Superior orbital fissure	—	Somatic motor to superior oblique m
Trigeminal V	V-1 Superior orbital fissure	Trigeminal	General sensory from skin of face, scalp, mucosa of oral and nasal cavities and pharynx
	V-2 Foramen rotundum	Masticator	Branchial motor to mm of mastication, anterior digastric, mylohyoid, tensor tympani, and tensor veli palatini mm
	V-3 Foramen ovale		
Abducens VI	Superior orbital fissure	Abducens	Somatic motor to lateral rectus m
Facial VII	Internal auditory meatus, facial canal, and stylomastoid foramen	Gustatory	Special sensory taste anterior two thirds of tongue
		Trigeminal	General sensory small part of external ear and external auditory meatus
		Facial	Branchial motor to mm of facial expression, stylohyoid, posterior belly of digastric, and stapedius mm
		Superior salivatory	Visceral motor (parasympathetic) to all major and minor glands of head except parotid gland
Vestibulocochlear VIII	Internal auditory meatus	Cochlear	Special sensory hearing
		Vestibular	Special sensory balance
		Gustatory	Special sensory taste: posterior third of tongue
		Trigeminal	General sensory: posterior third of tongue, pharynx, middle ear
		Solitarius	Visceral sensory from carotid body and sinus
		Ambiguus	Branchial motor to stylopharyngeus m
		Inferior salivatory	Visceral motor (parasympathetic) to parotid gland
Vagus X	Jugular foramen	Gustatory	Special sensory taste from laryngeal inlet area
		Trigeminal	General sensation from small area of external ear
		Solitarius	Visceral sensory from pharynx, larynx, gut to left colic flexure, bronchial tree, heart
		Dorsal vagal	Visceral motor (parasympathetic) to thoracic, abdominal viscera
Accessory XI (cranial)	Jugular foramen (joined to cranial nerve X)	Ambiguus	Branchial motor to mm of larynx, pharynx, soft palate
Accessory XI (spinal)	Jugular foramen	Accessory	Branchial motor to sternocleidomastoid, trapezius mm
Hypoglossal XII	Hypoglossal canal	Hypoglossal	Somatic motor to extrinsic and intrinsic mm of tongue

mm, Muscles; *m,* muscle; *ant,* anterior.

with bipolar cells, which, in turn, synapse with *ganglionic cells* of the innermost layer. Central processes of the ganglionic cells collect and leave the eyeball as the optic nerve. The nerve, or tract, leaves the orbit through the optic canal, and right and left nerves join at the *optic chiasma.* Here the fibers originating from the medial (nasal) half of the retina decussate; the fibers of the lateral (temporal) half of the retina do not decussate. The optic tract continues posteriorly from the chiasma, and this ends in the *lateral geniculate body* of the thalamus, where the

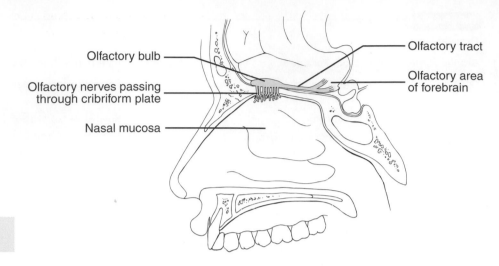

Figure 8-7 Olfactory nerve (cranial nerve I).

Olfactory bulb

Olfactory nerves passing through cribriform plate

Nasal mucosa

Olfactory tract

Olfactory area of forebrain

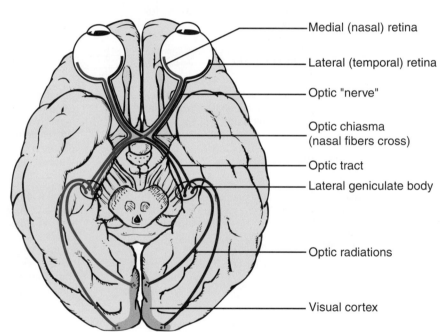

Medial (nasal) retina

Lateral (temporal) retina

Optic "nerve"

Optic chiasma (nasal fibers cross)

Optic tract

Lateral geniculate body

Optic radiations

Visual cortex

Figure 8-8 Optic nerve (cranial nerve II) and the optic pathway.

optic fibers synapse. Postsynaptic fibers pass posteriorly through optic radiations to the visual cortex in the occipital lobe of the cerebral hemispheres.

Cranial Nerve Test. In addition to standard eye tests for color perception and visual acuity, the visual fields are tested for blindness. Lesions may occur anywhere along the optic pathway and produce characteristic types of blindness.

Cranial Nerve III: Oculomotor Nerve

The oculomotor nerve arises from the interpeduncular fossa of the midbrain and passes forward to enter and traverse the cavernous sinus (*Figure 8-9*). The oculomotor nerve then enters the orbit through the superior orbital fissure.

Functional Components

1. **Somatic efferent fibers** originate from cell bodies of the *oculomotor nucleus* of the midbrain. Axons stream peripherally to supply the (1) levator palpebrae superioris muscle, (2) superior rectus muscle, (3) medial rectus muscle, (4) inferior rectus muscle, and (5) inferior oblique muscles of the eye.

2. ***Visceral* efferent (parasympathetic) cell bodies** occupy the *Edinger-Westphal nucleus* of the midbrain. Axons pass peripherally and synapse in the *ciliary ganglion*, and postsynaptic fibers supply the (1) ciliary muscles of the eye and (2) sphincter pupillae muscle of the eye.

Cranial Nerve Test. Lesions of the oculomotor nerve may reveal one or more of the following: (1) drooping of the

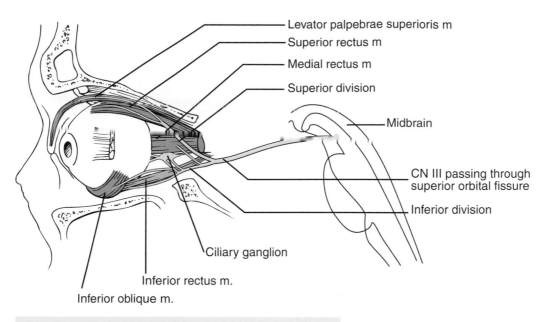

Figure 8-9 Oculomotor nerve (cranial nerve III) and branches.

upper lid (ptosis); (2) inability to move the eye upward, downward, and medially; (3) lack of pupil constriction when challenged with a light; and (4) inability to accommodate the eye for close vision.

Cranial Nerve IV: Trochlear Nerve

The trochlear nerve arises as a slender thread from the dorsal aspect of the midbrain and sweeps anteriorly under the cover of the free edge of the tentorium cerebelli (*Figure 8-10*). It pierces the dura of the triangular field, enters and traverses the cavernous sinus, and enters the orbit through the superior orbital fissure.

Functional Component. Somatic efferent cell bodies are found in the trochlear motor nucleus of the midbrain. Axons pass peripherally to supply only one muscle of the orbit—the superior oblique muscle.

Cranial Nerve Test. A lesion of the trochlear nerve shows no obvious dysfunction. The ability to turn the eye downward and laterally is hampered on the affected side and double vision (diplopia) results.

Cranial Nerve VI: Abducens Nerve

The abducens nerve is described out of sequence because it follows a course similar to those of cranial nerves III and IV (*Figure 8-11*).

The abducens nerve arises from the ventral aspect of the brainstem at the junction of the pons and the medulla. The nerve ascends on the clivus, pierces the dura, and enters the cavernous sinus. On passing through the sinus, the nerve enters the orbit through the superior orbital fissure.

Functional Component. Somatic efferent cell bodies of the abducens motor nucleus in the pons give rise to axons

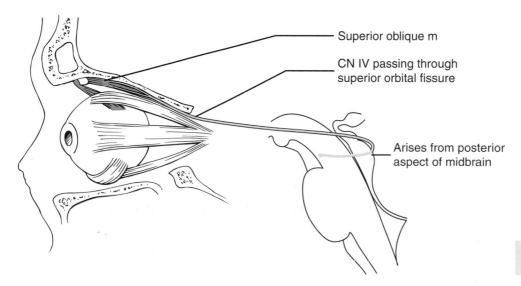

Figure 8-10 Trochlear nerve (cranial nerve IV).

371

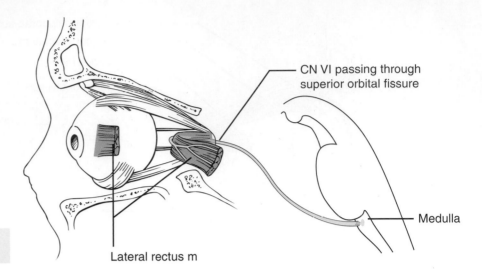

CN VI passing through superior orbital fissure

Medulla

Figure 8-11 Abducens nerve (cranial nerve VI).

Lateral rectus m

that travel peripherally to supply the lateral rectus muscle of the eye.

Cranial Nerve Test. A lesion of the nerve results in an inability to move the affected eye laterally (abduct) and in double vision (diplopia).

Cranial Nerve V: Trigeminal Nerve

The trigeminal nerve arises as a short, thick sensory trunk and a smaller motor component from the ventrolateral aspect of the pons (*Figure 8-12*, *Table 8-5*). The nerve passes anteriorly over the petrous temporal ridge and into a tunnel of dura (*trigeminal* or *Meckel's cave*) within the middle cranial fossa. Within the cave, the nerve flattens out as the large *trigeminal* (*semilunar*) *ganglion*, and this, in turn, gives rise to three divisions.

Functional Components

1. A **somatic afferent (exteroceptive) component** arises from cell bodies of the trigeminal ganglion. Central fibers pass to the pons to synapse with cell bodies of either the *pontene trigeminal (chief sensory) nucleus or the spinal trigeminal nucleus.* Peripheral fibers end as exteroceptive sense organs in the skin of the face, the oral and nasal mucosa, meninges, and conjunctiva of the eyelids.

2. A **somatic afferent (proprioceptive) component** arises from cell bodies of the *mesencephalic nucleus* of the pons. Central fibers pass to the nearby *principal sensory nucleus* or directly to the *motor nucleus of cranial nerve V*. Peripheral fibers end as proprioceptive endings within the periodontium, palatal mucosa, muscles of mastication, and temporomandibular joint.

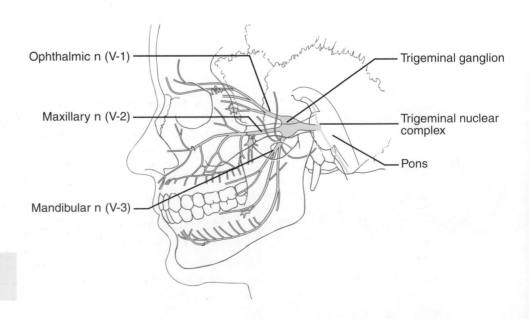

Ophthalmic n (V-1)

Maxillary n (V-2)

Mandibular n (V-3)

Trigeminal ganglion

Trigeminal nuclear complex

Pons

Figure 8-12 Trigeminal nerve (cranial nerve V) and its three divisions.

TABLE 8-5

Summary of the Cranial Parasympathetic Ganglia Associated with the Trigeminal Nerve

Ganglion	Location	Sensory Root	Parasympathetic Root	Sympathetic Root	Distribution
Ciliary	Orbit in interval between optic nerve and lateral rectus muscle	V-1 via ganglionic branches	CN III via its inferior branch	Internal carotid plexus via ophthalmic artery	**Sensory:** autonomic feedback from eyeball **Parasympathetic:** sphincter pupillae m, ciliary m **Sympathetic:** dilator pupillae m, blood vessels of eye
Pterygopalatine	Suspended from maxillary nerve in roof of pterygopalatine fossa	V-2 via ganglionic branches	CN VII via greater petrosal nerve and nerve of pterygoid canal	Internal carotid plexus via deep petrosal nerve and nerve of pterygoid canal	**Sensory:** mucosa of nasal cavity, paranasal air sinuses, superior pharynx, and hard and soft palates **Parasympathetic:** lacrimal gland via zygomatic nerve, mucous glands of nasal cavity, paranasal air sinuses, superior pharynx, and hard and soft palates **Sympathetic:** lacrimal gland and glands and vessels of the nasal cavity, paranasal air sinuses, superior pharynx, and hard and soft palates
Otic	Attached directly to medial aspect of stem of mandibular nerve as it passes through foramen ovale	V-3 via ganglionic branches	CN IX via tympanic nerve and plexus and lesser petrosal nerve	External carotid plexus via middle meningeal artery	**Sensory:** autonomic feedback from parotid gland **Parasympathetic:** parotid gland via auriculotemporal nerve **Sympathetic:** parotid gland and its blood vessels
Submandibular	Suspended from lingual nerve in floor of mouth	V-3 via lingual nerve	CN VII via chorda tympani and lingual nerves	External carotid plexus via lingual and facial arteries	**Sensory:** autonomic feedback from submandibular and sublingual glands and minor glands of floor of mouth **Parasympathetic:** submandibular and sublingual glands and minor glands of floor of mouth **Sympathetic:** submandibular and sublingual glands, minor glands of floor of mouth and glandular vessels

CN, Cranial nerve; *m*, muscle.

3. A **branchial efferent component** arises from cell bodies of the *motor trigeminal* nucleus of the pons. Axons travel peripherally with the third division of the trigeminal to supply the four muscles of mastication, the tensor tympani, tensor veli palatini, anterior belly of digastric, and mylohyoid muscles.

Branches

V-1 Ophthalmic Nerve (Sensory). The ophthalmic nerve passes through the superior orbital fissure and divides into three branches (*Figure 8-13*).

1. The **lacrimal nerve** travels anteriorly toward the lateral wall of the orbit. It receives hitchhiking secretomotor orbital branches of the pterygopalatine ganglion that are distributed to the lacrimal gland. The lacrimal nerve ends superficially as small sensory twigs to the lateral aspect of the upper eyelid.

2. The **frontal nerve** passes anteriorly just below the orbital roof. The frontal nerve divides into **supraorbital** and **supratrochlear nerves,** which pass as sensory branches to the upper eyelid, forehead, and scalp.

3. The **nasociliary nerve** curves toward the medial wall and gives off a number of branches: (1) **long ciliary branches** to the eyeball, (2) **ganglionic branches** to the ciliary ganglion, (3) **posterior** and **anterior ethmoidal nerves** to the ethmoidal air sinus and nasal cavity, and

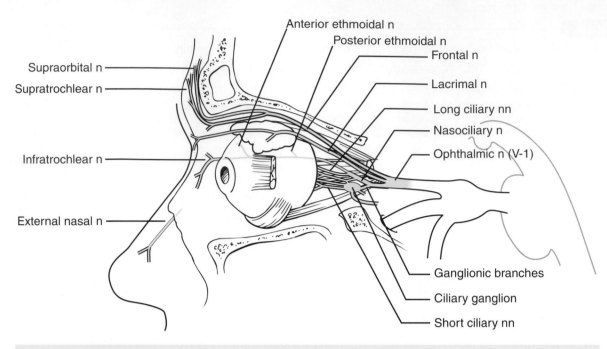

Figure 8-13 Ophthalmic division of trigeminal nerve (cranial nerve V-1).

(4) the **infratrochlear nerve** to the medial aspect of the upper eyelid and the lacrimal sac.

V-2 Maxillary Nerve (Sensory)

1. **Meningeal branches** arise within the middle cranial fossa to supply dura (*Figure 8-14*).
2. **Ganglionic branches** arise within the pterygopalatine fossa to enter the pterygopalatine ganglion as its sensory root.
3. **Posterior superior alveolar nerves** descend as several branches on the infratemporal surface of the maxilla. These enter the posterior superior alveolar foramina to supply the maxillary sinus and the roots of the maxillary molar teeth (except the mesiobuccal root of the first molar).
4. The **middle superior alveolar nerve** drops from the infraorbital portion of the maxillary nerve to supply the sinus mucosa, the roots of the maxillary premolars, and the mesiobuccal root of the first molar.
5. The **zygomatic nerve** branches from the maxillary nerve and passes anteriorly through the inferior orbital fissure to enter the orbit and passes along the lateral wall of the orbit and enters the zygomatic canal; within the canal, it bifurcates into the *zygomaticofacial nerve* supplying the skin overlying the zygomatic arch and into the *zygomaticotemporal nerve* supplying the skin of the anterior temple area.
6. The **anterior superior alveolar nerve** leaves the infraorbital portion of the maxillary nerve just before the infraorbital nerve issues onto the face; the alveolar branch descends through its own canal in the anterior wall of the maxillary sinus and sends branches to the sinus, a portion of the nasal septum, and the roots of the maxillary central, lateral, and canine teeth.
7. **Facial branches** radiate from the infraorbital nerve as it passes onto the face through the infraorbital foramen; the *inferior palpebral branches* supply the inferior eyelid, the *lateral nasal branches* supply the lateral aspect of the nose, and the *superior labial branches* stream down to supply the upper lip.
8. Branches arise from the **pterygopalatine ganglion** that carry sensory, sympathetic, and parasympathetic fibers to supply the lacrimal gland and mucosa of the superior pharynx, nasal cavity, maxillary sinus, oral cavity, and palate, These include the (1) secretory branches via the zygomatic nerve to the lacrimal gland, (2) greater palatine nerve supplying the hard palate distal to the canines, (3) lesser palatine nerve supplying the soft palate, (4) superior pharyngeal nerve supplying the roof of the pharynx, (5) nasopalatine nerve supplying the nasal septum and hard palate anterior to the canines, (6) posterolateral branches to the lateral wall of the nose, and (7) superior alveolar branches to the maxillary sinus.

V-3 Mandibular Nerve (Sensory and Motor). The mandibular nerve drops through the foramen ovale and divides into an anterior and a posterior trunk (*Figure 8-15*).

1. **Nervus spinosus** (*sensory*) arises from the main stem of the mandibular nerve and reenters the skull through the foramen spinosum. It helps to supply dura of the middle cranial fossa.
2. The **nerve to the medial pterygoid** (*motor*) supplies that muscle and also supplies motor fibers to the tensor

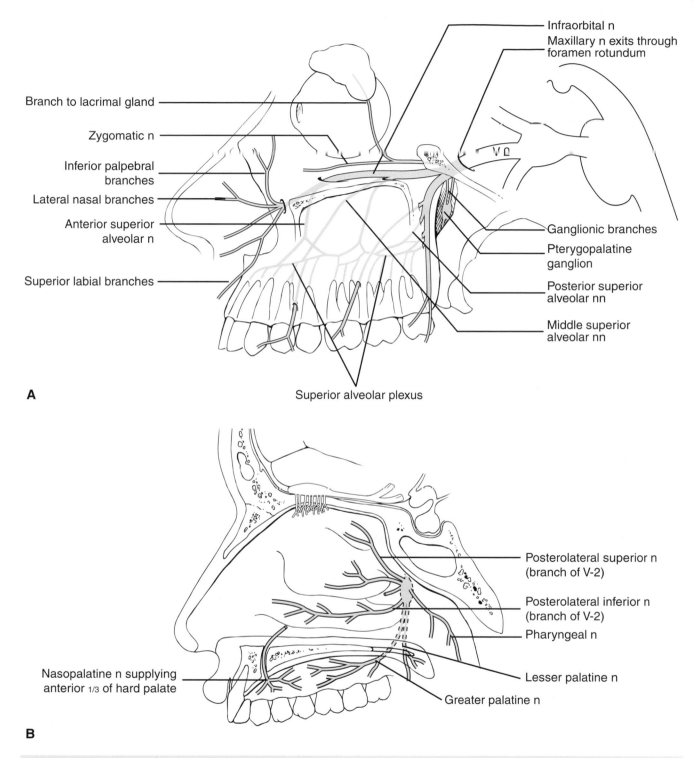

Branch to lacrimal gland

Zygomatic n

Inferior palpebral branches

Lateral nasal branches

Anterior superior alveolar n

Superior labial branches

Infraorbital n

Maxillary n exits through foramen rotundum

Ganglionic branches

Pterygopalatine ganglion

Posterior superior alveolar nn

Middle superior alveolar nn

Superior alveolar plexus

A

Posterolateral superior n (branch of V-2)

Posterolateral inferior n (branch of V-2)

Pharyngeal n

Nasopalatine n supplying anterior 1/3 of hard palate

Lesser palatine n

Greater palatine n

B

Figure 8-14 Maxillary division of the trigeminal nerve (cranial nerve V-2). **A,** Branches of the maxillary nerve. **B,** Branches of the pterygopalatine ganglion as seen from the medial or nasal aspect.

tympani and tensor veli palatini muscles. It arises from the stem of the mandibular nerve.

3. **Motor branches** arise from the anterior division to supply temporalis, masseter, and lateral pterygoid muscles.

4. The **(long) buccal nerve** (*sensory*) passes anteriorly and downward from the anterior division, pierces the temporalis tendon, and supplies the cheek and mandibular buccal gingiva.

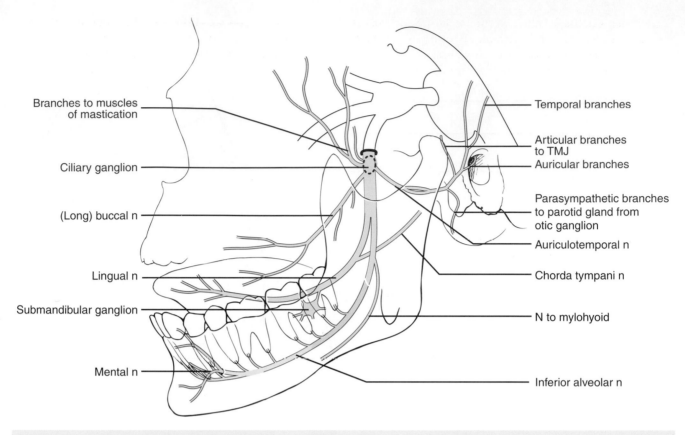

Branches to muscles
of mastication

Ciliary ganglion

(Long) buccal n

Lingual n

Submandibular ganglion

Mental n

Temporal branches

Articular branches
to TMJ

Auricular branches

Parasympathetic branches
to parotid gland from
otic ganglion

Auriculotemporal n

Chorda tympani n

N to mylohyoid

Inferior alveolar n

Figure 8-15 Mandibular division of trigeminal nerve (cranial nerve V-3).

5. The **auriculotemporal nerve** (*sensory*) arises from the posterior division and runs posteriorly as two roots that encircle the middle meningeal artery. The roots combine, pass deep to the lateral pterygoid muscle and temporomandibular joint, and then turn laterally and superiorly to emerge on the face between the jaw joint and the auricle. The nerve ascends onto the temple and lateral scalp. The auriculotemporal nerve sends sensory branches to the temporomandibular joint, auricle, external auditory meatus, and skin of the temple and lateral scalp. It also carries postsynaptic fibers of cranial nerve IX from the otic ganglion to the parotid gland.

6. The **lingual nerve** (*sensory*) arises deep to the lateral pterygoid muscle from the posterior division and travels anteriorly and inferiorly to emerge from under the inferior border of the lateral pterygoid muscle and then continues anteriorly along the surface of the medial pterygoid muscle. The lingual nerve enters the region of the floor of the mouth and here supplies sensory ganglionic fibers to the submandibular ganglion. It ends by supplying sensory fibers to mucous membrane of the floor of the mouth, mandibular lingual gingiva, and mucous membrane of the anterior two thirds of the tongue; the lingual nerve also carries hitchhiking fibers of the chorda tympani that are *special sensory taste* to the anterior two thirds of the tongue and

parasympathetic fibers to the sublingual and submandibular salivary glands and the minor mucous glands of the floor of the mouth.

7. The **inferior alveolar nerve** (*sensory and motor*) arises from the posterior division, travels inferiorly deep to the lateral pterygoid muscle, and, on reaching the inferior border of the muscle, turns laterally to enter the mandibular foramen.

Before entering the foramen, a slender *motor branch* is given off that passes downward and anteriorly to the submandibular region to supply the mylohyoid and the anterior bellies of the digastric muscles.

The inferior alveolar nerve passes through the mandibular canal, and, as it passes below the roots of the mandibular teeth, it sends sensory "twigs" to the apical foramina. In the region of the premolar, a *mental branch* is given off that turns laterally to emerge through the mental foramen onto the face. Here it divides to supply sensory branches to the skin of the chin, the mucous membrane and skin of the lower lip, and labial mandibular gingiva.

Cranial Nerve Test. A lesion of the trigeminal nerve may produce one or more of the following:

1. There may be anesthesia (lack of sensation) over the sensory distribution. The extent of involvement

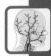

depends on the location of the lesion. Sensation is tested for light touch with a bit of cotton or facial tissue; pain perception is tested with a pin.

2. There may be paralysis of the muscles of mastication and flaccidity of the floor of the mouth and soft palate.

3. There may be sensitivity to high and loud sounds (hyperacusis) resulting from paralysis of the tensor tympani muscle of the middle ear.

Trigeminal Pain. The trigeminal nerve is the principal sensory nerve to the face and is responsible for the transmission of pain stimuli to the central nervous system. Pain elicited from dental operative procedures on hard and soft oral tissues is effectively controlled with local anesthesia (see Chapter 11, Section 1).

In addition, orofacial pain may arise from various oral diseases: (1) dental caries (generalized pain), (2) pulpitis and dentoalveolar abscess (localized pain), (3) impacted and infected wisdom teeth, (4) blocked or infected salivary ducts, (5) viral infections such as herpes simplex, (6) sinusitis, (7) spasm of the muscles of mastication, and (8) arthritis of the temporomandibular joint.

Occasionally, pain seems to originate from one location, but the actual source of pain is remote or is a different structure. For example, a maxillary sinusitis may manifest as a toothache of the maxillary posterior teeth. This occurs because the roots of the maxillary posterior teeth are in proximity to the maxillary sinus and both structures share the same nerve supply. Similarly, a painful, inflamed temporomandibular joint may be interpreted by the patient as an earache. Again, the structures are in proximity, and the external auditory meatus and the temporomandibular joint share a common nerve supply.

Cranial Nerve VII: Facial Nerve

The facial nerve arises as two distinct trunks from the lower border of the pons (*Figure 8-16*). The smaller of the two trunks is the **nervus intermedius** (a sensory and parasympathetic root), which joins the larger trunk (a motor root) as they both approach and enter the internal auditory meatus. The meatus leads into the petrous temporal bone and joins the facial canal. The facial nerve runs laterally within the facial canal, turns sharply at the genu (knee) to run posteriorly, and then drops inferiorly to exit through the stylomastoid foramen at the base of the skull. The nerve enters the substance of the parotid gland and then breaks up into five sets of branches. The genu of the nerve contains the sensory geniculate ganglion.

Functional Components

1. **Somatic afferent** fibers arise as a small component from cell bodies in the *geniculate ganglion* of the facial nerve. Central fibers pass back to the brainstem to synapse within the *principal sensory nucleus* of the trigeminal nerve. Peripheral fibers end as cutaneous receptors in the concha of the auricle.

2. **Special afferent (taste) fibers** originate from cell bodies within the *geniculate ganglion*. Central fibers pass back to the brainstem to synapse in the *nucleus of the solitary tract* of the medulla. Peripheral fibers end as taste receptors of the anterior two thirds of the tongue.

3. **Branchial efferent fibers** originate from cell bodies of the *facial motor nucleus* within the pons. Axons pass peripherally to supply (1) muscles of facial expression and the platysma, (2) the stylohyoid muscle, (3) the posterior belly of the digastric muscle, and (4) the stapedius muscle.

4. **Visceral efferent fibers** arise from cell bodies of the *superior salivatory nucleus* in the medulla. Axons pass peripherally to synapse in the following:
   A. The **pterygopalatine ganglion**: Postsynaptic fibers pass to the lacrimal gland and minor glands of the nasopharynx, auditory tube, palate, nasal cavity, and paranasal air sinuses.
   B. The **submandibular ganglion**: Postsynaptic fibers pass to the submandibular and sublingual salivary glands.

Branches

1. The **greater petrosal nerve** (*taste* and *parasympathetic*) arises from the genu of the facial nerve within the facial canal. The nerve passes anteriorly and medially through bone and exits through the superior hiatus on the anterior slope of the petrous temporal ridge in the middle cranial fossa. Here, it heads to the foramen lacerum, drops partially through, and then enters the pterygoid canal. At this point, it joins with the *deep petrosal nerve* (sympathetic) to form the **nerve of the pterygoid canal**. It travels through the canal and joins the pterygopalatine ganglion. Taste fibers eventually pass to the palate, and postsynaptic parasympathetic fibers go to the lacrimal gland and mucosa of the palate, nasopharynx, and nasal cavity.

2. The **nerve to the stapedius muscle** arises within the facial canal and is motor to the stapedius muscle of the middle ear.

3. The **chorda tympani nerve** (*parasympathetic* and *taste*) arises from the descending portion of the facial nerve within the facial canal. The chorda tympani passes through the middle ear between the medial aspect of the tympanic membrane and the handle of the malleus. It leaves the skull through the petrotympanic fissure to join the lingual nerve in the infratemporal region. Taste fibers are distributed to the anterior two thirds of the tongue via the lingual nerve. Parasympathetic fibers, on synapsing in the submandibular ganglion, supply the submandibular and sublingual salivary glands along with minor glands of the floor of the mouth.

4. **Suprahyoid** and **auricular motor branches** arise from the facial nerve after it emerges from the stylomastoid

foramen. The suprahyoid branches pass downward to supply the stylohyoid and posterior belly of the digastric muscles. The auricular branches pass upward to supply the auricular muscles.

5. **Facial branches** (*motor*) arise within the parotid gland as five main groups. These are temporal, zygomatic, buccal, mandibular, and cervical branches to the muscles of facial expression and the platysma muscle.

Cranial Nerve Test. Lesions of the facial nerve may cause (1) paralysis of the muscles of facial expression, (2) loss of taste sensation from the anterior two thirds of the tongue, and (3) decreased salivation.

Spontaneous inflammation of the facial nerve within the facial canal causes pressure on the nerve and a resultant facial paralysis (Bell's palsy) on the affected side. Early treatment with cortisone reduces the inflammation.

Cranial Nerve VIII: Vestibulocochlear Nerve
The vestibulocochlear nerve arises between the medulla and pons and enters the internal auditory meatus along

with the facial nerve within the petrous temporal bone (*Figure 8-17*). The **vestibular portion** ends on the semicircular canals; the **cochlear portion** ends on the cochlea of the inner ear.

Functional Components
1. **Special afferent** (*balance*) cell bodies are located within the *vestibular ganglion*, a swelling on the nerve in the internal auditory meatus. Central processes pass back to the medulla and pons to synapse in the *vestibular nucleus*. Peripheral processes end on the utricle, saccule, and ampulla of the semicircular canals.
2. **Special afferent** (*hearing*) cell bodies are found in the *spiral ganglion* of the cochlea. Central processes pass to the *cochlear nucleus* within the pons. Peripheral processes end on the spiral organ (of Corti) in the cochlea.

Cranial Nerve Test. Damage to the vestibular and/or cochlear portions of cranial nerve VIII results in (1) tinnitus (ringing or buzzing) or hearing impairment and (2) vertigo (dizziness) and loss of balance.

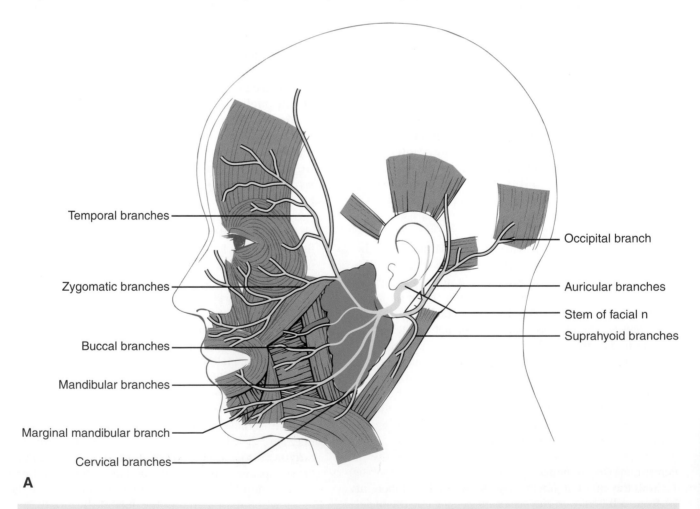

A

Figure 8-16 Facial nerve (cranial nerve VII). **A,** Motor branches to the muscles of facial expression.

Continued

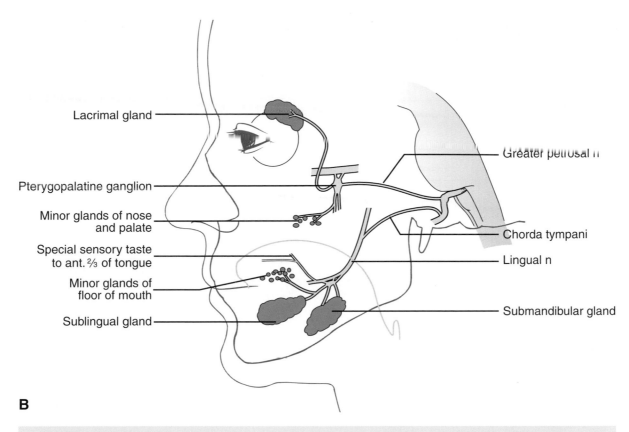

Lacrimal gland

Pterygopalatine ganglion

Minor glands of nose
and palate

Special sensory taste
to ant. ⅔ of tongue

Minor glands of
floor of mouth

Sublingual gland

Greater petrosal n

Chorda tympani

Lingual n

Submandibular gland

B

Figure 8-16 Cont'd. **B,** Visceral motor branches via trigeminal nerve to lacrimal, submandibular, and sublingual glands and minor glands of nasal and oral cavities.

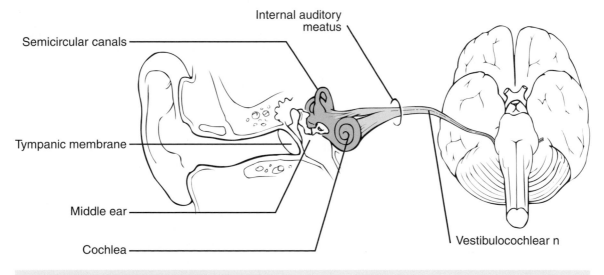

Semicircular canals

Internal auditory
meatus

Tympanic membrane

Middle ear

Cochlea

Vestibulocochlear n

Figure 8-17 Vestibulocochlear nerve (cranial nerve VIII).

Cranial Nerve IX: Glossopharyngeal Nerve

The glossopharyngeal nerve arises from the lateral aspect of the medulla as three or four rootlets (*Figure 8-18*). These rootlets merge and pass through the jugular foramen to exit the base of the skull. As the nerve passes through, it dilates as two swellings: the *superior* and *inferior glossopharyngeal ganglia*. The nerve descends to pass between the superior and middle constrictor muscles and enters the pharynx. It passes through the tonsillar bed and ends by plunging into the mucosa of the posterior third of the tongue.

Functional Components

1. **Somatic afferent cell bodies** are found in the *superior* and *inferior ganglia*. Central processes pass back to the

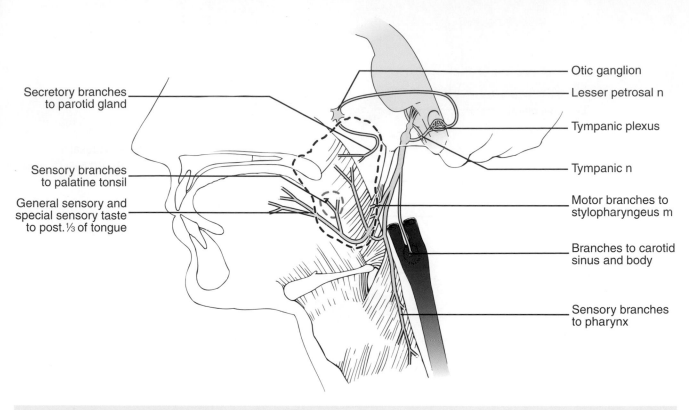

Secretory branches
to parotid gland

Sensory branches
to palatine tonsil

General sensory and
special sensory taste
to post. ⅓ of tongue

Otic ganglion

Lesser petrosal n

Tympanic plexus

Tympanic n

Motor branches to
stylopharyngeus m

Branches to carotid
sinus and body

Sensory branches
to pharynx

Figure 8-18 Glossopharyngeal nerve (cranial nerve IX).

brainstem to synapse with cell bodies of the *spinal trigeminal nucleus*. Peripheral processes end as general sensory receptors in the skin of the auricle and the mucous membrane of the posterior third of the tongue, pharynx, and middle ear.

2. A separate **visceral afferent** component exists for *chemoreception* and *baroreception*. The cell bodies are located in the *inferior ganglion*, and central processes travel to the brainstem to synapse in the *nucleus of the solitary tract* of the medulla. Peripheral processes end as chemoreceptors (oxygen) in the carotid body and baroreceptors (pressure) in the wall of the carotid sinus.

3. **Special afferent** (*taste*) cell bodies are located in the *inferior ganglion*. Central processes pass to the brainstem to synapse in the *nucleus of the solitary tract* (*gustatory portion*). Peripheral processes end as taste receptors in the mucosa of the posterior third of the tongue.

4. **Branchial efferent** cell bodies lie within the *nucleus ambiguus* of the medulla. Axons pass peripherally to supply only one muscle—the stylopharyngeus muscle.

5. **Visceral efferent** (*parasympathetic*) cell bodies reside in the *inferior salivatory nucleus* of the medulla. Axons pass peripherally to synapse in the *otic ganglion*; postsynaptic fibers are carried to the parotid gland by the auriculotemporal branch of V-3.

Branches

1. The **tympanic nerve** (*sensory and parasympathetic*) arises from the inferior ganglion and reenters the skull through the tympanic canal of the temporal bone. The canal leads to the middle ear, and here the nerve forms the *tympanic plexus* of the middle ear.

2. The **lesser petrosal nerve** is a branch of the tympanic plexus. It leaves the middle ear through a tiny canal and emerges through the inferior hiatus on the anterior slope of the petrous temporal ridge. The nerve passes directly to the foramen ovale, drops through, and synapses in the otic ganglion. Postsynaptic fibers are carried by the auriculotemporal nerve to the parotid gland.

3. **Carotid** (*sensory*) branches pass to the carotid sinus (baroreception) and to the carotid body (chemoreception).

4. The **nerve to the stylopharyngeus muscle** is the only motor branch of the glossopharyngeal nerve.

5. **Pharyngeal** (*sensory*) branches arise to help form the pharyngeal plexus along with vagal and sympathetic fibers.

6. **Tonsillar** (*sensory*) branches help supply the tonsillar and soft palate regions.

7. **Lingual** (*sensory*) branches pass to the mucosa of the posterior third of the tongue as general sensory and special sensory (taste) fibers.

Cranial Nerve Test. Impairment of the glossopharyngeal nerve could manifest as (1) loss of the pharyngeal gag reflex and (2) loss of taste from the posterior third of the tongue.

Cranial Nerve X: Vagus Nerve

The vagus nerve arises as eight to ten rootlets from the groove between the olive and the inferior cerebellar peduncle of the medulla (*Figure 8-19*). The rootlets converge and pass through the jugular foramen. The nerve dilates as two swellings: the *superior* and *inferior vagal ganglia*. The vagus nerve then descends through the neck within the carotid sheath and passes to the thorax, where it joins its opposite fellow to form the esophageal plexus. The plexus follows the esophagus through the diaphragm to the abdomen, and the vagus nerves reform as the *anterior* and *posterior vagal trunks*.

Functional Components

1. **Somatic afferent** cell bodies are located in the *superior* and *inferior vagal ganglia*. Central processes pass back

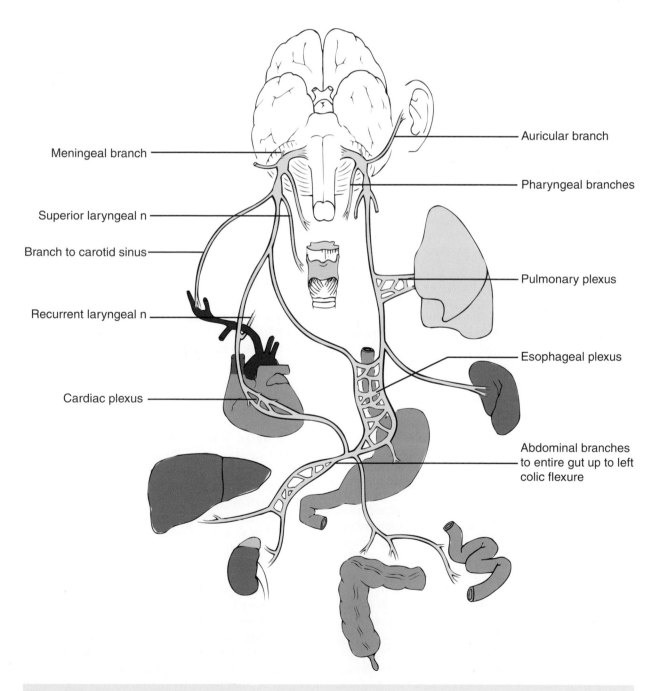

Figure 8-19 Vagus nerve (cranial nerve X).

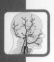

to synapse in the nucleus of the trigeminal spinal tract. Peripheral processes end as sensory receptors in (1) meninges of the posterior cranial fossa, (2) skin of the external auditory meatus, and (3) mucous membrane of the larynx.

2. **Visceral afferent** cell bodies are located in the inferior vagal ganglion. Central processes synapse in the nucleus of the tractus solitarius in the medulla. Peripheral processes end as receptors in the heart and bronchial tree and receptors in the gut and associated glands distal to the left colic flexure.

3. **Special afferent** (*taste*) cell bodies are found in the *inferior vagal ganglion*. Central fibers travel to the medulla to synapse in the *nucleus of the solitary tract* (*gustatory portion*). Peripheral fibers end as taste receptors around the inlet of the larynx and epiglottis.

4. **Branchial efferent** cell bodies are located in the motor *nucleus ambiguus* of the medulla. Axons group together as the *cranial root of the accessory nerve* (*cranial nerve XI*), which briefly joins the *spinal root* within the posterior cranial fossa and then disengages to join the fibers of the vagus nerve. This component supplies all the striated muscles supplied by branches of the vagus nerve: (1) superior, middle, and inferior constrictor muscles of the pharynx; (2) palatopharyngeus muscle; (3) levator veli palatini muscle; (4) palatopharyngeus muscle; (5) palatoglossus muscle; and (6) intrinsic muscles of the larynx.

5. **Visceral efferent** (*parasympathetic*) cell bodies lie within the *dorsal vagal nucleus* of the medulla. Axons pass peripherally to supply smooth muscle of (1) the bronchial tree, (2) the heart, (3) the stomach, and (4) the small and large intestine up to the left colic flexure.

These cell bodies also supply secretomotor fibers to glands of the respiratory system and digestive system.

Branches

1. **Meningeal sensory** branches arise from the superior vagal ganglion to supply the meninges of the posterior cranial fossa.

2. **Auricular** (*sensory*) branches arise from the superior vagal ganglion and travel to the ear to supply small portions of the external auditory meatus and lateral tympanic membrane.

3. The **pharyngeal branch** (*motor*) arises from the inferior ganglion and passes to the pharynx. It is motor to all the striated muscles of the pharynx and soft palate except the stylopharyngeus (cranial nerve IX) and tensor veli palatini (V-3).

4. **Carotid** (*sensory*) branches arise from the inferior vagal ganglion and pass to the walls of the carotid sinus. These branches are auxiliary to the carotid branches of cranial nerve IX.

5. The **superior laryngeal nerve** (*sensory* and *motor*) branches from the inferior vagal ganglion and descends in the neck. It divides into two branches: (1) the *internal laryngeal nerve*, which pierces the thyrohyoid membrane to supply sensation to the larynx above the vocal folds, and (2) the *external laryngeal nerve*, which is motor to the cricothyroid muscle of the larynx.

6. The **recurrent laryngeal nerve** (*sensory* and *motor*) turns upward around the subclavian artery on the right side and around the aorta on the left side to ascend in the neck and enters the larynx between the inferior constrictor and the esophagus. The nerve is sensory to the larynx below the vocal folds and motor to intrinsic muscles of the larynx.

7. **Cardiac branches** (*parasympathetic*) leave the vagus nerve in the neck and descend to the cardiac plexus in the thorax. The fibers synapse, and postsynaptic fibers pass to the heart and act to slow the heart and constrict coronary arteries.

8. **Pulmonary branches** (*parasympathetic*) are given off in the thorax, and these help form the anterior and posterior pulmonary plexuses. Vagal fibers synapse here, and postsynaptic fibers supply the smooth constrictor muscles of the bronchial tree.

9. The **esophageal plexus** (*parasympathetic*) is formed by a plexiform union of right and left vagus nerves. Fibers synapse here with ganglionic cells, and postsynaptic fibers go on to supply the smooth muscle and glands of the esophagus.

10. **Abdominal branches** arise from the reconstituted *anterior* and *posterior vagal trunks*. Vagal nerves within the abdomen synapse with secondary ganglionic cells in the walls of the viscera supplied (stomach and gut smooth muscle and glands as far distally as the left colic flexure).

Cranial Nerve Test. A patient with a vagal lesion may demonstrate (1) a paralysis of the soft palate and larynx on the affected side and (2) hoarseness and anesthesia of the larynx, permitting passage and aspiration of foreign bodies. Bilateral vagal damage would result in (1) rapid heartbeat (tachycardia), (2) decreased respiration, and (3) inability to speak and breathe because of paralysis of the vocal folds.

Cranial Nerve XI: Accessory Nerve

The accessory nerve forms from two roots (*Figure 8-20*). The **spinal root** arises from spinal filaments of segments C6 to C1, rises as a trunk through the foramen magnum, and briefly joins with the cranial root. The two roots part company, and the spinal root exits through the jugular foramen to enter the anterior and then posterior triangles of the neck.

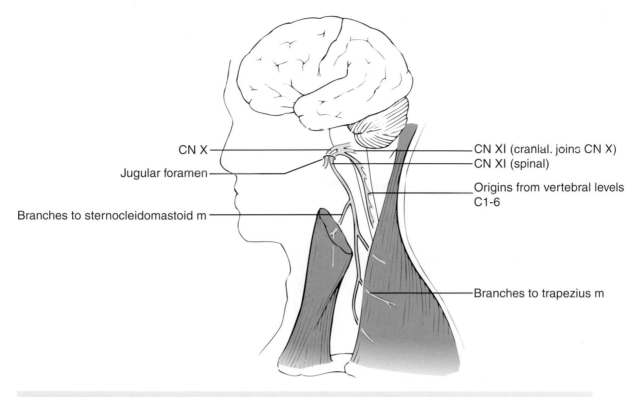

CN X

Jugular foramen

Branches to sternocleidomastoid m

CN XI (cranial. joins CN X)
CN XI (spinal)

Origins from vertebral levels
C1-6

Branches to trapezius m

Figure 8-20 Spinal accessory nerve (cranial nerve XI).

The **cranial root** arises as small filaments below the origin of the vagal fibers. It joins the spinal portion briefly, separates, and then joins the vagus nerve.

Functional Components. Only **branchial efferent** fibers are found within the spinal accessory nerve, but they arise from two sources.

1. The **cranial portion** arises from cell bodies of the *nucleus ambiguus* and was discussed previously as a functional component of the vagus nerve.
2. The **spinal portion** arises from cell bodies of the accessory nucleus located in the spinal cord at levels C1 to C6. These fibers are ultimately motor to the sternocleidomastoid and trapezius muscles.

Cranial Nerve Test. Possible sequelae to damage of the cranial root of the accessory nerve have been discussed with the vagus nerve. Damage to the spinal portion results in paralysis of the sternocleidomastoid and trapezius muscles and a drooping of the shoulder.

Cranial Nerve XII: Hypoglossal Nerve

The hypoglossal nerve arises as a series of 10 to 15 rootlets between the olive and pyramid of the medulla (*Figure 8-21*). The rootlets converge and pass through the hypoglossal canal to enter the anterior triangle of the neck. The

nerve descends in the neck and then loops anteriorly above the tip of the greater horn of the hyoid bone. It then disappears between the mylohyoid and hyoglossus muscles to enter the floor of the mouth.

Hitchhiking spinal fibers of the anterior primary rami of C1 follow the hypoglossal nerve briefly but leave to help supply infrahyoid strap muscles of the neck (see Figures 5-12 and 5-13).

Functional Component. Somatic efferent cell bodies of the *hypoglossal nucleus* in the medulla give rise to axons that supply all the intrinsic and extrinsic muscles of the tongue.

Cranial Nerve Test. A lesion of the hypoglossal nerve causes wrinkling and atrophy of the affected side of the tongue. Protrusion of the tongue deviates toward the paralyzed side.

CRANIAL AUTONOMIC NERVES

Cranial Sympathetic Nerves

A general description of the sympathetic nervous system is presented in Chapter 1, Section 7. The sympathetic trunk in the neck consists of a chain of three ganglia: **superior**, **middle**, and **inferior** cervical ganglia (*Figure 8-22*). The inferior ganglion may be fused with that of T1 as the large

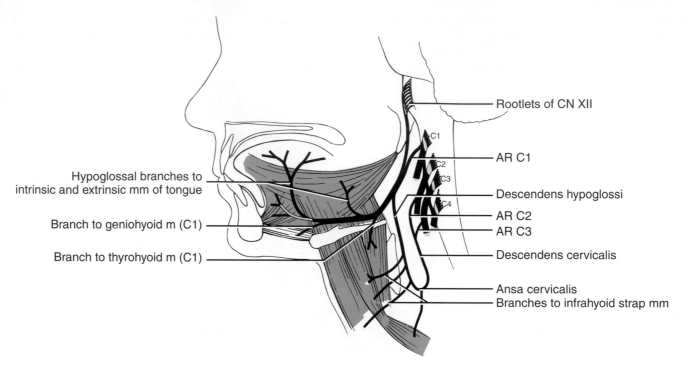

Rootlets of CN XII

AR C1

Hypoglossal branches to
intrinsic and extrinsic mm of tongue

Descendens hypoglossi

Branch to geniohyoid m (C1)

AR C2
AR C3

Branch to thyrohyoid m (C1)

Descendens cervicalis

Ansa cervicalis
Branches to infrahyoid strap mm

Figure 8-21 Hypoglossal nerve (cranial nerve XII).

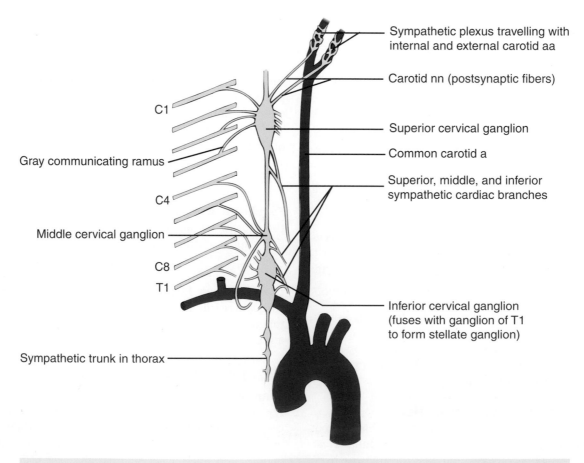

Sympathetic plexus travelling with
internal and external carotid aa

Carotid nn (postsynaptic fibers)

C1

Superior cervical ganglion

Gray communicating ramus

Common carotid a

Superior, middle, and inferior
sympathetic cardiac branches

C4

Middle cervical ganglion

C8

T1

Inferior cervical ganglion
(fuses with ganglion of T1
to form stellate ganglion)

Sympathetic trunk in thorax

Figure 8-22 Sympathetic nerve supply to the head and neck.

stellate ganglion. No cervical white communicating rami contribute to the ganglia, but gray rami are given off to each of the eight cervical spinal nerves. In addition, sympathetic cardiac fibers arise from the cervical sympathetic ganglia to descend to the thorax and supply the heart.

All the sympathetic supply to the head region arises from branches of the superior cervical ganglion. Primary neurons of cranial sympathetic fibers are located in the *intermediolateral horn of spinal cord levels T1 and T2.* Peripheral processes pass via ventral spinal roots to the sympathetic trunk. These fibers do not synapse and instead ascend to the superior cervical ganglion, where they finally synapse with secondary neurons. Postsynaptic fibers leave the ganglion as the **internal and external carotid nerves,** which form perivascular nerve plexuses on the internal and external carotid arteries. The arteries then distribute these sympathetic fibers to the head. The superior cervical ganglion also contributes small branches to cranial nerves IX, X, XI, and XII.

Structures Supplied. Sympathetic fibers of the head supply (1) skin—sweat glands, arterioles, and arrector pili muscles; (2) mucous membrane—arterioles and mucous glands; (3) orbital and cerebral vessels; (4) the dilator pupillae muscle; (5) a small tarsal portion of the levator palpebrae superioris muscle; and (6) the major salivary glands.

In addition, sympathetic fibers may play a more direct role in glandular secretion than generally thought. Although the parasympathetic division is traditionally taught as being secretomotor to salivary glands, it is now suspected that sympathetic fibers increase the viscosity of the saliva.

Horner Syndrome. Damage to the sympathetic trunk results in Horner syndrome. It is characterized by absence of sweating, vasodilation (flushing) of the skin, enophthalmos (sunken eyeball), ptosis (drooping eyelid), and double vision. Localized Horner syndrome is infrequently the result of a misdirected local anesthetic injection coming in contact with perivascular sympathetic fibers. The situation is temporary and passes quickly.

Cranial Parasympathetic Nerves

Cranial parasympathetic nerves originate from primary neurons of parasympathetic motor nuclei of the brainstem (*Figure 8-23*). Axons pass peripherally as functional components of cranial nerves III, VII, IX, and X. These parasympathetic fibers must synapse with secondary neurons at remote ganglia before they ultimately supply their effector organs.

In the head, the synapse occurs at one of four cranial parasympathetic ganglia: (1) ciliary, (2) pterygopalatine,

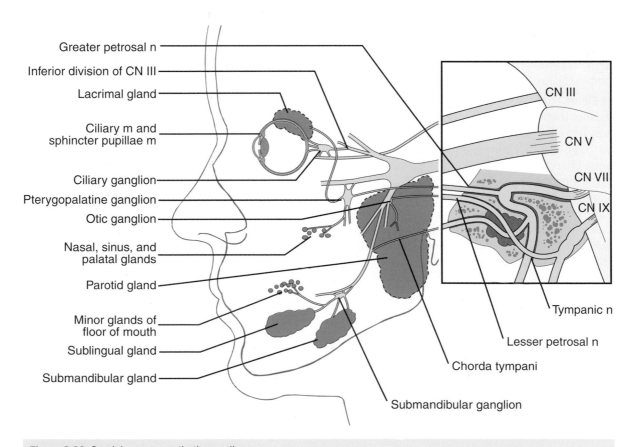

Figure 8-23 Cranial parasympathetic ganglia.

(3) otic, or (4) submandibular. In addition to a parasympathetic input that synapses with cell bodies, each ganglion receives sensory fibers from one of the three divisions of the trigeminal nerve and postsynaptic sympathetic fibers from the plexus of the nearest carotid arterial branch. The sensory and sympathetic fibers pass through the ganglion without synapsing (see *Table 8-5*).

Ciliary Ganglion

Location. The ciliary ganglion is located in the orbit in association with the nasociliary branch of the ophthalmic nerve (V-1). The ganglion lies in the interval between the lateral rectus muscle and the optic nerve behind the eyeball.

Incoming Fibers

1. **Parasympathetic fibers** arise from the *oculomotor nerve* (*cranial nerve III*) within the orbit, and these synapse in the ganglion.
2. **Sympathetic fibers** are from the sympathetic plexus of the internal carotid artery and the ophthalmic artery.
3. **Sensory fibers** are contributed by the nasociliary nerve, a branch of V-1.

Outgoing Fibers. Postsynaptic parasympathetic fibers are motor to the ciliary muscle and sphincter pupillae muscle of the eye. Sensory fibers go to the eyeball, and sympathetic fibers are vasoconstrictor to orbital vessels and motor to the dilator pupillae muscle.

Pterygopalatine Ganglion

Location. The pterygopalatine ganglion resides in the pterygopalatine fossa, hanging from the maxillary nerve as it traverses the fossa.

Incoming Fibers

1. **Parasympathetic fibers** originate from the *facial nerve* (*cranial nerve VII*) and travel via the greater petrosal nerve to synapse in the pterygopalatine ganglion.
2. **Sensory fibers** are received from the *maxillary nerve* (V-2) overhead.
3. **Sympathetic fibers** of the *internal carotid plexus* organize as the *deep petrosal nerve*, which, in turn, joins the *greater petrosal nerve* to form the *nerve of the pterygoid canal*; this nerve passes through the canal to join the ganglion in the pterygopalatine fossa.

Outgoing Fibers. Postsynaptic parasympathetic fibers are distributed to the lacrimal gland and minor glands of the nasal mucosa, palate, maxillary sinus, and pharyngeal roof. Sensory and sympathetic fibers are distributed to the same areas.

Otic Ganglion

Location. The otic ganglion is situated in the infratemporal region, adherent to the medial aspect of the stem of the mandibular nerve (V-3) as it passes through the foramen ovale.

Incoming Fibers

1. **Parasympathetic fibers** come from the *glossopharyngeal nerve* via the *lesser petrosal nerve*.
2. **Sensory fibers** arise directly from the stem of the *mandibular nerve* (V-3).
3. **Sympathetic fibers** come from the sympathetic plexus surrounding the *middle meningeal artery*.

Outgoing Fibers. The postsynaptic parasympathetic fibers travel with the auriculotemporal nerve to the parotid gland. Sensory and sympathetic fibers also pass to the gland.

Submandibular Ganglion

Location. The submandibular ganglion hangs from the lingual nerve as it loops across the lateral surface of the hyoglossus muscle in the floor of the mouth.

Incoming Fibers

1. **Parasympathetic fibers** arise from the facial nerve (cranial nerve VII) via the *chorda tympani branch*. The chorda tympani joins the lingual nerve and is carried by the nerve to the submandibular ganglion, where the parasympathetic fibers synapse.
2. **Sensory fibers** come directly from the *lingual branch of V-3*.
3. **Sympathetic fibers** are contributed by the plexuses about the *lingual* and possibly the *facial arteries*.

Outgoing Fibers. Postsynaptic parasympathetic fibers are secretomotor to the submandibular and sublingual salivary glands. Sensory and sympathetic components of the ganglion also pass to the glands and to mucous membrane and vessels of the mouth.

Review Questions

1. The external carotid artery ends by dividing into two terminal branches, the superficial temporal artery and the _____.
   a. occipital artery
   b. maxillary artery
   c. superior thyroid artery
   d. facial artery
   e. ascending pharyngeal artery

2. The pterygoid plexus of veins drains all of the following structures EXCEPT the _____.

   a. upper lip
   b. lower lip
   c. mandibular teeth
   d. upper eyelid
   e. lower eyelid

3. Infections and neoplasms (tumors) can spread through the lymphatic system. Choose one INCORRECT statement concerning lymphatic drainage of cranial structures.
   a. The upper lip drains to the submandibular nodes.
   b. The lower lip drains to the submental nodes.
   c. The maxillary teeth drain initially to the submandibular nodes.
   d. The tip of the tongue drains initially to the submandibular nodes.
   e. Vestibular gingivae of the maxillary and mandibular arches drain to the submandibular nodes.

4. Failure of the eye to turn outward (to the lateral or temporal side) along with double vision (diplopia) indicate possible damage to the _____.

   a. ophthalmic nerve
   b. abducens nerve
   c. oculomotor nerve
   d. optic nerve
   e. trochlear nerve

5. Branches of the maxillary nerve are sensory from all of the following areas EXCEPT the _____.

   a. mucosa of the maxillary air sinus
   b. mucosa of the soft palate
   c. mucosa of the hard palate
   d. mucosa of the nasal septum
   e. mucosa of the cheek

6. The facial nerve provides parasympathetic motor supply to all of the following glands EXCEPT the _____.

   a. lacrimal gland
   b. submandibular gland
   c. parotid gland
   d. sublingual gland
   e. minor glands of the nasal cavity

7. General sensation from the mucosa of the middle ear is conveyed by _____.
   a. CN VIII via cochlear portion
   b. CN V-3 via auriculotemporal nerve
   c. CN IX via tympanic nerve
   d. CN X via auricular branches
   e. Spinal nerves C2 and C3 via great auricular nerve

8. The intrinsic muscles of the larynx are supplied by _____.

   a. branchial efferent fibers of CN XI that join CN X
   b. branchial efferent fibers of CN IX
   c. somatic efferent fibers of CN IX
   d. somatic efferent fibers of CN X
   e. visceral efferent fibers of CN X

9. Inability to tense the soft palate would indicate a problem with _____.
   a. CN V-3
   b. CN IX
   c. CN X
   d. CN VII
   e. CN XI (cranial root)

10. Horner syndrome (damage to the cervical sympathetic trunk) results in all of the following EXCEPT _____.
    a. profuse sweating in the area of skin affected
    b. exophthalmos (protruding eyeball)
    c. vasoconstriction of skin vessels (blanching) in area affected
    d. double vision
    e. dilated pupil

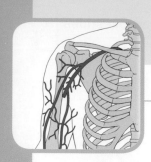

Chapter 9

The Upper Limb

1. Skeleton 388
2. Joints, Movements, and Muscles 394
3. Muscles 401
4. Axilla 414
5. Nerve Supply: The Brachial Plexus 415
6. Arterial Supply 418
7. Venous Return 420
8. Lymphatic Drainage 422

In the embryo, the limbs develop as outgrowths of the axial skeleton. The upper limb develops from body wall segments of the lower four cervical and first thoracic levels. Similarly, the lower limb develops from segments at the lumbosacral levels. As the limbs develop, they maintain the nerve and blood vessels of these levels, and this accounts for the axial source of nerve and blood supply to and from the limbs.

Functionally, the upper limb is designed for freedom of movement and prehension and is only loosely anchored to the axial skeleton. The lower limb, on the other hand, is engineered to bear the weight of the body during locomotion and standing and is thus rigidly attached to the axial skeleton. The upper limb comprises four components: the shoulder girdle, arm, forearm, and the hand.

1. Skeleton

SHOULDER (PECTORAL) GIRDLE

The shoulder girdle, or pectoral girdle, consists of two bones: the **scapula** (shoulder blade) and the **clavicle**

(collar bone) (*Figure 9-1*). The scapula is anchored to the posterosuperior surface of the thoracic cage by muscles. The clavicle is attached firmly to the manubrium of the sternum by the strong but movable sternoclavicular joint and to the scapula at the weaker acromioclavicular joint. The clavicle acts as a strut to keep the shoulders pointed laterally.

Scapula

Description. The **scapula** is a thin, triangular bone (*Figure 9-2*). Its concave anterior surface, is anchored by muscles to the posterior aspects of ribs 2 to 7. As a triangle, it possesses three sides: (1) a **vertebral (medial) border** that parallels the vertebral column, (2) an **axillary (lateral) border** that faces the axilla, and (3) a **suprascapular (superior) border.** The inferior angle is the apex of the triangle.

Features

1. A prominent **scapular spine** slashes across the convex posterior surface, dividing the posterior aspect into two fossae for muscle attachments: (1) the **supraspinous fossa,** above the spine, and (2) the **infraspinous fossa** below the spine.
2. The **acromion** is the club-shaped lateral expansion of the spine, which articulates with the clavicle at the *acromioclavicular joint.* The acromion can be palpated as the most lateral skeletal feature of the skeleton.
3. The **suprascapular notch** is a small notch on the superior border of the scapula that transmits the suprascapular nerve and vessels.
4. The **coracoid process** is a fingerlike extension that projects anteriorly and laterally from the superolateral border.
5. The **glenoid fossa** is a cup-shaped process at the superolateral angle just below the base of the coracoid process. It is lined with articular cartilage and articulates

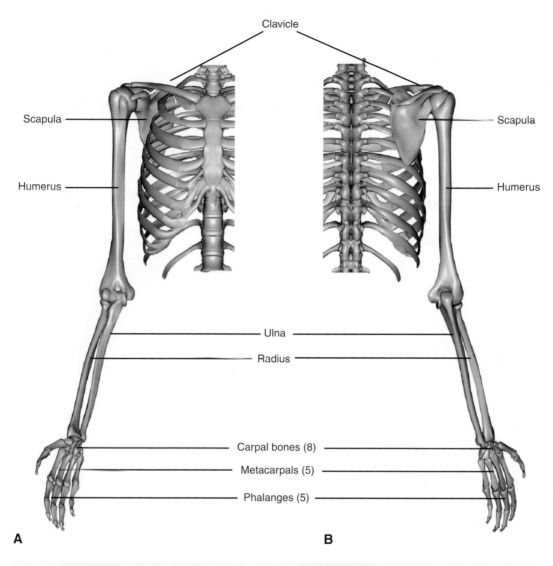

Clavicle

Scapula

Humerus

Scapula

Humerus

Ulna

Radius

Carpal bones (8)

Metacarpals (5)

Phalanges (5)

A

B

Figure 9-1 Skeleton of the right upper limb. **A,** Anterior view. **B,** Posterior view.

with the head of the humerus at the *glenohumeral* or *shoulder joint*.

6. The **subscapular fossa** is the concave anterior aspect of the scapula that is reciprocally shaped to the ribs.

Clavicle

Description. The **clavicle** is an elongated S-shaped bone that is subcutaneous and may be palpated over its entire length (*Figure 9-3*). The clavicle functions as a strut to prop the upper limb away from the body, affording the hand a greater range of positions, and transmits a portion of the weight of the upper limb through its sole articulation with the axial skeleton at the sternoclavicular joint.

Features

1. The **lateral end** is flattened for articulation with the acromion of the scapula at the relatively weak *acromioclavicular joint*.

2. The **medial end** is more bulbous, and it articulates with the manubrium at the strong *sternoclavicular joint*.

3. The clavicle features two **curvatures:** the medial half is bowed anteriorly; the lateral half is bowed posteriorly.

4. The **inferior aspect** is roughened by the attachment of **two ligaments:** the *coracoclavicular ligament* binds the clavicle to the coracoid process of the scapula; the *costoclavicular ligament* fixes the clavicle to the first rib.

ARM

Humerus

Description. The **humerus** is the only bone of the arm. It articulates superiorly with the scapula of the shoulder girdle and inferiorly with the radius and ulna of the forearm (*Figure 9-4*).

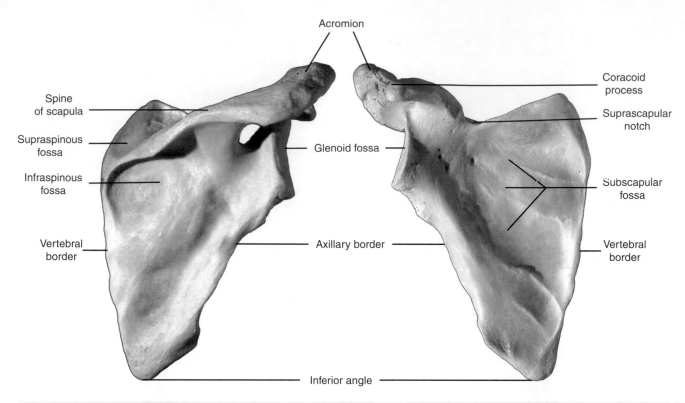

Acromion

Spine
of scapula

Supraspinous
fossa

Infraspinous
fossa

Vertebral
border

Glenoid fossa

Axillary border

Inferior angle

Coracoid
process

Suprascapular
notch

Subscapular
fossa

Vertebral
border

Figure 9-2 Right scapula. **A,** Posterior view. **B,** Anterior view.

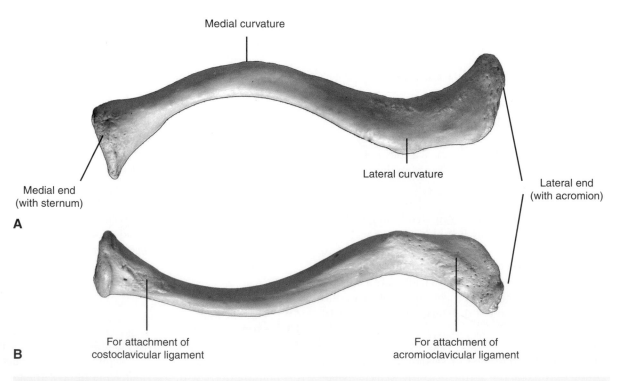

Medial curvature

Lateral curvature

Medial end
(with sternum)

Lateral end
(with acromion)

A

For attachment of
costoclavicular ligament

For attachment of
acromioclavicular ligament

B

Figure 9-3 Right clavicle. **A,** Superior view. **B,** Inferior view.

CLINICAL NOTES

Fractured Clavicle

The clavicle is the most commonly fractured bone in individuals less than 45 years old. A fall on the outstretched hand or a blow to the shoulder ultimately imparts its force to the clavicle. The sternoclavicular joint is generally strong enough to withstand the force, but the junction of the two curves of the clavicle is the weakest point and most vulnerable fracture site.

Absent or Rudimentary Clavicles

The clavicle is developmentally a membrane bone. *Cleidocranial dysostosis* is a condition that results in abnormal development of membrane bones in the skull and reduced or absent clavicles.

Features

1. A rounded **head** sits on its superomedial aspect for articulation with the glenoid fossa of the scapula.
2. The **greater** and **lesser tubercles** are prominences on the anterior aspect just below the head: the greater tubercle occupies a more lateral position; the lesser occupies a more anterior position—both tubercles provide attachment sites for muscles.
3. The humerus is distinguished by possessing two necks: the **anatomical neck** lies immediately below the head; the **surgical neck** is where the narrow shaft joins the wider superior upper portion of the humerus and marks the site where fractures of the humerus often occur.
4. The **intertubercular sulcus** (bicipital groove) lies between the greater and lesser tubercles; the tendon of the long head of the biceps muscle occupies the groove, and other muscles attach to the sides of the groove.

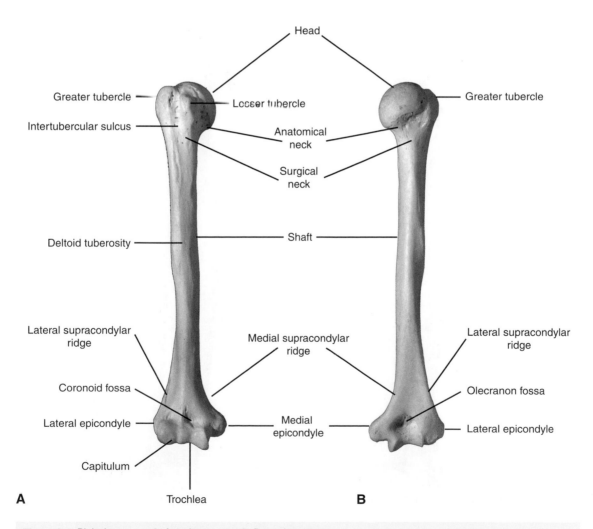

Figure 9-4 Right humerus. **A,** Anterior aspect. **B,** Posterior aspect.

5. The **deltoid tuberosity** is a bony elevation on the anterolateral aspect of the midshaft and marks the site for attachment of the deltoid muscle.

6. The **trochlea** is a spool-shaped process on the distal or inferior aspect that articulates with the ulna below.

7. The rounded **capitulum** is lateral to the trochlea, and it articulates with the radius below. Both trochlea and capitulum are also considered **condyles** or knuckle-like structures, which explains the terminology of the next two features.

8. The **epicondyles** are bony prominences immediately above the condyles (trochlea and capitulum); they can be readily palpated at the elbow and represent the widest diameter of the distal aspect of the humerus. The **medial epicondyle** is above the trochlea; the **lateral epicondyle** is above the capitulum; they represent sites for muscle attachments.

9. The **medial** and **lateral supracondylar ridges** extend upward from the medial and lateral epicondyles and provide attachment for muscles.

10. The **coronoid fossa** is on the anterior aspect immediately superior to the trochlea and accommodates the coronoid process of the ulna.

11. The **olecranon fossa** is on the posterior aspect above the trochlea and accommodates the olecranon of the ulna.

FOREARM

There are two long bones of the forearm, the **radius** and the **ulna.** In the anatomical position (palms facing forward or supine position), the radius is lateral and the ulna is medial. In the pronated position (palms facing posteriorly), the distal ends of the bones cross over, reversing their positions, and swing the distal radius to the medial side and the distal ulna to the lateral side.

Features of the Radius

1. The **head** of the radius at its proximal or superior end is disc-shaped, and it articulates with the capitulum of the humerus above and with the radial notch of the ulna medially (*Figure 9-5*).

2. The **radial tuberosity** is a projection on the medial surface just below the head; it is a site of muscle attachment.

3. The **lateral styloid process** is the pointed distal projection of the radius.

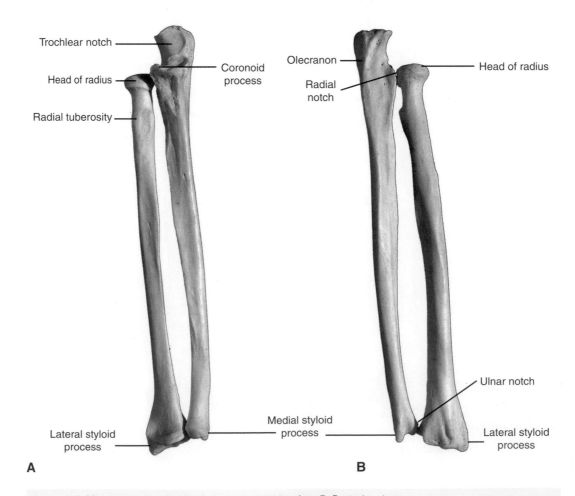

Trochlear notch

Head of radius

Radial tuberosity

Coronoid process

Olecranon

Radial notch

Head of radius

Lateral styloid process

Medial styloid process

Ulnar notch

Lateral styloid process

A

B

Figure 9-5 Ulna and radius of right forearm. **A,** Anterior view. **B,** Posterior view.

4. The **ulnar notch** is a shallow depression on the infero-medial aspect for articulation with the distal end of the ulna.

Features of the Ulna

1. The **trochlear notch** faces anteriorly on the proximal end of the ulna. It articulates with and curves around the trochlea of the humerus.
2. The **coronoid process** is the anteroinferior portion of the trochlear notch.
3. The **olecranon** is the superoposterior portion of the trochlear notch and forms the bony prominence of the elbow. The area between the coronoid process and the olecranon is thin and represents a potential site for fractures of the elbow.
4. The **medial styloid process** is the pointed distal projection of the ulna. Together with the lateral styloid process of the radius, the processes help to clamp the bones that make up the wrist.

THE WRIST AND HAND

Carpal Bones

Eight carpal bones make up the bones of the wrist (*Figure 9-6*). They are short, cuboidal bones and are arranged in two rows of four bones each to give a degree of flexibility of movement to the wrist. The bones are named rather fancifully by their shape.

Proximal Row. The proximal row of bones articulates directly or indirectly with the distal ends of the radius and the ulna. From lateral to medial, they are the **scaphoid** (canoe-shaped), **lunate** (moon-shaped), **triquetral** (three-sided), and **pisiform** (pea-shaped) bones. The pisiform bone does not participate in the wrist joint.

Distal Row. The **distal row** articulates with the proximal row superiorly and the metacarpals of the hand below. From lateral to medial, they are the **trapezium** (four-sided with two parallel sides), **trapezoid** (four-sided with no parallel sides), **capitate** (head-shaped), and **hamate** (hook).

Metacarpals

Five miniature long bones, or *metacarpals*, form the skeleton of the palm of the hand. Each metacarpal features an expanded **base** that articulates superiorly with the distal row of carpals and provides attachments for muscles. A rounded **head** on the distal end of the shaft articulates inferiorly with the phalanges of the fingers.

Phalanges

The phalanges are the bones of the fingers. Each finger has three phalanges: a **proximal phalanx** that articulates through its base with the inferior end of the metacarpal, a smaller **middle phalanx**, and a **small distal phalanx**. The thumb does not have a middle phalanx.

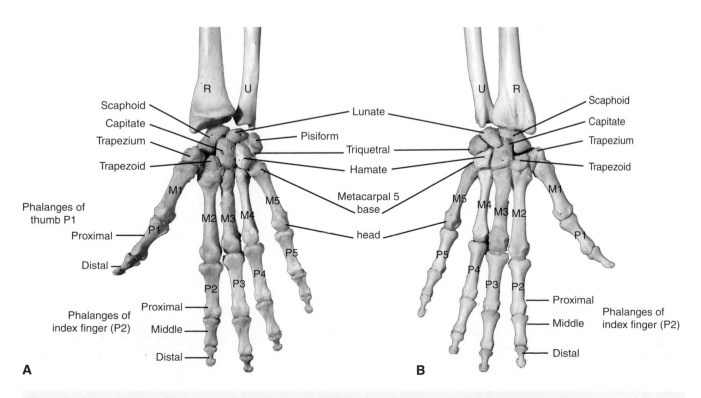

Figure 9-6 Bones of right hand and wrist. **A,** Anterior view. **B,** Posterior view. *M,* Metacarpal; *P,* phalanx; *R,* radius; *U,* ulna.

2. Joints, Movements, and Muscles

JOINTS OF THE PECTORAL GIRDLE

Features

Three joints contribute to the movements of the shoulder girdle: (1) the **sternoclavicular joint,** (2) the **acromioclavicular joint,** and (3) the **scapulothoracic joint** (*Figure 9-7*).

Sternoclavicular Joint

The sternoclavicular joint is an articulation between the spherical medial end of the clavicle and the manubrium of the sternum. It is a relatively strong joint, reinforced by extracapsular ligaments. In addition, an **intracapsular disc** is interposed between the bones. The disc divides the joint space into two compartments with movements unique to each compartment. This not only adds to the range of movements of the joint, but also increases the strength of the joint by preventing the clavicle from being driven medially by excessive medial force.

Acromioclavicular Joint

The lateral end of the clavicle articulates with the acromion of the scapula at this relatively weaker plane-type synovial joint.

Scapulothoracic Joint

The scapulothoracic "joint" is actually a moveable muscular anchorage of the scapula on the thoracic cage that allows for an increased range of movements of the upper limb.

CLINICAL NOTES

Shoulder Separation

Excessive medial force incurred by a fall or contact sport can cause the shoulder to separate. The acromion is medially displaced below the lateral end of the clavicle.

Movements

Although there may be some independent movements of the pectoral girdle, such as shrugging of the shoulders, most occur as coordinated movements with those of the arm. In addition, the muscles of the pectoral girdle act to stabilize the girdle for some upper limb functions such as lifting heavy objects. For this reason, the pectoral girdle joints will be considered as a unit participating in the following movements. There are six movements possible at the pectoral girdle.

Elevation is the drawing upward of the scapula, as in shrugging of the shoulders. The main muscles of elevation include the *levator scapulae* and the *trapezius* (upper fibers) muscles.

Depression is the lowering of the scapula and shoulder to the resting position through the pull of gravity. Forced depression is performed by the *pectoralis major*, *pectoralis minor*, *latissimus dorsi*, and *subclavius muscles*.

During **protraction,** the scapula is drawn upward and forward over the rib cage, placing the shoulders in a forward position. Muscles active in protraction include the

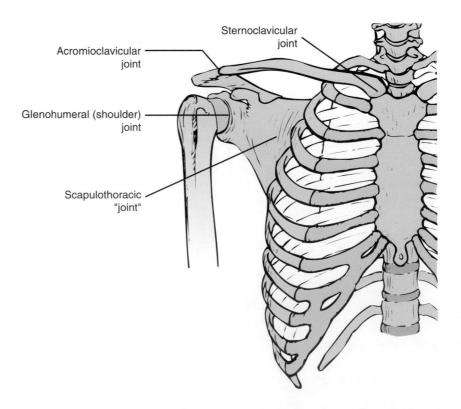

Figure 9-7 Joints of the pectoral girdle and shoulder.

levator scapulae, pectoralis major, pectoralis minor, and *serratus anterior muscles.*

Retraction is the resumption of the anatomical from the protracted position with the shoulders squarely back. The muscles that help retract the shoulders are the *trapezius,* the *latissimus dorsi,* and both *rhomboid muscles.*

In **upward rotation,** the scapula rotates about a midscapular axis in which the glenoid fossa points upward. The muscles responsible for upward rotation are the *trapezius* and *serratus anterior muscles.*

Downward rotation produces the opposite effect. The glenoid fossa and the tip of the shoulder are pulled downward by the actions of the *levator scapulae, rhomboids, latissimus dorsi, pectoralis major,* and *pectoralis minor muscles.*

GLENOHUMERAL JOINT

The glenohumeral, or shoulder, joint is an articulation between the spherical **head of the humerus** and the shallow depression of the **glenoid fossa** of the scapula (*Figure 9-8*). The shallow fossa is deepened only slightly by the **glenoid labrum,** a short fibrocartilage ring that encircles the rim of the fossa. The tendon of the long head of biceps

passes through the cavity of the joint en route to the intertubercular sulcus of the humerus.

The joint is a *ball-and-socket* configuration allowing three degrees of freedom and a considerable range of movement. Two factors contribute to this increased range: the shallow cuplike glenoid fossa and a fibrous articular capsule that is far more lax than those of other joints.

Movements
The glenohumeral joint is capable of six movements (*Figure 9-9*):

1. **Flexion** of the arm at the shoulder swings the upper limb anteriorly and superiorly in the sagittal plane from the anatomical position; this is accomplished by the *pectoralis major (clavicular head), deltoid (anterior fibers), coracobrachialis,* and *biceps muscles.*
2. **Extension** swings the arm back to the anatomical position; **hyperextension** swings the upper limb even farther posteriorly. Muscles that extend the arm include the *deltoid (posterior fibers), pectoralis major (sternal head), teres major, latissimus dorsi,* and *triceps (long head) muscles.*

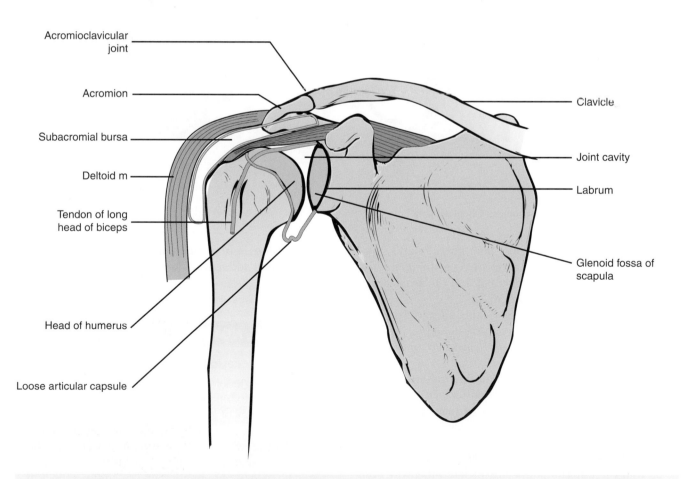

Figure 9-8 Anterior view of the right glenohumeral (shoulder) joint. The anterior capsule has been removed and the head of humerus displaced laterally to display the joint cavity. Note the shallow glenoid fossa.

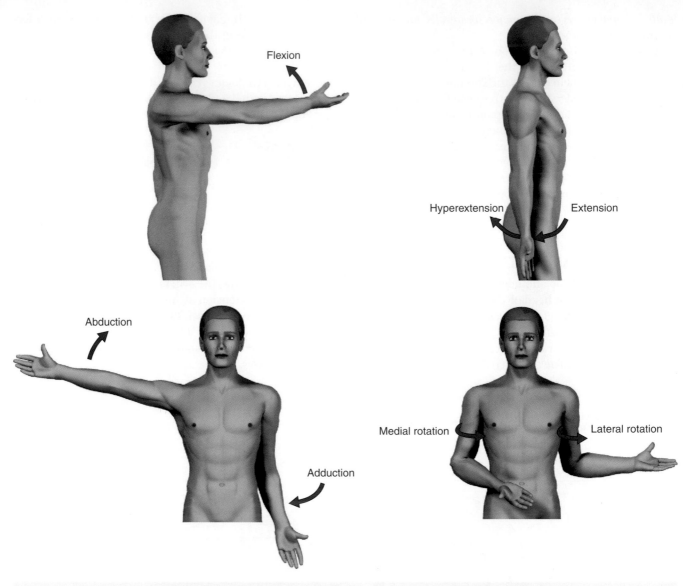

Figure 9-9 Movements of glenohumeral (shoulder) joint.

3. **Abduction** swings the upper limb laterally and superiorly away from the trunk in the coronal plane; the *supraspinatus* initiates abduction, and the *deltoid* (*middle fibers*) completes abduction.
4. **Adduction** swings the upper limb back toward the trunk through the actions of the *pectoralis major, latissimus dorsi, teres major, triceps* (*long head*), and *coracobrachialis muscles.*
5. **Medial rotation** is the rotation of the humerus around its long axis turning its anterior surface toward the median plane. This movement is performed by the *teres major, pectoralis major, latissimus dorsi, subscapularis,* and *deltoid* (*anterior fibers*) *muscles.*
6. **Lateral rotation** rotates the humerus about its long axis so that the anterior surface turns laterally away from the median plane; contributing muscles are *infraspinatus, teres minor,* and *deltoid* (*posterior fibers*).

Circumduction is a combination of flexion, extension, abduction, and adduction in a wide conical arc about the shoulder.

CLINICAL NOTES

Shoulder Dislocation

The shallow glenoid cavity and lax ligaments contribute to a greater range of shoulder movement but increase the risk of injury and dislocation. The head of the humerus is usually dislocated inferiorly below the glenoid fossa, where muscle support is weakest. The dislocated head may impinge on the axillary nerve, resulting in loss of sensation on the lateral aspect of the shoulder and atrophy of the deltoid muscle.

THE ELBOW (HUMEROULNAR) JOINT

Features

The elbow is a compound articulation between the distal end of the humerus and the proximal ends of the ulna and radius (*Figures 9-10* and *9-11*). The two sites of articulation take place between (1) the **trochlea of the humerus** and the **trochlear notch of the ulna** and (2) the **capitulum of the humerus and the radial head of the radius**. The joint capsule is lined by synovium and reinforced externally by radial (lateral) and ulnar (medial) collateral ligaments.

Movements

The elbow joint is basically a hinge-type joint allowing only two movements (*Figure 9-12*): **flexion**, or bending, is a movement that decreases the angle between the arm and forearm, and **extension** is a straightening movement that moves the limb back toward the anatomical position.

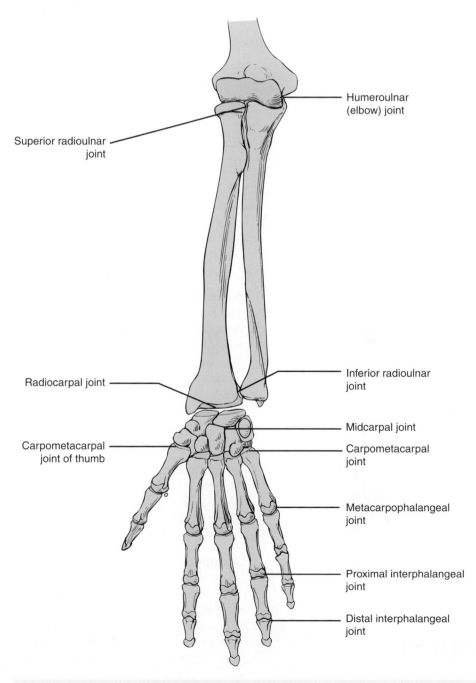

Figure 9-10 Joints of the elbow, wrist, and hand.

397

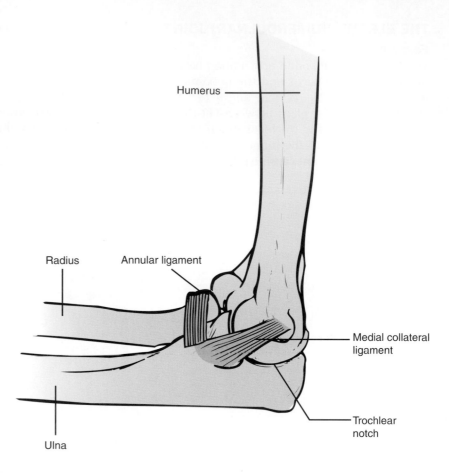

Humerus

Radius   Annular ligament

Medial collateral
ligament

Trochlear
notch

Ulna

Figure 9-11 Medial view of the flexed right elbow to display the humeroulnar joint and superior radioulnar joint.

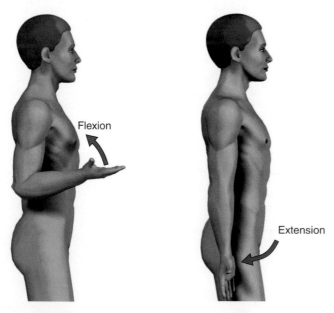

Flexion

Extension

Figure 9-12 Movements at the elbow joint.

THE RADIOULNAR JOINTS

Features

The radius and ulna articulate with each other at the **proximal** and **distal radioulnar joints.**

Superior Radioulnar Joint

The **head of the radius** is shaped like a thick, bony disc. Its superior border has already been described as articulating with the capitulum of the humerus in the elbow joint. The side of the disc revolves within the **radial notch of the ulna,** a shallow depression that seems to have been carved out for it on the lateral aspect of the coronoid process of the ulna. The head is held in place by an **annular ligament** that surrounds the head of the radius and holds it within the notch.

Distal Radioulnar Joint

The distal joint appears to be a reversal of the proximal joint. Here the **distal end of the ulna** is roughly disc-shaped, and it seems to have worn a facet for itself on the adjacent **ulnar notch of the radius.**

Movements

The forearm is capable of twisting around its long axis (*Figures 9-13* and *9-14*). The head of the radius spins within its annular ligament while the distal end of the ulna curves around the distal ulna from a lateral position to a medial position and back again. This results in two possible movements at these joints:

1. **Supination** is the turning of the forearm so that the palm faces anteriorly and the thumb points laterally in the

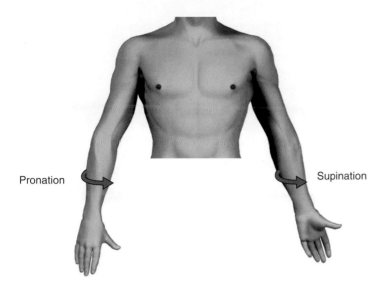

Pronation   Supination

Figure 9-13 Movements at the radioulnar joints. The right   f0070
forearm is pronated; the left forearm is supinated.

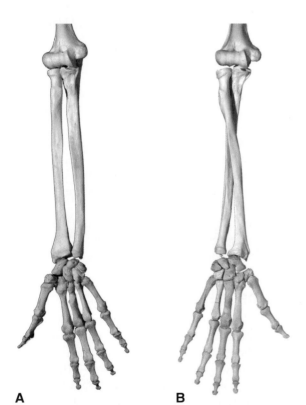

A   **B**

f0075   Figure 9-14 Skeleton of the right forearm, wrist, and hand.
A, Supine position. **B**, Prone position.

CLINICAL NOTES   b0025

A Sinister Twist   s0220

Supination is a more powerful action than pronation.   p1360
For this reason, screws and bottle caps are tightened
in a clockwise direction, taking advantage of the
stronger supinators of the forearm. This is designed
as an advantage for the majority who are right-handed
but not for the left-handed minority who are consigned
to use the weaker pronators of their dominant left
hands for these tasks. Left-handers, on the other
hand, have an advantage in unscrewing bottle caps.

WRIST JOINT (RADIOCARPAL AND   s0225
MIDCARPAL JOINTS)

Features   s0230

The wrist joint is the articulation between the forearm and   p1365
the carpal bones of the wrist (see *Figure 9-10*). The ulna is
separated from these bones by an articular disc so only the
radius makes contact with the distal row of carpals. The main
joint of the wrist is the biaxial, condyloid **radiocarpal joint.**
The **midcarpal joint** is a planar joint between the proximal
and distal rows of carpal bones. It contributes to the range of
movements at the wrist **carpometacarpal joints** between the
distal row and the bases of the medial four metacarpals.

Movements   s0235

The radiocarpal joint, aided by the midcarpal joint, is capa-   p1370
ble of four movements (*Figure 9-15*):

1. **Flexion** bends the wrist so that the palm faces upward   o0745
   from the anatomical position.
2. **Extension** straightens the wrist, and **hyperextension**   o0750
   bends the wrist back so that the palm faces downward
   from the anatomical position.

anatomical position; if this is performed while the elbow
is flexed, the palm faces upward as in accepting change.

o0740   2. **Pronation** is the turning of the palm inward and then
   backward from the anatomical position so that the
   palm faces posteriorly and the thumb points medially;
   if this is done while the elbow is flexed, the palm faces
   the ground.

399

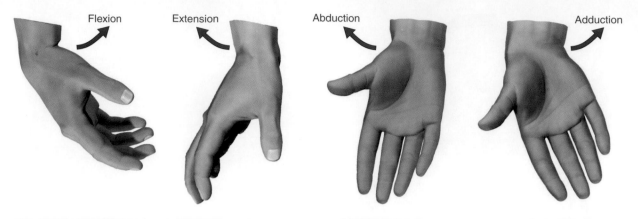

Flexion   Extension   Abduction   Adduction

Figure 9-15 Movements at the right wrist.

3. **Abduction** angles the hand away from the body.
4. **Adduction** angles the hand toward the body.

Circumduction is a combination of the above four movements in sequence, moving the hand about the forearm in a conical arc.

CARPOMETACARPAL JOINTS

The carpometacarpal joints vary from the extremely flexible joint of the thumb to the right second and third carpometacarpal joints. The fourth and fifth joints allow some hinge movement, and this contributes to the power grip. Hold a pen in the palm of your hand and grasp it lightly with your fingers. Tighten the grip, as in making a fist, and observe the hinge movement at the fourth and fifth joints on the back of your hand.

JOINTS OF THE FOUR FINGERS
Sets

Three sets of joints contribute to the movements of the fingers (see *Figure 9-10*):

1. **Metacarpophalangeal (MP) joints** are articulations between the distal ends of the metacarpals and the proximal ends of the proximal phalanges of the medial four digits. The joint surfaces are *condyloid*, allowing two degrees of freedom and a greater range of movement. The capsules of the joints are reinforced by collateral ligaments and further reinforced anteriorly by a dense connective tissue termed the ***palmar ligament.*** The four joints are joined to each other by **deep transverse ligaments.**
2. **Proximal interphalangeal (PIP) joints** are *hinge joints* between the proximal and middle phalanges, with one axis of rotation.
3. **Distal interphalangeal (DIP) joints** are articulations between middle and distal phalanges and, like the PIP joints, are *hinge joints* with one axis of rotation.

Movements

The fingers are capable of four movements (*Figure 9-16*):

1. **Flexion** at the MP joints bends the fingers toward the palm, and flexion at the PIP and DIP joints curls the fingers.
2. **Extension** at the MP, PIP, and DIP joints straighten the fingers so that they lie in the same plane as the palm.
3. **Abduction** takes place only at the MP joints; it is the movement of the fingers away from the median plane of the hand, that is, the fingers are spread apart in the coronal plane. The median plane of the hand is the long axis of the second finger.
4. **Adduction** occurs at the MP joints and is the movement of the fingers toward the median plane; that is, the fingers approximate with their sides touching.

JOINTS OF THE THUMB

The thumb is considered separately because its structure and function are slightly different from those of the other digits and these unique features contribute in a large way to the versatility of the hand (see *Figure 9-10*). The thumb is a short digit with only two phalanges. The thumb, including its metacarpal, is rotated at 90 degrees to the planes of the other digits, and it possesses a number of muscles dedicated solely to the movements of the thumb. Three joints contribute to the movements of the thumb:

1. The **first carpometacarpal joint** is an articulation between the trapezium and the distal end of the first metacarpal. It is a *saddle joint* that functions as a universal joint with three axes of rotation.
2. The **first metacarpophalangeal (MP) joint** is a *hinge joint* between the distal end of the first metacarpal and the proximal phalanx of the thumb.
3. The **interphalangeal joint** is a *hinge joint* between the proximal and distal phalanges of the thumb.

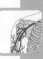

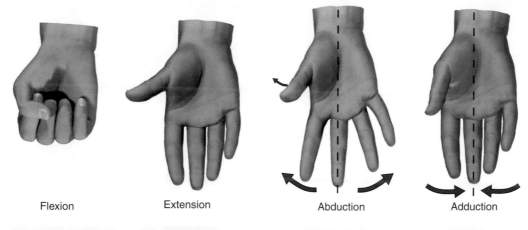

Flexion   Extension   Abduction   Adduction

Figure 9-16 Movements of the fingers and thumb of right hand at the carpometacarpal joints and interphalangeal joints.

The first **metacarpophalangeal** and the **interphalangeal joints** of the thumb were noted previously as hinge joints allowing for only two movements: (1) **flexion**, which *curls* the thumb, and (2) **extension**, which *straightens* the thumb. The **carpometacarpal joint,** however, allows three axes of rotation and, therefore, a greater range of movement (see *Figures 9-16* and *9-17*).

1. **Flexion** curls the thumb at a right angle to the other digits across the palm of the hand.
2. **Extension** straightens the thumb and carries it laterally away from the other digits.
3. **Abduction** moves the thumb away from the palm in a forward direction.
4. **Adduction** pulls the thumb back toward the palm and into the anatomical position.
5. **Opposition** rolls the thumb toward the palm so that the thumb pad faces and is capable of touching the finger pads of any of the four fingers—this movement makes the *precision grip* possible, in which an object such as a

pen or explorer is gripped between the tips of the index finger and the thumb.
6. **Reposition** moves the thumb back to the anatomical position.

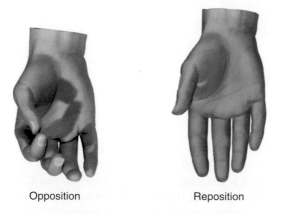

Opposition   Reposition

Figure 9-17 Opposition and reposition of the right thumb. NOTE: Thumb can oppose each of the flexed digits in turn.

3. Muscles

MUSCLE GROUPS OF THE UPPER LIMB

The muscles of the upper limb are grouped by regions: pectoral, superficial back, arm, forearm, and hand and wrist.

Muscles of the Pectoral Region and Lateral Chest Wall

The muscles in this group (except the subclavius) arise from the skeleton of the anterior and lateral chest wall (*Figure 9-18, Table 9-1*). The pectoralis major inserts into the humerus and the pectoralis minor, and serratus anterior muscles insert into the scapula. In general, they are responsible for movements of the pectoral girdle and shoulder and are supplied by collateral branches of the brachial plexus.

The **pectoralis major** is a large triangular muscle on the anterior chest wall that arises as two heads, one from the clavicle and the other from the sternum. Both heads insert into the humerus, with the clavicular head overlapping the sternal head. The muscle can *flex, medially rotate*, and *adduct* the arm. The pectoralis major is supplied by the *lateral* and *medial pectoral nerves*.

The **pectoralis minor** is a small triangular muscle that arises from the anterior chest wall deep to the pectoralis major muscle and attaches to the coracoid process of the scapula. In addition to *protraction of the scapula*, it *depresses* the scapula, *rotates it laterally* and, when the scapula is held stationary by other muscles, it *elevates* the ribs during forced inspiration. It is supplied by the *medial pectoral nerve*.

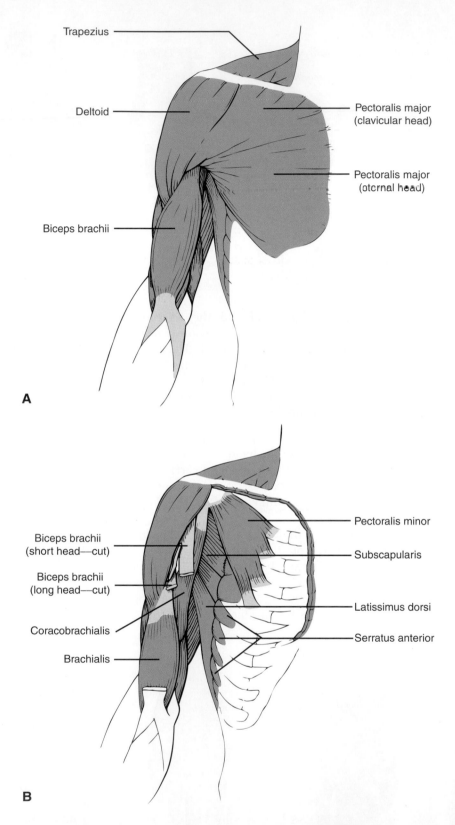

Figure 9-18 Muscles of the pectoral region and anterior right arm. **A,** Superficial. **B,** Deep.

The **subclavius** is a small, likely insignificant, muscle below the clavicle that receives its nerve supply from the *nerve to subclavius.*

The **serratus anterior** is a large, flat, powerful muscle that has a serrated or notched origin from the anterior chest wall and inserts into the vertebral border of the scapula. It *protracts* the scapula, rotates it medially, and helps *elevate* the ribs during forced inspiration when the scapula is held stationary by other muscles. The serratus anterior is supplied by the *long thoracic* nerve.

TABLE 9-1

Muscles of the Pectoral Region and Lateral Chest Wall

Muscle	Origin	Insertion	Action(s)	Nerve
Pectoralis major	Clavicle: medial third Sternum: body Costal cartilages of ribs 1 to 6	Humerus: greater tubercle	1. Flexes arm 2. Rotates arm medially 3. Adducts arm 4. Elevates ribs in forced inspiration	Lateral and medial pectoral
Pectoralis minor	Ribs 3 to 5: anterior surfaces	Scapula: coracoid process	1. Protracts scapula 2. Depresses scapula 3. Rotates scapula laterally (glenoid fossa up) 4. Elevates ribs during forced inspiration when the scapula is held stationary by other muscles	Medial pectoral
Subclavius	Rib 1 and its costal cartilage	Clavicle: inferior aspect	1. Depresses scapula 2. Protracts scapula	Nerve to subclavius
Serratus anterior	Ribs 1 to 9: anterosuperior surfaces	Scapula: anterior aspect of vertebral border	1. Protracts scapula 2. Rotates scapula medially (glenoid fossa down) 3. Elevates ribs during forced inspiration when scapula is held stationary by other muscles	Long thoracic

Muscles of the Superficial Back

The superficial group of back muscles is functionally upper limb muscles (*Figure 9-19*, *Table 9-2*). Their origins may be on the back, but their insertions are into the skeleton of the upper limb. Four muscles belong to this group, and their functions and nerve supplies are varied. As a group, they act to move the pectoral girdle or shoulder. All but the trapezius receive their motor supply from collateral branches of the brachial plexus.

The **trapezius** is a large, flat, triangular muscle covering the back of the neck and the upper half of the trunk. It forms a four-sided, diamond or trapezoidal shape along with its fellow of the opposite side. The fibers of the trapezius run in various directions, and it therefore has several functions. Its superior fibers act to *elevate* and *laterally rotate* the scapula, but its inferior fibers *depress* the scapula. The middle fibers help to *retract* the scapula. The trapezius also has a cervical portion that can move the head and neck (its functions are noted in Chapter 5). A major portion of the trapezius muscle receives its innervation from *cranial nerve XI* (*spinal accessory nerve*). A small supply comes from branches of the cervical plexus in the neck.

The **latissimus dorsi** is a large, flat muscle occupying the lower half of the back and extends from a broad-based origin on the back to insert into the humerus. It *adducts*, *extends*, and *medially rotates* the arm and is supplied by the *thoracodorsal nerve*.

The **levator scapulae** is a muscle that descends from the cervical vertebrae to the superior border of the scapula. As the name suggests, it elevates the scapula, but it also helps to medially rotate the scapula. It is supplied by the dorsal scapular nerve, a collateral branch of the brachial plexus.

The rhomboids are two muscles (major and minor) that run from the back of the neck into the vertebral border of the scapula. Because both function as a single unit, they are considered as a single entity. They act to *retract* and *medially rotate* the scapula. The rhomboids are supplied by the *dorsal scapular nerve*.

Muscles of the Shoulder

The muscles of the shoulder arise from the scapula and insert into the humerus (see *Figures 9-18* and *9-19* and *Table 9-3*). They not only provide movements at the shoulder joint, but also act to stabilize the joint. The deltoid and teres minor are innervated by the axillary nerve; the remainder are supplied by collateral branches of the brachial plexus.

The **deltoid** is a triangular muscle wrapped around the posterior, lateral, and anterior aspects of the shoulder, giving it a rounded appearance. The base of the triangle arises from the bones of the pectoral girdle; the apex inserts below into the humerus. The fibers are arranged in several planes, allowing the deltoid muscle to perform antagonistic movements. The anterior fibers *flex* and *medially rotate* the posterior fibers and *extend* and *laterally rotate* the arm at the shoulder. In addition, the middle fibers *abduct* the arm. The deltoid muscle is supplied by the *axillary nerve*.

The **teres major** is found just above the latissimus dorsi, running from the scapula to the humerus. Both muscles help form the inferior border of the posterior wall of the axilla. The teres major can *extend*, *medially rotate*, and *adduct* the arm. It is supplied by the *lower subscapular nerve*.

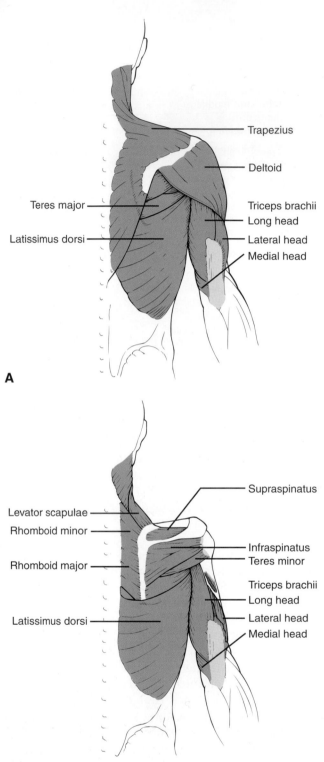

A

B

Figure 9-19 Posterior muscles of the right shoulder and arm. **A,** Superficial. **B,** Deep.

The **rotator cuff muscles** are four muscles that arise from the scapula and insert into the upper humerus and joint capsule as a common tendon or cuff. They contribute

to the stability of the glenohumeral joint through their tendinous insertions into the humerus and prevent dislocation of the shoulder under normal conditions. The rotator cuff muscles function as ligaments in a dynamic way by pressing the head of the humerus into the shallow glenoid fossa. The four muscles are the (1) *supraspinatus*, (2) *infraspinatus*, (3) *teres minor*, and (4) *subscapularis* (*SITS*).

The **supraspinatus muscle** arises from the supraspinous fossa, crosses the shoulder joint, and inserts into the greater tubercle of the humerus. It is an *abductor* of the arm at the shoulder and is supplied by the *suprascapular nerve*. The **infraspinatus muscle** arises from the infraspinous fossa, crosses the shoulder, and inserts into the greater tubercle of the humerus. It can *laterally rotate*, as well as *slightly adduct* the arm, and is supplied by the *suprascapular nerve*.

The **teres minor muscle** arises from the inferior lateral border of the scapula and inserts into the greater tubercle of the humerus. It is a *lateral rotator*, *extensor*, and *adductor* of the arm. The *axillary nerve* supplies motor branches to the teres minor.

The **subscapularis muscle** arises from the subscapular fossa of the scapula and inserts into the lesser tubercle of the humerus. It *medially rotates* the arm and is supplied by both the *upper* and *lower subscapular nerves*.

Muscles of the Arm

Anterior Muscles (Flexors). Three muscles lie within the anterior compartment of the arm and are responsible for the anterior bulge of the arm (see *Figure 9-18* and *Table 9-4*). All three muscles are supplied by the *musculocutaneous nerve*.

The **biceps brachii** has two heads, long and short. The tendon of the *long head* arises from the supraglenoid tubercle of the scapula, and takes a relatively long route through the glenohumeral joint and the intertubercular sulcus. The *short head* arises with the coracobrachialis

---

CLINICAL NOTES

Rotator Cuff Injuries

Throwing a ball forcefully, lifting a heavy weight, or direct trauma to the shoulder can result in rotator cuff tears, inflammation of the rotator cuff tendons (tendonitis), and decreased mobility and pain.

Bursitis of the Shoulder

The subacromial bursa is a synovial-lined sac that reduces friction between the supraspinatus tendon and the acromion above (see *Figure 9-8*). Inflammation of this bursa (bursitis) can result in considerable pain upon initial abduction of the arm.

TABLE 9-2

Muscles of the Superficial Back

Muscle	Origin	Insertion	Action(s)	Nerve
Trapezius	Vertebrae: all thoracic and cervical spines Ligamentum nuchae (membranous extension of cervical spines) Skull: superior nuchal line and inion	Scapula: spine and acromion Clavicle: superior lateral third	1. Upper fibers elevate scapula 2. Lower fibers depress scapula 3. Middle fibers retract scapula 4. Rotates laterally (glenoid fossa points up)	Cranial nerve XI: spinal accessory AR of C3-C4
Latissimus dorsi	Vertebrae: spines of T6 to T12 Os coxae: iliac crest Lumbodorsal fascia Ribs: lower 3 to 4	Humerus: floor of intertubercular sulcus	1. Adducts arm 2. Extends arm 3. Rotates arm medially	Thoracodorsal nerve
Levator scapulae	Vertebrae: transverse processes of C1 to C4	Scapula: superior aspect of vertebral border	1. Elevates scapula 2. Rotates scapula medially (glenoid fossa down)	Dorsal scapular
Rhomboids	Vertebrae: spinous processes of C7 to T5	Scapula: vertebral border	1. Retracts scapula 2. Rotates scapula medially (glenoid fossa down)	Dorsal scapular

AR, Anterior ramus

TABLE 9-3

Muscles of the Shoulder

Muscle	Origin	Insertion	Action(s)	Nerve
Deltoid	Clavicle: inferior lateral third Scapula: acromion and spine	Humerus: deltoid tuberosity	1. Abducts arm 2. Flexes arm 3. Rotates arm medially (anterior fibers) 4. Extends arm (posterior fibers) 5. Rotates arm laterally (posterior fibers)	Axillary
Teres major	Scapula: inferior angle	Humerus: medial lip of intertubercular sulcus	1. Extends arm 2. Medially rotates arm 3. Adducts arm	Lower subscapular
Rotator Cuff Muscles				
Supraspinatus	Scapula: supraspinous fossa	Humerus: greater tubercle	1. Abducts arm 2. Stabilizes shoulder joint	Suprascapular
Infraspinatus	Scapula: infraspinous fossa	Humerus: greater tubercle	1. Rotates arm laterally 2. Adduction (slight) 3. Stabilizes shoulder joint	Suprascapular
Teres minor	Scapula: inferior lateral border	Humerus: greater tubercle	1. Rotates arm laterally 2. Extends arm 3. Adducts arm 4. Stabilizes arm at shoulder	Axillary
Subscapularis	Scapula: subscapular fossa	Humerus: lesser tubercle	1. Rotates arm medially 2. Stabilizes shoulder joint	Upper and lower subscapular

from the coracoid process of the scapula. Both long and short heads blend into a common belly that traverses the anterior aspect of the elbow and inserts into the upper forearm allowing the biceps to *flex* the elbow. Because the long head spans the anterior aspect of the shoulder joint, it also functions as a weak *flexor* of the shoulder. In addition to flexion, the biceps is a strong *supinator* of the forearm.

TABLE 9-4

Muscles of the Arm

Muscle	Origin	Insertion	Action(s)	Nerve
Anterior (Flexors)				
Biceps brachii	Scapula (short head): coracoid process Scapula (long head): supraglenoid tubercle	Radius: both heads blend into common tendon that inserts into radial tuberosity	1. Major flexor of forearm at elbow 2. Strong supinator of forearm at superior radioulnar joint 3. Weak flexor of arm at shoulder	Musculocutaneous
Coracobrachialis	Scapula: coracoid process	Humerus: medial aspect of midshaft	1. Flexes arm 2. Adducts arm	Musculocutaneous
Brachialis	Humerus: anterior distal aspect	Ulna coronoid process	Major flexor of forearm at elbow	Musculocutaneous
Posterior (Extensors)				
Triceps brachii	Scapula (long head): infraglenoid tubercle Humerus (lateral head): posterolateral surface Humerus (medial head): posterior surface below the radial groove	Ulna: all three heads blend into a single tendon that inserts into the olecranon	Extends forearm at elbow	Radial
Anconeus	Humerus: lateral epicondyle	Ulna: olecranon along with triceps	1. Extends forearm at elbow 2. Aids in pronation of forearm	Radial

The **coracobrachialis** is a small muscle related in position to the short head of the biceps within the anterior compartment of the arm. It *flexes* and *adducts* the arm.

The **brachialis muscle** runs from the humerus to the upper part of the forearm across the anterior surface of the elbow. It is a powerful *flexor* of the elbow.

Posterior Muscles (Extensors). Two extensor muscles of the elbow occupy the posterior compartment of the arm (see *Figure 9-19*). They are both supplied by the *radial nerve.*

The **triceps brachii** is a powerful *extensor* with three heads that arise from one origin on the scapula and two on the humerus. The three heads fuse into one belly that spans the posterior aspect of the elbow joint and inserts into the ulna.

The **anconeus** (see *Figure 9-22*) is a small muscle that obliquely spans the posterior aspect of the elbow and blends with the triceps insertion. Some anatomists consider it a portion of the triceps brachii muscle.

Muscles of the Forearm

The forearm is crowded with muscles that move the wrist and fingers. To simplify matters, the muscles are arranged into anterior and posterior groups.

The **anterior group** occupies the anterior aspect of the forearm, forming its anterior bulge, and contains eight muscles. Of these, two are pronators of the forearm and six are *flexors* of the wrist and fingers. All but one muscle are supplied by the *median nerve.*

The **posterior group** arises from the posterior aspect of the forearm and contains 11 muscles. Of these, one is a *supinator* of the forearm, one is a *flexor* of the forearm, and the remainder are *extensors* of the wrist and fingers.

Anterior (Flexor and Pronator) Compartment. The eight muscles within the anterior forearm compartment occupy three layers: superficial, intermediate, and deep (*Figure 9-20, Table 9-5*).

Superficial Group. The superficial group consists of one pronator of the forearm and three flexors of the wrist that arise as a group from the medial epicondyle of the humerus.

The **pronator teres** runs obliquely downward and laterally and inserts into the shaft of the radius. It is active in *pronation* of the forearm and hand and is particularly active when resistance is encountered. It is supplied by the *median nerve.*

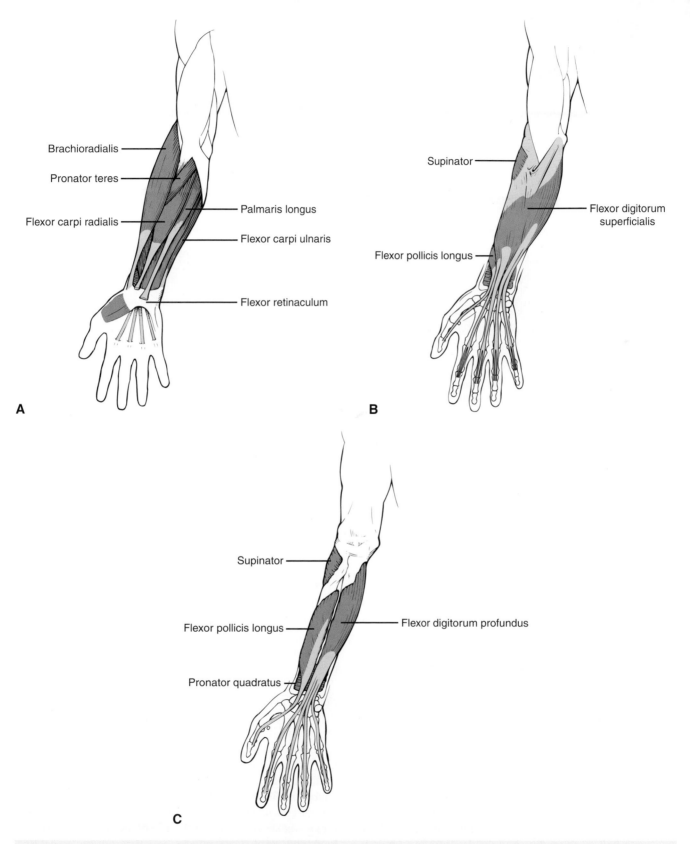

Figure 9-20 Anterior muscles of the right forearm. **A**, Superficial. **B**, Intermediate. **C**, Deep.

TABLE 9-5

Muscles of the Anterior Forearm Compartment

Muscle	Origin	Insertion	Action(s)	Nerve
Superficial				
Palmaris longus	Humerus: medial epicondyle via common flexor tendon	Palmar aponeurosis of hand Flexor retinaculum	Flexes hand at wrist	Median
Flexor carpi radialis	Humerus: medial epicondyle via common flexor tendon	Metacarpals: bases of 2nd and 3rd	1. Flexes hand at wrist 2. Abducts hand at wrist	Median
Flexor carpi ulnaris	Humerus: medial epicondyle via common flexor tendon Ulna: coronoid process	5th metacarpal, pisiform, and hamate bones	1. Flexes hand at wrist 2. Adducts hand at wrist	Ulnar
Pronator teres	Humeral head: medial epicondyle Ulnar head: coronoid process and medial aspect	Radius: lateral aspect of midshaft	Pronates forearm	Median
Intermediate				
Flexor digitorum superficialis	Humerus: medial epicondyle via common flexor tendon Radius: upper half of anterior shaft	Middle phalanges of all digits except thumb: palmar aspects	Flexes middle phalanges at proximal interphalangeal joints	Median
Deep				
Flexor pollicis longus	Ulna: coronoid process Interosseous membrane Radius: anterior surface of shaft	Distal phalanx of thumb: palmar side of base	Flexes thumb	Median
Pronator quadratus	Ulna: anterior distal surface of shaft	Radius: anterior distal aspect	Pronates forearm and provides power when pronating against resistance	Median
Flexor digitorum profundus	Ulna: medial and anterior aspect and adjacent interosseous membrane	Distal phalanges of all digits except thumb: bases	Flexes distal phalanges at distal interphalangeal joints	Ulnar and median

The **palmaris longus** runs down the anterior aspect of the forearm and inserts into the palmar aponeurosis of the hand and the flexor retinaculum of the wrist. It *flexes* the hand at the wrist and is supplied by the *median nerve*.

The **flexor carpi radialis** runs along the anterior aspect of the forearm, forms a long tendon, and inserts into the base of the second metacarpal. It is a *flexor* of the wrist and, because its insertion is on the radial side, acts as an *abductor* as well. It is supplied by the *median nerve*.

The **flexor carpi ulnaris** also runs along the anterior aspect of the forearm but its long tendon inserts on the ulnar side of the carpal bones of the hand. It *flexes* and *adducts* the wrist and is innervated by the *ulnar nerve*.

Intermediate Group. The **flexor digitorum superficialis** is the only muscle in this group. It arises from the common flexor tendon of the medial epicondyle of the humerus and the upper one half of the radius and divides into four tendons that cross the anterior surface of the wrist to insert into the middle phalanges of all four digits except the thumb. It acts as a *flexor* of the proximal interphalangeal joints, metacar-

pophalangeal joints, and the wrist joint and is supplied by the median nerve.

Deep Group. The deep group contains two more flexors of the digits and a deep pronator of the forearm. Their origins are more distal than those muscles of the superficial group.

The **flexor digitorum profundus** originates from the anterior aspect of the ulna and passes over the wrist as four tendons that insert into the distal phalanges of all digits except the thumb. It can flex the distal phalanges and the wrist and is supplied by the *median nerve* on its radial aspect and the *ulnar nerve* on its ulnar aspect. The flexor digitorum superficialis and flexor digitorum profundus are the muscles that enable the fingers to perform the *power grip*. The power grip is strongest when the wrist is bent back or hyperextended and is weakest when the wrist is bent forward or flexed. The long tendons of these muscles pass through the *carpal tunnel* below the *flexor retinaculum*. In the fingers, the flexor tendons travel in osseofibrous tunnels termed *flexor sheaths*. These tunnels keep the tendons applied to the

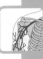

fingers and prevent bowstringing of the tendons. *Synovial sheaths* reduce friction within the tunnels (see *Figure 1-13*).

The **flexor pollicis longus** arises from both the ulna and radius. Its tendon passes over the wrist and inserts into the distal phalanx of the thumb. It is a *flexor* of the thumb and is supplied by the median nerve.

The **pronator quadratus muscle**, the deepest muscle of the forearm, runs transversely across the lower ends of the shafts of the radius and ulna. Its actions are on the radioulnar joints during all movements of *pronation*. As resistance is encountered, it is aided by the pronator teres. The pronator quadratus is supplied by the *median nerve*.

Flexor Retinaculum and the Carpal Tunnel. The carpal bones are arranged from lateral to medial in a ∪ with the concavity pointing forward (*Figure 9-21*). Four carpal bones form the walls of the ∪ with the pisiform and the hamate medially and the scaphoid and trapezium laterally. Attached to prominences of each of these bones is a strong ligament, the **flexor retinaculum**, which is about the size of a small postage stamp. It forms a roof over this carpal curvature, and the space below it is called the *carpal tunnel*. The tunnel is roughly the diameter of a thumb and contains the *flexor tendons* and the *median nerve*. The overlying flexor retinaculum holds the flexor tendons of the digits in place and keeps them from bowing outward.

Posterior (Extensor and Supinator) Compartment. The 11 muscles within the posterior forearm compartment occupy two layers: superficial and deep (*Figure 9-22* and *Table 9-6*). Their long tendons traverse the posterior aspect of the wrist and enter the dorsum of the hand. The **extensor retinaculum** is a fibrous transverse band that holds the extensor tendons in place and prevents their bowing

dorsally on extension. All the muscles within the posterior compartment are supplied by the *radial nerve*.

Superficial Group. The muscles of the superficial group arise as fleshy bellies from either the supracondylar ridge or lateral epicondyle of the humerus.

The **brachioradialis muscle** is an exception to the posterior compartment muscles. Unlike the other posterior muscles, it winds around the lateral aspect of the forearm to insert into the anterolateral surface of the radius. This allows it to function as a *flexor* of the forearm.

The **extensor carpi radialis longus muscle** extends from the lateral supracondylar ridge of the humerus, traverses the posterior aspect of the wrist, and inserts into the base of the second metacarpal. This allows it to not only *extend* the wrist but *abduct* it as well.

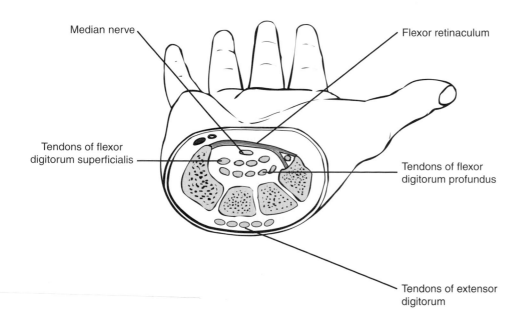

Figure 9-21 Transverse section through the right wrist to show the carpal tunnel and its contents.

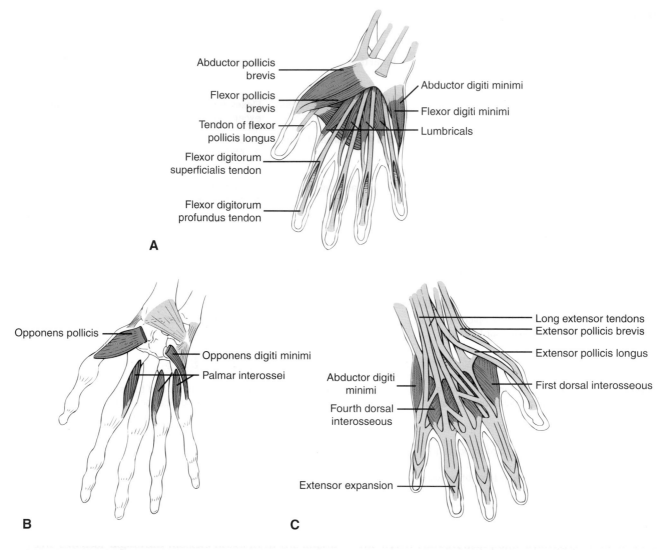

A

Abductor pollicis brevis

Flexor pollicis brevis

Tendon of flexor pollicis longus

Flexor digitorum superficialis tendon

Flexor digitorum profundus tendon

Abductor digiti minimi

Flexor digiti minimi

Lumbricals

B

Opponens pollicis

Opponens digiti minimi

Palmar interossei

C

Abductor digiti minimi

Fourth dorsal interosseous

Extensor expansion

Long extensor tendons

Extensor pollicis brevis

Extensor pollicis longus

First dorsal interosseous

Figure 9-23 Intrinsic muscles of the right hand. **A,** Superficial palmar. **B,** Deep palmar. **C,** Dorsal.

TABLE 9-7

Intrinsic Muscles of the Hand and Wrist

Muscle	Origin	Insertion	Action(s)	Nerve
Thenar Muscles				
Abductor pollicis brevis	Flexor retinaculum Scaphoid and trapezium carpal bones	Proximal phalanx of thumb: lateral aspect of base	Abducts thumb at right angles to palm through movement at metacarpophalangeal and carpometacarpal joints	Median
Flexor pollicis brevis	Flexor retinaculum Trapezium	Proximal phalanx of thumb: base (tendon contains a sesamoid bone)	Flexes proximal phalanx of thumb	Median and ulnar
Opponens pollicis	Flexor retinaculum Trapezium	1st metacarpal: lateral border	Draws tip of thumb to each tip of other digits	Median

Continued

TABLE 9-7

Intrinsic Muscles of the Hand and Wrist—cont'd

Muscle	Origin	Insertion	Action(s)	Nerve
Hypothenar Muscles				
Abductor digiti minimi	Pisiform bone Tendon of flexor carpi ulnaris	Proximal phalanx of 5th digit: medial aspect of base	Abducts 5th digit	Ulnar
Flexor digiti minimi brevis	Flexor retinaculum Hook of hamate	Proximal phalanx of 5th digit: ulnar aspect of base	Flexes 5th digit	Ulnar
Opponens digiti minimi	Flexor retinaculum Hook of hamate	5th metacarpal: ulnar aspect	Draws 5th metacarpal and little finger toward thumb	Ulnar
Other Muscles				
Palmaris brevis	Flexor retinaculum: medial aspect	Skin: ulnar side of palm	Creases skin of palm on ulnar side	Ulnar
Adductor pollicis	Transverse head 3rd metacarpal: dorsal aspect Oblique head Capitate 2nd and 3rd metacarpals: bases	Proximal phalanx of thumb: ulnar aspect of base	Adducts thumb Active in opposition	Ulnar
Lumbricals (4)	Flexor digitorum profundus tendons 1st and 2nd lumbricals arise from the radial aspects of index and middle fingers 3rd and 4th arise from adjacent sides of tendons of middle and ring fingers	Distal phalanges of the four fingers: bases and joins the extensor expansions of extensor digitorum muscle	Flex fingers at metacarpophalangeal joints Extend fingers at interphalangeal joints	Median nerve to two lateral muscles Ulnar nerve to two medial muscles
Dorsal interossei (4)	All four muscles Metacarpals: each muscle arises as two heads from adjacent or facing sides and dorsal aspects	First muscle Proximal phalanx of 2nd digit (index finger): radial side Second muscle Proximal phalanx of 3rd digit (middle) finger: radial side Third muscle Proximal phalanx of 4th digit (ring) finger: ulnar side Fourth muscle Proximal phalanx of 5th digit (little finger): ulnar side	Abduct fingers from median plane (2nd finger) of hand (DAB)	Ulnar
Palmar interossei (3)	First muscle 2nd metacarpal: ulnar side Second muscle 4th metacarpal: radial side Third muscle 5th metacarpal: radial side	1st into ulnar side of proximal phalanx of 2nd digit (index finger) 2nd into radial side of proximal phalanx of 4th digit (ring finger) 3rd into radial side of proximal phalanx of 5th digit (little finger)	Adduct digits toward median plane (2nd finger) of hand (PAD)	Ulnar

DAB, Dorsal abduct; *PAD*, Palmar adduct.

The **lumbricals** are four slender muscles resembling earthworms. They arise from the tendons of the flexor digitorum profundus in the palm of the hand and insert into lateral aspects of the extensor expansions of the four fingers. They flex the fingers at the meta- carpophalangeal joints and extend the fingers at the interphalangeal joints.

The **dorsal interossei** arise from adjacent sides of the metacarpals and insert into the extensor expansions and the proximal phalanges of the first, second, and third fingers. Along with the abductor digiti minimi, the four dorsal interossei *abduct*, or *spread*, the fingers from an axial line through the second finger.

The **palmar interossei** arise from the palmar aspects of the second, fourth, and fifth metacarpals and insert into the extensor expansions and proximal phalanges of all the fingers except the second finger. These muscles adduct the fingers, or close them toward the axial line, through the second finger. An easy way to remember the functions of the interossei is to remember the mnemonics DAB (**d**orsal **ab**duct) and PAD (**p**almar **ad**duct). In addition to these movements, all seven interossei help the lumbricals in flexing the metacarpophalangeal joints and extending the fingers at the interphalangeal joints.

4. Axilla

The **axilla** is described at this point because it contains the nerves and vessels that supply the upper limb; these structures will be described following the axilla. The axilla is a space that is classically described as a **pyramid** with a base composed of the skin and superficial fascia of the armpit. Its blunted, open apex is directed superiorly, rising to the level of the midclavicle, and it is the narrowed opening that serves as the gateway for vessels and nerves passing from the posterior triangle of the neck to the axilla (*Figure 9-24*).

BOUNDARIES

The axilla is bounded by three skeletal and muscular walls: (1) anterior, (2) medial, and (3) posterior (*Figure 9-25*). The anterior and posterior walls almost meet laterally but are separated by the intertubercular (bicipital) groove containing the tendon of the long head of the biceps.

The anterior wall consists of the **clavicle** superiorly and the **pectoralis major** and **pectoralis minor muscles.** The medial wall is the **lateral thoracic wall** covered by the **serratus anterior muscle.** The **posterior wall** is formed primarily by the scapula and the subscapularis muscle that covers its anterior surface. The teres major and latissimus dorsi muscles contribute to the inferior aspect of the posterior wall.

CONTENTS

The axilla contains portions of the **brachial plexus,** and the **axillary artery** and **vein.** These structures are surrounded by the axillary sheath, which encloses them as they pass

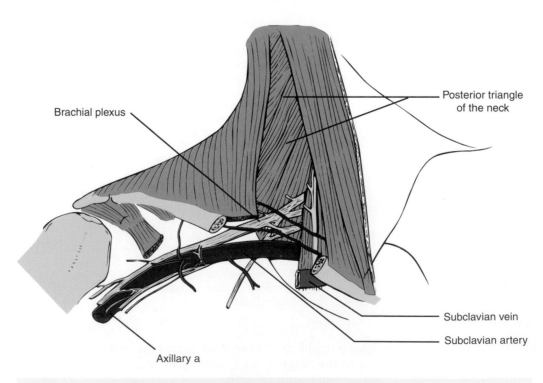

Brachial plexus

Posterior triangle
of the neck

Subclavian vein

Subclavian artery

Axillary a

Figure 9-24 Lateral aspect of the neck showing brachial plexus and subclavian vessels passing from posterior triangle of the neck to the axilla and upper limb.

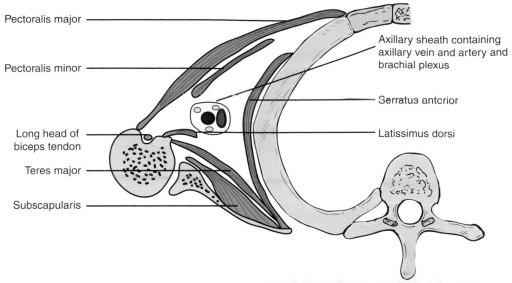

Figure 9-25 Transverse section through the right axilla viewed from below to show the boundaries and contents.

through the fat-filled axilla from the posterior triangle of the neck to the arm. In addition, an important group of axillary lymph nodes that receive lymph from the upper limb and the breast are present. Each of these structures is described in the following sections.

5.   Nerve Supply: The Brachial Plexus

The entire motor and sensory nerve supply to the upper limb is via the brachial plexus (*Figure 9-26*). The plexus originates as **five roots** from anterior rami of spinal nerves C5, C6, C7, C8, and T1. The roots unite to form **three trunks** in the following manner. The roots of C5 and C6 form the *upper trunk*; C7 forms the *middle trunk*; and C8 and T1 join to form the *lower trunk*. Each of the three trunks divides in two to form a total of **six divisions**. These then reunite to form **three cords**: *lateral, posterior,* and *medial.* The three cords each divide and ultimately form **five terminal branches.** The brachial plexus arises in the neck and passes downward under the clavicle and over the first rib to the axilla and then to the upper limb.

COLLATERAL BRANCHES

Several collateral branches arise from the roots, trunks, and cords (*Figure 9-27, Table 9-8*). These branches supply some muscles of the neck, upper limb girdle, and arm. There is also a cutaneous nerve supply to the arm and forearm.

CLINICAL NOTES

Brachial Plexus Injuries

There are two classic types of birth injuries to the brachial plexus that may occur during difficult deliveries. Typically, the damage is to the upper two roots of the brachial plexus or the lower two roots. Damage to the upper roots affects the muscles that move the shoulder and elbow. Damage to the lower roots affects the muscles of the forearm and the hand.

Erb's palsy can occur if the neck is severely flexed laterally and pulled, widening the angle between the head and the shoulder. This maneuver can tear C5 and C6, the upper roots of the plexus, with attendant loss of flexion, abduction, and lateral rotation of the arm at the shoulder, and loss of flexion at the elbow.

Klumpke's palsy can occur if forceful traction is applied to the shoulder during a breech delivery. Stretching of the arm upward can tear the lower roots (C8 and T1), with loss of flexion of the wrist and paralysis of the intrinsic muscles of the hand.

Injuries to Individual Branches

Any of the collateral or terminal branches may be damaged as a result of trauma, but the extent of the damage is entirely dependent upon the site of the lesion. Muscles proximal to a lesion are spared; muscles distal to the lesion are paralyzed. Use *Table 9-9* to determine the results of damage to each nerve, bearing in mind that, once a group of muscles is rendered paralyzed, the antagonist muscles act unopposed.

5. The **medial pectoral nerve** arises from the medial cord and supplies the pectoralis minor muscle and helps supply the *pectoralis major muscle.*

6. **Three motor branches** leave the posterior cord to supply muscles of the pectoral girdle. The branches are the **upper subscapular nerve** to the *subscapularis,* the **lower subscapular nerve** to the *subscapularis* and *teres major,* and the **thoracodorsal** nerve to the *latissimus dorsi muscle.*

7. Two long **cutaneous branches** arise from the distal end of the medial cord. These are the **medial cutaneous nerves of the arm** and the **forearm.**

TERMINAL BRANCHES

The six divisions of the brachial plexus ultimately join to form five terminal branches (see *Figures 9-27* and *9-28*). The branches are listed below, and the structures they supply are listed in *Table 9-9.*

1. The **musculocutaneous nerve** supplies three large flexor muscles of the anterior aspect of the arm, the *biceps brachii, coracobrachialis,* and *brachialis muscles;* it then continues down into the forearm as the **lateral cutaneous nerve of the forearm.**

2. The **median nerve** is a major motor nerve to the flexors and the pronators, overlying the anterior aspect of the forearm; it ends distally as cutaneous fibers to the lateral portion of the palm and palmar aspects of the thumb, first finger, second finger, and the lateral portion of the third finger.

3. The **ulnar nerve** is also motor to flexors, but chiefly to the smaller intrinsic muscles of the hand that are responsible for fine movements of the fingers; it ends as cutaneous branches to the medial aspect of the hand.

4. The **radial nerve** is large and must supply all the extensor muscles of the upper limb; in addition, it supplies cutaneous branches to skin of the posterior aspect of the arm, forearm, and the lateral aspect of the dorsum of the hand.

5. The **axillary nerve** is a small terminal branch that turns posteriorly near the shoulder joint to supply the joint and the deltoid area.

CUTANEOUS NERVES OF THE UPPER LIMB

The cutaneous nerves of the upper limb arise from both collateral and terminal branches of the brachial plexus, and their distributions are summarized in *Figure 9-29.*

6. Arterial Supply

The arterial supply to the upper limb is entirely from the **subclavian artery** and its various branches (*Figure 9-30*). The right subclavian artery arises from the **brachiocephalic**

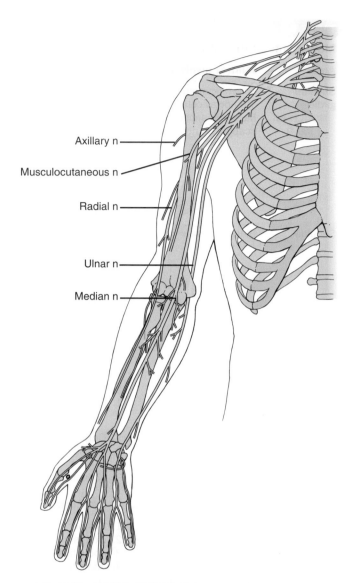

Figure 9-28 Distribution of terminal branches of the brachial plexus.

CLINICAL NOTES

Taking a Blood Pressure

Blood pressure is measured by pressing the brachial artery against the anterior shaft of the humerus with a pressure cuff to occlude the artery. A stethoscope is placed below the cuff in the cubital fossa, and the cuff pressure is slowly released. Two readings are taken as the pressure falls. The first reading is the *systolic pressure* and corresponds to the first audible sound as blood begins to pulse back through the brachial artery. The second reading, *diastolic pressure,* is noted when the brachial pulse is no longer audible.

TABLE 9-9

Branches of the Brachial Plexus

Nerve	Origin	Structures Supplied
Collateral Branches		
Long thoracic	Upper three roots (AR of C5, C6, and C7)	Motor: serratus anterior muscle
Dorsal scapular	Highest root (AR of C5)	Motor: rhomboid major and minor muscles
Suprascapular	Upper trunk	Motor: subclavius and infraspinatus muscles Sensory: the shoulder joint
Lateral pectoral nerve	Lateral cord	Motor: pectoralis major muscle posterior cord
Medial pectoral	Medial cord	Motor: pectoralis minor muscle and helps supply the pectoralis major muscle
Upper subscapular	Posterior cord	Motor: subscapularis
Lower subscapular	Posterior cord	Motor: subscapularis and teres major muscles
Thoracodorsal	Posterior cord	Motor: latissimus dorsi muscle
Terminal Branches		
Musculocutaneous	Lateral cord	Motor: coracobrachialis, biceps brachii, and brachial muscles Sensory: lateral aspect of forearm
Median	Lateral and medial cords	Motor: all flexor muscles of forearm (except flexor carpi ulnaris and ulnar aspect of flexor digitorum profundus), thenar muscles of the hand, and the lateral 2 lumbricals Sensory: lateral palm and digits 1, 2, and part of 3
Ulnar	Medial cord	Motor: flexor carpi ulnaris and ulnar side of flexor digitorum profundus of anterior forearm and hypothenar, adductor pollicis, all 7 interossei, and medial 2 lumbricals of hand
Radial	Posterior cord	Motor: triceps brachii, anconeus muscles of arm, and brachioradialis and extensor muscles of forearm Sensory: posterior of arm and forearm and dorsum of hand
Axillary	Posterior cord	Motor: teres minor and deltoid muscles Sensory: shoulder joint and skin below deltoid

AR, Anterior rami.

artery; the left subclavian artery arises directly from the aortic arch. On either side, the artery loops upward and laterally through the root of the neck and then descends over the first rib to enter the axilla.

The **subclavian artery**, on crossing the *first rib*, changes name to become the axillary artery. The branches of the subclavian artery were noted in Chapter 5, Section 4. The **axillary artery** traverses the axilla and gives off several collateral branches to the region that follow the collateral branches of the brachial plexus. It leaves the axilla by crossing over the tendon of the *teres major muscle* to enter the arm and changes name once more to become the **brachial artery.**

The **brachial artery** enters the arm from the medial aspect and assumes a position anterior to the humerus at its midlength. The artery gives several branches to muscles of the upper arm and descends to the anterior aspect of the elbow (cubital fossa). Here, the artery is in the midline between the biceps tendon laterally and the median nerve medially.

Below the elbow, the brachial artery bifurcates as the **radial** and **ulnar arteries.** The **radial artery** descends on the lateral aspect of the front of the forearm and passes through the wrist, where its *pulsations* may be felt at the base of the metacarpal of the thumb. The radial artery then enters the hand and loops medially as the *deep palmar arch.* The arch anastomoses medially with a branch of the ulnar artery. The **ulnar artery** descends on the medial aspect of the front of the forearm, passes through the wrist, and enters the hand. It loops laterally as the superficial palmar arch and anastomoses medially with a branch of the radial artery. **Digital arteries** arise from the palmar arches to supply the medial and lateral aspects of each finger.

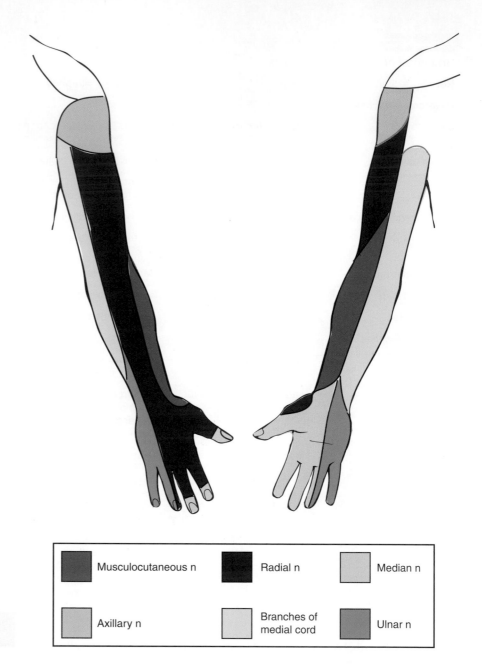

	Musculocutaneous n		Radial n		Median n
	Axillary n		Branches of medial cord		Ulnar n

Figure 9-29 Cutaneous innervation of the upper limb.

7. Venous Return

DEEP VEINS

The deep veins of the upper limb parallel the courses and share the names of the arterial supply. Often, more than one vein accompanies an artery, and these are called *venae comitantes*. The deep veins ultimately collect as the **axillary vein**, which ascends over the first rib to become the **subclavian vein** in the root of the neck (*Figure 9-31*).

SUPERFICIAL VEINS

The superficial, or cutaneous, veins of the upper limb are important because they are often used in venipuncture for collecting blood or performing an intravenous injection. Two sets of veins drain the upper limb: a deep set of veins and a superficial set. The venous drainage begins in the hand.

The **dorsal venous arch** of the hand lies below the skin of the dorsum and forms a pattern that varies among individuals. The dorsal venous arch receives tributaries from the fingers.

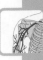

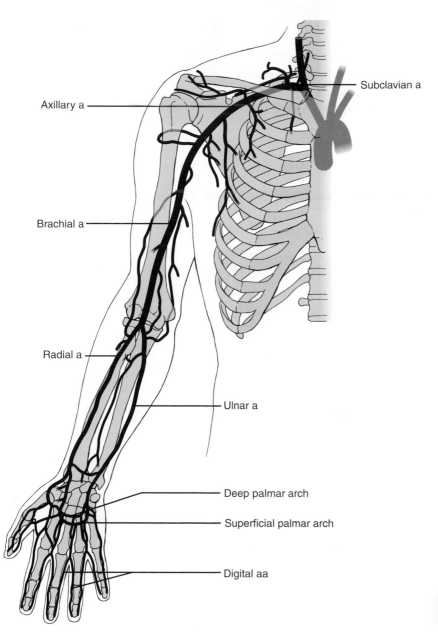

Axillary a

Subclavian a

Brachial a

Radial a

Ulnar a

Deep palmar arch

Superficial palmar arch

Digital aa

Figure 9-30 Arterial supply to the right upper limb.

CLINICAL NOTES

Venipuncture

Venipuncture is the entry into a vein with a needle for the purpose of either injecting intravenous solutions or for withdrawing blood. In most cases, the **median cubital vein** is chosen in the cubital fossa. A tourniquet is applied to the arm above the cubital fossa to occlude the venous return and distend the distal veins. For long-term intravenous drips, the **dorsal venous arch** on the back of the hand is the preferred site for venipuncture.

The **cephalic vein** drains the lateral aspect of the dorsal venous arch, spirals anteriorly at the wrist, and ascends on the lateral aspect of the arm and the forearm. In the arm, it comes to lie in the groove between the deltoid and pectoralis major muscles and then curves medially to plunge deeply into the axillary vein at the infraclavicular fossa.

The **basilic vein** arises from the medial aspect of the dorsal venous arch and ascends on the medial aspect of the forearm. As it traverses the cubital fossa, it receives direct communications from the cephalic vein through the **median cubital** and **median antebrachial veins**. The pattern of communication is variable among individuals. Halfway up the arm, the basilic vein turns deeply to join with and help form the **axillary vein**.

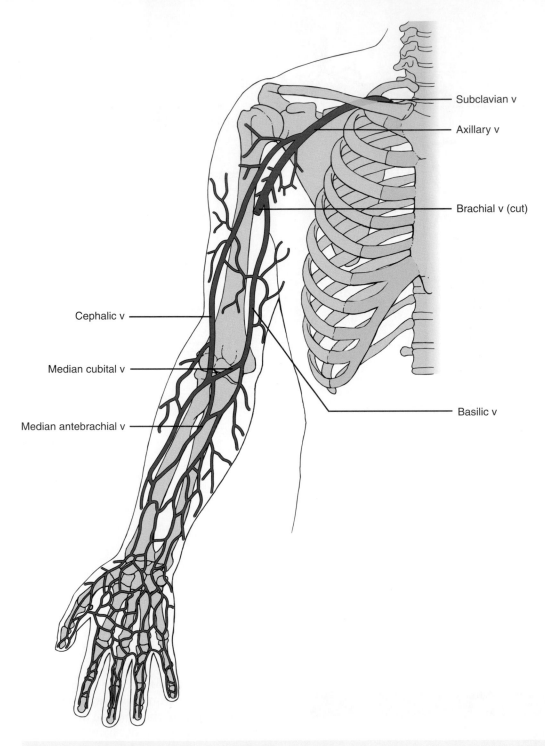

Figure 9-31 Venous return from the right upper limb.

8. Lymphatic Drainage

Like the venous drainage, there is a superficial and a deep set of lymph vessels that drain the upper limb (*Figure 9-32*). The superficial lymphatics form up from intricate plexuses on the hand and ascend to follow the basilic and cephalic veins. They ultimately drain to the *axillary lymph nodes* (lateral group). The **deep set** follows the radial, ulnar, brachial, and axillary veins and ultimately drains into the *axillary lymph nodes* (lateral group). The axillary nodes ultimately form up as the subclavian trunk, which, in turn, drains the upper limb lymph back into circulation at the confluence of the internal jugular and subclavian veins.

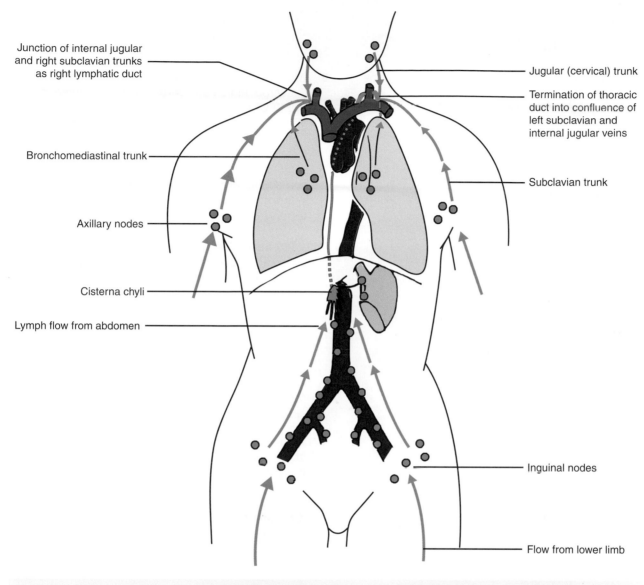

Junction of internal jugular and right subclavian trunks as right lymphatic duct

Jugular (cervical) trunk

Termination of thoracic duct into confluence of left subclavian and internal jugular veins

Bronchomediastinal trunk

Subclavian trunk

Axillary nodes

Cisterna chyli

Lymph flow from abdomen

Inguinal nodes

Flow from lower limb

Figure 9-32 Major groups of lymph nodes and trunks showing the scheme of the lymphatic flow back to the venous system.

Review Questions

1. The trochlea of the humerus articulates with the
_____.
a. olecranon of the ulna
b. trochlear notch of the ulna
c. proximal head of the radius
d. radial tuberosity of the radius
e. medial styloid process of the ulna

2. The shallow glenoid fossa is increased in depth by
_____.
a. the glenoid labrum
b. a joint meniscus
c. a joint disc
d. fat pads
e. synovial membranes

3. The pectoralis minor muscles attach to the
_____.
a. medial end of the clavicle
b. xiphoid process of the sternum
c. coracoid process of the scapula
d. acromion of the scapula
e. lesser tubercle of the humerus

4. All of the following muscles contribute to the
rotator cuff EXCEPT the _____.
a. deltoid muscle
b. teres minor muscle
c. supraspinatus muscle
d. infraspinatus muscle
e. subscapularis muscle

5. A muscle that functions as both a strong flexor
and a powerful supinator of the forearm is the
_____.
a. brachioradialis muscle
b. supinator muscle
c. coracobrachialis muscle
d. brachialis muscle
e. biceps brachii muscle

6. Which of the following statements concerning
the carpal tunnel and carpal tunnel syndrome is
CORRECT?
a. The tunnel is roughly the diameter of a thumb
and is roofed over by the extensor retinaculum.
b. Carpal tunnel syndrome is caused by forced and
prolonged extension of the wrist.
c. The ulnar nerve is compressed by inflamed
flexor tendons and sheaths.
d. Nerve compression may result in anesthesia
(lack of feeling) on the palmar aspect of the
fourth and fifth digits.
e. Nerve compression may result in a weakening
of the muscles responsible for opposition of the
thumb.

7. The cephalic vein terminates in the
_____.
a. axillary vein
b. brachial vein
c. dorsal venous arch
d. internal jugular vein
e. subclavian vein

8. Weakness of the hypothenar muscles would
indicate damage to the _____.
a. axillary nerve
b. musculocutaneous nerve
c. ulnar nerve
d. median nerve
e. radial nerve

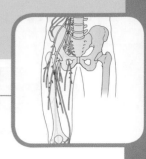

Chapter 10

The Lower Limb

1. Skeleton 425

2. Joints 429

3. Muscles 437

4. Nerve Supply: The Lumbar and
   Sacral Plexuses 444

5. Arterial Supply 450

6. Venous Return 453

7. Lymphatics 454

The lower limb can be compared to the upper limb, bearing in mind that, during development, both limbs rotate 90 degrees in opposite directions. This results in the big toe ending up on the medial side, whereas its upper limb equivalent, the thumb, is on the radial side. The bones, joints, and musculature of the lower limb are relatively larger and sturdier because they are modified for weight bearing and mobility.

1. Skeleton

PELVIC GIRDLE

The lower limb girdle consists of the right and left os coxae, the sacrum, and the coccyx (*Figure 10-1*). The bones of the pelvis were considered in Chapter 4, Section 1.

THIGH

Femur

Description. The femur is the only bone of the thigh (*Figure 10-2*). It is a large, long bone with a rounded head superiorly that articulates with the os coxae and two large knuckles, or condyles, that articulate inferiorly with the tibia.

Features

1. The **head** is somewhat spherical and fits in the cup-shaped acetabulum of the os coxae; approximately three fifths of the spherical head is covered with articular, hyaline cartilage except for a small pit, or fovea, for the attachment of the round ligament (*ligament teres*) of the head of the femur.

2. A **neck** fixes the head to the upper medial aspect of the shaft at an angle of about 130 degrees; at the junction of head and neck are two traction prominences or trochanters that serve as attachments for large lower limb muscles.

3. The **greater trochanter** is the larger of the two; it points superiorly, occupies a superolateral position, and can be palpated just below the skin in the hip region.

4. The **lesser trochanter** is a smaller projection that faces medially and posteriorly.

5. The **intertrochanteric line** is a ridge joining the bases of the two trochanters on the anterior aspect.

6. The **intertrochanteric crest** is a more prominent ridge seen from the posterior aspect that runs from the greater to the lesser trochanter.

7. The **shaft** of the femur angles downward medially and toward its distal end diverges to end as two large knuckles, or condyles.

8. The **medial** and **lateral condyles** of the femur are two large spherical structures that articulate below with the tibia.

9. A deep **intercondylar notch** separates the two condyles. Anteriorly the notch diverges into a smooth patellar fossa for articulation with the patella.

10. The **lateral** and **medial epicondyles** are small projections on the lateral and medial aspects of the condyles.

11. The **adductor tubercle** is another bony projection just above the medial epicondyle that can be palpated easily.

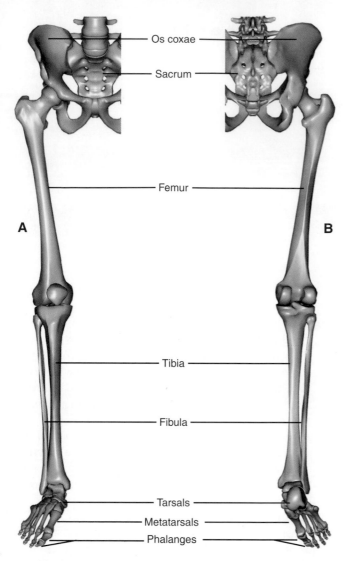

Os coxae

Sacrum

Femur

A

Tibia

Fibula

Tarsals

Metatarsals

Phalanges

Figure 10-1 Bones of the lower right limb. **A,** Anterior view. **B,** Posterior view.

B

12. The **linea aspera** is actually a double ridge on the posterior shaft that extends from the greater and lesser tubercles, converges as a fine double line, and then diverges inferiorly to pass to the medial and lateral epicondyles. It serves as a muscle attachment.

Patella

The patella is a sesamoid bone embedded within the tendon of the quadriceps femoris muscle (*Figure 10-3*). The anterior surface is roughened for the tendinous attachments to the quadriceps femoris muscle. The medial and lateral borders converge inferiorly as the apex. The posterior aspect of the patella is lined with articular cartilage that articulates with the trochlea of the femur. The articular surface is divided into several facets.

LEG

There are two long bones of the leg, the tibia on the medial aspect and the fibula on the lateral.

Tibia

Description. The tibia is relatively strong and massive because it bears all of the weight transmitted inferiorly from the femur and, in turn, transfers the weight to the ankle below (*Figure 10-4*).

Features
1. The **medial** and **lateral condyles** of the tibia are expanded knuckles that articulate with the femoral condyles superiorly through two flattened circular, articular surfaces; the medial condyle is the larger of the two.
2. The **intercondylar eminence** lies between the condyles superiorly.
3. An **articular facet** for the head of the fibular is a shallow, circular depression on the posterolateral aspect of the lateral condyle.
4. The **tibial tuberosity** is a prominent bony projection on the anterior aspect just below the condyles; it is palpable just below the anterior aspect of the kneecap, or patella, and it provides attachment for the patellar ligament.
5. The **shaft** of the tibia has a sharp anterior border that may be palpated because it is just below the skin (for this reason, it is vulnerable to painful bumps and bruises). Attached to the lateral or interosseous border of the shaft is an *interosseous membrane* that extends to the shaft of the fibula and provides an area for muscular attachment.
6. The **medial malleolus** is the medial prominence of the ankle.
7. The **inferior end of the tibia** articulates below with the talus of the ankle and laterally with the inferior end of the fibula.

Fibula

Description. The fibula is the thin lateral bone of the leg. It is not weight-bearing but does provide surface area for muscle attachments. It articulates superomedially with the tibia and inferomedially with the tibia and the talus.

Features
1. An expanded **head** sits atop the thin shaft of the fibula, and it articulates with the articular facet of the tibia described previously.
2. The **lateral malleolus** is the prominent lower end of the fibula that acts as a lateral splint to clamp the talus of the ankle laterally, whereas the medial malleolus of the tibia clamps it medially.

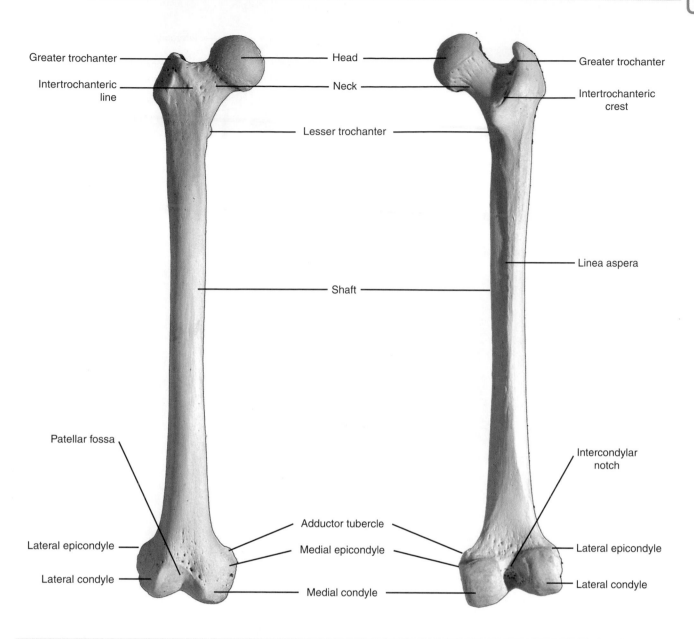

Greater trochanter

Intertrochanteric line

Head

Neck

Greater trochanter

Intertrochanteric crest

Lesser trochanter

Linea aspera

Shaft

Patellar fossa

Intercondylar notch

Lateral epicondyle

Adductor tubercle

Medial epicondyle

Lateral epicondyle

Lateral condyle

Medial condyle

Lateral condyle

Figure 10-2 Right femur. **A,** Anterior aspect. **B,** Posterior aspect.

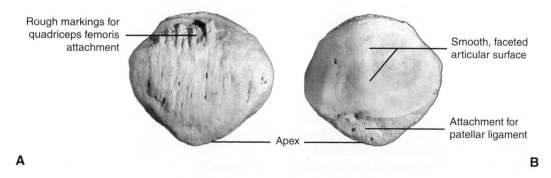

Rough markings for quadriceps femoris attachment

Smooth, faceted articular surface

Attachment for patellar ligament

Apex

A

B

Figure 10-3 Right patella. **A,** Anterior aspect. **B,** Posterior aspect.

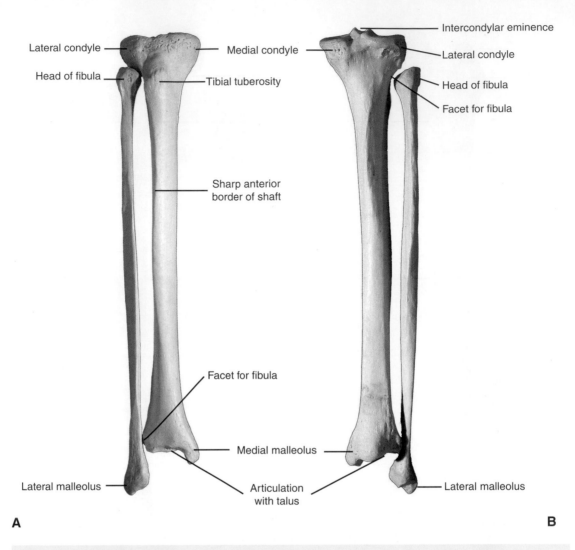

Lateral condyle

Head of fibula

Tibial tuberosity

Medial condyle

Sharp anterior
border of shaft

Facet for fibula

Medial malleolus

Lateral malleolus

Articulation
with talus

A

Intercondylar eminence

Lateral condyle

Head of fibula

Facet for fibula

Medial malleolus

Lateral malleolus

B

Figure 10-4 Right tibia and fibula. **A,** Anterior aspect. **B,** Posterior aspect.

ANKLE AND FOOT

Tarsal Bones

The tarsal bones in the ankle correspond to the carpal bones of the wrist, but there are seven tarsals in the ankle compared to eight carpals in the wrist (*Figure 10-5*). The tarsals occupy the posterior half of the foot. Two tarsals, the talus and calcaneus, are considerably larger, weight-bearing bones and comprise the entire posterior aspect of the foot.

Talus. The talus, or anklebone, consists of a body, a short neck, and a head. The **body** is clamped by and articulates with the fibula (lateral malleolus) and the tibia (medial malleolus). The body also articulates with the calcaneus below. A short neck attaches the body to a **head**, which articulates with the navicular bone anteriorly and the calcaneus inferiorly.

Calcaneus. The calcaneus, or heel bone, is the largest of the tarsal bones. It articulates with the body of the talus and the head of the talus. A bony shelf, or **sustentaculum tali**, helps to support the head of the talus. The posterior third of the talus projects backward beyond the ankle joint as the weight-bearing portion of the heel inferiorly. Superiorly this portion acts as a lever for extensor muscles.

Navicular. As the name suggests, the navicular bone is boat-shaped. The concavity of the boat faces posteriorly and articulates with the rounded head of the talus. The navicular bone articulates anteriorly with three cuneiform bones and laterally with the cuboid bone.

Cuneiforms. *Cuneiform* means wedge-shaped, and there are three of these bones arranged anterior to the navicular bone. The **medial cuneiform** articulates with the head

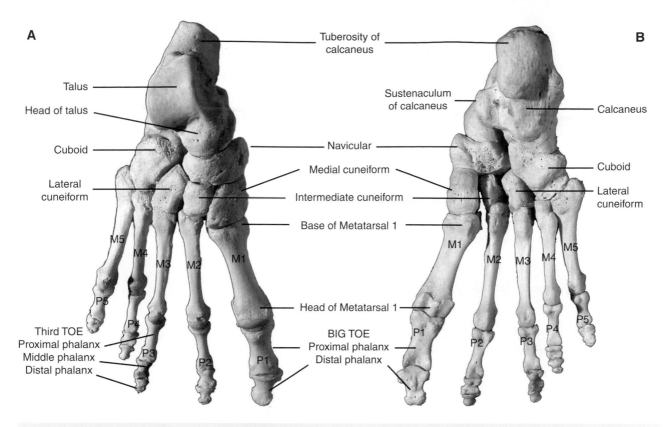

A

Tuberosity of calcaneus

Talus

Head of talus

Cuboid

Lateral cuneiform

Navicular

Medial cuneiform

Intermediate cuneiform

Base of Metatarsal 1

M5

M4

M3 M2

M1

P5

Head of Metatarsal 1

Third TOE
Proximal phalanx
Middle phalanx
Distal phalanx

P4

P3

P2

P1

BIG TOE
Proximal phalanx
Distal phalanx

B

Sustenaculum of calcaneus

Calcaneus

Cuboid

Lateral cuneiform

M1

M2 M3 M4

M5

P1

P2

P3

P4

P5

Figure 10-5 Bones of the right foot. **A,** Dorsal aspect. **B,** Plantar aspect. *M,* Metatarsal; *P,* phalanx.

of the first metatarsal, the **intermediate cuneiform** with the head of the second metatarsal, and the **lateral cuneiform** articulates with the third metatarsal.

Cuboid. The cuboid resembles a cube. Its posterior surface articulates with the calcaneus, and its anterior surface articulates with both the fourth and fifth metatarsals. The medial surface articulates with the lateral cuneiform.

Metatarsal Bones

There are five metatarsal bones that form the skeleton of the anterior sole of the foot. Metatarsals 1, 2, and 3 articulate with the three cuneiform bones; metatarsals 4 and 5 articulate with the cuboid bone.

Features. Each metatarsal features an expanded **base**, which articulates with the tarsals behind and provides attachments for muscles of the foot. A rounded **head** on the distal end of the shaft articulates anteriorly with the phalanges of the toes.

Phalanges. As in the hand, each toe consists of three phalanges: the **proximal, middle,** and **distal** phalanges. The sole exception is the first (big) toe. It has only two phalanges, proximal and distal.

2. | Joints

THE PELVIC GIRDLE
Features
Two joints anchor the pelvic girdle to the axial skeleton: (1) the sacroiliac joint and (2) the hip joint (*Figure 10-6*).

Sacroiliac Joint. The sacroiliac joint is a fairly rigid joint binding the ear-shaped, or auricular, surfaces of the sacrum to a reciprocally shaped area on the iliac portion of the os coxae. It has the features of two joints; it is a **synovial joint** anteriorly and a **fibrous joint** posteriorly.

Symphysis Pubis. The symphysis pubis is a midline joint between the pubic portions of the right and left os coxae. It is a typical symphysis in that the bony surfaces are lined with hyaline cartilage. Fibrous tissue binds the cartilaginous surfaces in the midline, forming a joint with little movement.

Movements
There is some movement in the sacroiliac joint that imparts some resilience as weight is transferred from the sacrum to the pelvis, but this resiliency tends to decrease with age. During pregnancy, the fibrous elements of both

429

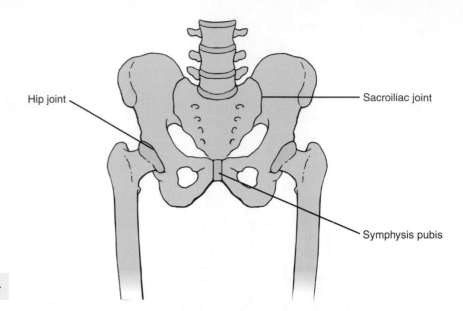

Figure 10-6 Joints of the pelvic girdle and hip.

the sacroiliac and the symphysis pubis joints become lax, allowing the pelvis to widen and facilitate passage of the head through the birth canal.

HIP JOINT

Features

The hip joint is an extremely stable yet moveable ball-and-socket joint (*Figure 10-7*). It is an articulation between the spherical **head of the femur** (ball) and the cup-shaped **acetabulum of the os coxae** (socket). The articular surface of the acetabulum is horseshoe-shaped. The concavity of the acetabulum is further deepened by the **acetabular labrum,** a fibrocartilage ring that encircles the rim of the fossa. A joint capsule surrounds the joint, affording it a fair degree of movement. The capsule is thickened and reinforced by three strong ligaments running from each component of the os coxae to the neck of the femur to

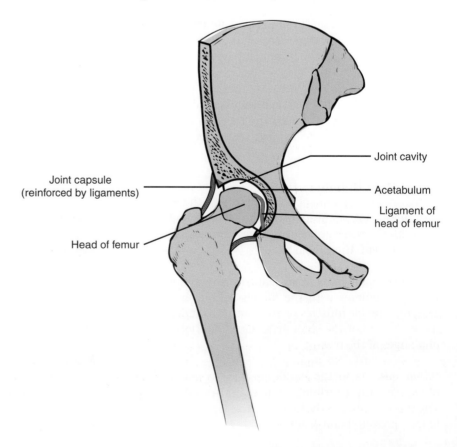

Figure 10-7 Coronal section through the right os coxae (hip bone) to display opened hip joint.

prevent dislocation of the joint. The ligaments include the **iliofemoral ligament** anteriorly, the **ischiofemoral ligament** posteriorly, and the **pubofemoral ligament** inferiorly and anteriorly. The **ligament of the head of the femur** is a rather weak ligament that runs from the lower end of the acetabulum to the fovea on the head of the femur. It may contain a small nutrient artery to the head of the femur.

Fracture of the Femoral Neck

Fractures of the femoral neck are more common in older people, particularly women suffering from osteoporosis. The nutrient arterial supply to the head of femur arises mainly from vessels that continue through the joint capsule as **retinacula**. Should the fracture damage these vessels, the head of the femur undergoes degeneration or **avascular necrosis**, a situation that necessitates surgical replacement.

Hip Replacement

Osteoarthritis of the hip is a degenerative disease that results in pain and limited movement to a point at which surgical hip replacement is the treatment of choice. The damaged elements of the joint, the femoral head and the acetabulum, are removed and replaced by inert prostheses.

Movements

The following movements are described in relation to the anatomical position (*Figure 10-8*). This assumes that the foot is moved from the ground with resultant movement of the femur at the hip. If the foot remains on the ground, however, the os coxae moves in relation to the femur. The hip joint is capable of six movements:

1. **Flexion** of the thigh at the hip swings the thigh anteriorly and superiorly in the sagittal plane from the anatomical position; this is accomplished by the *rectus femoris*, *sartorius*, *iliopsoas*, *pectineus*, and *adductor muscles*.
2. **Extension** swings the thigh back to the anatomical position; hyperextension swings the thigh even farther posteriorly. Muscles that extend the thigh include the *hamstrings*, *gluteus maximus*, and *adductor magnus muscles*.
3. **Abduction** swings the thigh laterally and superiorly away from the trunk in the coronal plane; the *gluteus medius*, *gluteus minimus*, *tensor fasciae latae*, *iliopsoas*, *piriformis*, and *sartorius muscles* abduct the thigh at the hip.
4. **Adduction** swings the thigh back toward the trunk through the actions of the *adductors* (*longus*, *brevis*, and

magnus), *pectineus*, *gracilis*, *gemelli*, *obturator internus*, and *obturator externus muscles*.

5. **Medial rotation** is the rotation of the thigh about its long axis turning its anterior surface toward the median plane; this movement is performed by the *glutei medius* and *minimus*, *adductors* (*longus*, *brevis*, and *magnus*), and *tensor fasciae latae* muscles.
6. **Lateral rotation** rotates the thigh about its long axis so that the anterior surface turns laterally away from the median plane; contributing muscles are the *gluteus maximus*, *iliopsoas*, *piriformis*, *obturator externus* and *internus*, *gemelli*, and *quadratus femoris*.

Circumduction is a combination of flexion, extension, abduction, and adduction in a wide conical arc about the hip.

THE KNEE JOINT

The knee joint is the largest and perhaps the most complicated joint in the body (*Figure 10-9*). It is classified as a synovial joint with interposing fibrocartilage discs, or menisci. The knee is really a complex of three joints: (1) between the lateral condyles of the femur and tibia, (2) between the medial condyles of the femur and the tibia, and (3) between the patella and the femur. The joints between the tibia and femur represent the *weight-bearing portion of the knee*. They are moveable, synovial joints that allow a combined hinge and sliding type movement and limited rotation. The joint between the patella and the femur allows a sliding type of movement.

The knee is susceptible to injuries that are work- and sports-related. In addition, genetic factors and the aging process may result in degenerative joint disease (primary osteoarthritis).

Features

Smooth, glassy **hyaline cartilage** coats the articular surfaces of the femoral and tibial condyles. When moistened with synovial fluid, the articulating surfaces move smoothly over each other. The condyles of the femur and the tibia are partially separated by two interposing fibrocartilaginous discs, or menisci, the **medial** and **lateral menisci**. Each meniscus is C-shaped, and a transverse ligament joins their anterior margins.

The **capsular ligament** or articular capsule is a thin, strong fibrous membrane that forms a sleeve around the knee, and it is strengthened considerably by **medial** and **lateral collateral ligaments** and overlying muscle tendons that help to stabilize the knee and limit movements of the knee to normal ranges. The medial meniscus is attached to the inner aspect of the medial collateral ligament. Contributing significantly to the stability of the knee are two strong, internal **anterior** and **posterior cruciate ligaments** that join the intercondylar areas of the

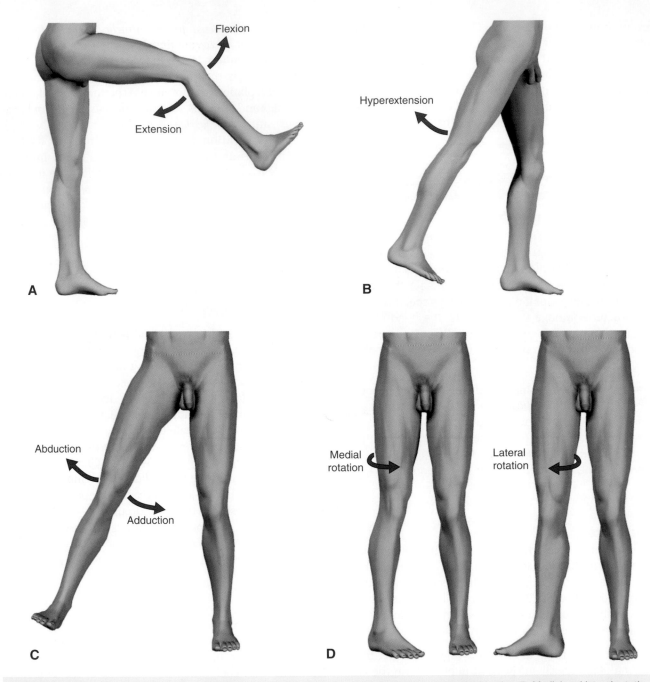

Figure 10-8 Movements at the hip joint. **A,** Flexion and extension. **B,** Hyperextension. **C,** Abduction and adduction. **D,** Medial and lateral rotation.

femur and the tibia. The ligaments are named according to their attachments on the tibia. The anterior cruciate ligament runs superiorly and posteriorly to prevent anterior displacement of the femur on the tibia. The posterior cruciate ligament runs anteriorly and superiorly to prevent posterior displacement of the femur on the tibia. A **synovial membrane** lines the inner aspect of the fibrous capsule to create an extensive chamber termed the *synovial cavity of the knee* that normally contains some synovial fluid for lubrication. The synovial membrane does not cover the articular surfaces of the tibia and femur. A number of muscles cross over the bones of the knee joint, and, where they do, enclosed, fluid-filled sacs, or **bursae**, act as lubricating devices, allowing free movement of the muscle over the joint. Of the bursae associated with the knee, three communicate directly with the synovial cavity and the remainder are separate compartments.

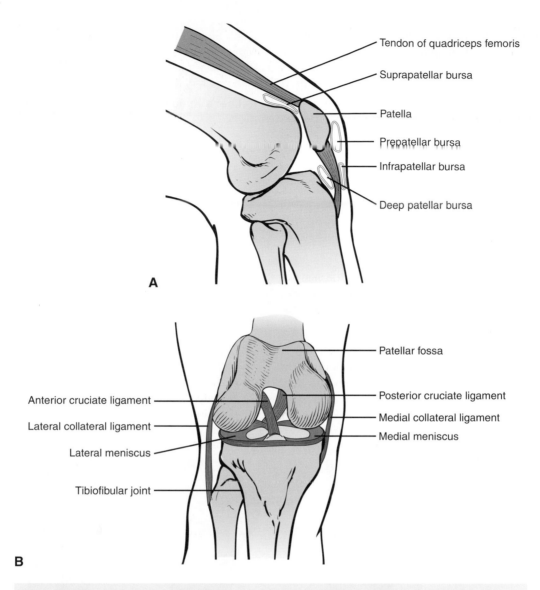

A

B

Figure 10-9 Internal features of the right knee. **A,** Lateral view. **B,** Anterior view with the knee flexed.

Labels (A): Tendon of quadriceps femoris; Suprapatellar bursa; Patella; Prepatellar bursa; Infrapatellar bursa; Deep patellar bursa

Labels (B): Patellar fossa; Posterior cruciate ligament; Medial collateral ligament; Medial meniscus; Anterior cruciate ligament; Lateral collateral ligament; Lateral meniscus; Tibiofibular joint

---

CLINICAL NOTES

Knee Injuries

The knee bears six to eight times an individual's body weight with each normal step and considerably more in running and jumping. For this reason, the knee is vulnerable to injury, particularly in the aged. Acute injuries occur suddenly when soft tissues of the knee are suddenly torn or damaged. Chronic injuries are the result of predisposing factors, overuse, and not following a good preventive program.

Tears of the Anterior Cruciate Ligament

This is the most common acute knee injury and is generally caused by a sudden, violent twisting or piv-

oting movement. An intact anterior cruciate ligament prevents excessive anterior movements of the tibia or subluxation. The patient may hear a pop as the ligament ruptures, and intraarticular bleeding may result in swelling. A physical examination will reveal a knee in which the tibia may be subluxated anteriorly. Some patients show minimal knee instability and require no treatment, but most (70%) require surgery.

Tears of the Menisci

Most tears of the menisci occur as sequelae to tears of the anterior cruciate ligament. Anterior subluxation of the tibia causes abnormal compression of the posterior third of the meniscus between the femur and tibia and a vertical or circumferential tearing of the meniscus. Treatment is usually by arthroscopic surgery, and, if at all possible, partial meniscectomies are performed rather than complete removal of the damaged meniscus.

Tears of the Medial Collateral Ligament

A violent blow to the lateral aspect of the knee can rupture the medial collateral ligament and displace or tear the medial meniscus because of its attachment to the ligament. Surgical repair was once routinely performed, but studies have shown that immobilization in a cast or hinge brace along with early movement and exercise is usually sufficient.

Occupational Bursitis

Continual occupational kneeling compresses the skin and underlying prepatellar and sometimes infrapatellar bursa against the patella. This chronic depression causes the small bursae to become inflamed and filled with fluid, with resultant swelling over the patella, or "water on the knee." Treatment consists of tensor bandages, ice, anti-inflammatory drugs, and moderation of movement.

Runner's Knee or Chondromalacia

It is a common problem in runners and is characterized by pain and clicking. A poorly balanced quadriceps femoris muscle tends to pull the patella laterally as it tracks through the femoral groove on flexion and extension. The patellar articular cartilage becomes damaged and roughened, and in long-term cases, the patella becomes misshapen. Treatment consists of tensor bandages, ice, anti-inflammatory drugs, and moderation of movement.

Knee Replacement

Like the hip joint, the knee can be replaced with a metal and plastic prosthesis to replace damaged femoral and tibial condyles.

Movements

1. **Flexion bends** the leg posteriorly and superiorly at the knee (*Figure 10-10*); the muscles that flex the knee include the *biceps femoris, semitendinosus* and *semimembranosus, gracilis, sartorius, gastrocnemius,* and *popliteus.*

2. **Extension** straightens the leg at the knee; extensors include the *quadriceps* and *tensor fasciae latae muscles.*

3. A slight **medial rotation** of the femur on the tibia takes place in the late stages of extension, which is referred to as the *screw-home movement* and is caused by the fact that

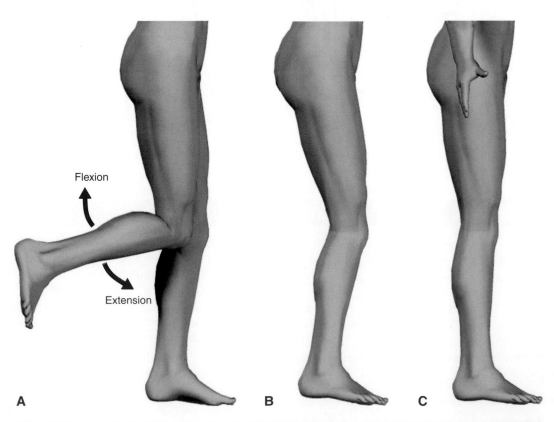

Figure 10-10 Movements of the knee. **A,** Flexion and extension. **B,** Initial extended knee. **C,** Fully extended knee (screw home).

the lateral femoral condyle reaches its extended position first, but the larger, more curved, medial femoral condyle moves slightly more to reach its fully extended and locked position. Flexion and extension of the knee joint take place between the femoral condyles and the superior aspects of the menisci. Rotation takes place between the inferior aspects of the menisci and the tibial condyles.

ANKLE JOINTS

Tibiofibular Joints

There is a **superior** and an **inferior joint** between the fibula and the tibia (*Figure 10-11*). The superior joint is synovial, allowing minimal compensatory movements for lateral ankle movements. The inferior joint is a strong, fibrous syndesmosis binding the tibia and fibula. An interosseous membrane joins the shafts of the two bones and provides for increased area for muscular attachments in the leg.

Talocrural (Ankle) Joint

Features. The distal ends of the **tibia** and **fibula** form a tight mortise into which the superior aspect of the **talus** fits, allowing pure hinge movements. It is a synovial joint with a fibrous capsule strengthened medially by the **deltoid (medial collateral) ligament** and laterally by the **lateral collateral ligament**. The talocrural joint is basically a *hinge joint*, allowing movement in a single plane.

Movements. The talocrural (ankle) joint is capable of two movements (*Figure 10-12*).

1. **Dorsiflexion** is the drawing up of the dorsum of the foot that allows the heel to strike the ground first in walking. The active muscles are extensor hallucis longus, extensor digitorum longus, and tibialis anterior.
2. **Plantarflexion** is the opposite movement that points the foot downward, with the sole or plantar surface of the foot pointing posteriorly, as in standing on the

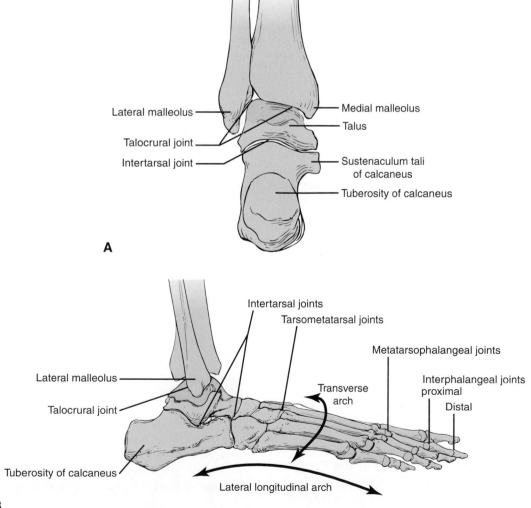

A

Lateral malleolus
Talocrural joint
Intertarsal joint
Medial malleolus
Talus
Sustenaculum tali of calcaneus
Tuberosity of calcaneus

B

Intertarsal joints
Tarsometatarsal joints
Metatarsophalangeal joints
Interphalangeal joints proximal
Distal
Transverse arch
Lateral malleolus
Talocrural joint
Tuberosity of calcaneus
Lateral longitudinal arch

Figure 10-11 Joints of the right ankle. **A,** Posterior view. **B,** Lateral view.

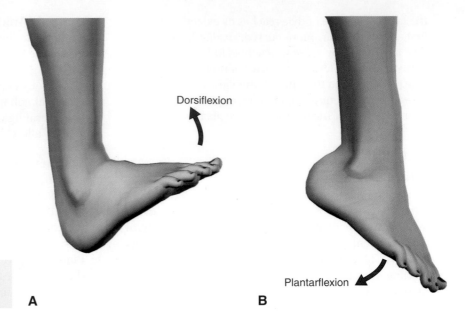

Figure 10-12 Movements of the right talocrural (ankle) joint. **A**, Dorsiflexion. **B**, Plantarflexion.

A

B

toes. Plantarflexors include the gastrocnemius, soleus, peroneus longus, plantaris, tibialis posterior, and peroneus brevis muscles.

Intertarsal Joints

Description. Although there are numerous joints between articular surfaces of the seven tarsal bones, only two, the **talocalcanean (subtalar)** and the **transverse tarsal joints**, add significantly to the range of movement at the ankle below the talus. The remaining intertarsal joints are of less importance, allowing some compensatory gliding movements.

Movements. In the movements of dorsiflexion and plantarflexion described previously, the talus moves together with the foot (*Figure 10-13*). During eversion and inversion described below, however, the talus moves with the bones of the leg.

1. **Eversion** is the movement at the intertarsal joints that turns the sole of the foot laterally, or outward. This movement is accomplished by the *fibularis longus, brevis,* and *tertius muscles.*
2. **Inversion** is the opposite movement that turns the sole medially, or inward. Invertors of the foot include the *tibialis anterior* and *posterior muscles.*

The Remaining Joints and Arches of the Foot

The remaining joints of the foot, including the **tarsometatarsal, metatarsophalangeal,** and **interphalangeal joints,** are similar to the joints of the hand, but their movements are far more restricted (see *Figure 10-11*). They are an integral part of a system of three major arches that provide the foot with the ability to sustain the weight of the body yet be sufficiently flexible to adapt to different terrains during standing and walking. There are two **longitudinal arches, medial** and **lateral,** and a **transverse arch.** The arches distribute the weight of the body between the calcaneus (heel) posteriorly and the heads of the first three metatarsals (ball of foot) anteriorly. Most of the anterior weight is borne by the head of the first metatarsal and the two sesamoid bones below it.

Four ligaments maintain the arches and provide some elasticity or spring. Their names fortunately describe their attachments, and they include the (1) plantar calcaneonavicular (spring) ligament, (2) long plantar ligament, (3) short plantar (calcaneocuboid) ligament, and (4) plantar aponeurosis that stretches from the tuberosity of the calcaneus to the bases of the metatarsals.

CLINICAL NOTES

Pott's Fracture

Violent or forced eversion of the ankle can result in this type of fracture. The extremely strong deltoid or medial ligament remains intact, but the tip of the medial malleolus to which it is attached fractures. This is accompanied by damage to the inferior tibiofibular joint and possibly a higher fracture of the fibula on the lateral side.

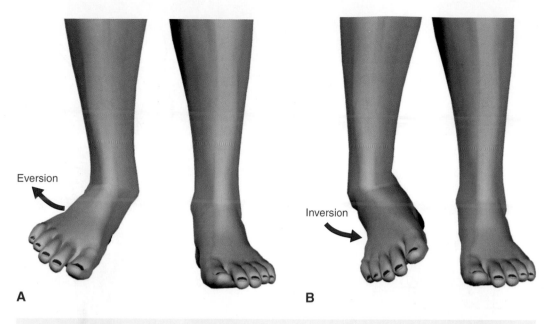

Figure 10-13 Movements of the intertarsal joints. **A**, Eversion. **B**, Inversion.

MOVEMENT OF THE LOWER LIMB JOINTS DURING WALKING

The hip, knee, ankle, and joints of the foot participate in movements that alternately support and propel the body forward during the two phases of walking. A stride is one complete cycle of walking that consists of a stance and a swing phase.

1. The **stance phase** occurs as the right foot, for example, is on the ground and assumes the weight. The phase begins when the right heel initially hits the ground (the heel strike) and ends with the push-off as the right foot goes up on its toes and pushes off to enter the swing phase.
2. The **swing phase** occurs as the right foot leaves the ground and swings forward to end once more with the right heel strike.

3. Muscles

In contrast to the upper limb, the lower limb is designed for support and locomotion and the muscles are accordingly more massive and less refined.

Because several lower limb muscles traverse more than one joint, it is convenient to group the muscles by region: (1) anterior thigh muscles, (2) posterior thigh muscles, (3) gluteal muscles, (4) anterior leg muscles, (5) lateral leg muscles, (6) posterior leg muscles, and (7) muscles of the foot.

ANTERIOR THIGH MUSCLES

The anterior group of thigh muscles includes *flexors of the hip* and *extensors of the knee* that are active during walking as the heel of the advancing foot is about to strike the ground. The *femoral nerve* supplies them all (*Figure 10-14, Table 10-1*).

Flexors of the Hip

The flexors of the hip arise from the os coxae and cross the anterior aspect of the hip joint to insert into the femur. The **iliopsoas muscle** (combined iliacus and psoas muscles) is the major flexor of the hip, but contributing to hip flexion are the **rectus femoris** and **sartorius muscles.**

Extensors of the Knee

The extensors of the knee traverse the anterior aspect of the knee and insert into the tibia. They include all components of the **quadriceps femoris muscle.** The **rectus femoris** is the only component to arise from the os coxae from the anterior inferior iliac spine. It traverses the hip joint, spans the anterior aspect of the thigh, and inserts as a narrowed tendon into the upper border of the patella. The patella, in turn, is attached by the strong patellar ligament to the tibial tuberosity of the tibia. The rectus femoris, therefore, really inserts via the patellar ligament into the tibia, allowing it to function as a powerful extensor of the knee. The remaining components of the quadriceps femoris are the **vastus lateralis, vastus medialis,** and **vastus intermedius muscles.** They originate from the anterior aspect of the upper femur

437

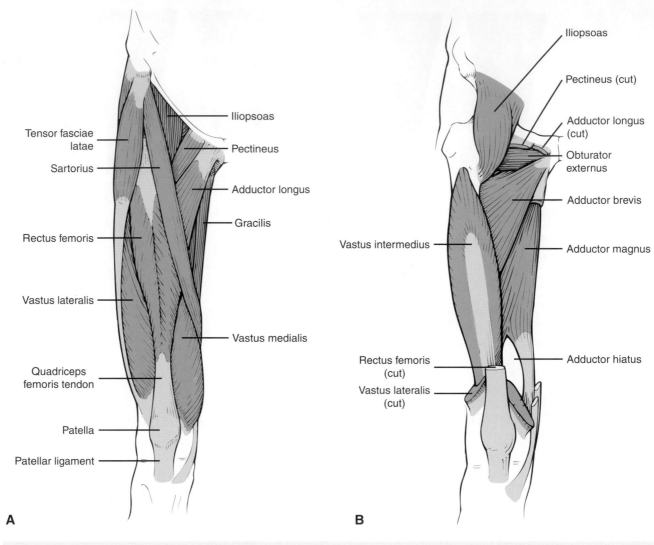

Figure 10-14 Anterior and medial muscles of the right thigh. **A,** Superficial. **B,** Deep.

and insert into the rectus femoris tendon. They act with the rectus femoris to extend the knee. The vastus medialis also acts to prevent lateral dislocation of the patella.

MEDIAL THIGH MUSCLES
Adductors of the Hip
The medial muscles of the thigh are also referred to as the *adductor mass* because they act in concert to adduct the thigh at the hip (see *Figure 10-14* and *Table 10-2*). They also help to hide the fact that the femur angles medially from hip to knee by filling in the angular interval with their mass. The adductors include the **pectineus, adductor longus, adductor brevis, adductor magnus, gracilis,** and **obturator externus muscles.** They arise from the pubic area of the os coxae and angle laterally into the femur,

allowing them to adduct the hip. In addition the muscles can also act as *flexors* and *medial rotators* of the hip. All the muscles are supplied by branches of the *obturator nerve* except for the pectineus, which receives branches from the *femoral nerve.*

Two Muscles that Differ
Two muscles are singled out as being different from the other adductors. The **adductor magnus** developed as a fusion of two muscles. The more anterior component behaves like the medial adductors and helps *flex the hip*; the posterior component is like the hamstrings and helps *extend the hip*. The **gracilis muscle** is the only member of the adductor group that, in addition to traversing the hip joint, spans the knee joint and attaches to the tibia. It can, therefore, help *flex the knee.*

TABLE 10-1

Anterior Muscles of the Thigh

Muscle	Origin	Insertion	Action(s)	Innervation
Iliopsoas				
A combination of iliacus and psoas major muscles	Iliacus portion Os coxae: iliac crest, ala of sacrum, and iliac fossa Psoas major portion Lumbar vertebrae: bodies and transverse processes	Femur: both muscles insert as a common tendon into the lesser trochanter	1. Single muscle: flexor of thigh at hip joint 2. Active during standing, keeping pelvis and body tilted forward	Anterior rami of L2, L3 Femoral nerve
Quadriceps Femoris				
Rectus femoris	Anterior inferior iliac spine and superior rim of acetabulum of os coxae	Tibia: tibial tuberosity via patellar ligament	1. Extends leg at knee 2. Helps in flexion of thigh at hip joint	Femoral nerve
Vastus lateralis	Lateral side of linea aspera, base of greater trochanter of femur	Tibia: tibial tuberosity via patellar ligament	Extends leg at knee	Femoral nerve
Vastus medialis	Medial aspect of linea aspera of femur	Tibia: tibial tuberosity via patellar ligament	Extends leg at knee	Femoral nerve
Vastus intermedius	Anterior and lateral aspects of femur	Tibia: tibial tuberosity via patellar ligament	Extends leg at knee	Femoral nerve
Sartorius	Anterior superior iliac spine of os coxae	Tibia: superior medial aspect	1. Flexes leg at knee 2. Helps in flexion of thigh at hip joint 3. Rotates thigh laterally at hip joint	Femoral nerve

MUSCLES OF THE GLUTEAL REGION

Larger Muscles

The **gluteus medius, gluteus minimus,** and the **tensor fasciae latae muscles** act as antagonists to the adductor muscles in that they are *abductors of the hip* and *lateral rotators*

(*Figure 10-15, Table 10-3*). They originate from the iliac crest of the os coxae, cross the hip joint, and insert into the femur except for the tensor fasciae latae, which continues across the knee joint and inserts into the tibia. These muscles are supplied by the *superior gluteal nerve.*

TABLE 10-2

Medial Muscles of the Thigh

Muscle	Origin	Insertion	Action(s)	Innervation
Pectineus	Os coxae: pectineal line on superior ramus of pubis	Femur: posterior aspect of below lesser trochanter	1. Adducts thigh at hip 2. Flexes thigh at hip 3. Rotates thigh medially at hip	Femoral nerve
Adductor longus	Os coxae: anterior aspect of pubis	Femur: medial aspect of linea aspera	1. Adducts thigh at hip 2. Aids in flexing thigh at hip	Obturator nerve
Adductor brevis	Os coxae: inferior ramus of pubic portion	Femur: above linea aspera	1. Adducts thigh at hip 2. Aids in flexing thigh at hip	Obturator nerve
Adductor magnus consists of two components: adductor and hamstring	Os coxae: inferior ramus of pubis and ischium	Femur: adductor portion: posterior aspect of shaft; hamstring portion: adductor tubercle	Adductor portion 1. Adducts thigh at hip 2. Rotates hip laterally Hamstring portion Extends thigh at hip	Adductor portion: obturator nerve Hamstring portion: sciatic nerve
Gracilis	Os coxae: inferior ramus of pubic portion	Tibia: superior medial aspect	1. Flexes leg at knee 2. Rotates thigh medially at hip 3. Adducts thigh	Obturator nerve

The **gluteus maximus** is different from the others in that it *extends the hip joint*, not so much during walking, but in rising from a sitting position or ascending the stairs. It is also a *lateral rotator of the hip*. It is supplied by the *inferior gluteal nerve*.

Smaller Muscles (Lateral Hip Rotators)

A number of smaller and deeper posterior muscles arise from the os coxae or sacrum and insert into the femur in a direction that allows them to laterally rotate the hip (see *Figure 10-15* and *Table 10-4*). These muscles include the **piriformis**, supplied by the *nerve to piriformis*, the **obturator internus**, and **superior gemellus**, supplied by the *nerve to obturator internus* and *superior gemellus*, and the **inferior gemellus** and **quadratus femoris**, supplied by the *nerve to inferior gemellus* and *quadratus femoris*.

POSTERIOR THIGH MUSCLES (HAMSTRINGS)

The hamstring muscles are *extensors of the hip* and *flexors of the knee* and are activated when the trailing foot is lifted from the ground during the act of walking (see *Figure 10-15* and *Table 10-5*). These muscles include the **semitendinosus, semimembranosus, biceps femoris,** and the **posterior portion of the adductor magnus muscles.** They arise from the ischium of the os coxae, pass over the posterior aspects of the hip and knee, and insert into the posterior aspects of the tibia and fibula. Motor branches of the *sciatic nerve* supply the hamstring muscles.

ANTERIOR LEG MUSCLES

The anterior leg muscle group arises from the anterior aspects of the tibia, fibula, and interosseous membrane;

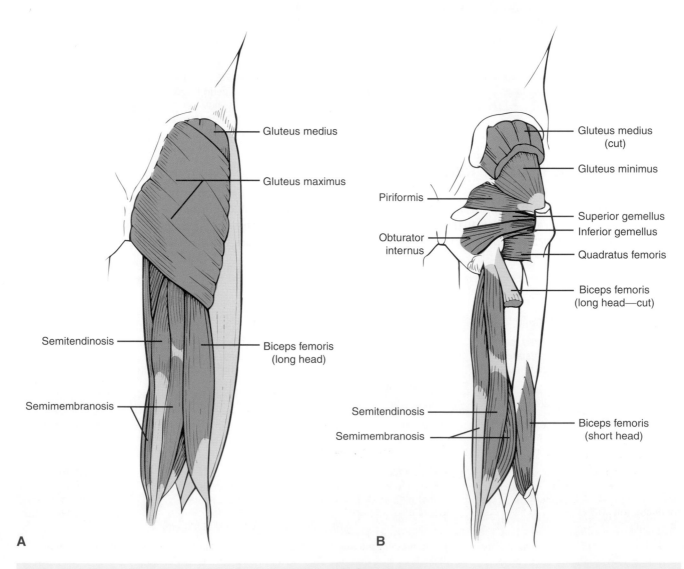

A **B**

Figure 10-15 Gluteal and posterior muscles of the right thigh. **A,** Superficial. **B,** Deep.

TABLE 10-3

Muscles of the Gluteal Region that Move the Hip

Muscle	Origin	Insertion	Action(s)	Innervation
Gluteus maximus	Os coxae: posterosuperior surface Sacrum: posterolateral aspect Coccyx	Femur: gluteal tuberosity Tibia: lateral condyle— inferior fibers of the gluteus maximus join the tensor fascia latae to form the iliotibial tract	1. Extends thigh at hip as in rising from a sitting position 2. Rotates thigh laterally at hip	Inferior gluteal nerve
Gluteus medius	Os coxae: outer aspect of iliac crest	Femur: greater trochanter	1. Abducts thigh at hip 2. Aids in medial rotation of thigh at hip	Superior gluteal nerve
Gluteus minimus	Os coxae: lateral aspect of ilium	Femur: greater trochanter	1. Abducts thigh at hip 2. Aids in medial rotation of thigh at hip	Superior gluteal nerve
Tensor fasciae latae	Os coxae: iliac crest and anterior superior iliac spine	Tibia: lateral condyle— joins inferior fibers of gluteus maximus to form the iliotibial tract	Abducts thigh at hip	Superior gluteal nerve
Deep Rotators of Thigh				
Piriformis	Sacrum: anterior lateral aspect	Femur: greater trochanter	1. Rotates thigh laterally at hip 2. Abducts thigh at hip	Nerve to piriformis (S1, S2)
Obturator internus	Os coxae: internal margins of obturator foramen and its membrane	Femur: greater trochanter	1. Rotates thigh laterally at hip 2. Abducts thigh at hip	Nerve to obturator internus and gemellus superior
Gemellus superior	Os coxae: ischial spine	Femur: greater trochanter	Rotates thigh laterally at hip	Nerve to obturator internus and gemellus superior
Gemellus inferior	Os coxae: ischial tuberosity	Femur: greater trochanter	Rotates thigh laterally at hip	Nerve to gemellus inferior and quadratus femoris
Quadratus femoris	Os coxae: ischial tuberosity	Femur: below greater trochanter	1. Rotates thigh laterally at hip 2. Adducts thigh at hip	Nerve to gemellus inferior and quadratus femoris
Obturator externus	Os coxae: external margin and membrane of obturator foramen	Femur: greater trochanter— trochanteric fossa	1. Rotates thigh laterally at hip 2. Adducts thigh at hip	Obturator nerve

traverses the anterior aspect of the ankle joint; and inserts into the dorsal surfaces of the bones of the foot (*Figure 10-16*, and see *Table 10-4*). The anterior muscles include the **tibialis anterior, extensor hallucis longus, extensor digitorum longus,** and **fibularis (peroneus) longus.** As a group, they *dorsiflex the foot* and *extend the toes* (the toes and foot curl upward). These actions occur when the heel of the leading foot strikes the ground in the act of walk-ing (heel strike). The *deep fibular nerve* supplies the anterior muscles of the leg.

LATERAL LEG MUSCLES

The **fibularis (peroneus) longus and brevis muscles** arise from the lateral surface of the fibula, and their tendons pass under the inferior end of the fibula (lateral malleolus)

TABLE 10-4

Anterior and Lateral Muscles of the Leg

Muscle	Origin	Insertion	Action(s)	Innervation
Anterior				
Tibialis anterior	Tibia: lateral condyle, lateral aspect of proximal two thirds muscular septum	Medial cuneiform 1st metatarsal: base	Dorsiflexes foot at ankle	Deep fibular nerve
Extensor hallucis longus	Fibula: anterior surface of middle half	Great toe: base of distal phalanx	1. Extends great toe at metatarsophalangeal joint 2. Dorsiflexes foot at ankle	Deep fibular nerve
Extensor digitorum longus	Tibia: lateral condyle Fibula: anterior aspect of upper three fourths Interosseous membrane	Lateral four toes: dorsal aspect of middle and distal phalanges	1. Extends lateral four toes at metatarsophalangeal joints 2. Dorsiflexes foot at ankle	Deep fibular nerve
Fibularis (peroneus) tertius	Fibula: inferior anterior surface	5th metatarsal: dorsal aspect of base	1. Dorsiflexes foot at ankle 2. Everts foot at ankle	Deep fibular nerve
Lateral				
Fibularis (peroneal) longus	Tibia: lateral condyle Fibula: lateral upper two thirds	1st metatarsal: base medial cuneiform—lateral surface	1. Plantarflexes foot at ankle 2. Everts foot at ankle	Superficial fibular nerve
Fibularis (peroneal) brevis	Fibula: lateral aspect	5th metatarsal: lateral base	1. Plantarflexes foot at ankle 2. Everts foot at ankle	Superficial fibular nerve

TABLE 10-5

Muscles of the Posterior Thigh (Hamstrings)

Muscle	Origin	Insertion	Action(s)	Innervation
Biceps femoris	Os coxae: long head—ischial tuberosity Femur: short head—lateral aspect of linea aspera	Fibula: head Tibia: lateral condyle	1. Flexes leg at knee 2. Extends thigh at hip 3. Laterally rotates leg at knee	Sciatic nerve via tibial branch to long head Sciatic nerve via common fibular one branch to short head
Semitendinosus	Os coxae: ischial tuberosity	Tibia: proximal medial aspect	1. Flexes leg at knee 2. Extends thigh at hip 3. Laterally rotates leg at knee	Sciatic nerve
Semimembranosus	Os coxae: ischial tuberosity	Tibia: posteromedial aspect	1. Flexes leg at knee 2. Extends thigh at hip 3. Laterally rotates leg at knee	Sciatic nerve

CLINICAL NOTES

Shin Splints

Overexertion during walking commonly causes pain in the anterior tibial region, which is known as *shin splints*. The overworked anterior compartment muscles become inflamed and edematous or swollen and painful to touch.

to insert into the foot allowing them to plantarflex and evert the foot at the ankle. The *superficial fibular nerve* supplies the lateral leg muscles.

POSTERIOR LEG MUSCLES

Superficial Group

The *gastrocnemius* and *plantaris muscles* arise from the inferoposterior aspect of the femur and cross the posterior surface of the knee and the posterior surface of the ankle to insert into the calcaneus as the calcaneal (Achilles)

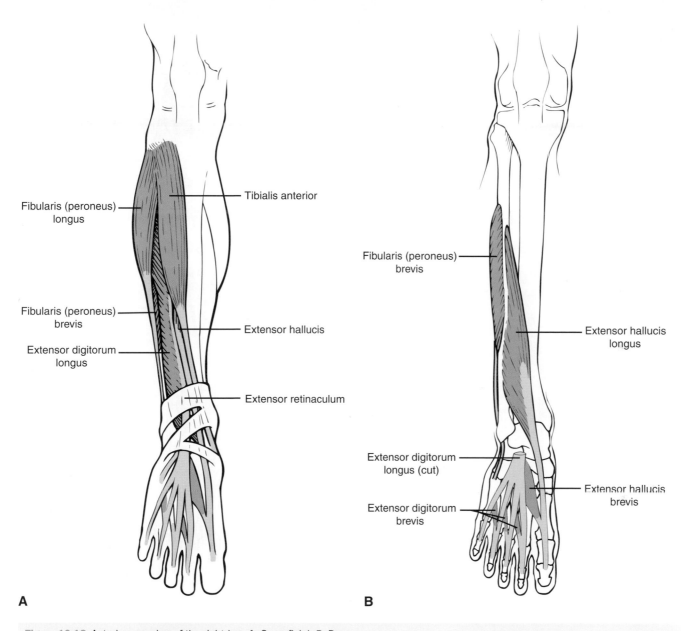

Fibularis (peroneus) longus

Fibularis (peroneus) brevis

Extensor digitorum longus

Tibialis anterior

Extensor hallucis

Extensor retinaculum

Fibularis (peroneus) brevis

Extensor digitorum longus (cut)

Extensor digitorum brevis

Extensor hallucis longus

Extensor hallucis brevis

A

B

Figure 10-16 Anterior muscles of the right leg. **A,** Superficial. **B,** Deep.

tendon (*Figure 10-17, Table 10-6*). They are in a position to *flex the knee* and *plantarflex the foot*. The **soleus muscle** arises from the posterior aspect of the tibia, fibula, and interosseous membrane and traverses only the ankle and then inserts with the others into the common calcaneal tendon. Its sole function, therefore, is *plantarflexion* of the foot. The motor nerve supply is the *tibial nerve*.

Deep Group

The **popliteus** is the only muscle of the group to originate from the femur. It crosses the posterior aspect of the knee and helps to flex the knee and rotates the leg medially on

initiation of flexion to unlock the knee. The **flexor hallucis longus** (flexor of the big toe) arises from the posterior surface of the fibula, the **flexor digitorum longus** (flexor of the toes) muscles arise from the posterior surface of the tibia, and both insert into the distal phalanges of the toes. They are able to *plantarflex* the foot and *flex* the toes. The **tibialis posterior muscle** arises from the posterior aspects of the tibia, fibula, and interosseous membrane crosses the posterior surface of the ankle joint and inserts into the bones of the foot in such a way that it is able to *plantarflex* the ankle and *invert* the foot. The muscles of the deep group, like the superficial group, are supplied by motor branches of the *tibial nerve*.

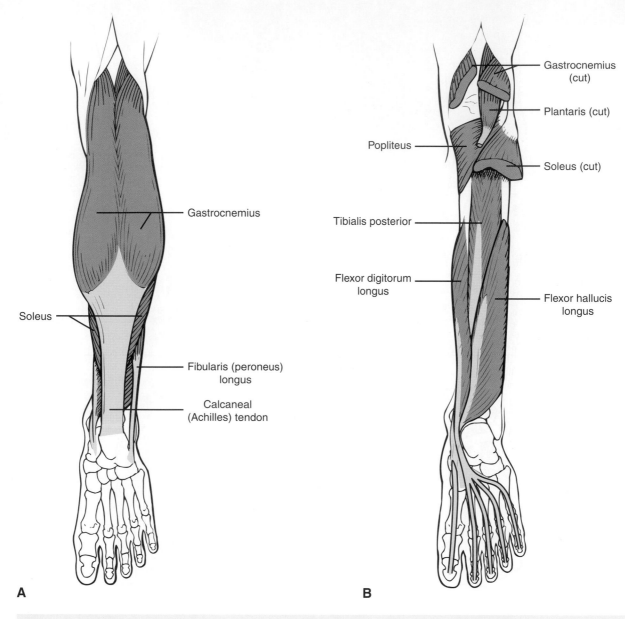

Figure 10-17 Posterior muscles of the right leg. **A,** Superficial. **B,** Deep.

MUSCLES OF THE FOOT

In contrast to the wide range of movements produced by the intrinsic muscles of the hand, the muscles of the foot are specialized for the purposes of bipedal locomotion and support (*Figure 10-18*; *Tables 10-7* and *10-8*). The names of the intrinsic muscles imply movements that are similar to those in the hand, but they are, in fact, modified as dynamic "ligaments" to support the architecture of the foot and help the foot to conform to the terrain while standing or in locomotion. Their precise attachments are not as important as their basic duty to maintain the arch of the foot. Their attachments and functions are listed in *Table 10-7*.

4. Nerve Supply: The Lumbar and Sacral Plexuses

The sensory and motor nerve supplies to the lower limb are from branches of the lumbar and sacral plexuses (*Figures 10-19* and *10-20*).

LUMBAR PLEXUS
Description
The lumbar plexus is formed by the anterior rami of spinal nerves L1, L2, L3, and L4, which issue from their

TABLE 10-6

Posterior Muscles of the Leg

Muscle	Origin	Insertion	Action(s)	Innervation
Superficial				
Gastrocnemius	Femur: posterior aspects of medial and lateral condyles	Calcaneus: through calcaneal (Achilles) tendon	1. Plantarflexes foot at ankle 2. Flexes leg at knee	Tibial nerve
Soleus	Tibia: medial border Fibula: head and upper shaft Interosseous membrane	Calcaneus: through calcaneal (Achilles) tendon	Plantarflexes foot at ankle	Tibial nerve
Plantaris	Femur: supracondylar ridge	Calcaneus: through calcaneal (Achilles) tendon	1. Plantarflexes foot at ankle 2. Flexes leg at knee	Tibial nerve
Deep				
Popliteus	Femur: lateral condyle	Tibia: posterior aspect of upper tibia	1. Flexes leg at knee 2. Rotates leg medially on initiation of flexion at knee	Tibial nerve
Flexor hallucis longus	Fibula: posterior two thirds Interosseous membrane	Great toe: base of distal phalanx	1. Flexes great toe 2. Plantarflexes foot at ankle	Tibial nerve
Flexor digitorum longus	Tibia: posterior aspect of shaft	Lateral four toes: plantar surfaces of base of distal phalanges	1. Flexes phalanges of lateral four toes at metacarpophalangeal joints 2. Plantarflexes foot at ankle	Tibial nerve
Tibialis posterior	Tibia: posterolateral surface Fibula: posterior surface Interosseous membrane: posterior surface	Navicular: tuberosity Cuneiforms: plantar surfaces Cuboid Talus Lateral four metatarsals: plantar surfaces	1. Plantarflexes foot at ankle 2. Plantarflexes foot at ankle	Tibial nerve

respective intervertebral foramina and enter the substance of the psoas muscle in the lower abdomen (*Table 10-9*). The roots combine to form the lumbar plexus, and this, in turn, gives rise to six branches that leave the lateral border of the psoas muscle.

Branches

1. The **iliohypogastric nerve** and the **ilioinguinal nerve** sweep anteriorly to supply skin and muscle of the lower portion of the anterior abdominal wall.
2. The **lateral femoral cutaneous nerve** is sensory to skin of the lateral aspect of the thigh.
3. The **genitofemoral nerve** supplies skin of the medial aspect of the thigh, scrotum or labium majus, and cremaster muscle.
4. The **femoral nerve** is a large branch of the lumbar plexus and passes below the midpoint of the inguinal ligament to enter the thigh, where it has an extensive distribution; the nerve supplies muscles and skin of

the anterior thigh and skin of the medial aspect of the leg.
5. The **obturator nerve** leaves the pelvis through the obturator foramen and goes to the medial aspect of the thigh to supply adductor muscles of the thigh.

SACRAL PLEXUS

Description

The sacral plexus arises from anterior rami of spinal nerves L4, L5, S1, S2, S3, and S4. These combine within the pelvis to form three main branches and several small branches (see *Figures 10-20* and *10-21*, and *Table 10-10*).

Branches

1. The **sciatic nerve** is the largest nerve in the body, and the entire sacral plexus seems to funnel into this one large nerve. It leaves the pelvis through the greater sciatic foramen below the piriformis muscle to enter the gluteal region deep to the gluteus maximus muscle.

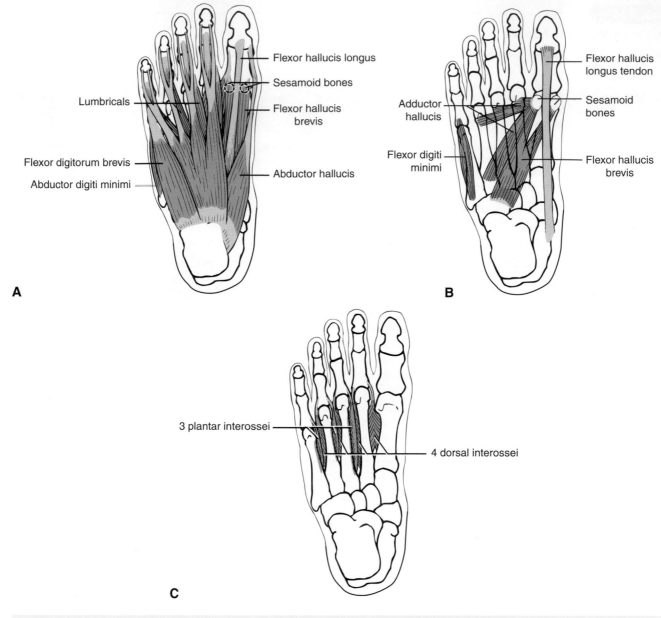

Figure 10-18 Intrinsic muscles of the right foot as seen from the plantar aspect. **A,** Superficial. **B,** Intermediate. **C,** Deep.

TABLE 10-7

Muscles of the Foot

Muscle	Origin	Insertion	Action(s)	Innervation
Layer 1				
Abductor hallucis	Calcaneus	Great toe: base of proximal phalanx	Abducts great toe	Medial plantar nerve
Flexor digitorum brevis	Calcaneus	Lateral four toes: middle phalanges	Flexes toes at proximal interphalangeal joints	Medial plantar nerve
Abductor digiti minimi	Calcaneus	Little toe: proximal phalanx	Abducts little toe	Lateral plantar nerve

TABLE 10-7

Muscles of the Foot—cont'd

Muscle	Origin	Insertion	Action(s)	Innervation
Layer 2				
Quadratus plantae lumbricals (4)	Calcaneus	Tendons: flexor digitorum longus	Flexes lateral four toes	Medial plantar nerve
	Tendons: flexor digitorum longus	Lateral four toes: bases of terminal phalanges along with tendons of flexor digitorum longus	1. Flex lateral four toes at metatarsophalangeal joints 2. Extend lateral four toes at interphalangeal joints	
Layer 3				
Flexor hallucis brevis	Cuboid: plantar surface Lateral cuneiform	Great toe: base of proximal phalanx	Flexes great toe at metatarsophalangeal joint	Medial plantar nerve
Adductor hallucis	Metatarsals 2, 3, 4: oblique head Metatarsophalangeal ligaments: transverse head	Great toe: base of proximal phalanx	1. Adducts great toe at metatarsophalangeal joint 2. Flexes toe at metatarsophalangeal joint	Lateral plantar nerve
Flexor digiti minimi	Metatarsal 5: base	Little toe: proximal phalanx	Flexes little toe at metatarsophalangeal joint	Lateral plantar nerve
Layer 4				
Dorsal interossei (4)	Metatarsals: adjacent sides of shafts	Lateral four toes: proximal phalanges	1. Abduct toes away from axis through 2nd toe at metatarsophalangeal joints 2. Flex metatarsophalangeal joints to prevent spreading of foot 3. Extend interphalangeal joints to prevent curling of toes	Lateral plantar nerve
Plantar interossei (3)	Metatarsals 3, 4, and 5: inferior aspects	Corresponding toes: medial aspects of bases of proximal phalanges	1. Adduct toes toward axis through 2nd toe at metatarsophalangeal joints 2. Flex metatarsophalangeal joints to prevent spreading of foot 3. Extend interphalangeal joints to prevent curling of toes	Lateral plantar nerve

TABLE 10-8

A Review of the Movements of the Lower Limb

Area	Joint(s) Involved	Movement	Muscles
Pelvic girdle	Sacroiliac	Little	—
Hip	Hip joint (femoroacetabular)	1. Flexion	Rectus femoris; sartorius; iliopsoas; pectineus; adductors longus, brevis, and magnus
		2. Extension	Hamstrings (semitendinosus, semimembranosus, biceps femoris), gluteus maximus, adductor magnus
		3. Abduction	Gluteus medius, gluteus minimus, tensor fasciae latae, iliopsoas, piriformis, sartorius
		4. Adduction	Adductors: longus, brevis, and magnus; pectineus; gracilis; gemelli; obturator internus; obturator externus
		5. Medial rotation	Glutei medius and minimus; adductor longus, brevis, and magnus; tensor fasciae latae
		6. Lateral rotation	Gluteus maximus, iliopsoas, piriformis, obturator externus and internus, gemelli, quadratus femoris

Continued

TABLE 10-8

A Review of the Movements of the Lower Limb—cont'd

Area	Joint(s) Involved	Movement	Muscles
Knee	Femorotibial	1. Flexion	Hamstrings (semimembranosus, semitendinosus, biceps femoris), gastrocnemius, gracilis, sartorius, plantaris, popliteus
		2. Extension	Quadriceps femoris (rectus femoris; vastus lateralis, medialis, intermedius)
		3. Medial rotation	Popliteus, sartorius, semimembranosus, semitendinosus
		4. Lateral rotation	Biceps femoris
	Superior tibiofibular	Little	—
Ankle	Ankle joint: talocrural (tibia, fibula, talus)	1. Plantarflexion	Gastrocnemius, soleus, peroneus longus, plantaris, tibialis posterior, peroneus brevis
	Intertarsal	2. Dorsiflexion	Extensor hallucis longus, extensor digitorum longus, tibialis anterior
		1. Plantarflexion	Peroneus longus, tibialis posterior, abductor digiti minimi, flexor digiti brevis, abductor hallucis, peroneus brevis, lumbricals, quadratus plantae, long flexor muscles of toes
		2. Inversion	Tibialis anterior and posterior
		3. Eversion	Peroneus longus, brevis, and tertius
Foot (toes)	Metatarsophalangeal and interphalangeal	1. Flexion	Flexor hallucis longus and brevis, flexor digiti longus and brevis and minimi brevis, quadratus plantae, lumbricals (metatarsophalangeal joints)
		2. Extension	Extensor hallucis longus, extensor digiti longus and brevis, lumbricals (interphalangeal joints)
		3. Abduction	Abductor hallucis, abductor digiti minimi, dorsal interossei
		4. Adduction	Adductor hallucis, plantar interossei

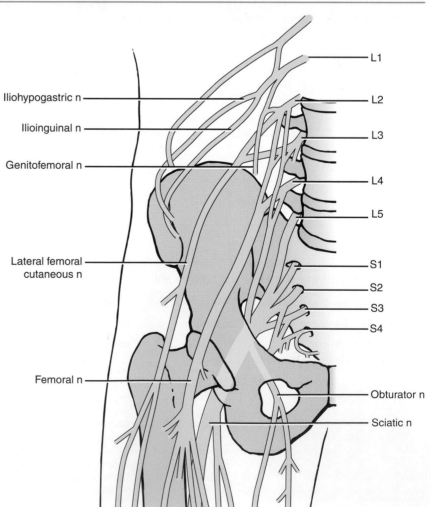

Figure 10-19 Lumbosacral plexus.

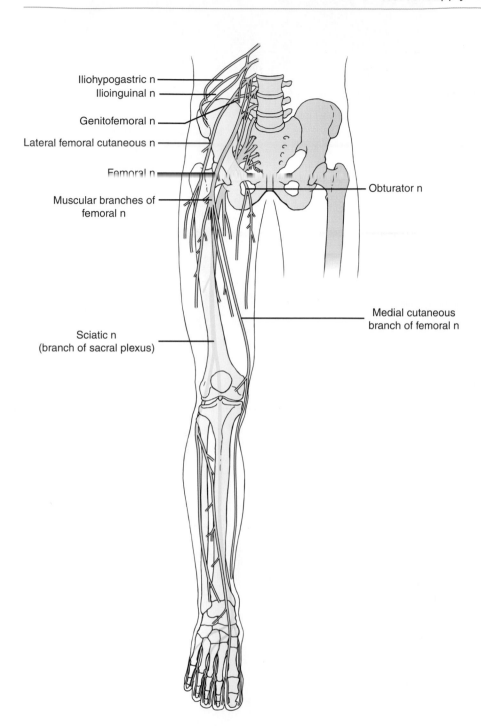

Iliohypogastric n

Ilioinguinal n

Genitofemoral n

Lateral femoral cutaneous n

Femoral n

Muscular branches of femoral n

Obturator n

Medial cutaneous branch of femoral n

Sciatic n (branch of sacral plexus)

Figure 10-20 Anterior view of right lower limb to show branches of lumbar plexus.

From here it runs straight down the back of the midline of the thigh, giving off motor branches to the hamstring muscles of the back of the thigh. Just above the back of the knee (popliteal space), it divides into two terminal branches:

A. The **common fibular (peroneal) nerve** takes a lateral course in the leg and divides to form the deep and superficial fibular nerves that supply muscles and skin of the lateral and anterior aspects of the leg and foot.

B. The **tibial nerve** passes to the back of the leg to supply muscles and skin. The nerve continues past the medial malleolus and supplies skin of the sole and intrinsic muscles of the foot.

2. The **pudendal nerve** passes to the pudendal region to supply muscles of the external genitalia, sphincter ani,

TABLE 10-9

Branches of the Lumbar Plexus

Nerve	Origin	Structures Supplied
Ilioinguinal	L1	Sensory: skin of lower anterior abdominal wall
Iliohypogastric	L1	Sensory: skin of groin, scrotum, or labia majora
Genitofemoral	L1, L2	Motor: cremaster muscle Sensory: skin of small area of medial thigh
Lateral femoral cutaneous	L2, L3	Sensory: skin of anterolateral aspect of thigh
Femoral	L2, L3, L4	Motor: flexors of hip and extensors of knee
Obturator	L2, L3, L4	Motor: adductor muscles of thigh
Lumbosacral trunk	L4, L5	Joins the sacral plexus

and sphincter urethrae. It is also sensory to skin of the perineum.

3. The **gluteal nerves** leave the pelvis through the greater sciatic notch to supply the gluteal muscles (maximus, medius, and minimus).

4. **Small branches** arise within the pelvis to supply some muscles and skin of the posterior aspect of the thigh.

CLINICAL NOTES

Gluteal Injections

A commonly used site for intramuscular injections is the gluteal region. The large sciatic nerve traveling through the area, however, is in danger of being punctured with the needle. To avoid the nerve, injections are given in the upper lateral quadrant of the buttock into the belly of the gluteus medius muscle (*Figure 10-22*).

5. Arterial Supply

The arterial supply to the pelvis and lower limb is derived from terminal branches of the abdominal aorta (*Figure 10-23*).

1. The **right** and **left common iliac arteries** arise as the terminal bifurcation of the abdominal aorta. Each common iliac artery divides into an external and an internal iliac artery within the false pelvis.

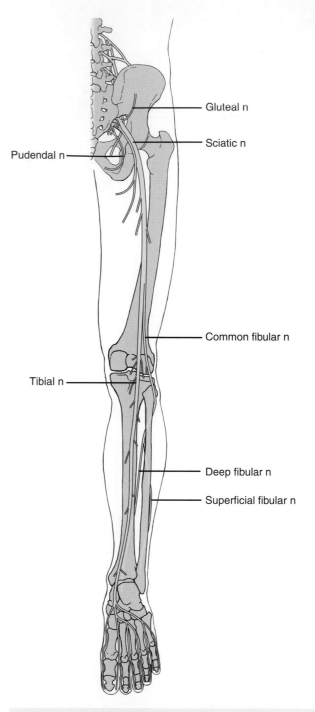

Figure 10-21 Posterior view of right lower limb to show branches of sacral plexus.

2. The **internal iliac artery** enters the true pelvis and supplies the gluteal region, the perineal region (including the anal canal and the external genitalia), and pelvic viscera (urogenital and gut).

3. The **external iliac artery** skirts the brim of the true pelvis and passes below the midpoint of the inguinal ligament to enter the thigh. At this point, the artery changes name to become the femoral artery.

TABLE 10-10

Branches of the Sacral Plexus

Nerve	Origin	Structures Supplied
Superior gluteal	L4-S3	Motor: gluteus medius and minimus mm
Inferior gluteal	L5-S2	Motor: gluteus maximus m
Small mm from pelvis to thigh	L4-S2	Motor: piriformis, quadratus femoris, superior and inferior gemelli, and obturator internus
Pudendal	S2-S4	Motor: perineal mm, voluntary (external) sphincters of urethra and anus, levator ani Sensory: skin of genitalia, distal end of rectum, and perianal skin
Perforating cutaneous	S2, S3	Sensory: skin of medial part of buttock
Posterior femoral cutaneous	S2, S3	Sensory: skin of buttock, posteromedial surface of thigh
Sciatic nerve	L4-S3	Motor: flexors of knee arising from the thigh, all mm in leg and foot Sensory: hip joint, skin of leg and foot
Tibial branch Common fibular branch		

m, Muscle; *mm*, muscles.

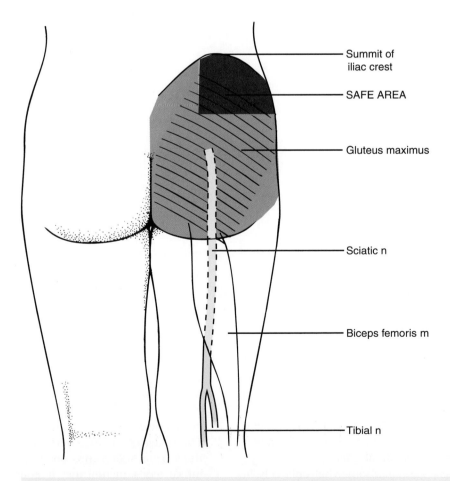

Figure 10-22 Position of the sciatic nerve in gluteal region. Safe area for intramuscular injections (distant from sciatic nerve) is in the superior lateral quadrant of the buttock.

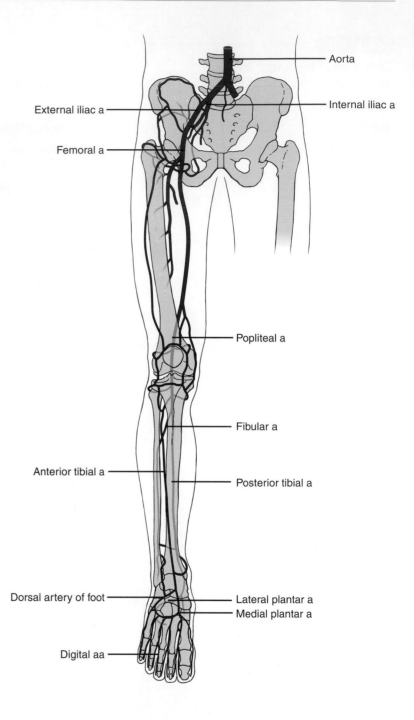

Aorta

External iliac a

Internal iliac a

Femoral a

Popliteal a

Fibular a

Anterior tibial a

Posterior tibial a

Dorsal artery of foot

Lateral plantar a

Medial plantar a

Digital aa

Figure 10-23 Arterial supply to the lower right limb. Anterior view.

4. The **femoral artery** supplies the entire lower limb through its various branches. Three large collateral branches are given off as the femoral artery descends in the thigh medial to the femur. The artery angles medially to pass behind the knee, where it changes name and becomes the popliteal artery.

5. The **popliteal artery** descends somewhat obliquely in the popliteal space and below the knee divides into the posterior and anterior tibial arteries.

6. The **posterior tibial artery,** the larger branch, descends on the posterior aspect of the leg and gives off (1) the fibular artery and (2) the medial and lateral plantar arteries as it enters the foot.

7. The **anterior tibial artery** passes anteriorly below the knee and descends on the anterior aspect of the interosseous membrane; it ends in the foot as the dorsal artery of the foot, and it anastomoses with the plantar branches of the posterior tibial artery.

6.   Venous Return

As in the upper limb, the venous return of the lower limb is via a deep and a superficial set of veins (*Figure 10-24*).

DEEP VEINS

The deep veins of the lower limb parallel the courses of the arteries. The veins assume the same names and ultimately collect as the **popliteal vein,** which emerges behind the knee as the **femoral vein.** The femoral vein ascends under the inguinal ligament, changes name to the **external iliac vein,** and then joins the **internal iliac vein** to form the **common iliac vein.** Right and left common iliac veins come together in the abdomen to form the **inferior vena cava.**

SUPERFICIAL VEINS

1   The **dorsal venous arch** of the foot receives blood from the toes. Arising from each side of the arch are two major cutaneous veins of the lower limb.

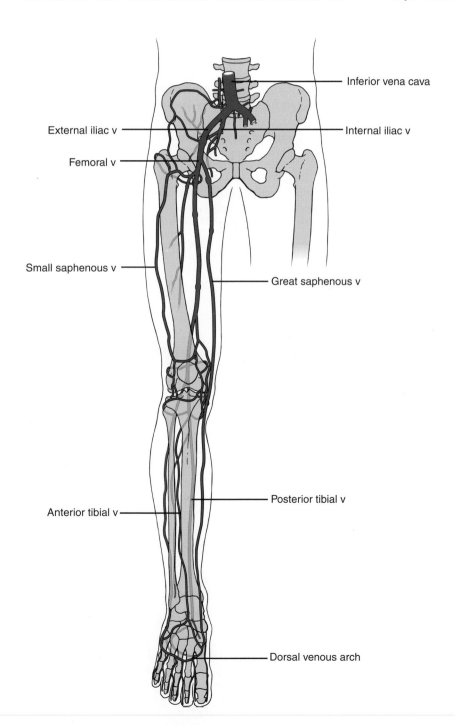

Inferior vena cava

External iliac v

Internal iliac v

Femoral v

Small saphenous v

Great saphenous v

Posterior tibial v

Anterior tibial v

Dorsal venous arch

Figure 10-24 Venous drainage of the lower limb. Anterior view.

CLINICAL NOTES

Varicose Veins

Communicating veins join the deep and saphenous veins, and these veins contain valves preventing backflow of blood toward the superficial saphenous veins. Breakdown of these valves allows blood to leak back to the superficial veins, causing them to dilate and become tortuous. Progressive degeneration of the superficial veins results and may cause ulcers of the leg.

Saphenous Cutdown

The great saphenous vein is often used to administer various agents intravenously. It is found immediately anterior to the medial malleolus. It is, therefore, relatively easy to find even though the vein may not be obvious superficially.

---

2. The **small saphenous vein** arises from the lateral aspect of the arch and ascends on the lateral aspect of the leg to the popliteal region to join the popliteal vein.
3. The **great saphenous vein** arises from the medial aspect of the dorsal venous arch of the foot and ascends on the medial aspect of the lower limb, receiving tributaries as it goes. Immediately below the pubic tubercle, it dives deeply through the fossa ovalis (an opening in the deep fascia) to enter the femoral vein.

7.   Lymphatics

SUPERFICIAL LYMPH NODES

Superficial structures of the lower limb are drained by lymphatic vessels that pass to superficial lymph nodes located in the superficial inguinal region and near the termination of the great saphenous vein (*Figure 10-25*). The efferents of the superficial lymph nodes, in turn, drain to the deep inguinal lymph nodes described next.

DEEP LYMPH NODES

Deep structures of the lower limb drain to deep lymph nodes located in the anterior compartment of the leg below the knee, the popliteal region behind the knee, and the deep inguinal nodes clustered around the proximal end of the femoral vein.

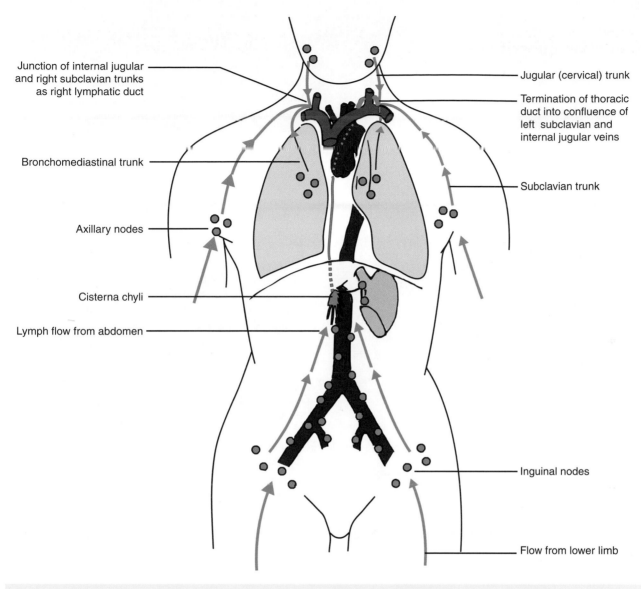

Junction of internal jugular and right subclavian trunks as right lymphatic duct

Bronchomediastinal trunk

Axillary nodes

Cisterna chyli

Lymph flow from abdomen

Jugular (cervical) trunk

Termination of thoracic duct into confluence of left subclavian and internal jugular veins

Subclavian trunk

Inguinal nodes

Flow from lower limb

Figure 10-25 Major groups of lymph nodes and trunks showing the scheme of lymphatic flow back to venous system.

Review Questions

1. The major flexor of the hip is the
   _____.
   a. adductor magnus muscle (anterior component)
   b. rectus femoris muscle
   c. sartorius muscle
   d. iliopsoas muscle
   e. vastus lateralis muscle

2. A tibia that can be subluxated anteriorly in relation to the femur within the knee joint indicates damage to the _____.
   a. anterior cruciate ligament
   b. posterior cruciate ligament
   c. medial collateral ligament
   d. lateral collateral ligament
   e. patellar ligament

3. The power required in extending the thigh when rising from a sitting position or when climbing the stairs is provided by the _____.
   a. tensor fasciae latae muscle
   b. gluteus medius muscle
   c. obturator internus muscle
   d. gluteus maximus muscle
   e. pectineus muscle

4. Which of the following statements concerning the hamstring muscles is FALSE?
   a. They are extensors of the hip and extensors of the knee.
   b. They mostly originate from the ischium of the os coxae.
   c. They include the semitendinosus and semimembranosus muscles.
   d. They are flexors of the knee.
   e. They are active when the trailing foot is lifted from the ground during the act of walking.

5. The muscle that rotates the knee medially to unlock it before flexion is the _____.
   a. gastrocnemius muscle
   b. vastus lateralis muscle
   c. biceps femoris muscle
   d. tibialis posterior muscle
   e. popliteus muscle

6. Which of the following statements concerning the muscles of the anterior compartment of the leg is FALSE?
   a. They are supplied by the deep fibular (peroneal) nerve.
   b. They act to dorsiflex the foot.
   c. They act to flex the toes.
   d. They are active as the leading foot strikes the ground during the act of walking.
   e. They can become inflamed when overactive and cause painful shin splints.

7. A gluteal intramuscular injection may be safely administered in the _____.
   a. upper medial quadrant
   b. lower medial quadrant
   c. upper lateral quadrant
   d. below the inferior margin of the gluteus maximus muscle
   e. lower lateral quadrant

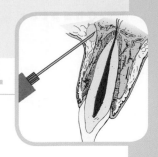

Chapter 11

Applied Anatomy

1. Anatomy of Local Anesthesia 457

2. Imaging 466

3. Fractures of the Face 473

4. Spread of Dental Infections 480

1. Anatomy of Local Anesthesia

This section is not intended as a comprehensive description of local anesthetic techniques, but it is instead intended to provide the student with an anatomical basis for a subsequent anesthetic course referenced by appropriate texts and handbooks about local anesthesia.

Pain control is a very important part of dental practice. Operative procedures require cutting through sensitive tooth structures, producing extreme discomfort and pain. Surgical procedures, such as tooth extraction, periodontal surgery, biopsies, and so on, also require a form of pain control.

General anesthetics affect the central nervous system and render the patient unconscious and incapable of feeling pain. General anesthesia, however, is potentially hazardous to the patient, and it is usually administered in a hospital environment.

Local anesthesia is the introduction, by injection, of an anesthetic fluid to a sensory peripheral nerve. The fluid diffuses through the nerve bundles to reach the individual nerve fibers and blocks the transmission of pain-perceived stimuli to the brain. It thus renders the territory supplied by the nerve void of sensation, or numb. This procedure is performed regularly and routinely in the dental office and is relatively safe because the patient remains awake.

A **topical anesthetic** is applied to the injection site to numb the subsequent penetration of the needle through the mucosa. In addition, before the release of the anesthetic, it is necessary to **aspirate**, or pull back on the plunger. If blood is not aspirated back into the syringe, this ensures that the tip of the needle has not entered a blood vessel and precludes inadvertent injection of the fluid into the bloodstream and the possibility of unwanted systemic reactions.

TYPES OF LOCAL ANESTHESIA

The two basic types of local anesthetic injections are local infiltration and nerve block.

Local Infiltration

Small areas of soft tissue or bone may be anesthetized by injecting a small amount of anesthetic fluid directly into the area (*Figure 11-1*). The fluid diffuses through a small, localized area and blocks the terminal nerve fibers there. Most maxillary teeth may be anesthetized in this manner. Anesthetic fluid is injected deep to the vestibular fold and deposited on the periosteum of the alveolar bone overlying the root apex (supraperiosteal injection). The fluid diffuses through the bone to reach and block the terminal nerve fibers at the apical foramen of the tooth. In general, a localized tooth block may be attempted on any tooth that has a vestibular alveolar plate of bone thin enough to permit diffusion of the solution to the apical nerves.

Nerve Block

Larger areas and several teeth may be anesthetized by blocking a main nerve; that is, the anesthetic solution is deposited adjacent to a main peripheral nerve. This will obviously produce a greater effect because the farther proximally a nerve is blocked, the greater the area anes-

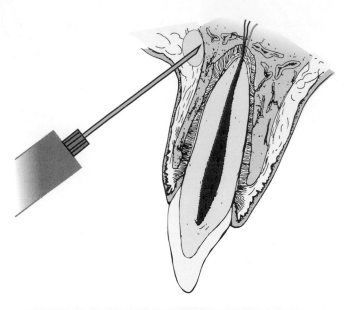

Figure 11-1 Local infiltration of individual teeth. The needle is inserted through vestibular fold, and anesthetic fluid is deposited over root apex. Fluid percolates through the thin alveolar bone to block terminal sensory nerves passing from root apex.

thetized. In the oral cavity, there are several areas where large peripheral nerves are accessible for nerve blocks.

LOCAL ANESTHESIA OF MAXILLARY STRUCTURES

Local Infiltration

Teeth. Each of the maxillary teeth may be individually anesthetized using local infiltration. The one tooth that may be a problem is the maxillary first molar, because the roots are covered by the zygomatic process of the maxilla. The anesthetic fluid does not always sufficiently diffuse through the bone, and if this is the case, a nerve block must be considered.

Injection Sites. The upper lip or the cheek is retracted to expose the vestibular fold and the root apex or root apices of the tooth involved, and this is noted as the penetration site (*Figure 11-2*). The needle is introduced through the vestibular mucosa with the bevel of the needle pointing toward the mucosa. The syringe is aspirated. The bevel of the needle should come to rest facing and on the periosteal surface of the vestibular alveolar bone directly overlying the root apex. The proper amount of fluid is slowly injected at the site, and the fluid percolates through the alveolar bone to reach and block the terminal branches of the maxillary nerve entering the apical foramen.

Complications. There are relatively few complications associated with local infiltration techniques.

1. **Penetration of the floor of the nose.** The root apices of the maxillary central incisors lie close to the floor of the nasal cavity. Improper alignment could result

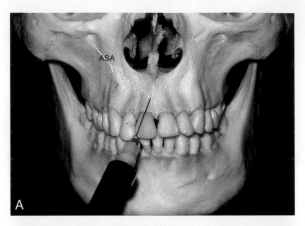

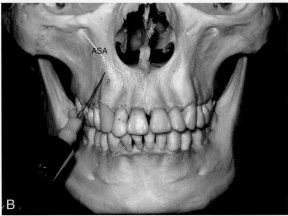

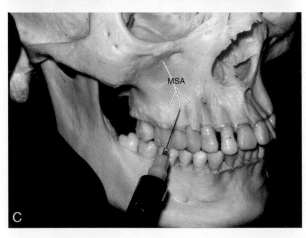

Figure 11-2 Placement of needle over the apex of maxillary right central incisor (**A**), maxillary right canine (**B**), and maxillary premolars (**C**) for local infiltration.

in the needle penetrating too far superiorly through the floor of the nasal cavity. If this happens, there is, of course, no effective anesthesia of the tooth and the patient will describe fluid trickling down the throat.

2. **Penetration of a blood vessel.** Infiltration at the site of the maxillary molars can result in penetration of a branch of the posterior superior alveolar vessels or, if delivered too high up, entry into the pterygoid plexus of veins, resulting in a pooling of blood, or hematoma.

Vestibular Gingivae and Mucosa. The vestibular mucosa and gingivae are automatically anesthetized along when the aforementioned infiltration techniques are used.

Palatal Gingiva and Mucosa. Anesthesia of the palatal gingiva and mucosa is not generally required in routine restorative procedures, but it is required for full crown preparation and surgical procedures.

Injection Sites. The injection sites for palatal local infiltration are at a point midway between the gingival crest of the tooth and the midline palatal raphé (*Figure 11-3*). This ensures that the needle will enter a relatively thick portion of the palatal mucosa to minimize pain.

Complications. Palatal injections can be painful because the mucosa of the hard palate is closely applied to bone. More pressure must be applied to force the solution under the tissue. To offset the pain of palatal injections, a topical anesthetic is absolutely necessary. In addition, pressure can be applied to the injection site with a cotton applicator before and after the injection to minimize the discomfort.

Block Anesthesia

Anterior and Middle Superior Alveolar Blocks (Infraorbital Block). The maxillary nerve enters the infraorbital groove in the floor of the orbit and changes its name to the infraorbital nerve. The maxillary nerve passes forward, giving off the middle superior and anterior superior alveolar nerves before exiting through the infraorbital foramen as facial branches (see *Figure 7-58*).

Nerves Blocked. The following nerves may be blocked with a single injection: (1) the terminal facial branches of the infraorbital nerve (superior labial, nasal, and inferior palpebral), (2) the anterior superior alveolar nerve, and (3) the middle superior alveolar nerve (usually).

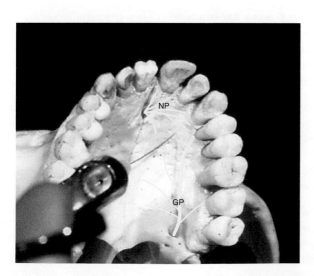

Figure 11-3 Placement of the needle for local infiltration of the palatal mucosa and palatal gingiva.

Injection Site. The site of injection is the mouth of the infraorbital canal (*Figure 11-4*). At this point, the middle superior and anterior superior alveolar nerves have branched from the main infraorbital nerve and are descending to their respective destinations. At the mouth of the canal, the terminal branches issue onto the face.

The infraorbital foramen lies on the facial aspect of the maxilla, approximately 0.5 to 1.0 cm below the midpoint of the inferior orbital margin. On a skull, the supraorbital, infraorbital, and mental foramina lie along a vertical line. In the living person, an imaginary line drawn through the palpable supraorbital foramen, pupil of the eye, and the crown of the maxillary second premolar tooth will pass through the infraorbital foramen. Immediately superior to the foramen is the origin of the levator labii superioris muscle, and below the foramen is the origin of the levator anguli oris muscle.

Complications

1. **Vascular penetration.** The terminal branches of the *infraorbital artery* and *vein* pass from the infraorbital foramen. Careful aspiration of the syringe during injection prevents inadvertent release of anesthetic agent into a blood vessel.
2. **Intraorbital injection.** Directly above the infraorbital foramen are the orbit and its contents. Inadvertent injection of anesthetic fluid into the orbit could result in temporary but unpleasant complications. The motor supply to the extraocular muscles may be blocked, causing *double vision*, or *diplopia*, or the optic nerve may be involved and result in *temporary blindness*.

Teeth Anesthetized. The pulps and periodontal ligaments of the maxillary central incisor, lateral incisor, canine, first premolar, and second premolar are anesthetized.

Other Tissues Anesthetized. In addition to the teeth just mentioned, the adjacent plate of labial alveolar bone, adjacent vestibular gingivae and alveolar mucosa, the skin and mucous membrane of the upper lip, the lateral aspect of the external nose, the skin and conjunctiva of the lower eyelid, and the anterior aspect of the maxillary sinus are anesthetized.

Posterior Superior Alveolar Block. The posterior superior alveolar nerve arises from the maxillary nerve just before it enters the infraorbital canal (see *Figure 7-58*). The nerve passes downward, along with corresponding branches of the maxillary artery, to the posterior or infratemporal surface of the maxilla.

Injection Site. The site of injection is the point where the posterior superior alveolar nerve enters the posterior superior alveolar foramen on the infratemporal surface of the maxilla (*Figure 11-5*). On the skull, this may be seen as several tiny foramina on the gently rounded, convex, posterior surface of the maxilla. In the living person, the

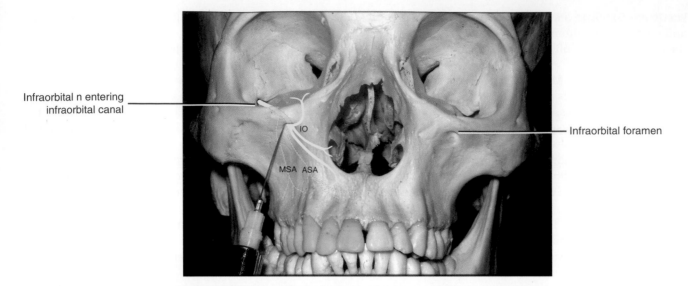

Infraorbital n entering infraorbital canal

Infraorbital foramen

IO

MSA ASA

Figure 11-4 Placement of the needle in infraorbital foramen for anterior and middle superior alveolar (infraorbital) nerve blocks.

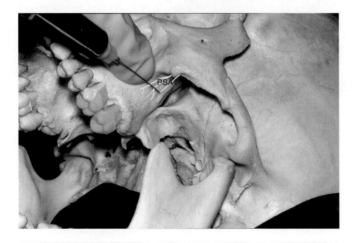

PSA

Figure 11-5 Placement of the needle for a posterior superior alveolar (*PSA*) nerve block.

area may be located by palpating the prominent zygomatic process of the maxilla in the vestibular fold. Posterior to this, the posterior surface of the maxilla may be palpated. If the mouth is opened too widely, the palpating finger is displaced by the coronoid process of the mandible and the attached temporalis tendon.

Complications

Vascular penetration: The needle could penetrate an accompanying posterior superior alveolar artery or vein. In addition, the pterygoid plexus of veins, a rich anastomosing network situated about the lateral pterygoid muscle, is slightly posterior to the injection site and relatively easy to penetrate with the needle. Aside from inadvertent injection of anesthetic fluid into the bloodstream, the peculiar nature of this injection site makes it particularly vulnerable to widespread intertissue hemorrhage, or **hematoma.** The area lateral to the site is filled with loose

areolar tissue, and puncture of a blood vessel fills the area with blood and produces a reddened swelling on the side of the face. This is traditionally attributed to a penetration of the pterygoid plexus of veins, but, judging by the speed with which the swelling takes place, it is more likely due to an arterial puncture. The hematoma goes through the same colorful stages as a healing black eye and is resolved in a few weeks.

Teeth Anesthetized. The pulps and periodontal ligaments of the maxillary first molar, second molar, and third molar are anesthetized. (Note: The **mesiobuccal aspect** of the first molar may be innervated by the *middle superior alveolar nerve*, and a separate injection is usually performed over the apical root of the second premolar to achieve complete anesthesia of the maxillary first molar.)

Other Tissues Anesthetized. Other tissues affected by this block are the buccal gingivae overlying the maxillary molars, the buccal plate of alveolar bone overlying the maxillary molars, and the bone and mucosa of the posterior portion of the maxillary sinus.

Nasopalatine Block. The nasopalatine nerve branches from the pterygopalatine ganglion and enters the nasal cavity through the sphenopalatine foramen (see *Figures 7-60* and *7-82*). It passes anteriorly and inferiorly along the nasal septum and exits onto the hard palate through the incisive foramen.

Nerves Blocked. The nasopalatine nerve branches from the pterygopalatine ganglion of the maxillary nerve. It passes medially through the sphenopalatine foramen to enter the nasal cavity, deflects downward and forward along the nasal septum and at the anterior aspect of the floor of the nose, then passes through the incisive canal to emerge on the oral aspect of the hard palate.

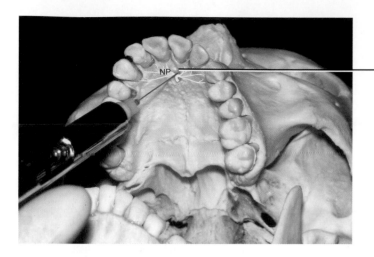

Incisive foramen

Figure 11-6 Placement of the needle in incisive foramen for a nasopalatine nerve block.

Injection Site. The injection site is the mouth of the incisive canal immediately posterior to the central incisor teeth (*Figure 11-6*). From the canal opening, branches of the nasopalatine nerve pass laterally and posteriorly. The right and left incisive canals merge on the palate as one incisive foramen. The opening on the dried skull is approximately 1.5 cm posterior to the alveolar crest between the central incisors. From this point, it funnels anteriorly behind the incisors. In the mouth, it lies in the midline immediately posterior to the incisive papilla. Topical anesthetic is used before injection. A very quick initial injection is performed just to one side of the incisive papilla. This eliminates the discomfort when the needle is subsequently placed into the incisive foramen through the incisive papilla.

Complications

1. **Vascular penetration:** Branches of the nasopalatine artery and vein accompany the nerve and should be avoided. Any injection in the hard palate is painful.
2. **Pain on injection:** The mucosa is tightly bound to the underlying bony palate, and, therefore, injections into the area should be administered slowly (see previous description concerning palatal infiltration).

Tissues Anesthetized. Because both right and left nerves emerge through a common midline opening, both nerves are anesthetized with the same injection. The tissues supplied are the palatal mucosa and lingual gingivae of the six anterior maxillary teeth and the lingual plate of alveolar bone and hard palate associated with the six anterior maxillary teeth.

Greater Palatine Block

Nerves Blocked. The greater palatine nerve arises from the pterygopalatine ganglion of the maxillary nerve. It drops through the greater palatine canal and descends to emerge on the posterior aspect of the hard palate (see *Figure 7-60*).

Injection Site. The injection site is the mouth of the greater palatine canal (*Figure 11-7*). At this point, the greater palatine nerve emerges on the hard palate between the second and third molars, about 1 cm superior to the margin of the palatal gingiva. From here the nerve passes anteriorly in a groove to supply structures of the palate. The groove and foramen may be palpated under the palatal mucosa.

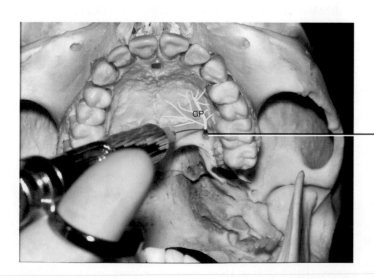

Greater palatine foramen

Figure 11-7 Placement of the needle in greater palatine foramen for a greater palatine nerve block.

461

Complications

Vascular penetration: Branches of the greater palatine artery and vein accompany the nerve, and these should be avoided. Again, this is a palatal injection, and it should be administered slowly to prevent stripping of the mucosa from the underlying bone.

Tissues Anesthetized. All the palatal mucosa of the side injected and lingual gingivae posterior to the maxillary canines and the underlying bone of the hard palate would be anesthetized.

Maxillary Block. Rarely, circumstances require a block of the entire maxillary nerve for extensive surgery or when traditional local anesthesia is contraindicated because of the presence of infection.

Injection Site. The only accessible point along the route of the maxillary nerve is where the nerve passes across the roof of the pterygopalatine fossa. This location may be approached several ways. The first is a high posterior, superior alveolar block. The technique previously described is used for this block, except that the needle is carried farther superiorly to the pterygopalatine fossa. The second is a greater palatine approach. The greater palatine foramen is entered with a needle and then followed superiorly to where the canal enters the pterygopalatine fossa. The third is an extraoral approach. The needle is passed through the skin of the face, through the mandibular notch of the mandible to the pterygopalatine fossa.

Tissues Anesthetized. A maxillary block results in anesthesia of half the maxillary dental arch and supporting structures, a major portion of the nasal cavity, half the palate, and the maxillary air sinus.

Complications

Vascular penetration: These procedures are performed rarely, and for good reason. Not only are branches of the maxillary blood vessels easily encountered, but the main vessels are vulnerable as well.

LOCAL ANESTHESIA OF MANDIBULAR STRUCTURES

Local Infiltration

In the pediatric patient, all deciduous teeth may be anesthetized using local infiltration. The mandibular first molars, however, are not easily anesthetized with this method. In the adult patient, infiltration may be attempted on the mandibular incisors but is not always successful. The labial and buccal plates of bone of the mandible are relatively thick and preclude successful local infiltration. In general, nerve blocks are used to anesthetize the mandibular dentition.

Block Anesthesia

Standard Inferior Alveolar Block. The inferior alveolar nerve arises from the posterior division of the mandibular nerve and passes inferiorly laterally, and slightly anteriorly toward the midpoint of the internal aspect of the ramus of

the mandible (see *Figure 7-53*). Here it enters the inferior alveolar canal, or mandibular canal, and travels anteriorly and medially in an arc below the roots of the mandibular teeth. It ends at the midline, as does its counterpart of the opposite side. At the level of the second premolar, the inferior alveolar nerve gives off the mental nerve, which passes through the mental foramen to emerge on the face.

Injection Site. The mouth of the mandibular canal is the site accessible for injection (*Figure 11-8*). It is situated on the medial aspect of the ramus of the mandible. On the dried skull, if one were to ignore the coronoid and condylar processes, the ramus is roughly rectangular, and two imaginary diagonal lines intersect approximately at the mandibular foramen. The opening is large and funnels down into the canal within the bone. The anterior border of the foramen is guarded by a variable-sized, tongue-shaped projection of bone called the *lingula*. An imaginary line drawn posteriorly from the molar occlusal plane would lie approximately 0.5 cm above the foramen.

In the mouth, location is rather difficult. Of all the routine injections attempted in the dental office, the inferior alveolar block is perhaps the most difficult to perform effectively. There is a higher degree of failure, and this is usually attributable to not following accepted techniques. There are, of course, individual variations in the locations of the mandibular foramen and its contents. One time-honored method of locating the area is to successively palpate a number of intraoral structures. The external oblique line is palpated in the buccal vestibule and followed posteriorly to where if ascends as the sharp anterior border of the ramus. This concavity is called by clinicians the *coronoid notch*. The finger is moved medially to engage the temporal crest (internal oblique ridge), and it remains in this position. The finger is now in the retromolar fossa with the fingernail pointing backward. A line is sighted from between the two premolar occlusal surfaces of the opposite side to the midpoint of the fingernail. The line continued posteriorly ends just above the mandibular foramen, at the point where the inferior alveolar nerve enters the canal.

Relationships at Injection Site

Lateral. The tip of the needle should rest on the bone of the mandibular ramus at the funnel-shaped opening of the mandibular foramen, just above the neurovascular bundle (*Figure 11-9*).

Inferior and Medial. A number of structures run laterally and inferiorly from the base of the skull to the ramus of the mandible. The inferior alveolar nerve and vessels pass from between the medial and lateral pterygoid muscles to run downward and laterally along the medial pterygoid muscle to the mandibular foramen. The needle tip lies just above and lateral to these structures as they enter the foramen. The medial pterygoid muscle continues down to the internal aspect of the angle. The sphenomandibular ligament extends from the spine of the sphenoid laterally and

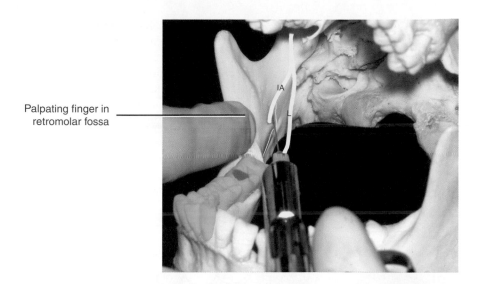

Palpating finger in retromolar fossa

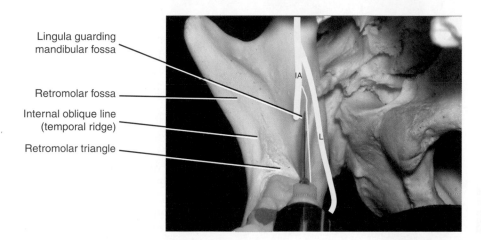

Lingula guarding mandibular fossa

Retromolar fossa

Internal oblique line (temporal ridge)

Retromolar triangle

Figure 11-8 Placement of the needle at mandibular foramen for inferior alveolar (*IA*) nerve block.

inferiorly to attach to the lingula. The needle tip should rest just above this attachment.

Anteriorly. The lingual nerve, at the level of the injection site, lies about 1 cm anteriorly and approximately 0.5 cm deeper than the inferior alveolar nerve. Use is made of this relationship for simultaneous injections for inferior alveolar and lingual nerve blocks.

Posteriorly. The encapsulated parotid gland lies posteriorly. The fibrous capsule of the deep portion of the gland attaches to the styloid process medially and the posterior border of the ramus of the mandible laterally. The capsule and gland balloon forward into the infratemporal region.

Complications. The inferior alveolar vessels, artery, and vein run with the nerve, and these should be avoided to prevent vascular penetration.

If the needle is directed too far posteriorly, it could penetrate the parotid gland capsule. Anesthetic fluid injected within the capsule quickly diffuses through the glandular tissue and anesthetizes the five main branches of the facial nerve contained within the gland. This results in a facial paralysis of the affected side, but the effects, fortunately, are transient.

Teeth Affected. All the mandibular teeth are anesthetized to the midline (pulps and periodontal ligaments).

Other Tissues Affected. The cheek and buccal gingivae receive no innervation from this nerve, and these tissues are therefore unaffected by an inferior alveolar nerve block. Similarly, the lingual gingivae are unaffected.

The mental branch of the inferior alveolar nerve, however, does supply soft tissues: the skin and mucous membrane of the lower lip (from the mental foramen anteriorly to the midline), labial alveolar mucosa and gingivae, and skin of the chin.

Gow-Gates Mandibular Nerve Block

Injection Site. The injection site for the Gow-Gates mandibular nerve block is considerably higher than that of the standard inferior alveolar. The needle tip in this method is placed in the infratemporal region below the insertion of the lateral pterygoid muscle at the anterior aspect of the condylar neck (*Figure 11-10*).

The injection parallels an external line extending from the intertragal (incisural) notch of the ear to the angle of

463

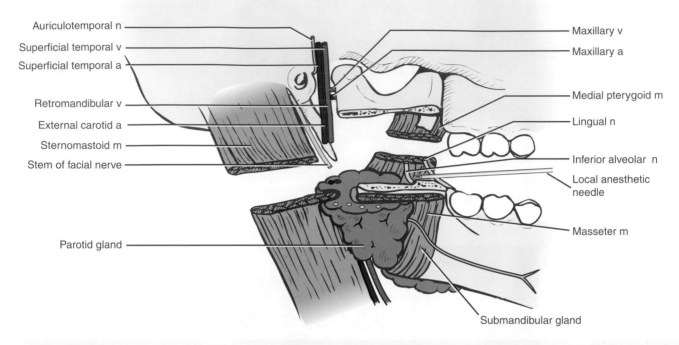

Figure 11-9 A horizontal section through parotid and infratemporal regions to show relationships of the inferior alveolar nerve at entrance of mandibular foramen.

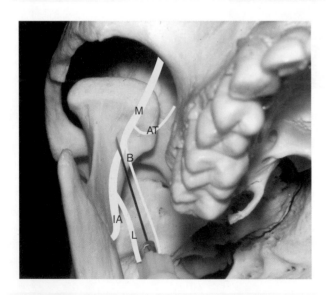

Figure 11-10 Placement of the needle for a Gow-Gates mandibular nerve block.

the mouth. The barrel of the syringe rests over the contralateral canine or the contralateral premolars if the mandibular rami are widely divergent. The needle is inserted through the mucosa distal to the maxillary second molar at the height of its mesiolingual cusp and with the opposite finger lined between the intertragal notch and angle of the mouth as a visual guide, the needle is advanced until

the condylar neck is reached (a depth of about 2.5 cm). The needle is retracted slightly and aspirated to prevent an intravascular injection.

Unlike the standard technique described a moment ago, the tip of the needle is remote from the main branches of the mandibular nerve. The Gow-Gates or high mandibular technique relies on a relatively large volume of anesthetic fluid to work. It is released into the infratemporal or pterygomandibular space and the patient is required to keep the mouth open for at least 30 seconds. This enables the fluid to permeate the area and flow around the nerves. The technique is purportedly more reliable and more comfortable than the standard inferior alveolar nerve block.

Complications. It is extremely important that careful aspiration be performed before release of the fluid. The needle ends up in the middle of the pterygoid plexus territory. In addition, the maxillary artery is close and may be punctured. In some cases, the maxillary artery lies superior to the lateral pterygoid muscle, making the artery even more vulnerable.

Nerves Blocked. The Gow-Gates technique blocks the (1) inferior alveolar nerve, (2) lingual nerve, (3) long buccal nerve, and (4) auriculotemporal nerve.

Teeth Affected. All the ipsilateral mandibular teeth (pulps and periodontal ligaments) are anesthetized to the midline.

Other Tissues Affected. Unlike the standard inferior alveolar block, the buccal and lingual nerves are concurrently anesthetized, obviating separate nerve blocks if anesthesia of these nerves is required as well. The auriculotemporal nerve is also affected but has no bearing on regular dental procedures. The patient should be warned, however, of numbness on the side of the head, because this technique may be new to some patients who have only experienced the standard inferior alveolar block.

p0360   Soft tissues anesthetized include (1) the chin, lower lip, and mandibular labial gingiva supplied by the inferior alveolar nerve via the mental branch; (2) the ipsilateral side of the tongue, floor of mouth, and mandibular gingiva via the lingual nerve; and (3) the ipsilateral cheek and mandibular buccal mucosa via the long buccal nerve.

s0280 ### Akenosi (Closed-Mouth) Mandibular Nerve Block
p0365 **Injection Site.** The injection site for this technique lies within the infratemporal or pterygomandibular space but between the site for the standard inferior alveolar block and the Gow-Gates mandibular block (*Figure 11-11*). It is a preferred technique when opening the mouth is either painful or limited.

p0370   The patient is asked to maintain the teeth in gentle occlusion, and the cheek is retracted and the injection site

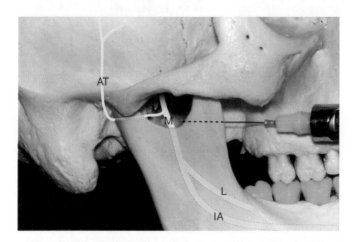

f0060   Figure 11-11 Placement of needle for an Akinosi mandibular nerve block.

is swabbed with topical anesthetic. The needle is advanced posteriorly through the maxillary vestibule, keeping the barrel of the syringe parallel to the maxillary occlusal plane and at the height of the mucogingival junction of the maxillary buccal segment. The needle is further advanced below the zygomatic process of the maxilla to pierce the mucosa of the retromolar fossa and penetrate to a depth of about 2.5 cm. After aspiration, the appropriate volume of fluid is deposited.

Complications. Penetration of the pterygoid plexus of veins or the inferior alveolar artery must be avoided with careful aspiration.   s0290 p0375

Nerves Blocked. The Akenosi technique blocks the (1) inferior alveolar nerve, (2) lingual nerve, (3) long buccal nerve, and occasionally (4) the auriculotemporal nerve.   s0295 p0380

Teeth and Soft Tissues Affected. The structures anesthetized by the Akenosi mandibular nerve block are identical to those affected by the Gow-Gates mandibular nerve block.   s0300 p0385

Mental and Incisive Block. The mental and incisive block procedure is administered occasionally when it is not desirable to anesthetize the entire inferior alveolar nerve (*Figure 11-12*).   s0305 p0390

Injection Site. The mental foramen is the mouth of a short canal that splits laterally from the main mandibular canal. The foramen is located on the facial aspect of the body of the mandible and overlies or is slightly anterior to the root apex of the second premolar tooth. The foramen opens upward and slightly posteriorly, which makes access to the foramen somewhat difficult unless the needle is bent slightly before the procedure. The foramen is approximately the midpoint of a vertical line between the gingival crest of the second premolar and the inferior border of the mandible.   s0310 p0395

Nerves Blocked. The **mental nerve** is blocked as it issues from the mental foramen. The **incisive branch** of the inferior alveolar nerve is merely the continuation of the nerve anteriorly from the mental foramen to the midline.   s0315 p0400

Complications. The mental artery and vein should be avoided.   s0320 p0405

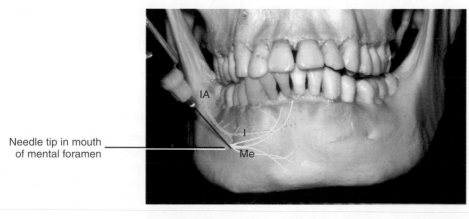

Needle tip in mouth of mental foramen

Figure 11-12 Placement of the needle at mental foramen for mental and incisive nerve blocks.   f0065

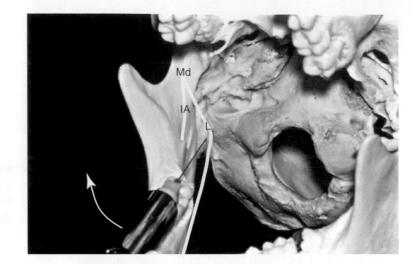

Figure 11-13 Positioning of the needle for a lingual nerve block subsequent to an inferior nerve block. The syringe is swung to same side, and fluid is released as syringe is slowly withdrawn to contact lingual nerve, which is more medial and anterior to the inferior alveolar nerve.

Teeth Affected. The mandibular canine, lateral incisor, and central incisor are affected (pulps, periodontal ligaments, and bone).

Other Tissues Anesthetized. Labial gingiva and alveolar mucosa, labial alveolar bone, skin and mucous membrane of the lip, and skin of the chin are anesthetized.

Lingual Block

Nerve Anesthetized. The lingual nerve is a branch of the posterior division of the mandibular nerve. It passes inferiorly along with the inferior alveolar nerve but pursues a more anterior and deeper course. It appears from between the medial and lateral pterygoid muscles and continues anteriorly to the floor of the mouth just deep to the root of the mandibular third molar.

Injection Site. As the injection is given for the inferior alveolar nerve, the lingual nerve is slightly deeper and anterior to the tip of the needle (see *Figure 11-9*). The syringe is shifted from the opposite side of the mouth to the same side. This has the effect of swinging the needle tip medially or deeper (*Figure 11-13*). The needle is then slowly withdrawn, and fluid is released as the needle passes by the lingual nerve. The lingual nerve is also accessible just deep to the lingual mucosa overlying the third mandibular molar root.

Tissues Anesthetized. The tissues affected are the mucosa of the anterior two thirds of the tongue, mucosa of the floor of the mouth, and lingual alveolar mucosa and gingivae of all the mandibular teeth to the midline.

Buccal (Long Buccal) Block. The buccal branch arises from the anterior division of the mandibular nerve and passes downward and laterally between the two heads of the lateral pterygoid muscle. It continues downward and forward, piercing the tendon of the temporalis muscle, and then emerges onto the cheek from under the cover of the ramus of the mandible (see *Figure 7-53*). At this point,

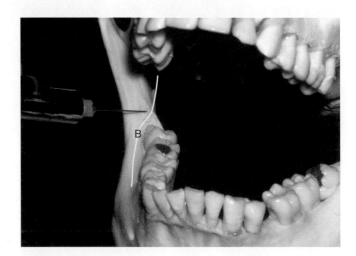

Figure 11-14 Placement of the needle in retromolar fossa for a long buccal nerve block.

the buccal nerve passes across the retromolar fossa before branching onto the cheek.

Injection Site. The retromolar fossa lies immediately behind the last mandibular molar, just under the mucosa (*Figure 11-14*).

Tissues Affected. The tissues affected are the skin and mucous membrane of the cheek and the buccal alveolar mucosa and gingivae of the mandibular molar region.

2. Imaging

Various imaging methods are used to display human anatomy in an attempt to distinguish normal from abnormal tissues. Techniques in current use are (1) radiology, which displays hard tissues such as bone and teeth; (2) magnetic resonance imaging, which displays soft tissues; (3) endoscopy, which uses a fiber optical system to visualize internal features of hollow organs or joint and body cavities; and (4) ultrasonography, which uses ultrasound to produce images of internal organs. In dentistry, radiology is used extensively, and magnetic resonance imaging is used as needed.

Dental practitioners must be able to read all images that are taken or ordered and be able to distinguish normal anatomy from abnormal or pathological. Failure to recognize any abnormality that may appear on the image may be deemed as negligence, and therefore a sound knowledge of anatomy is essential to interpret a radiograph. Image reading and interpretation are taught subsequently in radiology and pathology clinical courses.

RADIOLOGY

X-rays are similar to visible light rays and differ only in wavelength and frequency. Like visible light, they can produce an image on striking a photographic emulsion. However, the shorter wavelength of x-rays enables them to penetrate solid objects. The denser the object, the greater the amount of absorption. Tissues in the body are of varying densities and absorb (block) x-rays to a greater or lesser extent. This variation in blockage is transferred to the emulsion of a photographic film to produce a radiograph. The various shadows produced on the film range from white (blockage of all rays) to black (minimal blockage).

A **radiopaque tissue** is extremely *dense* and permits little or no passage of x-rays (they are absorbed). This shows as a *white area* on the developed radiographic film. A **radiolucent tissue**, conversely, is one that is not dense and permits passage of most x-rays. The result is a *black area* on the radiographic film.

The following structures or tissues are found in the human body. They are listed in increasing order of density, or radiopacity.

Traditional Radiographs (Plain Films)

Method. A photographic film is placed behind the subject, and x-rays are passed through the subject and allowed to

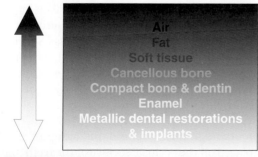

Radiolucent

Air
Fat
Soft tissue
Cancellous bone
Compact bone & dentin
Enamel
Metallic dental restorations & implants

Radiopaque

strike the film. The body tissues are of varying densities and allow the x-rays to pass through in varying amounts to expose the film. The film is then developed and interpreted. The resulting image is a two-dimensional representation of a three-dimensional subject, and, therefore, overlying structures are superimposed on underlying structures, making interpretation difficult without a sound knowledge of anatomy.

Projections, or Views. The view one sees in a radiograph is entirely dependent on the position of the patient relative to the film and the source of the x-rays. The x-ray beam diverges as it passes from the machine to the film. The farther a structure is from the film, the greater the magnification of the image. Thus the part of the body closest to the film shows the least magnification. Standard projections used in radiography are as follows:

1. An **anteroposterior (AP) projection is** one in which the subject is positioned with the back to the film—x-rays pass through the body from front to back; posterior structures show less magnification and are clearer on the resulting film than are anterior structures.
2. A **posteroanterior (PA) projection is** the opposite—the patient faces the film, and the x-rays pass through from back to front.
3. A **right lateral (RL) projection** is achieved by positioning the subject's right side against the film. Left-side structures appear as enlarged superimpositions on the film.
4. **Left lateral (LL) projections** are made with the subject's left side against the film.
5. **Oblique projections** are frequently used when superimposed structures make the viewing of a desired area or structure difficult—by turning the subject so that x-rays pass obliquely, intervening structures may be separated from the desired structure. For example, hold up two fingers (V sign) in front of one eye so that one finger visually hides the other. By moving your head to one side or the other, the two fingers move away from each other and are seen separately.

Tomographs (Sectional Films)

A conventional radiograph, as noted previously, contains superimposed images that are difficult to interpret. Tomography is a special technique that radiographically produces a section through the area of interest with no imposing overlying or underlying structures. There are three ways of achieving this.

Conventional Tomography. Conventional tomography is achieved by simultaneously moving the x-ray tube and the film in opposite directions during exposure. Images in the desired plane remain stationary and sharp, whereas images out of this plane move and are blurred on the film.

Computed Tomography (CT). Computed tomographic scanning uses a moving narrow x-ray beam that passes through the body through a predetermined plane. The beam moves in an arc about the body. The x-rays pass through the tissues in varying degrees, and this information is relayed to a computer for assimilation and reconstruction of the image on a monitor.

Cone Beam Computed Tomography. Cone beam computed tomography (CBCT) is a further refinement of CT that creates "slices" with no intermediate gaps. When reassembled the slices result in three-dimensional images that are highly accurate with no need to apply algorithms that artificially fill in the missing information, as is necessary when creating images reconstructed from ordinary computed tomographic scans. The result is a virtual anatomical reproduction that is accurate to within 0.10 mm, which is proving to be an invaluable diagnostic and treatment plan tool in dentistry, for example, during preoperative evaluation of impacted wisdom teeth, temporomandibular joints (TMJ) assessments, orthodontic treatment planning, endodontics, and particularly in the planning of sites and placements of dental implants. There are several sites in the dental arches that are at high risk by virtue of their close proximity to anatomical "danger zones," namely, the inferior alveolar canal and mental foramen in the mandible, and the incisive canal, maxillary paranasal sinus, and floor of nose in the maxilla. CBCT imaging minimizes inadvertent entry to these areas during dental implant surgical procedures.

MAGNETIC RESONANCE IMAGING

Unlike radiology, which uses ionizing radiation to expose a film or fluorescing screen, magnetic resonance imaging (MRI) makes use of a completely different technology. Hydrogen atoms behave like small magnets and spin randomly. An MRI unit consists of a powerful magnet and a source of radio waves (nonionizing radiation) from a secondary coil. When a patient is placed within the unit, the magnet realigns the hydrogen atoms so that their axes lie parallel to the direction of the external magnet. The radio waves are then applied from another angle, causing the hydrogen atoms to flip 180 degrees from their original positions. The radio waves are stopped, and the atoms realign to the external magnet. The energy released by this realignment or relaxation is electronically measured and makes use of the fact that hydrogen atoms in the various tissues behave differently and show varying speeds at which they

return to their original alignment. The rate at which the realignment takes place is called the *relaxation time* or T1. In addition, the time taken to dephase back to random spinning is measured as T2. The data are fed to a computer, which generates a two-dimensional image of a section through the tissues being examined. By manipulating parameters of the unit, the images can be either T1-weighted or T2-weighted. MRI provides excellent images of soft tissues but does not supply the precise detail of bone and dental tissues provided by traditional radiography. The use of MRI is presently limited to examination of the soft tissues of the TMJ and is extremely useful in determining internal disc derangement (see *Figures 7-43* and *7-46*).

IMAGING IN DENTISTRY
Intraoral Radiographs

Intraoral radiographs are ones in which the film packet is placed within the patient's mouth. Common radiographs of the jaws and teeth include the (1) bitewing radiograph, (2) periapical radiograph, and (3) occlusal radiograph.

Periapical Radiographs. Periapical radiographs provide a view of crowns, roots, alveolar bone, and some surrounding bony structures (*Figure 11-15*). For adults, a full-mouth series of 17 periapical and 4 bitewing radiographs is taken at initial visits at appropriate recall visits. Periapical radiographs are taken to assess or detect (1) periodontal disease (alveolar bone loss), (2) dentoalveolar and periodontal abscesses, (3) cysts and tumors, (4) fractures, (5) supernumerary teeth, (6) retained fractured root fragments, (7) foreign bodies, and (8) impacted third molars.

In addition, periapical radiographs are routinely taken before oral surgery to assess the size and shape of tooth roots and the proximity of maxillary roots to the maxillary sinus or mandibular roots to the mandibular canal. In endodontics, radiographs are indispensable in determining root canal length and proper degree of filling.

Bitewing Radiographs. Bitewing radiographs are taken at initial visits and at appropriate recall visits to provide a view of the maxillary and mandibular crowns of the posterior teeth in occlusion (see *Figure 11-18*). They are useful in detecting (1) occlusal caries, (2) interproximal caries, (3) recurrent caries under old restorations, (4) overhanging restoration margins, and (5) loss of alveolar bone height.

Occlusal Radiographs. Occlusal radiographs are films that are placed on the occlusal surface of the teeth and held by the patient closing gently on the film (*Figure 11-16*).

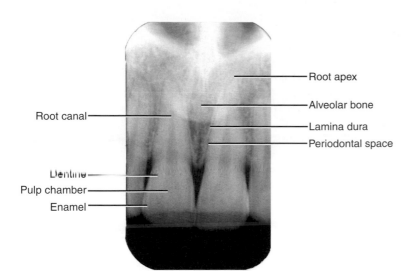

Root canal

Dentine
Pulp chamber
Enamel

Root apex
Alveolar bone
Lamina dura
Periodontal space

Figure 11-15 Periapical radiograph of the maxillary anterior segment.

They are routinely used to obtain radiographs of the anterior maxillary and mandibular segments in children in the primary dentition stage. They are also used to supplement and obtain alternate views of suspicious areas detected in a full-mouth series (described in the following section).

Full-Mouth Survey. A full-mouth radiographic survey includes periapical, bitewing, and occasionally occlusal films (*Figure 11-17*). A survey is taken at initial

Permanent central incisor

Intermaxillary suture

Deciduous central incisor

A

Symphysis menti

B

Figure 11-16 Occlusal radiograph of a 5½-year-old child. **A**, Maxillary anteriors. **B**, Mandibular anteriors. Crowns of a deciduous teeth are seen as well as developing permanent teeth. (Courtesy Dr. M. Pharoah.)

appointments and when needed or deemed necessary at subsequent recall visits. Children in the primary dentition stage (3 to 6 years of age) require 8 radiographs, children in the mixed dentition stage (7 to 12 years of age) require 12 radiographs, and adults require 21 radiographs.

Extraoral Radiographs

As the name suggests, extraoral radiographs are taken with the film positioned adjacent to the head.

Panoramic Radiographs. Panoramic x-ray units rotate an x-ray source and a film about the patient's head to produce a view of all the teeth of both arches, their roots, and both upper and lower jaws, which is similar to a full-mouth survey (*Figure 11-18*). There are both advantages and disadvantages to a panoramic radiograph, in contrast to a full-mouth survey. (1) A single panoramic film can be set up and exposed in minutes in comparison to the much longer time required to position and expose 21 individual periapical films; (2) the single extraoral film is better tolerated by patients in comparison to a series of intraoral films; (3) the panoramic film offers a complete view of the upper and lower jaws including the TMJ but lacks the fine anatomical detail of the teeth and supporting structures seen in periapical films; and (4) panoramic films are useful in edentulous patients or in situations that do not require the fine detail revealed in periapical films.

Cephalometric Radiographs. Complete head or cephalometric radiographs are used in orthodontic practice to help diagnose orthodontic problems, that is, whether the problem is one of malposed teeth (dentoalveolar) or malposed jaws in relation to each other and the cranial

469

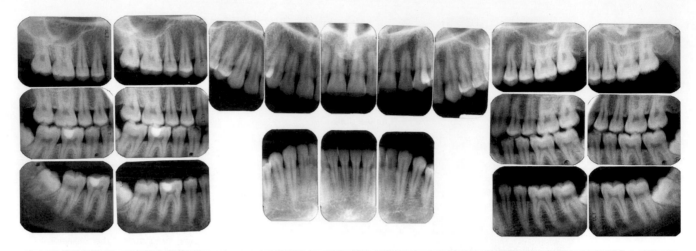

Figure 11-17 Full-mouth radiographic survey. *Upper row,* Maxillary periapicals; *lower row,* mandibular periapicals; *middle row,* bitewing radiographs. (Courtesy Dr. M. Pharoah.)

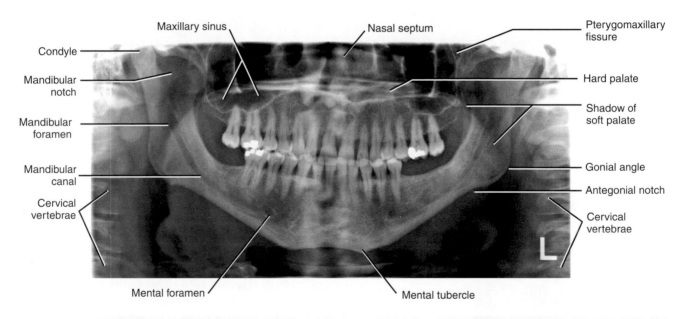

Maxillary sinus · Nasal septum · Pterygomaxillary fissure

Condyle

Mandibular notch

Mandibular foramen

Mandibular canal

Cervical vertebrae

Hard palate

Shadow of soft palate

Gonial angle

Antegonial notch

Cervical vertebrae

Mental foramen · Mental tubercle

Figure 11-18 Adult panoramic radiograph.

base (skeletal). Head radiographs are also used to assess the progress of treatment (before and after) and to predict eventual adult jaw sizes and relationships. The oral surgeon uses preoperative head radiographs to assess severe facial disharmonies in adults before surgical correction and postoperative radiographs to assess the progress of healing (*Figure 11-19*).

Alveolar Ridge Tomography. Sectional views through the maxillary and mandibular alveolar ridges are necessary for calculating an accurate depth for the surgical placement of a dental implant. A cone beam computed tomograph provides three-dimensional information that will be used to determine the implantation site and

the optimum depth for maximum support and to prevent the operator from inadvertently entering a danger area. Danger areas in the maxilla include the floor of the nasal cavity, the floor of the maxillary air sinus of the maxilla, and the incisive canal and contents (*Figure 11-20, A*). Danger areas of the mandible include the mandibular canal and mental foramen and their contents (*Figure 11-20, B*).

Other Areas and Structures of Clinical Interest

Maxillary Sinus (Antrum). Sinus radiographs are taken to assess (1) infection (sinusitis), (2) the presence of tumors or cysts, and (3) the location of fractured root fragments inadvertently pushed into the maxillary sinus.

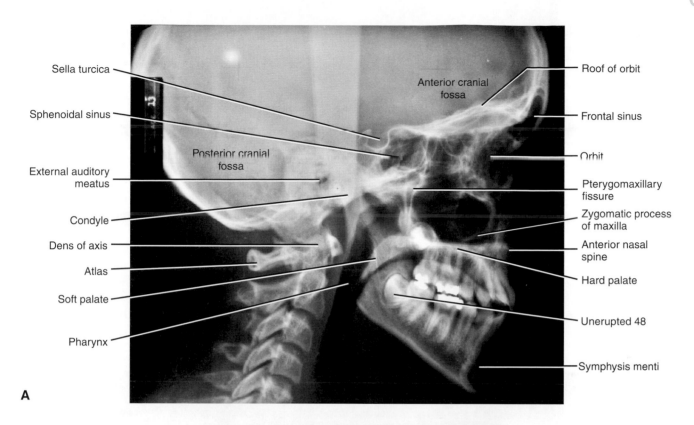

A

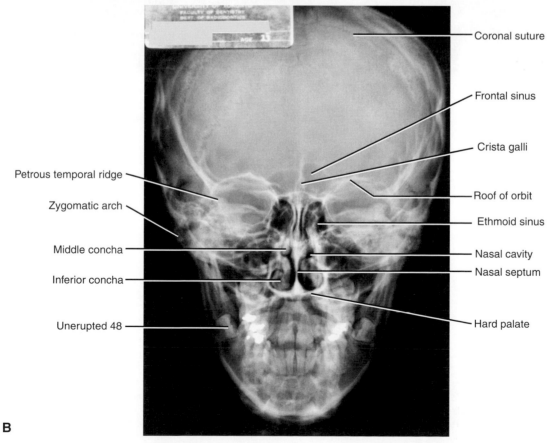

B

Figure 11-19 Full skull radiographs. **A,** Lateral projection. **B,** Posteroanterior (PA) projection. (Courtesy Dr. S. M. Fireman.)

The maxillary sinuses on normal extraoral radiographs are not clearly defined, and it is far more advantageous to use tomography or CT to view the sinuses (*Figure 11-21*).

s0480 p0590 *Hard Palate and Floor of Nasal Cavity.* The hard palate forms the roof of the oral cavity and the floor of the nasal cavity. This presents a hazard in oral surgery procedures that are undertaken in the anterior maxillary region. *Figure 11-22* is a core beam computed tomograph revealing an inverted supernumerary incisor that is dangerously close to the floor of the nasal cavity. In addition the scan reveals its proximity to the incisive canal.

s0485 p0595 *TMJ.* The TMJ may be depicted radiographically using a modified lateral technique with the head tilted (*Figure 11-23, A*). Even better views (*Figure 11-23, B to D*) are produced with tomographs of the joint. Radiographs of the joint are used to help diagnose joint pain (arthritis)

or joint dysfunction and for treatment plans that relate to TMJ surgery. Radiographs show the bony detail of the TMJ but do not reveal the disc and other soft tissue structures.

There are two ways to examine the disc tissue: p0600

1. **TMJ arthrography** is used to indirectly reveal an image o0080 of the disc. A radiopaque contrast medium is injected into one or both joint cavities to reveal disc morphology, position, and possible perforation (see *Figure 11-23, C*).
2. **TMJ MRI** is the best way to examine soft tissue of the o0085 joint and is useful in determining internal disc derangement (see *Figure 11-23, D*).

Salivary Glands (Sialographs). The duct and ductules s0490 of the parotid or submandibular gland may be studied by injecting a radiopaque medium into the orifice of the duct in the oral cavity. A radiograph is then taken in which

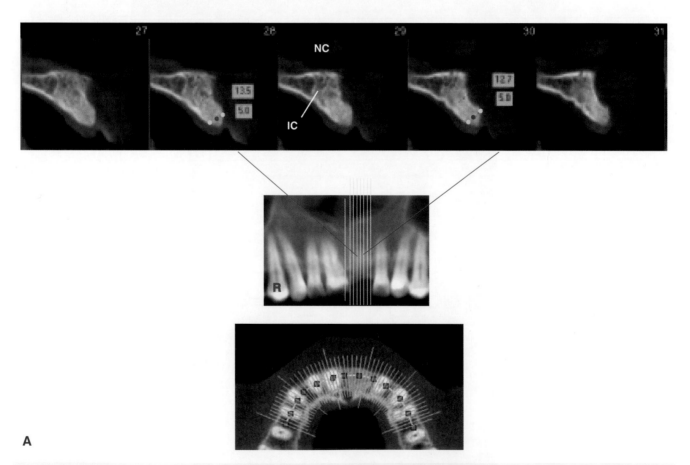

f0105 Figure 11-20 Cone beam computed tomographs (CBCT scans) to view edentulous areas of maxillary and mandibular dental ridges, to aid in correct placement of dental implants. The middle image in each case represents the "scout" and shows the paths of the sections (*yellow lines*). The top row of images displays the sagittal cuts through the alveolar ridge. The bottom image shows an axial (horizontal) cut through the area of interest. Distances between red dots represent maximum depth; distances between green dots represent maximum width. **A,** Maxillary anterior area. Note the danger areas, nasal cavity (*NC*) and incisive canal (*IC*).

Continued

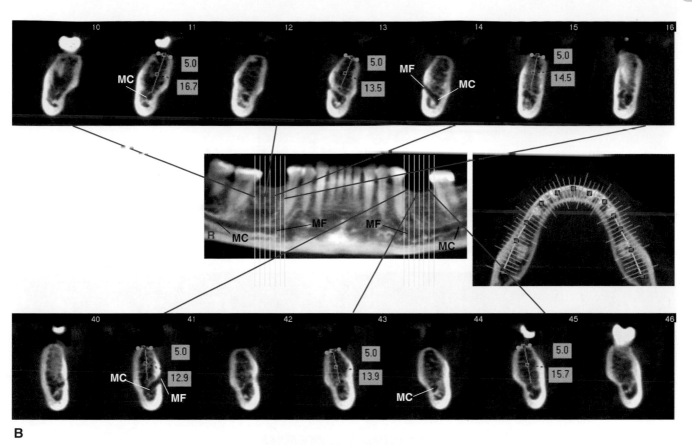

B

Figure 11-20 Cont'd. **B,** Mandibular posterior area. Note the danger areas, mandibular canal (*MC*) and mental foramen (*MF*). (Courtesy Dr. S. M. Fireman.)

the duct and ductules are clearly outlined and any glandular disturbances or blocking stones (sialoliths) may be detected (see *Figure 7-88*).

Hand and Wrist. We know from observation that children do not necessarily develop at the same rate. Children of the same chronological age may differ in their developmental ages; that is, a child may be average, advanced, or retarded in development.

A reliable method for determining the developmental age of a child is to assess the developing skeleton through radiographs and arrive at a skeletal age that closely reflects the child's developmental age. An economical area of assessment is the hand and wrist, because 30 developing centers may be assessed in a single radiograph of the hand and wrist (*Figure 11-24*). These centers closely parallel the development of the entire skeleton.

Atlases of skeletal age contain characteristic or modal radiographs of the hand and wrist for the entire age range (birth to adulthood). The standards are age- and sex-specific. The patient's radiograph is compared with the appropriate standards, and the closest match is said to be the patient's skeletal age.

3. Fractures of the Face

The bones of the upper face are hollow and light but are effectively buttressed against the cranial base to withstand relatively high pressures generated during mastication. Direct blows to the face, however, as in brawls or automobile accidents, commonly result in fractures of the facial bones.

CLASSIFICATION

1. A **simple fracture** is a break in the bone only and one that does not involve the skin externally or mucous membrane internally.

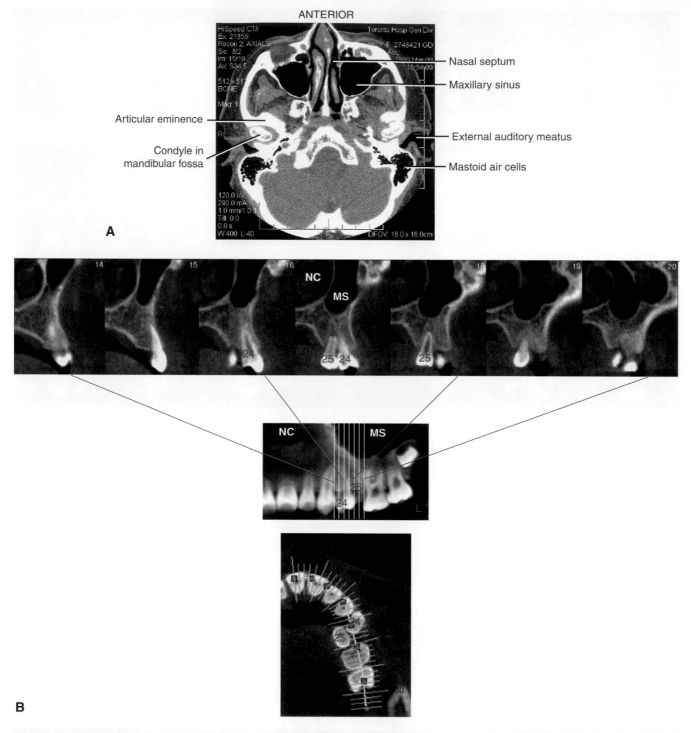

Figure 11-21 Radiographic imaging of maxillary air sinuses. **A,** Axial CT scan. **B,** CBCT scans. The middle image is the "scout" and shows the paths of the sections (*yellow lines*). Note the proximity of the unerupted third molar (*28*) to the maxillary sinus. The top row of images displays the coronal cuts through the alveolar ridge. The bottom image shows an axial (horizontal) cut through the area of interest. Note the lingually displaced bicuspid (*25*) and its relationship to the maxillary sinus (*MS*). (Courtesy Dr. S. M. Fireman.)

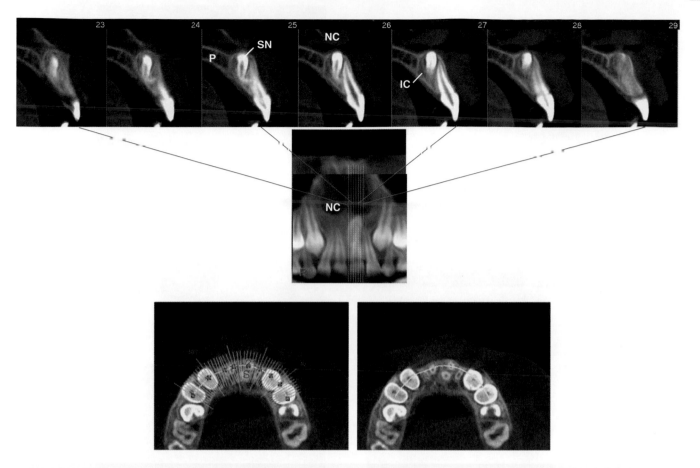

Figure 11-22 CBCT scan of anterior palatal region (*P*). The middle image is the "scout" and shows the paths of the sections (*yellow lines*). Note the proximity of a supernumerary tooth (*SN*) to the nasal cavity (*NC*) and to the incisive canal (*IC*). The top row of images displays the sagittal cuts through the alveolar ridge. The bottom images show an axial (horizontal) cut through the area of interest. (Courtesy Dr. S. M. Fireman.)

2. A **compound fracture** does involve the skin or mucous membrane; the resulting communication enhances the dangers of infection.

In addition, fractures may be single (one break) or multiple (more than one break). In a comminuted fracture, there are a number of small fragments at the fracture site. Facial fractures may be conveniently divided into those of the lower face (mandible) and the midface and upper face (the remaining facial bones).

Mandibular (Lower-Face) Fractures

The mandible is perhaps the most frequently fractured of all facial bones (*Figure 11-25*). The fracture may be single but is generally multiple (bilateral), and if a fracture is detected on one side, the contralateral side should be investigated for possible fracture.

Common Sites

1. In the **condylar neck,** the fracture may be unilateral, but it is frequently bilateral, especially if the blow is received on the chin. Usually the fracture line is below the joint capsule, and the condyle may or may not be dislocated.

2. In the **coronoid process,** fractures are generally single.

3. In the **mandibular ramus,** fractures extending from the mandibular notch to the angle occur infrequently because of the overlying padding of the masseter muscle.

4. In the **mandibular body,** fractures of the body frequently occur in line with the canine tooth because of its deep alveolus. Fracture lines also may extend from the third molar area to the antegonial region.

5. In the **alveolar process,** a portion of the alveolar process and one or more teeth may fracture away from the body of the mandible. This generally involves the anterior, more vulnerable segment.

Displacement of Fragments. Fragments may be noticeably displaced, causing an asymmetry of the face or a malocclusion of the teeth. The degree of displacement depends on the direction of the fracture lines and the muscle pull on the fragment.

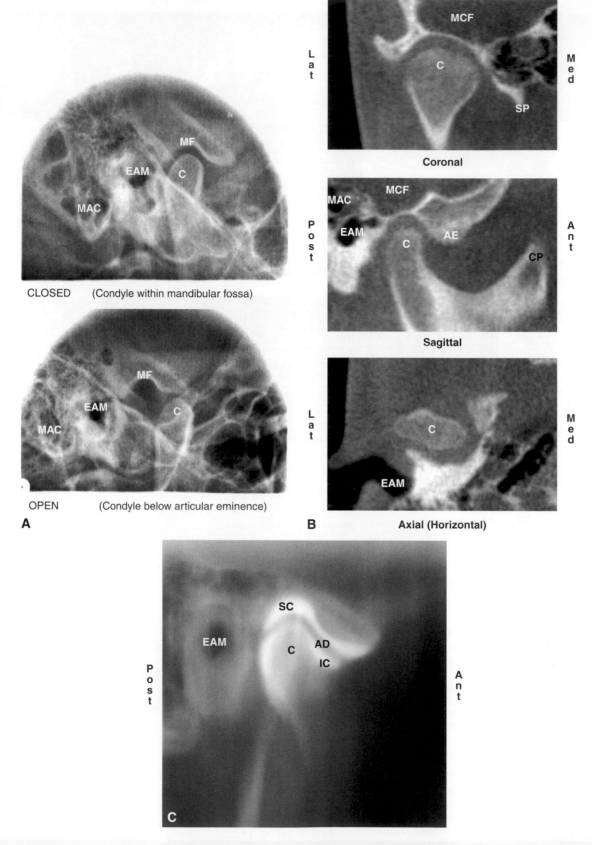

CLOSED (Condyle within mandibular fossa)

OPEN (Condyle below articular eminence)

A

Coronal

Sagittal

B Axial (Horizontal)

C

Figure 11-23 Various methods of TMJ imaging. **A,** Oblique lateral view. (Courtesy Dr. S. M. Fireman). **B,** CBCT scans, coronal, sagittal, and axial. (Courtesy Dr. S. M. Fireman) **C,** Lateral arthrograph following injections of radiopaque contrast medium into joint cavities. (Courtesy Dr. M. Pharoah).

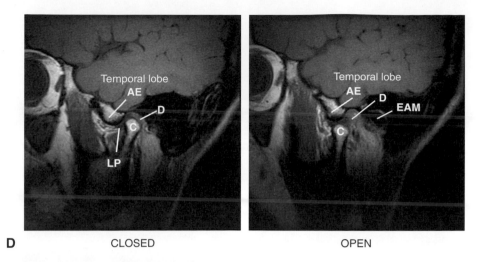

D   CLOSED   OPEN

Figure 11-23 Cont'd **D**, MRI showing sagittal section through the TMJ. *C,* condyle; *MF,* mandibular fossa; *CP,* coronoid process; *EAM,* external auditory meatus; *AE,* articular eminence; *MAC,* mastoid air cells; *MCF,* middle cranial fossa; *SC,* superior joint compartment; *IC,* inferior joint compartment; *AD,* articular disc; *LP,* lateral pterygoid muscle insertion. (Courtesy Dr. M. Pharaoh).

Unfavorable Fracture. An unfavorable fracture line angles upward, forward, and inward through the mandibular body. The posterior fragment is pulled upward and inward by the muscles of mastication, and the anterior fragment is pulled downward and backward by the suprahyoid muscles.

Favorable Fracture. A favorable fracture line angles upward, backward, and outward, and thus mechanically resists the upward drag of the muscles of mastication and the downward pull of the suprahyoid muscles. Severely displaced mandibular fractures may damage

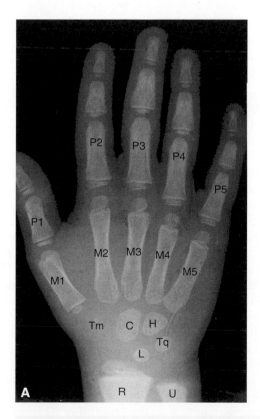
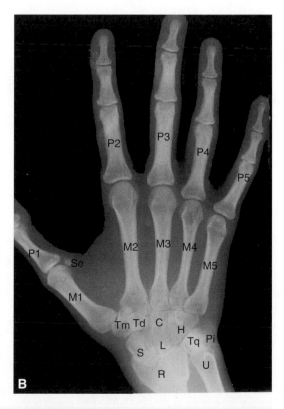

Figure 11-24 Hand and wrist radiographs. **A,** 4½-year-old boy. **B,** Adult. *C,* Capitate; *H,* hamate; *L,* lunate; *M,* metacarpal; *P,* phalanges; *Pi,* pisiform; *R,* radius; *S,* scaphoid; *Se,* sesamoid; *Td,* trapezoid; *Tm,* trapezium; *Tq,* triquetrum; *U,* ulna.

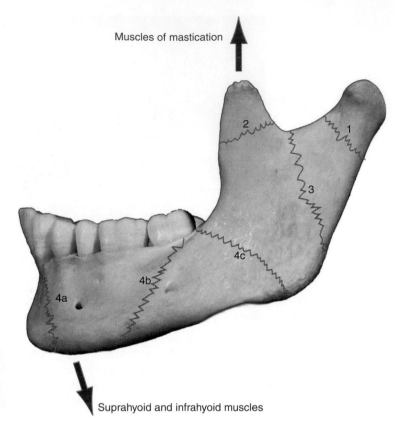

Muscles of mastication

Suprahyoid and infrahyoid muscles

Figure 11-25 Common sites for mandibular fractures. *1,* Represents a fracture through condylar neck; *2,* through coronoid process; *3,* through ramus; *4a,* through canine area of body; *4b,* favorable fracture of body; *4c,* unfavorable fracture of body.

the inferior alveolar nerve and result in anesthesia of the supplied areas.

Midface and Upper-Face Fractures

Localized Fractures. The nasal bones are commonly fractured because of their prominent position. The fracture is generally transverse, and displacement is usually to one side.

The zygomatic arches are also prominent facial features that are easily fractured and depressed. A break in the anterior root of the arch would involve the lateral wall of the orbit.

The orbital floor may be fractured indirectly as a result of a blow to the eye. The eyeball and orbital contents are forced back in the bony orbit, and, if the force is strong enough, the orbit fractures through the orbital floor, which is the thin orbital plate of the maxilla. The fracture opens a communication between the orbit above and the maxillary sinus below.

The alveolar process and several teeth may be separated from the body of the maxilla. This usually includes the vulnerable anterior segment.

Extensive Fractures. Fractures involving several bones of the mid and upper face were noted by LeFort as generally falling into one of three basic patterns (*Figure 11-26*).

LeFort I is a fracture line that extends over the apices of the maxillary teeth, through the base of the nasal septum,

and posteriorly through the pterygoid processes. Thus the teeth, alveolar processes, and palate are separated from the rest of the face. A variation is a unilateral break coupled with a fracture of the midsagittal suture.

LeFort II is a more complex fracture that involves the orbits and maxillary sinuses of both sides. The fracture line extends through the posterolateral wall of the maxillary sinus, through the floor of the orbit along the infraorbital canal, and through the zygomatic process of the maxilla. The line also extends upward on the medial wall of the orbit through the orbital plate of the ethmoid bone, the lacrimal bone, and then across the bridge of the nose. The displaced fragment includes the entire anterior and central portion of the face, the palate, and the alveolar processes and teeth.

LeFort III is an extremely complicated fracture that involves the orbits and the cranial base. The fracture line passes bilaterally through the zygomaticomaxillary suture, across the greater wing of the sphenoid in the lateral orbital wall, through the superior orbital fissure, and through the ethmoid bone, lacrimal bone, and maxilla at the bridge of the nose. The resulting fragment includes almost the entire face.

Rhinorrhea is the leakage of cerebrospinal fluid in breaks involving the cranial base. The cribriform plates may be damaged in the LeFort II or III types of fractures, and, if the meninges are torn, the cerebrospinal fluid leaks through the nose. Severely displaced fragments may involve and damage the infraorbital nerve and its branches.

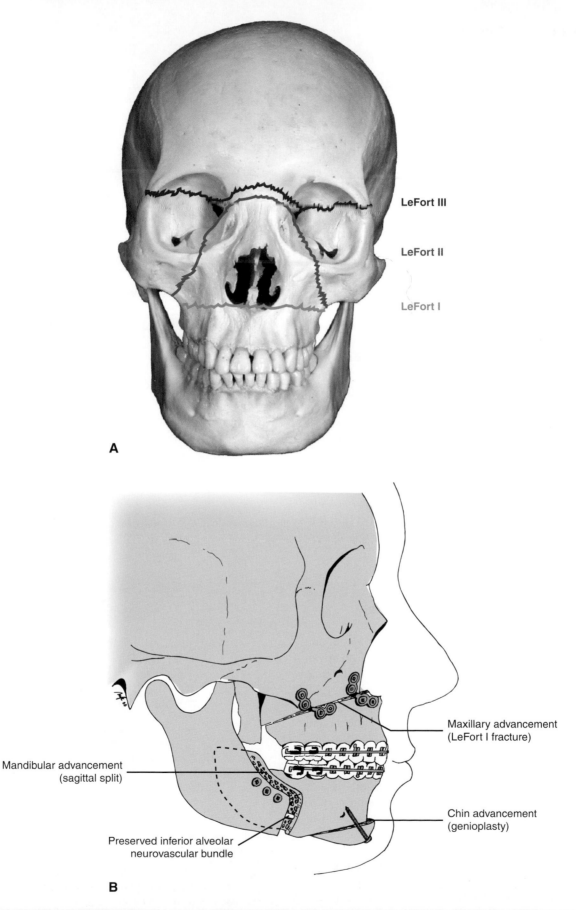

LeFort III

LeFort II

LeFort I

A

Mandibular advancement
(sagittal split)

Preserved inferior alveolar
neurovascular bundle

Maxillary advancement
(LeFort I fracture)

Chin advancement
(genioplasty)

B

Figure 11-26 **A**, LeFort classification of upper and midface fractures. **B**, Osteotomies of face. In this case, a LeFort I osteotomy allows advancement of separated maxillary fragment. A bilateral sagittal split through mandible allows advancement of detached mandibular body, and detached mental tuberosity allows advancement of chin (genioplasty). All three sites have been fixed in place following placement of detached segments in their new positions. (Courtesy Dr. M. Caminiti.)

SURGICAL TREATMENT OF FACIAL DISHARMONIES

The jaws may occasionally be fractured intentionally to treat severe facial disharmonies (see *Figure 11-26, B*). For example, a severely retrognathic mandible may be treated by strategic bilateral saw cuts in a vertical or oblique direction through the mandibular ramus, taking care to avoid the mandibular canal and its neurovascular bundle. The freed portion of mandible is then advanced to a predetermined position to improve the profile and the function.

A retrusion midface is treated by detaching the maxillary dental arch along the LeFort I fracture lines and then wiring the maxillary fragment into a more favorable esthetic and functional position.

4. Spread of Dental Infections*

Bacterial infections of the oral cavity commonly arise from an odontogenic source, and, like infection anywhere else in the body, they can be potentially life-threatening. Fortunately, antibiotics and effective dental care delivery have drastically reduced the frequency of orofacial infections. However, widespread infection resulting from dental abscesses does occur in the dental practice, and the dentist must have a thorough knowledge of the sources of dental infection and the anatomical pathways by which they may spread from one region to another.

PRIMARY SITES OF INFECTION

Pulpal Chamber of Tooth (Dentoalveolar Abscess)

The most commonly infected area is the dental pulp, and the usual insult to the dental pulp is the result of an invading carious lesion. A carious lesion extending to the pulp infects the pulpal tissues and produces inflammation (pulpitis) and localized pain. Normal reactionary swelling of the pulpal tissues within the rigid confines of the pulp chamber and root canal chokes off the nutrient blood vessels, and the pulp dies (pulpal necrosis). The necrotic, infected pulpal remains fester and produce an exudate that builds up pressure and escapes through the root apex into the surrounding alveolar bone (*Figure 11-28*). The pain may be temporarily relieved by drilling a hole through the crown of the tooth, to allow the exudate to drain to the oral cavity.

Periodontal Structures (Periodontal Abscess)

Destruction of the periodontium and alveolar bone (periodontitis) leads to the formation of soft tissue and bony

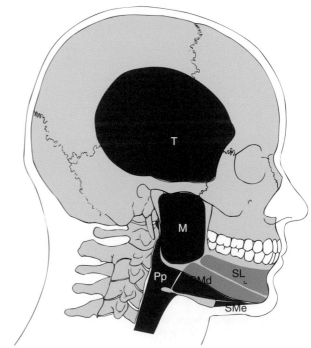

B

Figure 11-27 Fascial spaces of head. **A,** Superficial and parotid fascial spaces. *B,* Buccal region of superficial space; *C,* canine region of superficial space. **B,** Deep fascial spaces. *M,* Submasseteric portion of masticator space; *Pp,* parapharyngeal space; *SL,* sublingual; *Smd,* submandibular; *Sme,* submental; *T,* temporal portion of masticator space. **A,** Vital tooth. **B,** Dentoalveolar abscess.

---

* Written with contributions from Dr. Simon Weinberg and Dr. Bruce Pynn.

pockets about the necks and roots of the teeth. Because the pockets cannot be adequately cleansed by the patient, food debris and bacteria accumulate and form a periodontal abscess. These abscesses generally drain to the oral cavity but may spread to neighboring tissues.

SECONDARY SITES

Alveolar bone is secondarily infected from the root apex of the abscessed tooth and forms a dentoalveolar abscess. If the diseased tooth is treated by root canal therapy or if the tooth is extracted, the abscess generally resolves. If left untreated, the abscess may remain in a quiescent chronic stage, or it may become acute and begin to spread through the bone.

Spread of infection is generally along the line of least resistance. It may extend through the medullary cavity of the bone, or, more frequently, it erodes the cortical alveolar bone and elevates the periosteum. Then it may burst through the periosteum to overlying soft tissues and point into the oral cavity as a dentoalveolar abscess or gum boil; or the infection may remain subperiosteal, stripping away periosteum from the bone as it spreads.

TERTIARY SITES

On escape from the bone, infection invades the soft tissues, setting up an inflammatory process (cellulitis). Clinically the area appears poorly localized, reddened, indurated, and tender to palpation. Usually the most localized infections break through the buccal or labial alveolar mucosa and drain to the oral vestibule. The infection may also spread, however, in virtually any direction—buccal, lingual into adjoining soft tissues, or even externally to the skin. This type heals spontaneously following extraction or root canal treatment, with or without curettage of the abscess. On the other hand, the infection may spread along fascial planes to areas termed *fascial spaces*.

Fascia

General concepts concerning fascia are presented in Chapter 1, Section 8, and the deep fascia of the neck (Chapter 5, Section 1) should be reviewed. Superficial fascia (subcutaneous tissue) is found immediately below the skin and contains a variable amount of fat interspersed between the connective tissue fibers. In the face, the superficial muscles of facial expression are contained within this layer. Deep fascia contains less fat, is more organized, and surrounds deeper structures, such as bone, muscle, viscera, and neurovascular bundles.

Fascial spaces between deep structures contain loose areolar tissue. These are potential spaces only and are opened up only during surgery in the living or dissection in the cadaver. Infection in a fascial space can also displace the loose areolar tissue, creating a tertiary site of infection. If unchecked, the area fills up and the infection then may invade a neighboring fascial space.

Fascial Spaces
Superficial Spaces
Boundaries. The superficial fascia of the face is bounded superficially by skin; deeply by the facial aspects of the mandible, buccinator muscle, and the maxilla; superiorly by the zygomatic arch and infraorbital margin; inferiorly by the lower border of the mandible; and posteriorly by the parotid region (*Figure 11-27, Table 11-1*).

Contents. The area contains (1) fat; (2) lymph nodes; (3) muscles of facial expression; (4) facial vein and artery; (5) infraorbital nerve, artery, and vein; (6) mental nerve artery and vein; and (7) the branches of the facial nerve.

The superficial fascial space is further divided by the bony attachments of the muscles of facial expression. Thus,

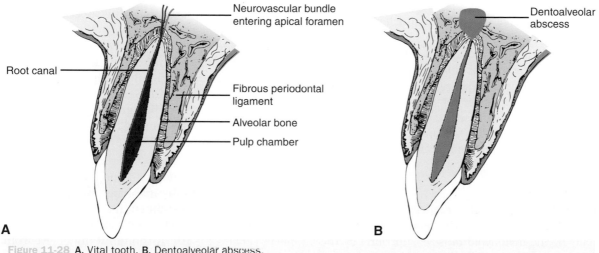

Root canal

Neurovascular bundle entering apical foramen

Fibrous periodontal ligament

Alveolar bone

Pulp chamber

Dentoalveolar abscess

A

B

Figure 11-28 **A,** Vital tooth. **B,** Dentoalveolar abscess.

TABLE 11-1

Infections Involving the Major Fascial Spaces of the Head

Potential Fascial Space	Odontogenic Source of Infection	Communications	Symptoms
Superficial Infraorbital or canine	Maxillary anteriors	Buccal space Cavernous sinus via venous communications	Firm or fluctuant mass along lateral border of nose, may extend up to medial angle of eye and periorbital area
Buccal	Maxillary molars and premolars Mandibular molars and premolars	Infraorbital, masticator, parapharyngeal spaces	Large, tender swelling of cheek May extend from philtrum of lip to parotid region May extend superiorly to eye and involve eyelids
Submandibular	Mandibular molars	Sublingual, submental, parapharyngeal spaces	Firm, painful swelling in submandibular region, dysphagia
Submental	Mandibular anteriors	Submandibular spaces on either side	Hard midline swelling under chin
Sublingual	Mandibular premolars, molars	Submandibular, parapharyngeal spaces	Elevated tongue with decreased mobility, swollen floor of mouth, dysphagia
Masticator (including infratemporal, massceteric, and temporal spaces)	Mandibular 3rd molars	Parapharyngeal, retropharyngeal	Pain, muscle trismus, swollen tonsillar pillars
Parapharyngeal and retropharyngeal	Maxillary molars Mandibular molars	Submandibular, submandibular, sublingual, masticator, and tonsillar spaces, mediastinum	Pain and muscle trismus, swollen soft palate with deviated uvula, dysphagia, inability to palpate angle of mandible

infection tends to localize in the cheek (**buccal space**), upper lip, lower lip, or infraorbital (**canine space**) region (*Figure 11-29*).

Parotid Region. Dental infections do not normally enter this region, but the gland may be infected via bacterial invasion along the parotid duct. The parotid region is entirely filled with the parotid salivary gland, which, in turn, is encapsulated with a thick fibrous glandular capsule. The capsule tends to keep infection localized.

Boundaries. The parotid region is bounded superficially by skin, deeply by the styloid process and attached muscles, superiorly and inferiorly by glandular capsule, posteriorly by the sternocleidomastoid muscle, and anteriorly by the posterior border of the mandibular ramus and the stylomandibular ligament, which balloons anteriorly into the infratemporal region deep to the ramus.

Contents. The parotid region contains (1) the parotid gland, (2) the facial nerve and its branches, (3) the external carotid artery and its terminal branches, and (4) the retromandibular vein.

Submandibular Region

Boundaries. The submandibular region is bounded laterally by superficial fascia and the body of the mandible, medially by the mylohyoid muscle, superiorly by the mylohyoid line, and inferiorly by the hyoid bone.

Contents. The area contains (1) the submandibular gland, (2) lymph nodes, (3) the hypoglossal nerve, (4) the nerve to the mylohyoid, and (5) the facial artery and submental branch.

Communications. The submandibular region may connect with (1) the superficial space, (2) the sublingual region, (3) the parotid region, and (4) the masticator region.

Sublingual Region (Floor of Mouth)

Boundaries. The area is bounded laterally by the body of the mandible, medially by the base of the tongue, inferiorly by the mylohyoid muscle, and superiorly by mucosa of the floor of the mouth.

Contents. The area contains (1) the sublingual gland, (2) the deep submandibular gland and duct, (3) the lingual nerve and submandibular ganglion, (4) the lingual artery and branches, and (5) the hypoglossal nerve.

Communications. The sublingual region may communicate with (1) the submandibular region or (2) the masticator region.

Ludwig's Angina. Ludwig's angina is an aggressive, rapidly spreading cellulitis involving bilateral sublingual, submandibular, and submental spaces, which can further spread down into the neck via the parapharyngeal spaces (*Figure 11-30*). Although it may arise from any mandibular tooth, the second and third mandibular

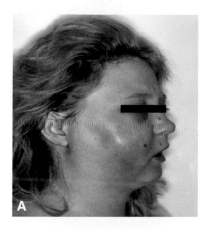

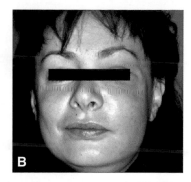

Figure 11-29 Infection of the superficial fascial space. **A**, Canine or infraorbital space. **B**, Buccal space. (Courtesy Dr. M. Caminiti.)

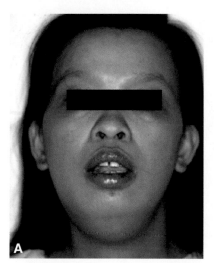

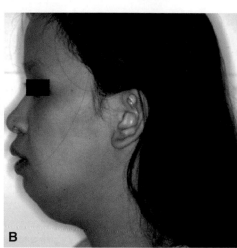

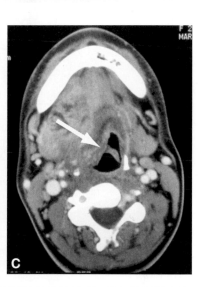

Figure 11-30 Ludwig's angina, a massive and potentially dangerous bilateral infection of the submental, sublingual, and submandibular regions. **A**, Anterior view. **B**, Left lateral view. **C**, CT image through upper cervical region showing impingement of the infected mass on the airway. (Courtesy Dr. M. Caminiti.)

molars account for most cases, because the roots of these teeth extend below the level of the attachment of the mylohyoid muscle. The neck and floor of mouth may become so swollen that breathing may be compromised, necessitating the creation of an artificial airway.

Tonsillar Region

Boundaries. The tonsillar area is bounded anteriorly by the palatoglossus muscle, posteriorly by the palatopharyngeus muscle, laterally by the pharyngobasilar fascia, and medially by the oropharyngeal mucosa (*Figure 11-31*).

Contents. The area contains (1) the palatine tonsil, (2) the glossopharyngeal nerve, and (3) tonsillar and ascending palatine branches of the facial artery.

Communications. The tonsillar region may communicate with (1) the submucosa of the soft palate, (2) the submandibular region, and (3) the sublingual region.

Masticator Space. The masticator region lies on either side of the mandibular ramus and is formed by cervical fascia,

which ascends from the neck and splits at the inferior mandibular border to envelop the area (see *Figure 11-31*).

Boundaries. The masticator region is bounded laterally by the lateral portion of the cervical fascia, which ascends over the masseter muscle, blending with the fascia of the muscle. The fascia tacks to the zygomatic arch and continues upward to blend with the dense temporalis fascia a few centimeters above the arch. The fascia continues superiorly and attaches to the superior temporal line on the side of the skull. Medially, the deep fascial component ascends deep to the mandibular ramus and deep to the medial pterygoid muscle to attach to the base of the skull. Posteriorly, the area is separated from the parotid region by the stylomandibular ligament, which balloons forward, encroaching on the masticator space. Anteriorly, the masticator fascia binds to the anterior border of the ramus and the temporalis tendon. A portion of the fascia continues anteriorly to fuse with the buccopharyngeal fascia covering the buccinator muscle. Superiorly, the area is limited by the roof of the infratemporal fossa and

483

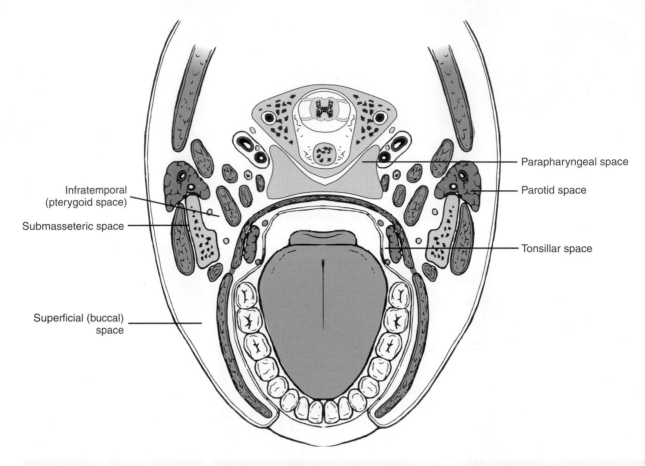

Infratemporal
(pterygoid space)

Submasseteric space

Superficial (buccal)
space

Parapharyngeal space

Parotid space

Tonsillar space

Figure 11-31 Horizontal section through the oral cavity to demonstrate parapharyngeal, tonsillar, and masticator regions. Also shown are submasseteric and infratemporal (pterygoid) regions of the masticator region.

the superior attachment of the temporalis muscle. *Figure 11-32* shows a patient with an infected masticator space.
Contents. The masticator area contains (1) the mandibular ramus and the TMJ, (2) four muscles of mastication, (3) the mandibular nerve and its branches, (4) the maxillary

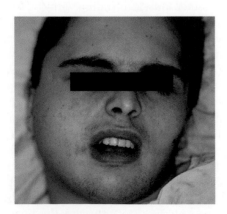

Figure 11-32 Infection of masticator space with spread into masseteric and temporal spaces. (Courtesy Dr. M. Caminiti.)

artery and its branches (parts 1 and 2), (5) the pterygoid plexus of veins and its tributaries, and (6) the chorda tympani nerve.
Communications. The masticator area may communicate with (1) the parapharyngeal space, (2) the parotid region, (3) the sublingual region, (4) the submandibular region, (5) the cavernous sinus via emissary veins through the foramen ovale, and (6) the orbit via veins passing through the inferior fissure.
Subdivisions. The masticator region may be divided as the infratemporal or pterygoid space medial to the ramus and the masseteric-temporal space lateral to the ramus (see *Figure 11-31*).

Parapharyngeal Area
Boundaries. The parapharyngeal area is a cervical, areolar-filled space between the visceral unit of the neck anteriorly, the vertebral unit posteriorly, and the sternocleidomastoid muscle laterally. Its posterior component, the retropharyngeal space, extends from the base of the skull superiorly down to the superior mediastinum of the thorax.

Contents. The paraphayngeal area contains (1) the carotid sheath and its contents and (2) the deep cervical chain of lymph nodes.

Communications. The parapharyngeal area is potentially dangerous, for, if infected, the entire area may be involved, creating difficulty in speaking and swallowing. Infection may spread inferiorly through either the danger space or retropharyngeal space down the neck and into the thorax, involving the mediastinum (mediastinitis) (*Figure 11-33*).

PATHWAYS OF DENTAL INFECTION

More often than not, dentoalveolar abscesses extend into the oral cavity through the oral vestibule, where they are easily drained. In addition, there are a number of alternative routes through which infections may spread to various fascial spaces of the head and neck.

From the Maxillary Incisors

1. The **oral vestibule** is the usual site of perforation (*Figure 11-34*); infection is limited superiorly by the bony attachment of the orbicularis oris muscle.
2. Infection may track superiorly to perforate the **floor of the nose** and involve the nasal cavity.
3. The spreading infection may track backward through the medullary cavity of the **palate**; this occurs frequently with abscessed lateral incisors. Probing in the mouth what seemed to have been a small abscess on the radiograph can be a startling experience—the abscess may extend posteriorly through the palate for a considerable distance and erode the bony floor of the nose.
4. Infection may track above the orbicularis oris attachment to enter the superficial space of the lip.

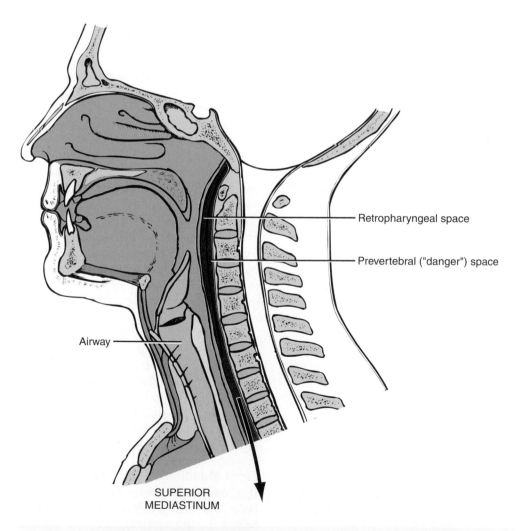

Retropharyngeal space

Prevertebral ("danger") space

Airway

SUPERIOR
MEDIASTINUM

Figure 11-33 Sagittal section through the head, neck, and upper chest to demonstrate spread of infection or air through the neck to the mediastinum.

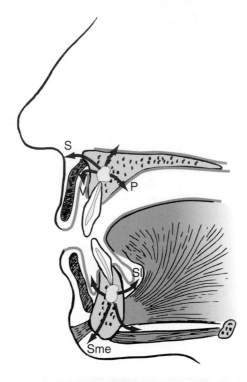

Figure 11-34 Sagittal section through the oral cavity to show possible routes of infection from abscesses of anterior teeth. *N*, Nasal cavity; *P*, palate; *S*, superficial fascial space; *Sl*, sublingual space; *Sme*, submental space; *V*, vestibule.

From the Maxillary Canine

The canine tooth, because of its long root, may pose slightly different problems involving the infraorbital region. The most common pathway is through the labial alveolar plate of bone and through the vestibular mucosa. The attachment of the levator labii superioris muscle limits upward invasion.

If the infection perforates bone above the levator anguli oris origin, infection invades the superficial fascia of the **infraorbital (canine)** area, involving the lower eyelid and closure of the lids. Infection does not usually enter the orbit, but it may by tracking back along the infraorbital canal. Clinically a firm or fluctuant mass appears along the lateral border of the nose that may extend to include the medial aspect of the eye and periorbital area (see *Figure 11-29, A*). Infections in this region may spread to the cavernous sinus via the facial venous system or extend posteriorly and superiorly to the buccal space and then to the deep temporal space.

The infection may pass upward and medially to enter the floor of the **nasal cavity.**

The **maxillary sinus** may be involved through its anterior wall if the sinus is large and in proximity to the canine root.

From Maxillary Premolars and Molars

The maxillary attachment of the buccinator muscle determines the pathway of potential spread. If the abscess perforates the buccal plate of the alveolar process below the buccinator attachment, infection drains to the **vestibule** (see *Figure 11-34*).

If the infection breaks through above the buccinator attachment, the **superficial fascia** of the cheek is involved. The swelling may be extensive, ranging from the inferior border of the mandible to the zygomatic arch (see *Figure 11-29, B*).

Abscesses over the lingual or palatal roots tend to be self-limiting but may break through the dense bone and **palatal mucosa.** Infrequently, infection from involved maxillary molars and premolars tracks upward to involve the maxillary sinus through the antral floor. In extreme cases, antral infections, in turn, may involve the orbit superiorly.

Posterior spread would lead to the infratemporal portion of the **masticator space.** Posterior spread from the third molar may involve the **tonsillar region** and the soft palate.

From Mandibular Anterior Teeth

Abscesses at the apices of the mandibular anteriors tend to perforate the labial alveolar plate above the orbicularis oris and mentalis attachments and point to the oral vestibule through the vestibular mucosa. If the abscess perforates the alveolus below the muscle attachments of the mentalis and orbicularis oris muscles, invasion of the superficial fascia of the **lower lip** and **chin** occurs.

Infection may penetrate lingually to enter the **sublingual region.** The abscess may point through lingual alveolar mucosa or may continue posteriorly to invade the floor of the mouth. Invasion of this area is generally due to lymphatic spread. The submental lymph nodes drain the mandibular incisor teeth. Infection may track backward along the **medullary cavity of the mandibular body.** The invasion may be quite extensive and destructive.

From Mandibular Premolars and Molars

Infections tend to penetrate through the buccal alveolar plate and point through the buccal alveolar mucosa (*Figure 11-35*). If the infection perforates below the mandibular buccinator attachment, the **superficial fascial area of the cheek** would be involved.

Infection may track lingually, and if it perforates below the mylohyoid attachment, the **submandibular region** is involved. The parapharyngeal areas posteriorly and inferiorly may be secondarily involved.

If the infection breaks through above the mylohyoid attachment, the infection may point through the lingual alveolar mucosa or extend medially to involve the entire **floor of the mouth,** causing the tongue to be clinically elevated.

From Mandibular Third Molars

It is common for impacted third molars to erupt only partially and communicate with the oral cavity through a breach in the overlying gingival tissues. Oral bacteria and food often accumulate beneath this soft tissue cover, resulting in inflammation and infection of the pericoronal

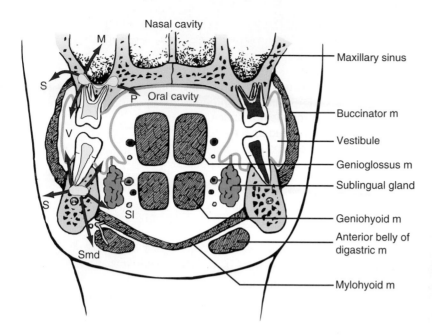

Figure 11-35 Coronal section through the molar region to demonstrate possible routes of infection from abscesses of posterior teeth. *P,* Palate; *S,* superficial fascial space; *sl,* sublingual space; *Smd,* submandibular space; *V,* vestibule.

tissues (**pericoronitis**) and the formation of a **pericoronal abscess.** Infection from this area may spread to a number of sites: the (1) submandibular region, (2) sublingual region, (3) masticator space (deep to the infratemporal portion or externally to the masseteric region), (4) parapharyngeal space, (5) tonsillar bed and soft palate, and (6) superficial fascia of the cheek (see *Figures 11-31* and *11-35*).

From Cervicofacial Emphysema
Emphysema of the head and neck occurs when air gains entry into fascial spaces and becomes trapped. The entry of air occurs following a breaching or opening of the mucosa usually in conjunction with the inappropriate use of a high-speed air turbine or compressed water/air syringe. Some dentists rely on the air turbine to rapidly remove bone during tooth removal or use the air syringe to dry operative fields. Air, under pressure, enters the tissues and inflates the potential fascial planes. The tissues, when palpated, crackle to the touch.

Emphysema is a swelling of the tissues caused by trapped air. Invasion of the tissues is generally through a wound in the buccal mucosa followed by hard blowing (e.g., brass musicians and glassblowers). The trapped air may also track to neighboring areas, such as the submandibular region or sublingual region. The air may also migrate down the neck via the parapharyngeal space, causing respiratory difficulty, and/or enter the mediastinum, resulting in **mediastinal emphysema** (see *Figure 11-33*). Patients should be promptly referred for appropriate medical imaging if cervicofacial emphysema is suspected.

Review Questions

1. After an inferior alveolar nerve block, all of the mandibular teeth on that side and all of the following soft tissues are anesthetized EXCEPT the _____.
   a. buccal mandibular gingiva
   b. labial mandibular gingiva
   c. skin of the lower lip
   d. mucosa of the lower lip
   e. skin of the chin

2. A local anesthetic has been injected into the mouth at the right infraorbital foramen to perform an infraorbital or anterior superior alveolar nerve block. All of the following areas or structures will be anesthetized EXCEPT the _____.
   a. conjunctiva and skin of the lower eyelid
   b. skin of the lateral aspect of the external nose
   c. skin overlying the zygomatic bones
   d. skin and mucosa of the upper lip
   e. anterior maxillary teeth

3. A patient has a fractured mandible. There is no protrusion of bone through the skin, but an intraoral inspection reveals involvement of the mucous membrane, and a radiograph reveals a fracture line that is reproduced in the diagram at the right. The most complete classification of this fracture would be _____.
   a. simple favorable
   b. compound favorable
   c. simple unfavorable
   d. compound unfavorable
   e. unfavorable comminuted

4. Infection from a partially erupted third molar is LEAST likely to spread to the _____.
   a. masticator space
   b. parotid space
   c. sublingual space
   d. submandibular space
   e. parapharyngeal space

5. Ludwig's angina is a massive infection of the _____.
   a. cavernous sinus
   b. orbit
   c. masticator space
   d. canine space
   e. submandibular, sublingual, and submental spaces

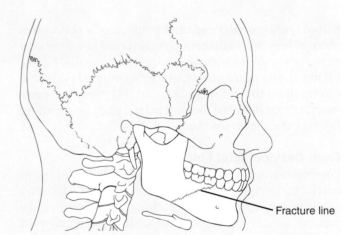

Fracture line

Review Questions Answer Key

Chapter 1
1. b
2. a
3. c
4. e
5. e
6. a
7. d
8. a
9. e
10. d
11. e

Chapter 2
1. e
2. b
3. a
4. a
5. b
6. d
7. b

Chapter 3
1. b
2. e
3. a
4. e
5. b
6. d
7. b
8. a
9. b
10. a
11. e
12. d

Chapter 4
1. e
2. a
3. b
4. a
5. e
6. a
7. b
8. b
9. e
10. c
11. f
12. d
13. b

Chapter 5
1. a
2. a
3. d
4. d
5. b
6. c
7. b
8. a
9. a
10. d

Chapter 6
1. d
2. a
3. c
4. a
5. b
6. c
7. e
8. a
9. e
10. b

Chapter 7
1. e
2. a
3. b
4. a
5. b
6. a
7. d
8. a
9. e
10. c
11. d
12. c
13. b
14. e
15. c
16. c
17. c
18. a
19. d
20. b
21. e
22. e
23. b

Chapter 8
1. b
2. d
3. d
4. b
5. e
6. c
7. c
8. a
9. e
10. d

Chapter 9
1. b
2. a
3. c
4. a
5. e
6. e
7. a
8. c

Chapter 10
1. d
2. a
3. d
4. a
5. e
6. c
7. c

Chapter 11
1. a
2. c
3. d
4. b
5. e

Index

Note: Page numbers followed by *f* refer to figures; page numbers followed by *t* refer to tables; page numbers followed by *b* refer to boxes.

A

Abdomen, 87
  aponeuroses of, 91–92
  blood and nerve supply to, 101
  deep fascia of, 91
  divisions of, 88–89, 90*f*
  nerves of, 103–104
  skeleton of, 87–88, 88*f*
  superficial fascia of, 91
Abdominal aorta, 81–82, 101–102, 101*f*
Abdominal viscera, 30, 104
Abdominal walls, 89
  anterolateral, 89–96
  inferior, 97–99, 98*f*
  posterior abdominal wall, 97, 97*f*
  superior abdominal wall, 96–97, 97*f*
Abducens nerve (cranial nerve VI), 30, 30*t*,
      251–253, 259, 369*t*, 371–372,
      372*f*
Abductor digiti minimi muscle, 411, 412*f*,
      412*t*, 446*t*
Abductor hallucis muscle, 446*t*
Abductor pollicis brevis muscle, 410–411,
      412*f*, 412*t*
Abductor pollicis longus muscle, 410, 410*f*,
      411*t*
Abscess(es), 309
  dentoalveolar, 332, 480, 480*f*
  pericoronal, 486–487
  periodontal, 480–481
Absent or rudimentary clavicle, 391
Accessory hemiazygos vein, 83
Accessory meningeal artery, 289
Accessory nerve (cranial nerve XI), 147,
      153–154, 254, 382–383
  cranial root, 316–317, 369*t*, 383
  functional components of, 383
  spinal root, 30, 30*t*, 140, 369*t*, 382–383,
      383*f*
Accessory nipples or breasts, 59
Accessory salivary glands, 327
Accommodation reflex, 263

Acetabular labrum, 430–431
Acetabulum, 430–431
Acromioclavicular joint, 394, 394*f*
Acromion, 388
Acute pancreatitis, 120
Acute peritonitis, 121
Adam's apple (thyroid prominence),
      134–136
Adductor brevis muscle, 438, 439*t*
Adductor hallucis muscle, 446*t*
Adductor longus muscle, 438, 439*t*
Adductor magnus muscle, 438 439,
      439*t*, 440
Adductor mass, 438
Adductor pollicis muscle, 411–413,
      412*t*
Adductor tubercle, 425–426
Adenoiditis, 339
Adenoids, 302, 339
Adipose tissue, 32–33
Aditus, 342, 350
Afferent fibers, 15, 23
Age, bone or skeletal, 8
Airway obstruction
  clearing, 348
  upper airway, 347
Akenosi (closed mouth) mandibular nerve
      block, 465, 465*f*
Alar cartilage, 235
Alar fascia, 136–138
Alar ligaments, 161
Alar space, 138–139
Alimentary canal, 104–121, 105*f*
Allergic reactions, 294, 347–348
Alveolar mucosa, 310, 332
Alveolar process, 199, 211, 475
Alveolar ridge tomography, 470, 472*f*
Alveoli, 64, 66
Ampulla, 119, 125–126
Anal canal, 112–113, 114*f*
Anal columns, 113
Anal triangle, 99
Anal valves, 113

Anatomical cuts and planes, 2*f*, 3
Anatomical position, 2–3, 2*f*
Anatomy
  applied anatomy, 1, 457–487
  classification of functional
      components based on tissue
      origins, 24
  clinical anatomy, 1
  developmental, 2
  gross anatomy, 1
  imaging, 2
  of local anesthesia, 457
  neuroanatomy, 1–2
  study of, 1
  surface, 2
Anconeus muscle, 406, 406*t*, 410*f*
Anesthesia
  block
    infraorbital block, 459
    of mandibular structures, 462–466
    of maxillary structures, 459–462
  dental, 223–224
  epidural, 47, 48*f*
  local, 153, 287, 295
    anatomy of, 457
    inadvertent intravascular injections,
      291
    of mandibular structures, 462–466
    of maxillary structures, 458–462
    types of, 457–458
  spinal, 47, 48*f*
Angina, Ludwig's, 482–483, 483*f*
Angina pectoris, 77, 78–79
Angioplasty, coronary, 77
Angular artery, 225
Angular cheilosis, 234
Angular vein, 226
Ankle joint, 435–437, 435*f*
  movements of, 447*t*
  skeleton of, 428–429
Annulus ovalis, 71
Ansa cervicalis, 147, 147*f*, 148
Antegonial notch, 211 212, 212*f*

Anterior abdominal wall, 89–96
  blood and nerve supply of, 95–96
  layers of, 91–92, 91f
  muscles of, 91–92, 92t, 93f
  surface features of, 89–91, 90f
Anterior arch, 313
Anterior auricular muscle, 229t, 236
Anterior clinoid process, 180, 181f, 182f, 195
Anterior communicating artery, 250–251
Anterior condylar canal, 183, 189
Anterior cranial fossa, 180
Anterior cruciate ligament, 431–434
Anterior cruciate ligament tears, 433
Anterior cutaneous nerve of the neck, 147
Anterior ethmoidal artery, 262
Anterior ethmoidal canal, 214t
Anterior ethmoidal foramen, 171
Anterior ethmoidal nerve (cranial nerve V-1),
      260, 300–301
Anterior intercostal arteries, 62
Anterior jugular arch, 142, 153
Anterior jugular vein, 142, 142f, 153
Anterior mediastinum, 79
Anterior palatal region, 475f
Anterior palate clefts, 319
Anterior spinal artery, 46–47, 250
Anterior superior alveolar artery, 331–332
Anterior superior alveolar nerve, 294, 331,
      374
    block of, 459, 460f
    nasal branch of, 301
Anterior teeth, mandibular, 486
Anterior temporal nerve, 286
Anterior tibial artery, 452–453
Anterior tympanic artery, 288–289
Antero-inferior cerebellar arteries, 250
Anterolateral abdominal wall, 89–96
Antibiotics, prophylactic, 76
Anvil (incus), 352
Aorta, 79–83
Aortic arch, 80–81
Aortic sinus, 76, 80
Aortic valve, 74
Apical ligament, 161
Aponeuroses, 12, 91–92, 238
Appendices epiploicae, 111
Appendicitis, 111
Appendix, 111
Applied anatomy, 1, 457–487
Aqueous humor, 263
Arachnoid granulations, 242
Arachnoid mater, 45–46, 242
Arcades, 110
Arch of the aorta, 358
Arcuate arteries, 122
Arcuate line, 92
Arm
    bones of, 389–392
    medial cutaneous nerve of, 418
    muscles of, 404–406, 406t
Arterial anastomoses, 17–18
Arterial circle (of Willis), 249–251, 252f
Arteries, 16–17. See also specific arteries
    anterior intercostal, 62
    antero-inferior cerebellar, 250
    arcuate, 122

Arteries (Continued)
  bronchial, 66–67
  cerebellar, 250
  cerebral, 251
  communicating, 250–251
  coronary, 76–77
  cutaneous, 225–227
  deep temporal, 289–290
  digital, 419–420
  distributing or muscular, 16
  elastic, 16, 17f
  end, 18
  of eyeball, 264
  of face, 224–225, 224f
  of head and neck, 358, 359f, 360t
  helicine, 127–128
  intercostal, 46–47, 62, 62f, 97
  interlobar, 122
  lumbar, 101
  masseteric, 290
  muscular, 16
  of neck, 145–146
  obliterated umbilical, 19
  phrenic, 97
  posterior cerebral, 250
  posterior ciliary, 262
  posterior intercostal, 62
  posterior spinal, 46–47
  posteroinferior cerebellar, 250
  pterygoid, 290
  renal, 102, 122–123
  spinal, 46–47
  suprarenal, 102
  umbilical, 19
  vesicular, 122–123
Arterioles, 16–17
Arteriovenous anastomoses, 17
Arthritis, 276
Arthrography, TMJ, 472, 476f
Articular capsule, 272, 272f
Articular cartilage, 4, 10
Articular discs, 10, 10f, 272–274, 274f
Articular eminence, 193, 271–272, 271f
Articulated spine, 39–42, 41f
Aryepiglottic ligaments, 342
Aryepiglottic muscle, 344
Aryepiglotticus muscle, 344t
Arytenoid cartilage, 341
Ascending aorta, 80
Ascending cervical artery, 156
Ascending colon, 111–112, 113f
Ascending lumbar veins, 102
Ascending palatine artery, 319
Ascending pharyngeal artery, 146
Aspiration of foreign objects, 66
Association areas, 246
Association tracts, 246
Asthma, bronchial, 68
Astigmatism, 264
Atlantoaxial joint, 160f, 161, 161f
Atlanto-occipital joint, 159–161, 160f,
      161f
Atlas vertebrae (C1), 38–39, 40f, 160f
Atria, 16
Atrioventricular node, 72, 77–78
Atrioventricular orifice, 16

Atrioventricular sulcus, 70
Atrioventricular valves, 16
Auditory area, 246
Auditory (pharyngotympanic) canal, 193
Auditory tube, 350
Auditory (pharyngotympanic) tube, 349,
      353–354
Auricle, 221, 236, 236f, 349
Auriculotemporal nerve (cranial nerve V-3),
      223, 236, 238, 275, 286, 376
Auscultation of heart sounds, 74–76, 75f
Autonomic nervous system, 23
    of abdomen, 103–104, 104f
    central nervous system origins of, 25–30
    cranial autonomics, 383–386
    motor (visceral efferent) nervous system,
        25–30
    sensory (visceral afferent) nervous system,
        30
Axilla, 414, 414f, 415f
Axillary artery, 154
Axillary nerve, 155, 418, 419t
Axillary nodes, 20
Axillary vein, 154, 420, 421–422
Axis vertebrae (C2), 39, 40f, 160f
Axon terminals, 21
Axons, 21–22
Azygos vein, 83, 83f

B

B cells, 19
Back, 37–49
    bones of, 37, 38f
    muscles of, 47, 403, 405t
        deep (innermost) group, 49
        deep (intrinsic) muscles, 49, 50f, 49,
            51t
        intermediate, 47–49, 50f, 49
        minor deep muscles, 49
        responsible for back movements, 52t
        superficial, 47, 49f
        that participate in respiration, 60–62,
            61t
    skeletal parts of, 37
    skeleton of, 37, 38f
    surface features of, 43, 44f
Back pain, 42, 43f
Back strain, 49
Bacterial endocarditis, subacute, 76
Balance, 352, 353
Ball-and-socket joints, 11
Basal ganglia, 247
Basilar artery, 156, 163, 250
Basilar sinus, 244, 363t
Basilic vein, 421–422
Basiocciput, 189
Bell's palsy, 232
Biceps brachii muscle, 404–406, 406t
Biceps femoris muscle, 440, 442t
Bilateral synovial joints, 42
Bile, 118
Biliary apparatus, 110f, 118–119
Birth, 19
Bitewing radiography, 468
Bladder, 123–124, 126f
Block anesthesia

infraorbital block, 459
of mandibular structures, 462–466
of maxillary structures, 459–462
Blood, 15–16, 118
Blood coagulating factors, 118
Blood flow, 70–71, 72f
Blood platelets, 16
Blood pressure, taking, 394
Blood vessels, 15–18. *See also specific types, specific vessels*
of heart, 76–77, 76f
major, 17f
in orbit, 261–262
walls of, 16, 16f
Body cavities, 31, 35, 35f
Body coverings, 31, 34f
Bone(s), 4–8. *See also specific bones*
carpal, 393, 393f
classification of, 5–6
depressions and openings in, 7–8
development of, 8
facial, 199–213, 218–219
flat bones, 6
of foot, 429f
functions of, 4–5
fusion of, 217–218
of hand, 393–394, 393f
irregular, 6
long bones, 5–6, 6f, 7f
of lower limb, 426f
metatarsal bones, 429
of neurocranium, 184–199
raised markings or elevations on, 7
sesamoid, 6
short bones, 6
of skull, 184
surface features of, 6–8
tarsal bones, 428–429
of wrist, 393f
Bone grafts, 88
Bone or skeletal age, 8
Bone remodeling, 8
Bony auditory (pharyngotympanic) tube, 214t
Bony fossae, 269
Bony labyrinth, 352
Bony palate, 177
Boutons, 21
Brachial artery, 419
Brachial plexus, 31, 155, 155f, 415, 416f
collateral branches, 415–418, 416f, 419t
terminal branches, 416f, 418, 418f, 419t
Brachial plexus injuries, 415
Brachialis muscle, 406, 406t
Brachiocephalic artery, 80–81, 154, 418–419
Brachiocephalic vein, 154, 358
Brachioradialis muscle, 409, 410f, 411t
Brain, 23, 244–249
blood supply to, 249–251, 252f
functional areas of, 245–246, 246f
internal features of, 246–247, 247f
lobes of, 244–245, 245f
Brainstem, 247–249, 248f
Branchial structures, 24

Breast, 58–59
accessory nipples or breasts, 59
carcinoma of, 59
Breathing
mechanics of, 67–68
nasal, 301
Bregma, 173, 175f, 176
Broca's (motor speech) area, 245–246
Bronchi, 65–66, 79
left, 65
right, 65
Bronchial arteries, 66–67
Bronchial artery, 65
Bronchial asthma, 68
Bronchial tree, 65–66
Bruxism, 276
Buccal artery, 225, 290
Buccal mucous membrane, 234–235
Buccal nerve, 375–376
Buccal nerve (long buccal) block, 466, 466f
Buccal sucking fat pad, 235
Buccal vestibule, 311, 312f
Buccinator muscle, 227–231, 229t, 230f, 234–235
Buccopharyngeal fascia, 136
Bulbospongiosus muscle, 127
Bulbourethral glands, 126
Bulla ethmoidalis, 302
Bundle of His, 77–78
Bursae, 431–434
Bursitis
occupational, 434
of shoulder, 404
Bypass, coronary, 77

C
Calcaneus, 428
Calcarine sulcus, 245
Calculi (stones), 328
gallstones, 119
supragingival, 328
urinary, 124
Calyces, 122
Camper's fascia, 91, 91f
Canal (bony), 7
Canaliculi, 116–117
Cancer
breast carcinoma, 59
oral, 309
Canine fossa, 169f, 171, 199–200
Canine ridge, 169f, 199
Canine teeth, maxillary, 486
Capillaries, 17
lymph capillaries, 19–20
precapillary sphincters, 16–17
Capitate, 393
Capitulum, 392
Capsular ligaments, 10, 431–434
Carcinoma
of breast, 59
oral, 309
Cardiac arrest, 79
Cardiac dysrhythmias, 79
Cardiac ischemia, 77
Cardiac muscle, 15
Cardiac nerves, 78–79

Cardiac notch, 64–65
Cardiac plexus, 78, 84
Cardiovascular system, 15–16, 15f
Carina, 65
Carotid body, 145
Carotid canal, 193, 214t, 254
Carotid periarterial plexus, 29
Carotid pulse, 145
Carotid sheaths, 138
Carotid sinus, 145
Carotid sympathetic plexus, 255
Carotid triangle, 141
Carpal bones, 393, 393f
Carpal tunnel, 404f, 409
Carpal tunnel syndrome, 409
Carpometacarpal joint, 399, 400
Cartilage, 4
articular, 4, 10
arytenoid, 341
auditory, 4
corniculate cartilage, 341–342
costal, 4
cricoid, 134–136, 341
cuneiform, 342
elastic, 4
fibrocartilage, 4, 10
growth of, 4
hyaline, 4
respiratory, 4
thyroid, 133, 340–341
types of, 4
Cartilaginous joints
primary, 9–10, 9f
secondary, 9f, 10
Cartilaginous rings, 65
Caruncle, 236
Cataract, 264
Cavernous sinus, 242–244, 254–255, 255f, 363t
Cavernous sinus thrombosis, 226
CBCT. *See* Cone beam computed tomography
Cecum, 111, 113f
Celiac ganglion, 103, 104f, 107–108
Celiac trunk, 102
Cementum, 328
Central nervous system, 23
autonomic motor (visceral efferent) components of, 25–30
autonomic (visceral) nerve origins in, 25–30
autonomic sensory (visceral afferent) components of, 30
functional components of, 23
Central sulcus, 244
Central tendon, 96
Cephalic vein, 421
Cephalometric radiography, 469–470, 471f
Cerebellum, 249
Cerebral aqueduct, 249
Cerebral arteries, 251
Cerebral cortex, 244–246
Cerebral hemispheres, 244–247, 249
Cerebral peduncles (crura cerebri), 247
Cerebrospinal fluid (CSF), 44–45, 250f
Cerebrospinal fluid rhinorrhea, 302

Cerebrospinal tap, 48*f*
Cerebrovascular accident, 251
Cerumen, 349
Cervical fascia
    deep, 136–138
    superficial fascia, 136
Cervical pleura, 63
Cervical plexus, 31, 147–148, 148*f*
Cervical skeleton, 133–134, 134*f*
Cervical vertebrae, 38–39, 40*f*, 136
    atypical features of, 38–39, 40*f*
    C7, 39
    typical features of, 38, 40*f*
Cervical vertebral unit, 136
Cervical viscera, 158–159
Cervicofacial emphysema, 487
Cheeks (buccae), 221, 227–231, 234–235, 235*f*
    mucosa of, 312*f*
    muscles of, 227–231, 229*t*
    visual inspection of, 310
Chest, 59
Chest wall, 58
    muscles of, 401–403
    surface landmarks of, 59, 60*f*
Chiasmatic groove, 194
Children, 468–469, 469*f*
Chin, 221
    infection of, 486
    muscles of, 229*t*, 231
Cholecystectomy, 119
Chondroblasts, 4
Chondrocytes, 4
Chondromalacia, 434
Chorda tympani, 286, 350, 354–355, 377
Chordae tendineae, 72, 74
Choroid, 262
Choroid plexus, 249
Chyle, 19–20
Cilia, 236
Ciliary ganglion, 261, 261*f*, 373*t*, 386
Ciliary glands, 236-237
Circulation, 54
    changes at birth, 19
    collateral, 17–18
    fetal, 18–19, 18*f*
    lymphatic, 20, 21*f*
Cisterna chyli, 83–84
Classification of functional
            components based on tissue
            origins, 24
Clavicle, 389, 390*f*
    absent or rudimentary, 391
    fractured, 391
Cleft lip and palate, 319
Clinical anatomy, 1
Clitoris, 130, 130*f*
Clivus, 182
Coccygeal plexus, 31
Coccygeus muscle, 98
Coccyx, 39
Cochlea, 349, 352
Cochlear nerve, 353
Cochlear window, 352
Collecting tubules, 125

Colon, 111–115
    arterial supply, 114–115
    features and parts of, 111–113, 113*f*
    position of, 111
Colon wall, 113
Colonoscopy, 114
Columella, 233
Commissural or bridging fibers, 246
Common bile duct, 118
Common carotid artery, 138, 145, 145*f*, 358, 360*t*
Common facial vein, 142, 142*f*, 226–227, 363*t*
Common fibular (peroneal) nerve, 449
Common hepatic artery, 107
Common hepatic duct, 118
Common iliac vein, 453
Communicating arteries, 250–251
Communicating vein, 142, 142*f*, 153
Compressor nares, 235–236
Computed tomography (CT), 468
    cone beam, 468
        alveolar ridge tomography, 470, 472*f*
        of anterior palatal region, 475*f*
        of maxillary air sinuses, 474*f*
        of TMJ, 476*f*
    of maxillary air sinuses, 474*f*
Conchal crest, 202, 204
Condylar neck fractures, 475, 478*f*
Condyle, 7, 212
    of the mandible, 269–271, 270*f*
    relationship of disc to, 272–274, 274*f*
Condyloid joints, 11–12
Cone beam computed tomography, 468
    alveolar ridge tomography, 470, 472*f*
    of anterior palatal region, 475*f*
    of maxillary air sinuses, 474*f*
    of TMJ, 476*f*
Congenital torticollis, 140
Conjunctiva, 238
Conjunctival sac, 236
Conjunctivum, 236
Constrictor pupillae muscle, 262
Contraction
    isometric, 13
    isotonic, 13
    types of, 13
Coracobrachialis muscle, 406, 406*t*
Coracoid process, 388
Cornea, 262
Corniculate cartilage, 341–342
Coronal plane, 2*f*, 3
Coronal suture, 175*f*, 176
Coronary angioplasty, 77
Coronary arteries, 76–77
Coronary atherosclerosis, 77
Coronary bypass, 77
Coronary ligament, 116
Coronary sinus, 71–72, 77
Coronary sulcus, 70
Coronary veins, 77
Coronoid fossa, 392
Coronoid notch, 213, 310–311
Coronoid process, 173, 212, 212*f*, 393
Coronoid process fractures, 475, 478*f*
Corpora quadrigemina, 247
Corpus callosum, 244–246

Corpus spongiosum, 127
Corrugator muscle, 229*t*, 231
Costal cartilage, 4
Costal margin, 59, 60*f*
Costal pleura, 63
Costal slips, 96
Costocervical trunk, 156, 360*t*
Costochondral joints, 58
Costodiaphragmatic recess, 64
Costomediastinal recess, 64
Costovertebral joints, 57
Cranial accessory nerve (cranial nerve XI), 316–317, 369*t*, 383
Cranial facial cavities, 184
Cranial ganglia, 260–261
Cranial nerve I (olfactory nerve), 30, 30*t*, 251, 368, 369*t*, 370*f*
Cranial nerve II (optic nerve), 30, 30*t*, 251, 259, 368–370, 369*t*, 370*f*
Cranial nerve III (oculomotor nerve), 30, 30*t*, 251, 255, 258–259, 369*t*, 370–371, 371*f*
Cranial nerve IV (trochlear nerve), 30, 30*t*, 251, 255, 259, 369*t*, 371, 371*f*
Cranial nerve V (trigeminal nerve), 251, 369*t*, 372–377, 372*f*
    branches of, 373–376
    cranial parasympathetic ganglia associated with, 373*t*
    cutaneous distribution of, 31, 33*f*
    functional components of, 30, 30*t*, 372–373
    ophthalmic division, 373–374, 374*f*
Cranial nerve V-1 (anterior ethmoidal nerve), 300–301
Cranial nerve V-1 (ophthalmic nerve), 221–222, 251, 255, 260*f*, 373–374
Cranial nerve V-1 (supraorbital nerve), 222, 238, 373
Cranial nerve V-1 (supratrochlear nerve), 222, 238, 373
Cranial nerve V-2 (maxillary nerve), 221–222, 251, 255, 340, 374, 375*f*
Cranial nerve V-2 (maxillary nerve) block, 462
Cranial nerve V-3 (mandibular nerve), 221–222, 223–224, 251, 284–287, 285*f*, 374–376, 376*f*
Cranial nerve V-3 (mandibular nerve) block
    Akenosi (closed mouth) block, 465, 465*f*
    Gow-Gates block, 463–465, 464*f*
Cranial nerve VI (abducens nerve), 30, 30*t*, 251–253, 259, 369*t*, 371–372, 372*f*
Cranial nerve VII (facial nerve), 253, 265, 354–355, 369*t*, 377–378, 378*f*
    branches of, 377–378
    functional components of, 30, 30*t*, 377
Cranial nerve VIII (vestibulocochlear nerve), 30, 30*t*, 253–254, 353, 369*t*, 378–379, 379*f*
Cranial nerve IX (glossopharyngeal nerve), 254, 321, 324, 340, 379–381, 380*f*
    branches of, 380–381
    functional components of, 30, 30*t*, 379–380

Cranial nerve X (vagus nerve), 103–104, 138, 157, 254, 316–317, 321, 340, 347, 369t, 381–382, 381f
  branches of, 382
  functional components of, 30, 30t, 381–382
Cranial nerve XI (accessory nerve), 147, 153–154, 254, 382–383
  cranial root, 316–317, 369t, 383
  functional components of, 383
  spinal root, 30, 30t, 140, 369t, 382–383, 383f
Cranial nerve XII (hypoglossal nerve), 30, 30t, 254, 324–325, 369t, 383, 384f
Cranial nerves, 23, 24–25, 251–254, 253f, 368–383, 369t
  autonomic nerves, 383–386
  functional components of, 30, 30t, 368
  origins of, 26, 27–28
  parasympathetic nerves, 385–386, 385f
  sympathetic nerves, 383–385
Cranial vault region, 171–173, 214t
Cranial venous sinuses, 242–244, 243f
Cranium, 167
  neurocranium, 167
  viscerocranium, 167
Cremaster muscle, 95
Crest (bony), 7
Cricoarytenoid joint, 342
Cricoid cartilage, 134–136, 341
Cricopharyngeus muscle, 334
Cricothyroid membrane, 342
Cricothyroid muscle, 344, 344t
Cricothyroid space, 134–136
Cricothyrotomy, 348
Crista galli, 180, 181f, 182f
Crista terminalis, 71
Cross section, 3
Cruciate ligament, 161–162
Crura cerebri (cerebral peduncles), 247
Cryptorchidism (undescended testes), 95–96
CSF. See Cerebrospinal fluid
CT. See Computed tomography
Cuboid, 429
Cuneiform cartilage, 342
Cuneiforms, 428–429
Cutaneous arteries, 225–227
Cutaneous nerves
  of face, 221–224, 223f
  of neck, 153
  spinal, 31, 33f
  veins that accompany, 225–227
Cystic artery, 107
Cystic duct, 118
Cysts, thyroglossal, 158

D

Dacryocystitis, 264
Dacryostenosis, 264
Dartos muscle, 95
Deciduous teeth, 311–312, 330f
Deep artery of the penis, 127–128
Deep auricular artery, 288
Deep cardiac plexus, 148
Deep cervical fascia, 136–138

Deep facial vein, 226
Deep fascia, 34f, 35
  of abdomen, 91
  cervical, 136–138
  of face, 221
  functions of, 35
Deep inguinal ring, 95
Deep investing fascia, 136
Deep lymph nodes
  of lower limb, 454
  parotid, 364, 365t
Deep petrosal nerve, 294
Deep temporal arteries, 289–290
Deep transverse ligaments, 400
Deep veins
  of head and neck, 362f
  of upper limb, 420
Deglutition, 334–336
Deltoid (medial collateral) ligament, 435
Deltoid muscle, 403, 404f, 405t
Deltoid tuberosity, 392
Dendrites, 21–22
Dens, 39
Dental accidents, 347
Dental anesthesia, 223–224
Dental blood supply, 331–332
Dental caries, 309
Dental infection(s)
  pathways of, 485–487, 486f, 487f
  spread of, 480, 485f
Dental nerve supply, 331
Dental ridges, 470, 472f
Dental surfaces, 328–331
Dental tissues, 328
Denticulate ligament, 45
Denticulate sutures, 8–9
Dentine, 328
Dentinal tubules, 328
Dentistry
  imaging in, 468–473
  restorative, 309
Dentition, 330f
  development of, 218–219
  numerical symbols for, 311–312, 313f
Dentoalveolar abscess, 332, 480, 480f
Depressor anguli oris muscle, 227, 229t
Depressor labii inferioris muscle, 227, 229t
Dermatomes, 33f
Dermis, 32–33, 34f
Descending (thoracic) aorta, 80, 81–82, 82f, 101
Descending colon, 112
Descending palatine artery, 297, 319
Development
  of bones, 8
  of facial bones, 218–219
  of gut (alimentary canal), 99–101, 100f
  of liver, 99–100
  of long bones, 7f
  of mandible, 218–219
  of maxilla, 218
  of pancreas, 99–100
  of paranasal air sinuses, 301
  of peritoneum, 99–101, 100f
  postnatal, 2

Development (Continued)
  prenatal, 2
  of skull, 213, 218f
  of temporal bone, 219
  of testes, 94f
Developmental anatomy, 2
Diaphragm, 61t, 62
  blood supply of, 97
  functions of, 96–97
  insertion of, 96
  nerve supply of, 97
  structures passing through, 96
  thoracic, 96
Diaphragma sellae, 240–242, 241f
Diaphragmatic pleura, 63
Diaphyses, 5–6
Diarthrodial joints, 8
Diencephalon, 244, 247
Digastric fossa, 212–213, 212f
Digastric muscle
  anterior belly of, 143–144, 144t
  posterior belly of, 143, 144t
Digastric notch, 176f, 177, 193
Digital arteries, 419–420
Dilator nares, 235–236
Dilator pupillae muscle, 262
DIP joints. See Distal interphalangeal joints
Diploë, 6
Diploic veins, 244, 363t
Disc derangement
  internal, 276
  with reduction, 276
  without reduction, 276
Discomalleolar (Pinto's) ligament, 274
Discs, articular, 10, 10f
Dislocated ribs, 58
Dislocation
  of shoulder, 396
  of temporomandibular joint, 276
Distal interphalangeal (DIP) joints, 400
Distal phalanx, 429
Distal radioulnar joint, 398
Distributing or muscular arteries, 16
Dorsal artery of the penis, 127–128
Dorsal interossei, 412f, 412t, 413–414, 446t
Dorsal nasal artery, 224, 262
Dorsal scapular nerve, 417, 419t
Dorsal venous arch, 420–421, 453–454
Dorsum sellae, 180, 181f, 182f, 194
Dry mouth (xerostomia), 328
Ductus arteriosus, 18–19
Ductus deferens, 125–126
Ductus (vas) deferens, 95
Ductus venosus, 18–19
Duodenal ulcers, 108
Duodenum, 105, 108–109, 109f
  arterial supply to, 109
  parts of, 108–109
  peritoneal attachments, 109
  position of, 108
  venous return from, 109
  wall of, 109
Dura mater, 45, 46, 240–242
Dysphagia, pharyngeal, 336
Dysphasia, esophageal, 79

E

Ear, 349
  external ear, 221, 236, 236f, 349, 349f
  external ear muscles, 229t
  inner ear, 349, 349f
  internal ear, 352–353
  internal ear infection, 354
  lymphatic drainage of, 368
  middle ear, 193, 349, 349f, 351f
  middle ear cavity (tympanic cavity), 350–352
  middle ear ossicles, 213, 351f, 352
  parts of, 349–355
  skeleton of, 349
Eardrum (tympanic membrane), 349–350
Earlobe, 236, 236f
Efferent fibers, 15, 23
Ejaculation, 128
Ejaculatory duct, 125–126
Elastic arteries, 16, 17f
Elastic cartilage, 4
Elbow (humeroulnar) joint, 397–398, 397f, 398f
Electrocardiography, 78
Ellipsoid joints, 11
Embryology, 2
Emissary veins, 244, 363t
Emphysema, 68
  cervicofacial, 487
  mediastinal, 487
  surgical, 138
Enamel, 328
End arteries, 18
Endocarditis, subacute bacterial, 76
Endocardium, 70
Endochondral ossification, 8
Endodontics, 309
Endolymph, 352
Endometrium, 129
Endomysium, 12, 12f
Endoneurium, 23–24
Endotracheal intubation, 348, 348f
Epicardium, 70
Epicondyle, 7, 392
Epidermis, 32, 34f
Epididymis, 125
Epidural anesthesia, 47, 48f
Epidural (extradural) space, 242
Epiglottis, 340, 341
Epimysium, 12, 12f
Epineurium, 23–24
Epiphyseal plate, 8
Episiotomy, 130
Epistaxis (nosebleed), 302
Epithalamus, 247
Epitympanic recess, 350
Erb's palsy, 415
Erector spinae muscle, 49, 51t
Erythrocytes, 16
Esophageal dysphasia, 79
Esophageal plexus, 382
Esophagus, 79, 105, 136, 158
  blood supply to, 79
  lymphatic drainage of, 368
  nerve supply to, 79
  thoracic, 79

Ethmoid bone, 180, 197–199, 197f, 198f
Ethmoid labyrinth, 199
Ethmoidal crest, 202, 204
Ethmoidal foramen, 180, 214t
Ethmoidal notch, 184
Ethmoidal sinuses, 307, 307f, 308f
Ethmoidal spine, 194
Ethmoidal sulcus, 214t
Expiration, 67–68
  forced, 67–68
  quiet, 67
Extensor carpi radialis brevis muscle, 410, 410f, 411t
Extensor carpi radialis longus muscle, 409–410, 410f, 411t
Extensor carpi ulnaris muscle, 410f, 411t
Extensor digiti minimi muscle, 410, 410f
Extensor digitorum longus muscle, 440–441, 442t
Extensor digitorum muscle, 410, 410f, 411t
Extensor hallucis longus muscle, 440–441, 442t
Extensor indicis muscle, 410, 410f, 411t
Extensor pollicis brevis muscle, 411t, 412f
Extensor pollicis brevis tendon, 410, 410f
Extensor pollicis longus muscle, 410, 410f, 411t, 412f
Extensor retinaculum, 409, 410f
External auditory meatus, 179, 191, 349
External carotid artery, 145–146, 267, 359f, 360t
External carotid nerve, 385
External cerebral vein, 363t
External ear, 221, 236, 236f, 349, 349f
  features of, 236, 236f
  muscles of, 229t
External genitalia, female, 130, 130f
External iliac artery, 450
External iliac vein, 453
External intercostal muscle, 61t
External intercostal muscles, 60
External jugular vein, 142, 142f, 152–153, 154, 226, 358, 363t
External nasal artery, 224
External nasal nerve, 223, 262
External nose, 221, 235–236, 235f
External oblique line, 211, 212f
External oblique muscle, 91–92, 92t, 93f
External occipital crest, 37, 177, 187
External occipital political regulations, 187
External occipital protuberance, 37
External sphincter ani, 113
Extradural hemorrhage, 240
Extradural (epidural) space, 46, 242
Extraocular muscles
  actions on movements of eyes, 259f
  motor nerves to, 258–259
  nerve supply of, 259
Extraoral radiography, 469–470
Extraperitoneal layer, 92
Extrapyramidal motor system, 247
Eye muscles, 229t, 231
Eyeball (oculus bulbi), 262–264, 263f
  blood supply to, 264
  movements of, 258
  muscular actions of, 259f
  nerve supply to, 264

Eyelashes, 236
Eyelids (palpebrae), 236–238
  blood supply, 238
  features of, 236–238, 237f
  layers of, 236–238, 237f
  sensory nerve supply, 238

F

Face, 221
  arteries of, 224–225, 224f
  deep fascia of, 221
  features of, 233–238
  foramen of, 214t
  fractures of, 473
  lymphatic drainage of, 367f
  mandibular (lower-face) fractures, 475–478
  mid-face fractures, 478–480
  motor nerves of, 231–233
  osteotomy of, 479f, 480
  pulse points on, 225
  regions of, 221, 222f
  sensory (cutaneous) nerves of, 221–224, 223f
  skin of, 221
  superficial fascia (tela subcutanea) of, 221
  upper-face fractures, 478–480
  veins of, 225–227
Facial artery, 146, 149–150, 226f, 340
  branches of, 225
  ligation of, 225
Facial bones, 199–213, 218–219
Facial disharmonies, 480
Facial expression, 35, 228f
Facial hematoma, 291
Facial muscles, 35, 227–231, 228f, 229t
Facial nerve (cranial nerve VII), 231–233, 253, 265, 354–355, 369t, 377–378, 378f
  branches of, 354–355, 377–378
  functional components of, 30, 30t, 377
Facial paralysis, 232, 233f, 268
Facial skeleton, 167
Facial vein, 142, 142f, 150, 225–227, 226f, 363t
Falciform ligament, 116
False ribs, 54–57
False vocal folds, 342
Falx cerebelli, 240, 241f
Falx cerebri, 240, 241f
Fascia, 31, 33–35, 34f
  alar, 136–138
  buccopharyngeal, 136
  deep, 34f, 35
    of abdomen, 91
    cervical, 136–138
    of face, 221
    functions of, 35
  deep investing fascia, 136
  infections in, 481
  myofascial pain syndrome, 282
  of neck, 136–139, 137f
  pharyngobasilar, 334
  pretracheal (visceral), 136
  prevertebral, 136
  superficial, 35, 136

Fascia (Continued)
  of abdomen, 91
  cervical, 136
  of face, 221
  functions of, 35
  infections in, 481, 483f, 486
  transversalis fascia, 92
  visceral (pretracheal), 136
Fascial clefts, 35
Fascial planes, 35
Fascial spaces, 481–485, 481f, 482t
Fat cells, 32–33
Female breast, 58, 59f
Female genital system, 128–131, 128f
Female genitalia, external, 130, 130f
Female pelvis, 131, 131f
Femoral artery, 452
Femoral neck fracture, 431
Femoral nerve, 445, 450t
Femoral vein, 453
Femur, 425–426, 427f
Fetal circulation, 18–19, 18f
Fetal skull, 217f
Fibrocartilage, 4, 10
Fibromyalgia, 282
Fibrous joints, 8–9, 9f
Fibula, 426–428, 428f
Fibularis (peroneus) brevis muscle, 441–442,
    442t
Fibularis (peroneus) longus muscle, 441–442,
    442t
Fibularis (peroneus) tertius muscle, 442t
Filiform papillae, 319
Filum terminale, 45
Fimbria, 128–129
Fimbriated folds, 314
Fingers
  joints of, 400
  movements of, 400, 401f
First carpometacarpal joint, 400
First metacarpophalangeal joint, 400
First rib, 54–57, 56f
Fissure, 8
Flat bones, 6
Flexor carpi radialis, 407f, 408, 408t
Flexor carpi ulnaris, 407f, 408, 408t
Flexor digiti minimi brevis muscle, 411, 412t
Flexor digiti minimi muscle, 446t
Flexor digitorum brevis muscle, 446t
Flexor digitorum longus muscle, 443–444,
    445t
Flexor digitorum profundus, 407f, 408–409,
    408t
Flexor digitorum profundus tendon, 412f
Flexor digitorum superficialis, 407f, 408,
    408t
Flexor digitorum superficialis tendon, 412f
Flexor hallucis brevis muscle, 446t
Flexor hallucis longus muscle, 443–444,
    445t
Flexor pollicis brevis muscle, 410–411, 412f,
    412t
Flexor pollicis longus, 407f, 408t, 409
Flexor retinaculum, 407f, 409
Flexor sheaths, 408–409
Floating kidney, 121

Floating ribs, 57
Focusing (lens accommodation), 263
Folia, 249
Foliate papillae, 320
Fontanelles, 218
Food obstruction, upper airway, 347
Foot
  arches of, 436–437
  bones of, 428–429, 429f
  joints of, 436–437
  movements of, 447t
  muscles of, 444, 446f, 446t
Foramen, 7
Foramen cecum, 158, 180, 181f, 214t, 244,
    319
Foramen lacerum, 180–182, 181f, 182f,
    195, 214t
Foramen magnum, 176f, 177, 180, 181f,
    182–183, 182f, 187–188, 214t
Foramen ovale, 71, 181f, 182, 182f, 195,
    214t
Foramen rotundum, 181f, 182, 182f, 195,
    214t, 291
Foramen spinosum, 179, 181f, 182, 182f,
    195–196, 214t
Forearm, 398, 399f
  lateral cutaneous nerve of, 418
  medial cutaneous nerve of, 418
  muscles of, 406–410, 407f, 408t, 410f,
    411t
  skeleton of, 392–393
Forehead, 221
Forehead muscles, 229t, 231
Foreign objects
  aspiration of, 66
  lodging of, 79
  upper airway obstruction, 347
Fossa, 7
Fossa ovalis, 71
Fourth ventricle, 249
Fracture(s)
  classification of, 473–480
  compound, 475
  extensive, 478–480
  of face, 473
  favorable, 477–478, 478f
  of femoral neck, 431
  LeFort I, 478, 479f
  LeFort II, 478, 479f
  LeFort III, 478, 479f
  localized, 478
  mandibular (lower-face), 475–478, 478f
  mid- and upper-face, 478–480, 479f
  Pott's fracture, 436
  unfavorable, 477, 478f
  upper and mid-face, 478–480, 479f
Fractured clavicle, 391
Fractured ribs, 58
Frankfort plane, 167
Frontal bone, 180, 184–185, 185f, 186f
Frontal eminences, 175f, 176
Frontal lobe, 244–245
Frontal nerve, 259, 373
Frontal process, 199
Frontal sinuses, 304f, 307f, 308, 308f
Frontalis muscle, 229t, 231

Full skull radiography, 469–470, 471f
Fungiform papillae, 319–320

G
Gallbladder, 118
Gallstones, 119
Ganglion
  celiac, 103, 104f, 107–108
  ciliary, 261, 261f, 373t, 386
  definition of, 23
  hay fever, 294
  inferior cervical, 157
  middle cervical, 157–158
  otic, 287, 288f, 373t, 386
  pterygopalatine, 294–296, 295f, 296f,
    373t, 374, 377, 386
  spiral, 353
  submandibular, 322–324, 325f, 326–327,
    373t, 377, 386
  superior cervical, 158
Gastric ulcers, 108
Gastrocnemius muscle, 442–443, 445t
Gastrocolic ligament, 107, 107f
Gastroduodenal artery, 107
Gastroesophageal reflux disease, 106
Gastrointestinal system, 105f
Gastrophrenic ligament, 107
Gastrosplenic ligament, 107, 107f, 120
Gemellus inferior muscle, 441t
Gemellus superior muscle, 441t
General concepts, 1–35
General sensory (somesthetic) area, 245
Genial tubercles, 212f, 213
Genioglossus muscle, 320, 320t
Geniohyoid muscle, 144, 144t
Genital system
  female, 128–131, 128f
  male, 125–128, 125f
Genitofemoral nerve, 445, 450t
Gingivae (gums), 332
  local anesthesia of, 459
  lymphatic drainage of, 367
  nerve and blood supply to, 332–333
  palatal, 459
  vestibular, 459
  visual inspection of, 310, 312f
Gingivitis, 333
Ginglymus, 12
Glabella, 168, 169f, 184
Glaucoma, 264
Glenohumeral (shoulder) joint, 394f,
    395–397, 395f, 396f
Glenoid fossa, 388–389, 395
Glenoid labrum, 395
Glenoid tubercle, 173, 191
Glomerulus, 121
Glossoepiglottic folds, 340
Glossopharyngeal nerve (cranial nerve IX),
    254, 321, 324, 340, 379–381, 380f
  branches of, 380–381
  functional components of, 30, 30t,
    379–380
Glottis, 342
Gluteal injections, 450, 451f
Gluteal muscles, 439–440, 440f, 441t
Gluteal nerves, 450

Gluteus maximus, 440, 441*t*
Gluteus medius, 439–440, 441*t*
Gluteus minimus, 439–440
Gomphosis, 9, 9*f*
Gonial angle, 173, 211, 212*f*
Gow-Gates mandibular nerve block, 463–465, 464*f*
Gracilis muscle, 438–439, 439*t*
Grafts, bone, 88
Gray matter, 23
   brain, 244, 247, 247*f*
   spinal cord, 44
Great auricular nerve, 147, 153, 236
Great cardiac vein, 77
Great saphenous vein, 454
Greater occipital nerve, 163, 238
Greater omentum, 106, 107, 107*f*
Greater palatine artery, 319
Greater palatine canal, 177, 214*t*, 291
Greater palatine foramen, 204, 214*t*, 316
Greater palatine nerve, 294, 318
Greater palatine nerve block, 461–462, 461*f*
Greater petrosal hiatus, 191–193
Greater petrosal nerve, 294, 354, 377
Greater splanchnic nerve, 103, 104*f*
Greater trochanter, 425
Greater tubercle, 391
Groove or sulcus, 7
Gross anatomy, 1
Growth, 8. *See also* Development
Gubernaculum, 94–95
Gums (gingivae), 332
Gut (alimentary canal), 104–121, 105*f*
   development of, 99–101, 100*f*
   lymphoid tissue of, 20
Gynecomastia, 59
Gyri, 244–246, 245*f*

H

Hamate, 393
Hammer (malleus), 352
Hamstrings, 440, 442*t*
Hamulus, 179, 196
Hand
   bones of, 393–394, 393*f*
   imaging of, 473, 477*f*
   joints of, 397*f*
   muscles of, 410–414, 412*f*, 412*t*
Hard palate, 313–316
   imaging of, 472, 475*f*
   surface features of, 313, 314*f*
Haustra, 111
Hay fever ganglion, 294
Head and neck, 221–355
   arteries of, 358, 359*f*, 360*t*
   deep veins of, 362*f*, 363*t*
   distribution of postganglionic sympathetic fibers to, 29
   fascial spaces of, 481–485, 481*f*
   lymph nodes of, 358, 365*t*
   lymphatic drainage of, 137*f*, 358
   muscles responsible for movements of, 164*t*
   supervicial veins of, 362*f*, 363*t*
   sympathetic nerve supply to, 383–385, 384*f*

Head and neck *(Continued)*
   sympathetic supply to, 158
   systemic anatomy of, 358–386
   veins of, 358, 362*f*, 363*t*
Hearing, 353
Hearing organ, 352
Heart, 16, 69–79
   blood flow through, 70–71, 72*f*
   blood vessels of, 76–77, 76*f*
   conducting system of, 77, 78*f*
   entrances and exits to, 70–71, 72*f*
   features of, 70
   innervation of, 77–79
   shape and position of, 69
   surfaces of, 70, 70*f*, 71*f*
Heart block, 78–79
Heart chambers
   disposition of, 69–70
   internal features of, 71–74
Heart murmur, 67
Heart sounds, 74–76, 75*f*
Heart valves
   auscultation of, 74–76
   damaged, 76
Heart wall, 70
Heartbeat
   extrinsic modification of, 78
   intrinsic control of, 77–78
Heartburn, 79
Heat regulation, 33
Helicine arteries, 127–128
Hematoma
   facial, 291
   with posterior superior alveolar block, 460
Hemopoiesis, 4
Hemorrhage
   extradural, 240
   intracranial, 240
   subarachnoid, 240
   subdural, 240
Hemorrhoids, 113, 114, 116
Hepatic artery, 107, 116
Hepatic flexure, 111–112
Hepatic veins, 102, 116
Herniated disc, 42, 43*f*
Herpes labialis, 234
Hiatus hernia, 106
Hiatus semilunaris, 301–302
Highest nuchal line, 177, 187
Hilum, 65
Hinge (ginglymus) joints, 12
Hip bone (os coxae), 87–88, 89*f*
Hip joint, 430–431, 430*f*
   adductors of, 438
   flexors of, 437
   gluteal muscles that move, 441*t*
   movements at, 431, 432*f*, 447*t*
Hip replacement, 431
Histology, 1
Hollow spaces, 244
Horizontal plane, 3
Horner syndrome, 385
Horner's syndrome, 158
Humeroulnar joint, 397–398, 398*f*
Humerus, 389–392, 391*f*
Hyaline cartilage, 4, 431

Hydrocele, 96
Hymen, 129–130
Hyoepiglottic ligament, 341
Hyoglossus muscle, 320, 320*t*
Hyoid bone, 133, 135*f*, 167, 213
Hyperopia, 264
Hypoglossal canal, 179*f*, 181*f*, 182*f*, 183, 190*f*, 214*t*
Hypoglossal nerve (cranial nerve XII), 30, 30*t*, 147, 147*f*, 149, 254, 324–325, 369*t*, 383, 384*f*
Hypophyseal (pituitary) fossa, 180, 181*f*, 182*f*, 194–195
Hypophysis cerebri, 247
Hypothalamus, 247
Hypothenar muscles, 411, 412*t*

I

ID. *See* Internal disc derangement
Ileocecal orifice, 111
Ileocecal valve, 111
Ileum, 105, 109–111
   features of, 112*f*
   peritoneal attachments, 110
   position of, 109–110
Iliocostalis muscle, 49, 51*t*
Iliofemoral ligament, 430–431
Iliohypogastric nerve, 95, 103, 445, 450*t*
Ilioinguinal nerve, 95, 103, 445, 450*t*
Iliopsoas muscle, 98*t*, 437, 439*t*
Ilium, 87
Imaging, 466–467, 468–473
Imaging anatomy, 2
Incisive canal, 177, 214*t*
Incisive crest, 203
Incisive foramen, 203, 214*t*, 316
Incisive fossa, 199, 211, 212*f*
Incisive papilla, 313
Incisors, maxillary, 485–486
Incus (anvil), 352
Infection(s)
   from cervicofacial emphysema, 487
   dental
      pathways of, 485–487, 486*f*, 487*f*
      spread of, 480, 485*f*
   in fascia, 481
   in fascial spaces, 481–485, 482*t*
   of infraorbital (canine) area, 486
   internal ear, 354
   of lower lip and chin, 486
   of masticator space, 483–484, 484*f*, 486
   in maxillary sinus, 486
   of nasal cavity, 486
   oral, 309
   orbital, 308
   of palatal mucosa, 486
   in parapharyngeal area, 484–485, 485*f*
   of parotid gland, 268
   in parotid region, 482
   of periodontal structures, 480–481
   primary sites, 480–481
   of scalp, 239
   secondary sites, 481
   spread of, 226

Infection(s) *(Continued)*
  in sublingual region, 486
  in sublingual region (floor of mouth),
    482–483
  in submandibular region, 482, 486
  in superficial fascia, 481, 483f, 486
  tertiary sites, 481–485
  in tonsillar region, 483
Inferior abdominal wall, 97–99, 98f
Inferior abdominal wall muscles, 98t
Inferior alveolar artery, 289
Inferior alveolar nerve, 287, 376, 462–463,
    464f
  mental and incisive block, 465
  standard block, 462–463
Inferior cervical ganglion, 157
Inferior colliculi, 247
Inferior concha, 167, 207–210, 209f, 299
Inferior constrictor muscle, 334, 336t
Inferior epigastric artery, 95–96
Inferior gemellus muscle, 440
Inferior gluteal nerve, 451t
Inferior hemiazygos vein, 83, 83f
Inferior labial artery, 225
Inferior meatus, 299
Inferior mesenteric artery, 99, 102, 115
Inferior mesenteric vein, 115, 116
Inferior nuchal line, 37, 177, 187
Inferior oblique muscle, 258, 258t
Inferior orbital fissure, 169f, 170, 173, 196,
    201, 214t, 291
Inferior pancreaticoduodenal artery, 109, 120
Inferior pancreaticoduodenal vein, 109, 120
Inferior papillae, 237
Inferior petrosal hiatus, 214t
Inferior petrosal sinus, 244, 363t
Inferior petrosal sulcus, 182, 214t
Inferior phrenic artery, 101
Inferior phrenic veins, 102
Inferior rectus muscle, 258, 258t
Inferior sagittal sinus, 242–244, 363t
Inferior thyroid artery, 156, 158, 347, 363t
Inferior thyroid vein, 158
Inferior vena cava, 71, 82, 102–103, 103f,
    116, 118f
Inferior vesical artery, 124
Infraglottic cavity, 343
Infrahyoid lymph nodes, 365t, 366
Infrahyoid muscles, 143, 143f, 144t, 320
Infraorbital (canine) area, 486
Infraorbital artery, 225, 297
Infraorbital block, 459
Infraorbital canal, 201–202, 214t, 291
Infraorbital foramen, 169f, 170, 199,
    201–202, 214t
Infraorbital groove, 291
Infraorbital nerve, 223, 293–294, 301
Infraorbital sulcus or groove, 201–202
Infraspinatus muscle, 404, 404f, 405t
Infraspinous fossa, 388
Infratemporal crest, 196
Infratemporal fossa, 269, 269f
Infratrochlear nerve, 222–223, 238, 260
Infundibulum, 128–129
Inguinal canal, 92–94, 125–126
Inguinal hernia, 96

Inguinal nodes, 20
Inguinal region, 92–95
Inion, 37, 177, 187
Injection(s)
  gluteal, 450, 451f
  inadvertent intravascular injections, 291
  intraorbital, 459
  pain on, 461
Injection sites
  for Akenosi (closed mouth) mandibular
    nerve block, 465, 465f
  for anterior and middle superior alveolar
    nerve block, 459, 460f
  for Gow-Gates mandibular nerve block,
    463–464
  for greater palatine nerve block, 461–462,
    461f
  for lingual nerve block, 466, 466f
  for local anesthesia of maxillary structures,
    458, 458f, 459, 459f
  for maxillary block, 462
  for mental and incisive block, 465, 465f
  for nasopalatine nerve block, 461, 461f
  for posterior superior alveolar nerve block,
    459–460, 460f
  for standard inferior alveolar block, 462,
    463f
Injury
  brachial plexus injuries, 415
  knee injuries, 433
  rotator cuff injuries, 404
Inner ear, 349, 349f, 353f
Inspiration, 67, 67f
Insulin, 120
Intercavernous sinuses, 244
Intercondylar eminence, 426
Intercostal arteries, 46–47, 62, 62f, 97
Intercostal blood vessels, 62–63
Intercostal muscles, 60, 61t, 62f
  external, 60, 61t
  innermost, 60, 61t
  internal, 60, 61t
Intercostal nerves, 62–63, 62f, 84
Intercostal space, 60f
Intercostal veins, 62
Interlobar arteries, 122
Interlobular ducts, 118
Intermediate cuneifrom, 428–429
Intermediolateral horns, 27
Internal auditory meatus, 181f, 182f, 183,
    191, 214t
Internal carotid artery, 145, 249–250,
    254–255, 359f, 360t
Internal carotid nerve, 385
Internal cerebral vein, 363t
Internal disc derangement (ID), 276
Internal ear, 193, 352–353
Internal ear infection, 354
Internal iliac artery, 450
Internal iliac vein, 102, 453
Internal intercostal muscles, 61t
Internal jugular vein, 138, 146, 146f, 154,
    226–227, 358, 363t
Internal laryngeal nerve, 148
Internal oblique crest, 310–311
Internal oblique line, 213

Internal oblique muscle, 92, 92t
Internal occipital crest, 183, 188
Internal occipital protuberance, 181f, 183,
    188
Internal pudendal artery, 127–128
Internal sphincter ani, 113
Internal thoracic artery, 156
Interphalangeal joint, 400–401, 436
Interspinales muscle, 51t
Intertarsal joints, 436, 437f
Intertransversarii muscle, 51t
Intertrochanteric crest, 425
Intertubercular sulcus, 391–392
Interventricular foramina, 249
Interventricular sulcus, 70
Intervertebral disc
  herniated disc, 42, 43f
  loss of vertical dimension of, 42, 43f
Intervertebral foramina, 37
Intervertebral joints, 42–43
Intestinal glands (of Lieberkühn), 110
Intracranial hemorrhage, 240
Intramembranous ossification, 8
Intraoral radiography, 468–469
Intraorbital injection, 459
Intravascular local anesthesia, 291
Intubation, endotracheal, 348, 348f
Iris, 262
Ischemia, 77
Ischiocavernosus muscle, 127
Ischiofemoral ligament, 430–431
Ischiorectal fossa, 99
Ischium, 87
Islets of Langerhans, 120
Isthmus, 128–129

J

Jaundice, 119
Jaws, 171
  improper relationships, 310
  nerve supply to, 333
Jejunum, 105, 109–111
  features of, 112f
  peritoneal attachments, 110
  position of, 109–110
Joint cavity, 10
Joints, 8. *See also specific joints*
  ankle joint, 435–437, 435f
  between articular facets, 42
  ball-and-socket, 11
  biaxial, 11–12
  bilateral synovial, 42
  between bodies, 42
  carpometacarpal joint, 399, 400
  cartilaginous
    primary, 9–10, 9f
    secondary, 9f, 10
  condyloid, 11–12
  costochondral, 58
  costovertebral, 57
  diarthrodial, 8
  of elbow, 397–398, 397f
  fibrous, 8–9, 9f
  of fingers, 400
  of foot, 436–437
  of hand, 397f

Joints(s) *(Continued)*
    hinge (ginglymus), 12
    hip joint, 430–431, 430*f*
    intervertebral, 42–43
    knee joint, 431–435
    of larynx, 342
    of lower limb, 429
    movements during walking, 437
    multiaxial, 10–11
    of pectoral girdle, 394–395, 394*f*
    pivot, 12
    plane, 12
    radioulnar joints, 398–399
    saddle or ellipsoid, 11
    of spine, 42–43
    sternocostal, 57–58
    of suboccipital region, 159–162
    synarthrodial, 8
    syndesmosis type, 42–43
    synovial, 10–12, 10*f*
    between thoracic vertebrae, 57–58
    of thumb, 400–401
    tibiofibular, 435
    uniaxial, 12
    wrist joint, 397*f*, 399–400
Jugular foramen, 180, 181*f*, 182*f*, 183, 189,
        191, 214*t*
Jugular notch, 54, 59, 60*f*, 134–136
Jugular processes, 189
Jugulodigastric lymph nodes, 365*t*
Juguloomohyoid lymph nodes, 365*t*

K

Kidneys, 109*f*, 121–122
    blood supply to, 121, 122, 122*f*
    features and parts of, 121, 123*f*
    floating kidney, 121
    position of, 121
    structure and function of, 121–122
Klumpke's palsy, 415
Knee injuries, 433
Knee joint, 431–435
    extensors of, 437–438
    internal features of, 431, 433*f*
    movements of, 434–435, 434*f*, 447*t*
    runner's knee, 434
Knee replacement, 434
Kyphosis, 42

L

Labia majora, 130, 130*f*
Labia minora, 130, 130*f*
Labial frenectomy, 234
Labial frenula, 234, 310
Labial mucocele, 234
Labial veins, 226
Labiomental groove, 233
Lacerations, 239
Lacrimal apparatus, 238, 264–265, 265*f*
Lacrimal artery, 224, 262
Lacrimal bone, 206, 207*f*
Lacrimal bones, 167
Lacrimal fossa, 184
Lacrimal gland, 264, 354
Lacrimal hamulus, 206

Lacrimal nerve, 223, 238, 259–260, 373
Lacrimal sac, 265
Lactation, 59
Lacus lacriminalis, 236
Lambda, 176, 176*f*
Large intestine, 105, 111–115
    arterial supply to, 111*f*
    peritoneal attachments, 113–114
    sections of, 113*f*
    venous return from, 115
Laryngeal inlet, 342
Laryngeal pharynx, 336–340, 338*f*
Larynx, 136, 340
    blood supply, 347–349
    functions of, 340
    interior of, 342–343, 343*f*
    joints of, 342
    ligaments of, 342, 343*f*
    lumen of, 342–343
    lymphatic drainage of, 368
    movements of muscles of, 346–347, 346*f*
    muscles of, 343–347, 344*t*, 345*f*
    nerve supply, 347
    skeleton of, 135*f*, 340–342, 341*f*
Lateral chest wall muscles, 401–403
Lateral collateral ligament, 435
Lateral cricoarytenoid muscle, 344, 344*t*
Lateral cruciate ligament, 431–434
Lateral cuneifrom, 428–429
Lateral epicondyle, 392, 425
Lateral femoral cutaneous nerve, 445, 450*t*
Lateral hip rotators, 440
Lateral longitudinal arches, 436
Lateral malleolus, 426–428
Lateral menisci, 431
Lateral pectoral nerve, 417–418, 419*t*
Lateral pterygoid muscle, 280*t*, 282–283,
        283*f*, 284*f*
Lateral pterygoid plate, 196
Lateral rectus muscle, 258, 258*t*
Lateral sinus, 363*t*
Lateral styloid process, 392–393
Lateral sulcus, 244
Lateral thyrohyoid ligaments, 342
Lateral ventricles, 249
Latissimus dorsi muscle, 47, 403, 405*t*
Least splanchnic nerve, 103
LeFort I fracture, 478, 479*f*
LeFort II fracture, 478, 479*f*
LeFort III fracture, 478, 479*f*
Left ascending lumbar vein, 83
Left atrioventricular valve, 74
Left atrium, 69–70, 74, 74*f*
Left brachiocephalic vein, 82, 83*f*
Left bronchi, 65
Left bronchial tree, 66
Left common carotid artery, 81
Left common iliac artery, 101, 450–452
Left common iliac vein, 102
Left coronary artery, 76, 77, 80
Left external iliac artery, 101
Left gastric artery, 107–108
Left gastric vein, 108
Left gastro-omental artery, 107–108
Left gastro-omental vein, 108
Left heart, 16

Left hepatic duct, 118
Left inferior alveolar nerve, 331
Left internal iliac artery, 101
Left maxilla, 177
Left palatine bone, 177
Left pleural cavity, 58
Left pulmonary vein, 74
Left recurrent laryngeal nerve, 84
Left subclavian artery, 81
Left temporal bone, 177, 180
Left transverse sulcus, 188
Left ventricle, 18–19, 69–70, 74, 75*f*
Leg. *See also* Lower limb
    anterior leg muscles, 440–441, 442*t*,
        443*f*
    lateral leg muscles, 441–442, 442*t*
    posterior leg muscles, 442–444, 444*f*,
        445*t*
Lens, 263
Lens accommodation (focusing), 263
Lesions, 234
Lesser occipital nerve, 147, 153, 236, 238
Lesser omentum, 106–107, 107*f*, 116
Lesser palatine artery, 319
Lesser palatine canal, 177, 214*t*, 291
Lesser palatine foramen, 204, 214*t*, 316
Lesser palatine nerve, 294, 318
Lesser petrosal hiatus, 193
Lesser petrosal nerve, 287, 380
Lesser splanchnic nerve, 103
Lesser trochanter, 425
Lesser tubercle, 391
Leukocytes, 16
Levator anguli oris muscle, 227, 229*t*
Levator ani muscles, 98, 98*t*
Levator costarum muscles, 60–62, 61*t*
Levator labii superioris muscle, 227, 229*t*
Levator palpebrae superioris muscle, 237,
        257, 258*t*
Levator scapulae muscle, 47, 151*t*, 152, 163*f*,
        164, 403, 405*t*
Levator veli palatini muscle, 316, 318*t*
Lieberkühn, intestinal glands of, 110
Ligament teres, 116
Ligaments
    capsular, 10
    of larynx, 342
    of peritoneum, 99
    vocal, 342
Ligamentum venosum, 116
Linea aspera, 426
Linea or line, 7
Lingual artery, 146, 150, 325–326
Lingual frenulum, 314, 319
Lingual nerve, 286–287, 321–324, 376
Lingual nerve block, 466, 466*f*
Lingual tonsils, 20
Lingual vein, 150
Lingula, 64–65, 212*f*, 213
Lips, 221, 233–234, 233*f*
    cleft lip and palate, 319
    lesions of, 234
    lower lip infection, 486
    lymphatic drainage of, 367
    muscles of, 227, 229*t*
    visual inspection of, 310

Liver, 105, 115–119
  blood flow to, 116
  development of, 99–100
  features of, 115–116
  metabolic functions, 117–118
  peritoneal attachments, 116
  structure and function of, 116–118, 117f
  surfaces of, 115–116
  venous return from, 116, 118f
Local anesthesia, 287, 295
  anatomy of, 457
  block anesthesia
    of mandibular structures, 462–466
    of maxillary structures, 459–462
  inadvertent intravascular injections, 291
  by local infiltration, 457–458, 458f
    of mandibular structures, 462
    of maxillary structures, 458–459
  of mandibular structures, 462–466, 463f
  of maxillary structures, 458–462, 458f, 459f
  types of, 457–458
Local infiltration, 457–458, 458f
  complications of, 458–459
  of mandibular structures, 462
  of maxillary structures, 458–459
Long bones, 5–6
  blood supply to, 6, 7f
  development of, 7f
  features of, 5–6, 6f
Long buccal nerve, 286, 375–376
Long buccal nerve block, 466, 466f
Long sphenopalatine nerve, 301
Long thoracic nerve, 417, 419t
Longissimus muscle, 49, 51t
Longitudinal arches, 436
Longitudinal section, 3
Longus capitis muscle, 162t, 163f, 164
Longus colli muscle, 162t, 163f, 164
Loop of Henle, 121
Lordosis, 42
Low back pain, 42, 43f
Lower limb, 425–454
  anterior leg muscles, 440–441, 442t, 443f
  arterial supply to, 450–453, 452f
  bones of, 425, 426–428, 426f
  deep lymph nodes of, 454
  deep veins of, 453
  joints of, 429
  lateral leg muscles, 441–442, 442t
  lymphatics of, 454, 455f
  movements of, 447t
  movements of joints during walking, 437
  muscles of, 437
  nerve supply to, 444
  posterior leg muscles, 442–444, 444f, 445t
  skeleton of, 425
  superficial lymph nodes of, 454
  superficial veins of, 453–454
  venous drainage of, 453, 453f
Lower lip infection, 486
Lower motor neurons, 24, 232
Lower subscapular nerve, 418, 419t
Ludwig's angina, 482–483, 483f
Lumbar arteries, 101
Lumbar attachments, 96

Lumbar plexus, 31, 103, 444–445, 449f, 450t
Lumbar splanchnic nerve, 30, 103, 104f
Lumbar veins, 102
Lumbar vertebrae, 39, 40f
Lumbosacral plexus, 448f
Lumbosacral trunk, 450t
Lumbrical muscles, 412f, 412t, 413
Lumpectomy, 59
Lunate, 393
Lung emphysema, 68
Lung resection, 68
Lungs, 64–65
  blood supply to, 66–67
  fissures and lobes, 64–65
  nerve supply to, 67
  pigmented, 68
  surfaces and borders of, 64, 64f, 65f
Lymph, 19, 19f
Lymph capillaries, 19–20
Lymph flow, 20
Lymph nodes, 20, 20f
  deep, of lower limb, 454
  deep cervical vertical chain, 365t, 366–367
  deep parotid, 364, 365t
  deep ring of, 365–366, 365t
  of head and neck, 358, 365t
  infrahyoid, 365t, 366
  jugulodigastric, 365t
  juguloomohyoid, 365t
  major groups, 423f
  mastoid (retroauricular), 365, 365t
  occipital, 365, 365t
  paratracheal, 365t, 366
  prelaryngeal, 365t, 366
  pretracheal, 365t, 366
  retropharyngeal, 365–366, 365t
  submandibular, 149, 360–364, 365t
  submental, 359–360, 365t
  superficial, of lower limb, 454
  superficial parotid, 364, 365t
  superficial ring of, 358–365, 365t
Lymph vessels, 20
Lymphatic circulation, 20, 21f
Lymphatic system, 15–16, 19–20
  functions of, 20
  of head and neck, 358
  large vessels of, 20
  of lower limb, 454
  of upper limb, 422, 423f
Lymphocytes, 120
Lymphoid tissues, 20

M

Magnetic resonance imaging, 468, 472, 476f
Major duodenal papilla, 109
Male genital system, 125–128, 125f
Male pelvis, 127f, 130–131, 131f
Malleolus, 7
Malleus (hammer), 352
Malocclusion, 310
Mandible, 167, 210–213, 211f, 212f
  centric occlusion, 275
  condyles of, 269–271, 270f
  development of, 218–219

Mandible (Continued)
  external oblique ridge of, 310–311
  movements of, 276–279, 277f
  reference positions of, 275
  rest position, 275
Mandibular anterior teeth, 486
Mandibular arch, 333f
Mandibular canal, 213, 214t
Mandibular dentition, 169f
Mandibular foramen, 212f, 213, 214t
Mandibular fossa, 173, 179, 191, 193
Mandibular (lower-face) fractures, 475–478, 478f
Mandibular lingual gingivae, 333
Mandibular molars, 486
Mandibular nerve (cranial nerve V-3), 221–222, 223–224, 251, 284–287, 285f, 374–376, 376f
Mandibular nerve (cranial nerve V-3) block
  Akenosi (closed mouth) block, 465, 465f
  Gow-Gates block, 463–465, 464f
Mandibular notch, 212
Mandibular premolars, 486
Mandibular process, 269–271
Mandibular structures
  block anesthesia of, 462–466
  cone beam computed tomography (CBCT) scans of, 470, 472f
  local anesthesia of, 462–466
  local infiltration of, 462
Mandibular teeth, 212f, 331
Mandibular third molars, 486–487, 487f
Mandibular vestibular gingivae, 332–333
Manubrium, 54
Masillary tuberosity, 200
Masseter muscle, 279, 280t, 281f, 284f
Masseter nerve, 286
Masseteric arteries, 290
Mastectomy, 59
Mastication, 228–230, 275–279
  accessory muscles of, 283
  muscles of, 279–284, 280t
Masticator region, 269, 483, 484f
Masticator space, 269
Masticator space infection, 483–484, 484f, 486
Mastoid foramen, 214t, 244
Mastoid (retroauricular) lymph nodes, 365, 365t
Mastoid process, 173, 177, 191
Mastoiditis, 354
Maxilla, 167, 171, 199–203, 200f, 201f
  development of, 218
  zygomatic process of, 169f, 174, 199, 201f, 310–311
Maxillary arch, 333f
Maxillary artery, 146, 225, 267, 287–290, 292f, 340
Maxillary canine teeth, 486
Maxillary dentition, 169f
Maxillary hiatus, 202, 303–304
Maxillary incisors, 485–486
Maxillary lingual (palatal) gingivae, 332
Maxillary molars, 486
Maxillary nerve (cranial nerve V-2), 221–222, 223, 251, 255, 291–296, 293f, 340, 374, 375f

Maxillary nerve (cranial nerve V-2) block, 462
Maxillary premolars, 486
Maxillary sinus, 202, 302–306, 304f, 305f
  drainage of secretions from, 306
  imaging of, 470–472, 474f
  infection in, 486
  nerve and blood supply to, 306–308
  size and shape variations, 306, 306f, 307f
Maxillary sinusitis, 306
Maxillary structures
  block anesthesia of, 459–462
  cone beam computed tomography (CBCT) scans of, 470, 472f
  injection sites for local infiltration of, 458, 458f
  local anesthesia of, 458–462
  local infiltration of, 458–459, 458f
  periapical radiography of, 468, 469f
Maxillary teeth, 177, 331, 331f
Maxillary tubercle, 174, 200
Maxillary vein, 267, 290–291, 332, 363t
Maxillary vestibular gingivae, 332
Meckel's (trigeminal) dural cave, 251
Medial angular process, 184
Medial collateral ligament, 435
Medial cruciate ligament, 431–434
Medial cruciate ligament tears, 434
Medial cuneiform, 428–429
Medial epicondyle, 392, 425
Medial longitudinal arches, 436
Medial malleolus, 426
Medial menisci, 431
Medial pectoral nerve, 418, 419t
Medial pterygoid muscle, 280t, 281–282, 282f, 284f
Medial pterygoid nerve, 285–286
Medial pterygoid plate, 196
Medial rectus muscle, 258, 258t
Medial styloid process, 393
Median antebrachial vein, 421–422
Median cricothyroid ligament, 342
Median cubital vein, 421–422
Median nerve, 418, 419t
Median plane, 2f, 3
Median sacral artery, 101–102
Median sacral vein, 102
Mediastinal emphysema, 487
Mediastinal pleura, 63
Mediastinitis, 138
Mediastinum, 58, 68–69, 68f, 80f, 81f, 125
  anterior, 79
  divisions of, 68, 68f
  middle, 68, 68f, 69–79
  superior and posterior, 79–84
Medulla oblongata, 248–249
Medullary rays, 121–122
Membranous labyrinth, 352–353
Meningeal spaces, 46, 242
Meninges, 45–46, 239–242, 239f
  blood supply to, 242
  sensory nerve supply to, 242
Meningitis, 46, 240
Meniscal tears, 433–434
Meniscus, 431
Mental and incisive block, 465–466, 465f

Mental artery, 225
Mental foramen, 169f, 171, 173, 211, 212f, 213, 214t
Mental nerve, 224, 287
Mental protuberance, 169f, 211, 212f
Mental spine, 212f, 213
Mental tubercles, 211, 212f
Mentalis muscle, 229t, 231
Mesencephalon, 244
Mesentery, 99, 110
Mesoappendix, 113–114
Metacarpals, 393
Metacarpophalangeal (MP) joints, 400
Metatarsal bones, 429
Metatarsophalangeal joint, 436
Metencephalon, 244
Micturition, 124
Midbrain, 247
Midcarpal joint, 399
Middle cardiac vein, 77
Middle cervical ganglion, 157–158
Middle colic artery, 115
Middle concha, 299
Middle constrictor muscle, 334, 336t
Middle cranial fossa, 180–182, 182f
Middle ear, 193, 349, 349f, 351f
Middle ear cavity (tympanic cavity), 350–352
Middle ear ossicles, 213, 351f, 352
Middle meatus, 299
Middle meningeal artery, 289, 363t
Middle phalanx, 393–394, 429
Middle superior alveolar artery, 331–332
Middle superior alveolar nerve, 293–294, 331, 374
Middle superior alveolar nerve block, 459, 460f
Middle temporal nerve, 286
Middle thyroid vein, 158
Midline symphysis menti, 211
Milk lines, 59
Minor duodenal papilla, 109
Missing teeth, 309–310, 311
Mitral valve, 74
Molar glands, 234–235
Molars
  mandibular molars, 486
  mandibular third molars, 486–487, 487f
  maxillary, 486
Motor nerves
  to extraocular muscles, 258–259
  of face, 231–233
  of neck, 153–155
  to upper limb muscles, 154
Motor neurons, 21, 22f
  lower, 24
  upper, 24
Motor speech (Broca's) area, 245–246
Mouth, 221
  floor of, 321–327, 324f, 326f
  infections in floor of, 482–483, 486
  muscles of, 227, 229t
MP joints. See Metacarpophalangeal joints
MRI. See Magnetic resonance imaging
Mucobuccal fold, 234–235, 310
Mucolabial fold, 310

Mucosa
  alveolar, 310, 332
  of cheek, 312f
  palatal, 316, 459
  respiratory, 314–316
  vestibular, 459
Mucous glands, palatal, 316
Mucous membrane, 31
Multifidus muscle, 49, 51t
Muscle(s). See also specific muscles
  of abdomen, 91–92
  accessory extrinsic muscles of respiration, 60
  actions of, 13
  anterior leg muscles, 440–441, 442t, 443f
  anterior thigh muscles, 437–438, 438f, 439t
  of arm, 404–406, 406t
  of back, 47, 60–62, 61t, 403, 405t
  cardiac, 15
  of cheeks, 227–231, 229t
  of chin, 229t, 231
  of external ear, 229t
  of eye, 229t
  of face, 227–231, 229t
  of facial expression, 35, 228f
  of foot, 444, 446f, 446t
  of forearm, 406–410, 407f, 408t, 410f, 411t
  of forehead, 229t, 231
  of gluteal region, 439–440, 440f, 441t
  of hand, 410–414, 412f, 412t
  intercostal, 60
  of larynx, 343–347, 344t
  lateral leg muscles, 441–442, 442t
  of lips, 227, 229t
  of lower limb, 437
  of mastication, 279–284, 280t
  medial thigh muscles, 438–439, 439t
  of mouth, 227, 229t
  of nose, 229t, 231
  of orbit, 256–258, 257f, 258t
  of pectoral region, 401–403, 402f, 403t
  of penis, 127
  pennate, 13, 14f
  of pharynx, 334–336, 335f, 336t
  posterior leg muscles, 442–444, 444f, 445t
  posterior thigh muscles, 440, 440f, 442t
  postvertebral, 162t
  prevertebral, 162t
  rectangular or strap, 13, 14f
  responsible for back movements, 52t
  of shoulder, 403–404, 404f, 405t
  skeletal, 12–15
  smooth, 15
  of soft palate, 316–317, 317f, 318t
  sphincter, 13, 14f
  of suboccipital region, 162–163
  superficial, 35, 47, 49f
  of thorax, 59–62, 61t
  of tongue, 320–321
  of upper limb, 401
  vertebral, 162–163, 162t
  voluntary versus involuntary, 15
  of wrist, 412t

Muscular arteries, 16
Muscular system, 12
Musculocutaneous nerve, 155, 418, 419*t*
Musculophrenic artery, 62, 97
Myelencephalon, 244
Mylohyoid muscle, 144, 144*t*
Mylohyoid nerve, 149, 287
Mylohyoid ridge, 212*f*, 213
Mylohyoid sulcus, 213
Myocardial infarction, 77
Myocardium, 70
Myofascial pain syndrome, 282
Myometrium, 129
Myopia, 264

N

Nasal bone, 167, 171, 206–207, 208*f*
Nasal breathing, 301
Nasal cavity, 167, 297, 298*f*, 304*f*
    arterial supply to, 301, 303*f*
    autonomic nerve supply to, 301
    boundaries, 299–300
    foramen of, 214*t*
    functions of, 297
    imaging of floor of, 472, 475*f*
    infection of, 486
    lymphatic drainage of, 368
    nerve supply to, 300–301, 300*f*
    skeletal components of lateral wall, 299,
        299*f*
    veins of, 301
Nasal conchae, 171
Nasal crest, 203, 204–205, 299–300
Nasal margin, 184, 199
Nasal obstruction, 302
    chronic, 302
    occasional, 302
Nasal septum, 299–300, 299*f*
Nasal spine, 184
Nasal veins, 226
Nasalis muscle, 229*t*, 231
Nasion, 169*f*, 171
Nasociliary nerve, 260, 307–308, 373–374
Nasolacrimal duct, 171, 214*t*, 265
Nasolacrimal sulcus, 202
Nasolacrimal system, 264–265
Nasopalatine nerve, 294–295, 301, 317–318
Nasopalatine nerve block, 460–461, 461*f*
Nasopharynx, 336–339, 338*f*, 368
Navicular, 428
Neck, 133–164. *See also* Head and neck
    anterior triangle of, 140, 141*f*
    arteries of, 145–146
    coverings of, 136
    cutaneous nerves of, 153
    fascial coverings, 136–139, 137*f*
    infrahyoid muscles of, 143, 143*f*, 144*t*
    key muscles of, 139, 139*f*
    motor nerves of, 153–155
    muscular triangle, 140–141
    nerves of, 147–148, 147*f*, 153, 153*f*,
        157–158
    posterior triangle of, 140, 150–151,
        152*f*, 154*f*
    postvertebral muscles of, 162*t*
    potential fascial spaces, 138–139

Neck *(Continued)*
    prevertebral muscles of, 162*t*, 163–164,
        163*f*
    regions of, 139–140
    root of, 155, 156*f*
    skeleton of, 133
    submandibular triangle of, 141–142,
        148–150, 150*f*
    superficial nerves of, 142
    superficial veins of, 142, 142*f*
    suprahyoid muscles of, 143–145, 144*t*
    surface anatomy of, 134–136, 135*f*
    veins of, 146–147
    vertebral muscles of, 162–163, 162*t*
    visceral unit of, 136
Neck triangles, 140
Nephrons, 121, 123*f*
Nerve block, 457–458
    Akenosi (closed mouth) mandibular nerve
        block, 465, 465*f*
    anterior superior alveolar nerve block, 459,
        460*f*
    Gow-Gates mandibular nerve block,
        463–465, 464*f*
    greater palatine block, 461–462
    infraorbital block, 459
    lingual nerve block, 466, 466*f*
    long buccal nerve block, 466, 466*f*
    for mandibular structures, 462–466
    maxillary block, 462
    for maxillary structures, 459–462
    mental and incisive block, 465–466, 465*f*
    middle superior alveolar nerve block, 460*f*
    nasopalatine nerve block, 460–461,
        461*f*
    posterior superior alveolar nerve block,
        459–460, 460*f*
    standard inferior alveolar nerve block,
        462–463
Nerve plexuses, 31, 32*f*
Nerves. *See also specific nerves*
    of abdomen, 103–104
    of orbit, 258–261
    of suboccipital region, 163
    of thorax, 84
Nervous system, 20–21
    autonomic nervous system, 23
    central nervous system, 23
    parasympathetic division, 23, 26–27, 27*f*
    peripheral nervous system, 23
    somatic nervous system, 23
    sympathetic division, 23, 27–29, 28*f*, 29*f*
    terms, 22–23
    visceral (autonomic) nervous system, 23
Nervus intermedius, 354, 377
Nervus spinosus, 286, 374
Neurilemma (Schwann) cells, 23–24
Neuroanatomy, 1–2
Neurocranium, 167
    bones of, 184–199
    contents of, 238
Neuroglia, 20–21, 22
Neurons, 20–22
    motor neurons, 21, 22*f*
    sensory neurons, 21–22, 22*f*
Nipples, accessory, 59

Nose
    external anatomy of, 221, 235–236, 235*f*
    functions of, 297
    muscles of, 229*t*, 231
Nosebleed (epistaxis), 302
Notch (bony), 7–8
Nucleus, 23
Nucleus cuneatus, 249
Nucleus gracilis, 249

O

Obccipital lobe, 244–245
Oblique plane, 2*f*, 3
Oblique vein, 77
Obliquus capitis inferior muscle, 162, 162*t*
Obliquus capitis superior muscle, 162, 162*t*
Obliterated umbilical arteries, 19
Obturator externus muscle, 438, 441*t*
Obturator internus muscle, 440, 441*t*
Obturator nerve, 445, 450*t*
Occipital artery, 146, 238
Occipital bone, 177, 180, 187–189, 189*f*,
    190*f*
Occipital condyle, 177, 180
Occipital groove, 177
Occipital lymph nodes, 365, 365*t*
Occipital sinus, 244, 363*t*
Occipitalis muscle, 229*t*
Occipitofrontalis (epicranius) muscle, 238
Occiput, 37, 177
Occlusal radiography, 468–469, 469*f*
Occupational bursitis, 434
Oculomotor nerve (cranial nerve III), 30,
    30*t*, 251, 255, 258–259, 369*t*,
    370–371, 371*f*
Oculus bulbi (eyeball), 262–264
Odontoblasts, 328
Odontoid process, 39
Olecranon, 393
Olecranon fossa, 392
Olfactory area, 246
Olfactory bulbs, 251
Olfactory foramina, 214*t*
Olfactory nerve (cranial nerve I), 30, 30*t*,
    251, 368, 369*t*, 370*f*
Olfactory tract, 251
Omentum, 99
Omohyoid muscle, 143, 144*t*
Oögonia, 128
Ophthalmic artery, 224–225, 260*f*,
    261–262
Ophthalmic nerve (cranial nerve V-1),
    221–223, 251, 255, 259–260,
    260*f*, 373–374
Ophthalmic veins, 262
Opponens digiti minimi muscle, 411, 412*f*,
    412*t*
Opponens pollicis muscle, 410–411, 412*f*,
    412*t*
Optic canal, 170, 180, 195, 214*t*
Optic chiasma, 251
Optic foramen, 169*f*, 214*t*
Optic nerve (cranial nerve II), 30, 30*t*, 251,
    259, 368–370, 369*t*, 370*f*
Optic tracts, 251
Oral cancer, 309

Oral cavity, 104, 167, 308–309, 324*f*
  features of, 311*f*
  foramen of, 214*t*
  structures and areas of, 314
  vestibule and vestibular gingivae of,
    310–311, 312*f*
  visual inspection of, 310–314
Oral infections, 309
Oral medicine and pathology, 309
Oral surgery, 306
  for improper jaw relationships, 310
  tooth removal, 309
Oral-antral fistula, 306
Orbicularis oculi muscle, 229*t*, 231, 237
Orbicularis oris muscle, 227, 229*t*
Orbit
  blood vessels in, 261–262
  contents of, 256–265
  muscles of, 256–258, 257*f*, 258*t*
  nerves of, 258–261
Orbital area, 221
Orbital cavity, 256, 256*f*
  foramen of, 214*t*
  skeleton of, 256
Orbital infection, 308
Orbital plates, 184
Orbital process, 203–204
Orbital septum, 237–238, 265*f*
Orbits, 167
Orofacial pain, 377
Oropharynx, 336–339, 338*f*
Orthodontics, 231, 310
Os coxae (hip bone), 87–88, 89*f*
Ossicles, 213, 351*f*, 352
Ossification
  endochondral, 8
  intramembranous, 8
  primary center of, 13
  secondary centers of, 13
Osteotomy, 479*f*, 480
Ostia, 194, 301
Otic ganglion, 287, 288*f*, 373*t*, 386
Otitis externa, 354
Otitis media, 354
Otoscope, 350, 350*f*
Outer ear, 349
Ovarian artery, 102, 122–123
Ovaries, 128

P

Pacemakers, 78–79
Pain
  on injection, 461
  low back pain, 42, 43*f*
  myofascial pain syndrome, 282
  orofacial, 377
  referred, 306
  shin splints, 442
  trigeminal, 377
Palatal gingiva, 316, 459, 459*f*
Palatal mucosa, 316
  infection of, 486
  local anesthesia of, 459, 459*f*
Palatal mucous glands, 316
Palatal muscles, 316–317
Palatal process, 199, 203

Palatal raphé, 313
Palatal rugae, 313
Palate
  arteries, 318–319, 318*f*
  blood and sensory nerve supply to,
    317–319, 318*f*
  cleft lip and palate, 319
  sensory nerves, 317–318, 318*f*
Palatine bones, 167, 202–205, 203*f*, 204*f*
Palatine tonsils, 20, 237, 302, 313, 368
Palatinovaginal canal, 177–179, 214*t*
Palatoglossal arch, 313, 339
Palatoglossus muscle, 316
Palatopharyngeal arch, 313, 339
Palatopharyngeus muscle, 316, 318*t*, 334, 336*t*
Palmar interossei, 412*f*, 412*t*, 414
Palmar ligament, 400
Palmaris brevis muscle, 412*t*
Palmaris longus, 407*f*, 408, 408*t*
Palpebrae (eyelids), 236–238
Palpebral commissures, 236
Palpebral fissure, 236
Pampiniform plexus, 95
Pancreas, 105, 109*f*, 119–120
  arterial supply to, 120
  development of, 99–100
  endocrine portion, 120
  exocrine portion, 120
  features and parts of, 119
  structure and function of, 120
  venous drainage from, 120
Pancreatic duct, 110*f*
Pancreatitis, 120
Panoramic radiography, 469, 470*f*
Papillary muscles, 72, 74
Paralysis
  facial, 232, 233*f*, 268
  tongue, 321
Paranasal air sinuses, 184, 194, 301–308,
    304*f*
  development of, 301
  drainage from, 301–302
  lymphatic drainage of, 368
Parapharyngeal area, 484–485, 484*f*, 485*f*
Parasympathetic nerves
  of abdomen, 103–104
  cranial, 385–386, 385*f*
Parasympathetic nervous system, 23, 26–27,
    27*f*, 30, 103–104
Parathyroid glands, 158
Paratracheal lymph nodes, 365*t*, 366
Parietal bone, 185–187, 187*f*, 188*f*
Parietal eminence, 187
Parietal foramen, 175*f*, 177, 214*t*, 244
Parietal lobe, 244–245
Parietal peritoneum, 99
Parietal pleura, 63
Parietal serous pericardium, 69
Parieto-occipital sulcus, 244
Parotid duct, 235, 267
  blocked, 268
  orifice of, 311
Parotid gland, 267–269, 327*t*
  blood supply to, 267
  infections of, 268
  nerve supply to, 267–269

Parotid region, 265, 266*f*, 268*f*
  boundaries of, 265
  contents of, 265–269
  infections in, 482
  skeleton of, 265
Parotitis, 268
Pars flaccida, 350
Patella, 426, 427*f*
Peau d'orange (orange peel), 59
Pectinate muscles, 71
Pectineus muscle, 438, 439*t*
Pectoral girdle, 388–389, 394–395, 394*f*
Pectoral muscles, 401–403, 402*f*
Pectoralis major muscle, 401, 402*f*, 403*t*
Pectoralis minor muscle, 401–402, 402*f*,
    403*t*
Pelvic cavity, 87, 88
Pelvic girdle, 425, 429–430, 430*f*, 447*t*
Pelvic splanchnic nerves, 104
Pelvic viscera
  distribution of postganglionic sympathetic
    fibers to, 30
  relationships of, 130–131, 131*f*
Pelvis
  female, 131, 131*f*
  male, 127*f*, 130–131, 131*f*
Penis, 126–128
  blood and nerve supply to, 127–128
  bulb of, 127
  components of, 126, 127*f*
  glans of, 127
Pennate muscles, 13, 14*f*
Peptic ulcers, 108
Periapical radiography, 468, 469*f*
Pericardial sac, 69
Pericardiophrenic artery, 97
Pericardium, parietal serous, 69
Pericoronal abscess, 486–487
Pericoronitis, 486–487
Perilymph, 352
Perimysium, 12, 12*f*
Perineum, 98–99
Perineurium, 23–24
Period, 129
Periodontal abscess, 480–481
Periodontal disease, 309
Periodontal ligament, 332
Periodontal structures, 480–481
Periodontics, 309
Periodontitis, 309, 333
Periosteum, 238
Peripheral nerves, 23–31, 24*f*
  definition of, 23
  function of, 24
  somatic, 24–25, 25*f*
  structure of, 23–24, 24*f*
Peripheral nervous system, 23
Peritoneal cavity, 99
Peritoneal reflections, 120–121
Peritoneum, 92, 99, 99*f*, 119–120, 119*f*, 121
  development of, 99–101, 100*f*
  ligaments of, 99
  nomenclature of, 99
  parietal, 99
  visceral, 99, 104, 106
Peritonitis, 111, 121

Petrosal nerves, 255–256
Petrotympanic fissure, 179, 214*t*
Petrous temporal ridge, 191
Phalanges, 393–394, 429
Pharyngeal dysphagia, 336
Pharyngeal gaps, 336, 337*f*
Pharyngeal plexus, 148, 340
Pharyngeal recess, 339
Pharyngeal tonsils, 20, 302, 339
Pharyngeal tubercle, 179
Pharyngobasilar fascia, 334
Pharyngotympanic tube, 214*t*, 349, 353–354
Pharynx, 104–105, 136, 333–334
    blood supply to, 340
    functional areas of, 336–339, 338*f*
    interior of, 336–340
    laryngeal, 336–340, 338*f*
    lymphatic drainage of, 368
    muscles of, 334–336, 335*f*, 336*t*
    nasopharynx, 336–339, 338*f*
    nerve supply to, 340
    oropharynx, 336–339, 338*f*
    walls of, 334
Philtrum, 233
Phonation, 340
Phrenic arteries, 97
Phrenic nerve, 84, 97, 147, 154
Pia mater, 45, 242
Pigmented lungs, 68
Piles, 114
Pinto's (discomalleolar) ligament, 274
PIP joints. *See* Proximal interphalangeal joints
Piriform recess, 340
Piriformis muscle, 440, 441*t*
Pisiform, 393
Pivot joints, 12
Plane joints, 12
Plantar interossei, 446*t*
Plantaris muscle, 442–443, 445*t*
Plasma, 16
Plate, 7
Platysma muscle, 136, 138*f*, 151*t*
Pleura, 63–64
    cervical, 63
    costal, 63
    diaphragmatic, 63
    mediastinal, 63
    parietal, 63
    visceral, 63–64
Pleural cavities, 63, 63*f*
Plica semilunaris, 236
Plicae circulares, 110
Pneumatic bones, 301
Pneumothorax, 68
Pons, 247–248
Pontine nuclei, 247–248
Popliteal artery, 452
Popliteal vein, 453
Popliteus muscle, 443–444, 445*t*
Porta hepatis, 115–116
Portal system, 102–103
Portal vein, 102, 116
Portosystemic anastomosis, 114, 116
Postcentral gyrus, 244, 245
Postcentral sulcus, 244

Posterior abdominal wall, 97, 97*f*, 98*t*
Posterior arch, 313
Posterior auricular artery, 146, 236, 238
Posterior auricular muscle, 229*t*, 239
Posterior auricular vein, 142, 142*f*, 226
Posterior cerebral arteries, 250
Posterior choanae, 177
Posterior ciliary arteries, 262
Posterior clinoid process, 180, 181*f*, 182*f*, 195
Posterior communicating artery, 250–251
Posterior condylar canal, 189, 244
Posterior cranial fossa, 180, 182–183
Posterior cricoarytenoid muscle, 344, 344*t*
Posterior cruciate ligament, 431–434
Posterior ethmoidal artery, 262
Posterior ethmoidal canal, 214*t*
Posterior ethmoidal foramen, 171
Posterior ethmoidal nerve, 260
Posterior femoral cutaneous nerve, 451*t*
Posterior intercostal arteries, 62
Posterior lacrimal crest, 206
Posterior longitudinal ligament, 162
Posterior mediastinum, 79–84
Posterior nasal apertures, 177
Posterior nasal spine, 177, 204
Posterior palate clefts, 319
Posterior septal artery, 297
Posterior spinal arteries, 46–47
Posterior superior alveolar artery, 297, 331–332
Posterior superior alveolar foramen, 174, 200, 214*t*
Posterior superior alveolar nerve, 293, 374
Posterior superior alveolar nerve block, 459–460, 460*f*
Posterior temporal nerve, 286
Posterior tibial artery, 452
Posteroinferior cerebellar arteries, 250
Posterosuperior lateral nasal nerves, 301
Postglenoid tubercle, 173, 191
Postvertebral muscles, 162*t*
Pott's fracture, 436
Preaortic ganglia, 103
Precentral gyrus, 244, 245–246
Precentral sulcus, 244
Prelaryngeal lymph nodes, 365*t*, 366
Premolars
    mandibular, 486
    maxillary, 486
Prenatal development, 2
Prepuce, 127
Pretracheal (visceral) fascia, 136
Pretracheal lymph nodes, 365*t*, 366
Prevertebral fascia, 136
Prevertebral muscles, 162*t*, 163–164, 163*f*
Primary motor area, 245–246
Primary palate clefts, 319
Primary visual area, 245
Procerus muscle, 229*t*, 231
Process (bony), 7
Projection fibers, 246–247
Promontory, 350–352
Pronator quadratus muscle, 407*f*, 408*t*, 409
Pronator teres, 406–408, 407*f*, 408*t*

Prostate enlargement, 126
Prostate gland, 126
Prostatic urethra, 126
Prosthodontics, 309–310
Proximal interphalangeal (PIP) joints, 400
Proximal phalanx, 393–394, 429
Pterion, 173
Pterygoid arteries, 290
Pterygoid canal, 196, 214*t*, 291
    artery of, 297
    nerve of, 377
Pterygoid fossa, 196, 212, 212*f*
Pterygoid notch, 196
Pterygoid plexus of veins, 290–291, 290*f*, 332, 363*t*
Pterygoid processes, 195*f*, 196
Pterygomandibular raphé, 227–228
Pterygomaxillary fissure, 173–174
Pterygopalatine fissure, 291
Pterygopalatine fossa, 291, 292*f*
    contents of, 291–297
    location and terminology for, 291
    skeletal review, 291
Pterygopalatine ganglion, 294–296, 295*f*, 296*f*, 373*t*, 374, 377, 386
Pubis, 87–88
Pubofemoral ligament, 430–431
Pudendal nerve, 449–450, 451*t*
Puillary light reflex, 263–264
Pulmonary artery, 65
Pulmonary plexus, 84
Pulmonary valve, 72–74
Pulmonary vein, 65
Pulp chamber, 328
Pulpitis, 309
Pulse points, 225
Punctum, 264–265
Pyloric sphincter, 105, 106*f*
Pylorus, 105, 106*f*
Pyramid, 350
Pyramidal decussation, 248–249
Pyramidal motor system, 245–246
Pyramidal process, 174, 204
Pyramidal tracts, 245–246
Pyramids, 248–249

Q

Quadrangular membrane, 342
Quadratus femoris, 437–438, 439*t*, 440, 441*t*
Quadratus lumborum, 98*t*
Quadratus plantae lumbricals, 446*t*

R

Radial artery, 419–420
Radial nerve, 155, 418, 419*t*
Radial tuberosity, 392
Radiocarpal joint, 399, 400*f*
Radiography
    bitewing, 468
    cephalometric, 469–470, 471*f*
    extraoral, 469–470
    full mouth surveys, 469, 470*f*
    full skull, 469–470, 471*f*
    hand and wrist, 473, 477*f*

Radiography (Continued)
  intraoral, 468–469
  of maxillary air sinuses, 470–472, 474f
  occlusal, 468–469, 469f
  panoramic, 469, 470f
  periapical, 468, 469f
  sinus, 470–472
  traditional (plain films), 467
Radiology, 467–468
  tomography (sectional films), 467–468
  traditional radiography (plain films), 467
Radioulnar joints, 398–399, 399f
Radius, 392–393, 392f
Rectal examination, 114
Rectum, 105, 112–113, 114f
Rectus abdominis muscle, 92, 92t, 93f
Rectus capitis anterior muscle, 162t, 163f
Rectus capitis lateralis muscle, 162t, 163f, 164
Rectus capitis posterior major muscle, 162t, 163
Rectus capitis posterior minor muscle, 162–163, 162t
Rectus femoris muscle, 437–438, 439t
Rectus sheath, 92
Recurrent laryngeal nerve, 157, 347, 382
Red nucleus, 247
Referred pain, 306
Reflux, gastroesophageal, 106
Refractive correction, 264
Refractive errors, 264
Refractive surgery, 264
Regional approach, 1
Renal arteries, 102, 122–123
Renal artery, 122
Renal colic, 124
Renal columns, 121–122
Renal corpuscle, 121
Renal cortex, 121
Renal medulla, 121
Renal papilla, 121–122
Renal pelvis, 122
Renal pyramids, 121
Renal veins, 122
Respiration, 54, 96–97
  accessory extrinsic muscles of, 60
  back muscles that participate in, 60–62, 61t
  phases of, 67
Respiratory cartilage, 4
Respiratory mucosa, 314–316
Respiratory tract, 65, 66f
Restoration of missing teeth, 309–310
Restorative dentistry, 309
Rete testis, 125
Reticular formation, 249
Retina, 262–263
Retromandibular vein, 142, 142f, 226–227, 265–267, 332, 363t
Retromolar fossa or triangle, 213, 310–311
Retroperitoneal viscera, 99
Retropharyngeal lymph nodes, 365–366, 365t
Retropharyngeal space, 138, 340
Rhinitis, 302
Rhinorrhea, 302, 478–480

Rhomboid muscles, 47, 405t
Rib fracture, 58
Rib separation, 58
Ribs, 54–57
  articulation of, 57, 57f, 58f
  components of, 54
  dislocated, 58
  false, 54–57
  first rib, 54–57, 56f
  floating, 57
  true, 54
  types of, 54
  typical, 54, 56f
Right ascending lumbar vein, 83
Right atrioventricular valve, 71, 72
Right atrium, 18–19, 69–70, 71–72, 73f, 358
Right auricle, 71
Right brachiocephalic vein, 82, 83, 83f
Right bronchi, 65
Right bronchial tree, 65–66
Right clavicle, 390f
Right colic artery, 115
Right colic flexure, 111–112
Right common carotid artery, 80–81
Right common iliac artery, 101, 450–452
Right common iliac vein, 102
Right coronary artery, 76–77, 80
Right external iliac artery, 101
Right gastric artery, 107–108
Right gastric vein, 108
Right gastro-omental artery, 107–108
Right gastro-omental vein, 108
Right heart, 16
Right hepatic duct, 118
Right inferior alveolar nerve, 331
Right internal iliac artery, 101
Right lymphatic duct, 157
Right maxilla, 177, 201f
Right palatine bone, 177, 203f, 204f
Right pleural cavity, 58
Right pulmonary vein, 74
Right recurrent laryngeal nerve, 84
Right subclavian artery, 80–81
Right temporal bone, 177, 180, 191f, 192f
Right transverse sulcus, 188
Right ventricle, 69–70, 72–74, 73f
Rima glottidis, 342
Risorius muscle, 227, 229t
Rostrum, 194
Rotator cuff injuries, 404
Rotator cuff muscles, 404, 405t
Rotatores muscle, 49, 51t
Round ligament, 95
Ruffini corpuscles, 10
Rugae, 106
Runner's knee, 434
Ruptured tympanic membrane, 354

S

Sacral plexus, 31, 103, 232, 445–450, 450f, 451t
Sacroiliac joint, 429
Sacrum, 39, 41f
Saddle or ellipsoid joints, 11
Sagittal plane, 2f, 3

Sagittal suture, 175f, 176
Saliva, 327
Salivary glands, 327, 327t
  accessory, 327
  imaging of, 472–473
  nerve supply to, 327
Salpingopharyngeal fold, 339
Salpinx, 339
Saphenous cutdown, 454
Sarcolemma, 12
Sarcoplasm, 12
Sartorius muscle, 437, 439t
Scalene muscles, 164
Scalenus anterior muscle, 151t, 152, 163f
Scalenus medius muscle, 151t, 152, 163f
Scalenus posterior muscle, 151t, 152, 163f
Scalp, 221, 238, 239f
  detachment of, 239
  infections of, 239
  lacerations to, 239
Scaphoid, 393
Scaphoid fossa, 196
Scapula, 388–389, 390f
Scapulothoracic joint, 394, 394f
Scarpa's fascia, 91, 91f
Schwann cells, 23–24
Sciatic nerve, 445–449, 451f, 451t
Sciatica, 42
Sclera, 262
Scoliosis, 42
Scrotum, 95
Secondary palate clefts, 319
Sella turcica, 180, 194
Semicircular canals, 349, 352
Semimembranosus muscle, 440, 442t
Seminal vesicles, 125–126
Seminiferous tubules, 125
Semispinalis muscle, 49, 51t
Semitendinosus muscle, 440, 442t
Sensory (cutaneous) nerves, 221–224
Sensory neurons, 21–22, 22f
Sensory speech (Wernicke's)area, 245–246
Separated ribs, 58
Septal cartilage, 235, 299
Serous body cavities, 35, 35f
Serratus anterior muscle, 402–403, 402f, 403t
Serratus posterior inferior muscle, 47–49, 61t, 62
Serratus posterior superior muscle, 47–49, 61t, 62
Sesamoid bones, 6
Sexual dimorphism, 219
Shin splints, 442
Shock wave lithotripsy, 124
Short bones, 6
Short gastric artery, 107–108
Short gastric vein, 108
Short sphenopalatine nerves, 301
Shoulder
  bursitis of, 404
  dislocation of, 396
  muscles of, 403–404, 404f, 405t
  separation of, 394
Shoulder (pectoral) girdle, 388–389, 394–395, 394f

Sialography, 328, 329f, 472–473
Sight, 368–370
Sigmoid colon, 112
Sigmoid sinus, 242, 363t
Sigmoid sulcus, 183, 191
Sinoatrial node, 72, 77
Sinus radiography, 470–472
Sinusoids, 17
Skeletal age, 8
Skeletal muscle, 12–15
  architecture of, 13
  blood and nerve supply to, 14–15
  nomenclature for, 12
  origins and insertions, 13
  parts of, 12–13, 12f
Skeleton, 4
  of abdomen, 87–88, 88f
  of ankle and foot, 428–429
  appendicular, 5, 5f
  of arm, 389–392
  axial, 5, 5f
  of back, 37, 38f
  cervical, 133–134, 134f
  of ear, 349
  facial, 167
  of forearm, wrist, and hand, 392–393, 399f
  of larynx, 135f
  of lower limb, 425
  of neck, 133
  of orbital cavity, 256
  of parotid region, 265
  thoracic, 54–58, 55f
  of upper limb, 388, 389f
  of vertebral unit, 133
  of visceral unit, 133–134
Skin, 31–33, 34f
  of face, 221
  functions of, 33
  as mechanical envelope, 33
  as organ, 33
  thick, 31
  thin, 31
Skull, 167, 168f
  basal or inferior view, 177–180, 178f
  bones of, 184
  fetal, 217f
  frontal view of, 167–171, 169f
  full skull radiography, 469–470, 471f
  fusion of bones, 217–218
  intermediate area, 179f
  internal aspect of, 180–183, 181f
  key sections through, 183–184, 183f
  lateral view, 171–174, 172f, 174f
  posterior view of, 37, 176f, 177
  postnatal development of, 213, 218f
  radiography of, 469–470, 471f
  superior view of, 174–177, 175f
Skull foramina, 213
Small distal phalanx, 393–394
Small intestine, 112f
  arterial supply to, 110, 111f
  venous drainage from, 110–111
Small intestine wall, 110
Small saphenous vein, 454
Smell, 301, 368

Smooth muscle, 15
Soft palate, 313–314, 316–319
  functions of, 317
  muscles of, 316–317, 317f, 318t
  structures of, 316
  surface features of, 313, 314f
Soleus muscle, 442–443, 445t
Somatic nervous system, 23
  of abdomen, 103
  peripheral nerves, 24–25, 25f
Somatic structures, 24
Somesthetic (general sensory) area, 245
Spasmodic torticollis, 140
Speech areas, 245–246
Spermatic cord, 92–95, 125–126
  contents of, 95
  formation of, 94–95, 94f
  layers of, 95
Spermatozoa, 125
Sphenoethmoidal recess, 299
Sphenoid bone, 177, 180, 193–197, 194f, 195f
Sphenoidal air sinuses, 307f, 308, 308f
Sphenoidal crest, 194
Sphenoidal notch, 204
Sphenoidal process, 204
Sphenomandibular ligament, 274
Sphenopalatine artery, 297
Sphenopalatine foramen, 204, 214t, 291
Sphincters, 13, 14f
  external sphincter ani, 113
  internal sphincter ani, 113
  precapillary, 16–17
  pyloric, 105, 106f
Spinal accessory nerve (cranial nerve XI), 30, 30t, 140, 369t, 382–383, 383f
Spinal anesthesia, 47, 48f
Spinal cord, 23, 43, 45f, 46f
  blood supply to, 46–47
  central canal of, 44–45
  cervical portion of, 136
  coverings (meninges), 45–46, 48f
  external features of, 43–44, 45f
  internal features of, 44–45, 47f
  location and length, 43
  protection for, 46
  sulci and fissures on, 44
  swellings of, 43–44
Spinal nerves, 23, 24, 25, 30–31, 44, 46f
  cutaneous distribution (dermatomes) of, 31, 33f
  nomenclature of, 31, 31f
  origins of, 26, 26f
Spinal tap, 46
Spinalis muscle, 49, 51t
Spine (bony), 7
Spine (vertebral)
  abnormal curvatures of, 42
  articulated spine, 39–42, 41f
  joints of, 42–43
  movements of, 49, 50f
  muscles responsible for movements of, 52t
Spiral ganglion, 353
Spiral organ of Corti, 353
Splanchnic nerves, 28–29, 30
  lumbar, 30
  pelvic, 104

Spleen, 20, 105, 109f, 120
  blood supply to, 120
  features and parts of, 120
  structure and function of, 120
Splenectomy, 121
Splenic artery, 107, 120
Splenic vein, 120
Splenius capitis muscle, 151–152, 151t
Splenius muscle, 24, 51t
Splenorenal ligament, 120
Squama, 187, 189–190
Squamotympanic fissure, 179, 193
Squamous cell carcinoma, 234
Squamous sutures, 8–9
Stapedius muscle, 352
Stapes (stirrup), 352
Sternal angle, 54, 59, 60f
Sternal slips, 96
Sternoclavicular joint, 394, 394f
Sternocleidomastoid muscle, 139, 139f, 140, 151t
  actions of, 140
  insertions, 140
  nerve supply to, 140
  origins of, 140
Sternocostal joints, 57–58
Sternohyoid muscle, 143, 144t
Sternothyroid muscle, 143, 144t
Sternum, 54, 55f
Steroid hormones, 124
Stirrup (stapes), 352
Stomach, 105–108
  arterial supply to, 107–108, 108f
  features of, 105–107, 106f
  peritoneal coverings and attachments, 106, 107f
  position of, 105
  venous return to, 108
Stomach wall, 106
Straight sinus, 242, 363t
Strap muscles, 13, 14f
Stroke (cerebrovascular accident), 251
Styloglossus muscle, 320, 320t
Stylohyoid muscle, 144, 144t
Styloid process, 180, 193
Stylomandibular ligament, 274
Stylomastoid foramen, 180, 193, 214t
Stylopharyngeus muscle, 334, 336t
Subarachnoid hemorrhage, 240
Subarachnoid space, 46, 242
Subclavian artery, 154–156, 154f, 358, 418–419
Subclavian vein, 154, 154f, 156, 358, 420
Subclavius muscle, 402, 403t
Subcostal nerve, 84
Subcutaneous tissue, 35
Subdural hemorrhage, 240
Subdural space, 46, 242
Sublingual artery, 326–327
Sublingual fossa, 212f, 213
Sublingual gland, 326–327, 327t
Sublingual infections, 482–483, 486
Sublingual ridge, 314
Submandibular ducts, 314, 326, 328
Submandibular fossa, 212f, 213

Submandibular ganglion, 322–324, 325*f*, 326–327, 373*t*, 377, 386
Submandibular gland, 149, 326, 327*t*
Submandibular infections, 482, 486
Submandibular lymph nodes, 149, 360–364, 365*t*
Submandibular triangle, 141–142, 148–150, 150*f*
Submental lymph nodes, 359–360, 365*t*
Submental triangle, 142
Suboccipital nerve, 163
Suboccipital region, 159, 160*f*
    muscles of, 162–163
    nerves of, 163
Subscapular fossa, 389
Subscapularis muscle, 404, 405*t*
Substantia nigra, 247
Sulci, 44, 244, 245*f*
Sulcus, 7
Sulcus terminalis, 319
Superciliary arches, 168
Superficial fascia (tela subcutanea), 35, 136
    of abdomen, 91
    cervical, 136
    of face, 221
    functions of, 35
    infections in, 481, 483*f*, 486
Superficial inguinal ring, 92–94
Superficial lymph nodes
    of lower limb, 454
    parotid, 364, 365*t*
Superficial temporal artery, 146, 225, 236, 238, 267, 275
Superficial temporal vein, 265–267, 332, 363*t*
Superficial veins, upper limb, 420–422
Superior abdominal wall, 96–97, 97*f*, 98*t*
Superior alveolar foramen, 291
Superior alveolar plexus, 293
Superior and posterior mediastinum, 79–84
Superior auricular muscle, 229*t*, 236
Superior cervical ganglion, 158
Superior colliculi, 247
Superior concha, 199, 299
Superior constrictor muscle, 334, 336*t*
Superior epigastric artery, 62, 95–96, 156
Superior gemellus muscle, 440
Superior gluteal nerve, 451*t*
Superior hemiazygos vein, 83
Superior labial artery, 225
Superior laryngeal nerve, 382
Superior meatus, 299
Superior mesenteric artery, 99, 102, 110, 114–115
Superior mesenteric vein, 115, 116
Superior nuchal line, 37, 177, 187
Superior oblique muscle, 258, 258*t*
Superior orbital fissure, 169*f*, 170, 182, 182*f*, 196, 214*t*
Superior palpebral margin, 236
Superior pancreaticoduodenal artery, 107, 109, 120
Superior pancreaticoduodenal vein, 120
Superior papillae, 236
Superior petrosal hiatus, 214*t*

Superior petrosal sinus, 244, 363*t*
Superior petrosal sulcus, 182, 214*t*
Superior radioulnar joint, 398
Superior rectus muscle, 257–258, 258*t*
Superior sagittal sinus, 242, 363*t*
Superior sagittal sulcus, 185, 188
Superior thyroid artery, 146, 158, 347
Superior thyroid vein, 158
Superior vena cava, 71, 82–83, 358
Superior vesical artery, 124
Supination, 399
Supinator muscle, 410, 410*f*, 411*t*
Supraciliary arch, 169*f*
Supraclavicular nerves, 147, 153
Supragingival calculus, 328
Suprahyoid muscles, 143–145, 144*t*
Supramastoid crest, 191
Suprameatal triangle, 191
Supraorbital artery, 224, 238, 262
Supraorbital foramen, 168–170, 169*f*, 184, 214*t*
Supraorbital nerve (cranial nerve V-1), 222, 238, 373
Supraorbital notch, 168–170, 169*f*, 184, 214*t*
Suprarenal arteries, 102
Suprarenal cortex, 124, 124*f*
Suprarenal glands, 124–125
Suprarenal medulla, 124, 124*f*
Suprascapular artery, 154–155, 156
Suprascapular nerve, 417, 419*t*
Suprascapular notch, 388
Suprascapular vein, 152–153
Supraspinatus muscle, 404, 404*f*, 405*t*
Supraspinous fossa, 388
Suprasternal notch, 54, 59, 60*f*
Suprasternal space (of Burns), 136
Supratrochlear artery, 224, 238, 262
Supratrochlear nerve (cranial nerve V-1), 222, 238, 373
Suprrahyoid muscles, 320
Surface anatomy, 2
Surgery
    for facial disharmonies, 480
    oral, 306
Surgical emphysema, 138
Sustentaculum tali, 428
Sutures, 8, 8*f*, 218
    denticulate, 8–9
    serrated, 8–9
    squamous, 8–9
    types of, 8–9
Swallowing, 334–336, 337*f*
Swellings, spinal cord, 43–44
Sympathetic nervous system, 23, 30, 103
    of abdomen, 103, 104*f*
    cranial nerves, 383–385
    distribution of postganglionic sympathetic fibers, 29
    origins and distributions, 27–29, 28*f*, 29*f*
    supply to head, 158
Sympathetic trunk, 157–158, 157*f*
Symphysis, 9*f*, 10
Symphysis menti, 212*f*, 218
Symphysis pubis, 429
Synapses, 21, 22, 22*f*

Synaptic cleft, 22
Synarthrodial joints, 8
Synchondroses, 9–10, 9*f*
Syndesmosis, 9, 9*f*, 42–43
Synovial bursae and sheaths, 13–14, 14*f*
Synovial joints, 10–12, 10*f*
    bilateral, 42
    blood and nerve supply to, 10
    classification of, 10–12, 11*f*
Synovial membrane, 10, 274–275, 431–434
Synovium, 274–275
Systemic approach, 1

T

T cells, 19
Talocalcanean (subtalar) joint, 436
Talocrural joint, 435–436, 436*f*
Talus, 428
Tarsal bones, 428–429
Tarsal glands, 237
Tarsal plates or tarsi, 238
Tarsi, 237–238
Tarsometatarsal joint, 436
Taste area, 245
Taste buds, 320
Teeth, 171, 311–312, 327–333
    abscess of, 309
    arterial supply to, 331–332
    block anesthesia for, 459, 460, 463, 464, 465, 466
    deciduous, 311–312, 330*f*
    external features of, 328, 330*f*
    local anesthesia for, 457–458, 458*f*
    local infiltration of, 457–458, 458*f*
    lymphatic drainage of, 367
    mandibular
        anatomy of, 212*f*, 331
        block anesthesia for, 463, 464, 465, 466
    maxillary
        anatomy of, 177, 331
        block anesthesia for, 459, 460
        local anesthesia of, 458–459, 458*f*
    missing, 309–310, 311
    nerve supply to, 333
    numerical symbols and quadrants, 311–312, 313*f*
    pulpal chamber of, 480
    removal of, 309
    supporting structures for, 332–333
    visual inspection of, 311–313
Tegmen tympani, 350
Tela subcutanea, 91
Telencephalon, 244
Temples, 221
Temporal bone, 189–193, 271–272, 271*f*
    articular eminence of, 271–272, 271*f*
    development of, 219
    zygomatic process of, 172*f*, 173, 189–191, 270*f*, 271–272
Temporal crest, 213, 310–311
Temporal fossa, 173, 269, 269*f*
Temporal lobe, 244–245
Temporalis muscle, 279–281, 280*t*, 281*f*, 284*f*

Temporomandibular joint (TMJ), 269–275, 270*f*, 275*f*
  accessory ligaments, 274, 275*f*
  blood supply of, 275
  dislocation of, 276
  imaging of, 472, 476*f*
  internal features of, 272, 273*f*
  movements at, 275–276
  nerve supply of, 275, 275*f*
  with perforated disc, 276, 277*f*
Temporomandibular joint (TMJ) arthrography, 472, 476*f*
Temporomandibular joint (TMJ) MRI, 472, 476*f*
Temporomandibular ligament, 272, 272*f*
Tendons
  common, 12–13
  cylindrical, 12
  intermediate, 12–13
  linear, 12
Teniae coli, 111
Tensor fasciae latae muscle, 439–440, 441*t*
Tensor palate nerve, 286
Tensor tympani muscle, 350, 352
Tensor tympani nerve, 286
Tensor veli palatini muscle, 316, 318*t*
Tentorium cerebelli, 240–242, 241*f*
Teres major muscle, 403–404, 404*f*, 405*t*
Teres minor muscle, 404, 404*f*, 405*t*
Terminology, 2
  dental surfaces, 328–331
  nervous system, 22–23
  nomenclature of peritoneum and peritoneal cavity, 99
  nomenclature of spinal nerves, 31, 31*f*
  numerical symbols for dentition and quadrants, 311–312, 313*f*
  pterygopalatine fossa, 291
  skeletal muscle nomenclature, 12
  terms of relationship, 3–4, 3*f*, 4*t*
Testes, 125
  development and descent of, 94*f*
  undescended, 95–96
Testicular artery, 95, 102, 122–123
Testicular vein, 95
Testosterone, 125
Thalamus, 247
Thenar muscles, 410–411, 412*t*
Thigh, 425–426
  anterior thigh muscles, 437–438, 438*f*, 439*t*
  deep rotators of, 441*t*
  medial thigh muscles, 438–439, 439*t*
  posterior thigh muscles, 440, 440*f*, 442*t*
Third molars, mandibular, 486–487, 487*f*
Third occipital nerve, 163, 238
Third ventricle, 249
Thoracic (descending) aorta, 80, 81–82, 82*f*
Thoracic diaphragm, 96, 98*t*
Thoracic duct, 83–84, 83*f*, 156–157
Thoracic esophagus, 79
Thoracic inlet, 54
Thoracic muscles, 59–62, 61*t*
  action of, 59
  extrinsic, 59–60
Thoracic skeleton, 54–58, 55*f*

Thoracic vertebrae, 39, 57
  features of, 39, 57, 57*f*
  joints between, 57–58
Thoracic wall, 58
  skeletal landmarks, 59
  surface features of, 58–59
Thoracodorsal nerve, 418, 419*t*
Thorax, 54–84
  distribution of postganglionic sympathetic fibers to, 29–30
  divisions of, 58
  nerves of, 84
  veins of, 82, 83*f*
Thumb
  joints of, 400–401
  movements of, 401, 401*f*
  opposition and reposition of, 401*f*
Thymus gland, 20, 84
Thyroarytenoid muscle, 344, 344*t*
Thyrocervical trunk, 154, 156, 360*t*
Thyrocricoid joint, 342
Thyroepiglotticus muscle, 344, 344*t*
Thyroglossal cysts, 158
Thyroglossal duct, 158
Thyrohyoid membrane, 342
Thyrohyoid muscle, 143, 144*t*
Thyrohyoid space, 134–136
Thyroid cartilage, 133, 340–341
Thyroid gland, 136, 158, 159*f*
Thyroid ima artery, 158
Thyroid notch, 340–341
Thyroid prominence (Adam's apple), 134–136, 340
Thyroxine, 158
Tibia, 426, 428*f*
Tibial nerve, 449
Tibial tuberosity, 426
Tibialis anterior muscle, 440–441, 442*t*
Tibialis posterior muscle, 443–444, 445*t*
Tibiofibular joints, 435
Tic douloureux (trigeminal neuralgia), 224
TMJ. *See* Temporomandibular joint
Toes, 447*t*
Tomography (sectional films), 467–468
  alveolar ridge tomography, 470, 472*f*
  computed tomography (CT), 468
  cone beam computed tomography, 468
  conventional tomography, 467–468
Tongue, 319–321
  accessory muscles of, 320, 323*f*
  actions of, 321
  extrinsic muscles of, 320, 320*t*, 323*f*
  functions of, 319
  intrinsic muscles of, 320–321
  lymphatic drainage of, 367–368, 368*f*
  motor nerve supply to, 321
  mucosa of dorsum of, 319–320
  muscles of, 320–321
  paralyzed, 321
  parts and surfaces of, 319
  sensory nerve supply to, 321
  surface features of, 313–314, 315*f*, 322*f*
  visual inspection of, 313–314
Tongue tie, 321
Tonsillar crypts, 313
Tonsillar region, 483, 484*f*

Tonsillectomy, 339
Tonsillitis, 339
Tonsils, 20
  lingual, 20
  palatine, 20, 237, 302, 313, 368
  pharyngeal, 20, 302, 339
Tooth abscess, 309
Tooth removal, 309
Torticollis (wry neck), 140
  congenital, 140
  spasmodic, 140
Torus palatinus, 319
Trabeculae carneae, 72, 74
Trachea, 79, 136, 158–159, 368
Tract, 23
Transversalis fascia, 92
Transverse arch, 436
Transverse arytenoid muscle, 344, 344*t*
Transverse cervical artery, 154, 156
Transverse cervical nerve, 142, 142*f*, 153
Transverse cervical vein, 152
Transverse colon, 112
Transverse facial artery, 267
Transverse mesocolon, 112, 113–114
Transverse or horizontal plane, 2*f*, 3
Transverse sinus, 242
Transverse sulcus, 183, 187
Transverse tarsal joint, 436
Transversospinalis muscle, 49, 51*t*
Transversus abdominis muscle, 92, 92*t*, 93*f*
Trapezium, 393
Trapezius muscle, 47, 139, 139*f*, 140, 151*t*, 403, 404*f*, 405*t*
  actions of, 140
  insertions of, 140
  nerve supply to, 140
  origins of, 140
Trapezoid bone, 393
Trauma, 289
Triceps brachii muscle, 406, 406*t*
Tricuspid valve, 71, 72
Trigeminal (Meckel's) dural cave, 251
Trigeminal nerve (cranial nerve V), 251, 369*t*, 372–377, 372*f*
  branches of, 373–376
  cranial parasympathetic ganglia associated with, 373*t*
  cutaneous distribution of, 31, 33*f*
  functional components of, 30, 30*t*, 372–373
  mandibular division, 374–376, 376*f*
  maxillary division, 374, 375*f*
  ophthalmic division, 373–374, 374*f*
Trigeminal neuralgia (tic douloureux), 224
Trigeminal pain, 377
Trigone of the bladder, 124
Triquetral, 393
Trochanter, 7
Trochlea, 392
Trochlear nerve (cranial nerve IV), 30, 30*t*, 251, 255, 259, 369*t*, 371, 371*f*
Trochlear notch, 393
True ribs, 54
True vocal folds, 342
Trunk, 29
Tubercle, 7
Tuberculum sellae, 194

Tuberosity, 7
Tunica adventitia, 16, 16*f*
Tunica albuginea, 125
Tunica intima, 16, 16*f*
Tunica media, 16, 16*f*
Tunica vaginalis, 95
Tympanic canal, 193, 214*t*
Tympanic cavity (middle ear cavity), 350–352
Tympanic membrane (eardrum), 349–350, 350*f*
  inspection of, 350, 350*f*
  ruptured, 354
Tympanic nerve, 380
Tympanic plate, 179

U

Ulcers
  duodenal, 108
  peptic, 108
Ulna, 392, 392*f*, 393
Ulnar artery, 419–420
Ulnar nerve, 155, 418, 419*t*
Ulnar notch, 393
Umbilical arteries, 19
Umbilical vein, 18–19
Undescended testes (cryptorchidism), 95–96
Upper airway obstruction, 347
Upper limb, 388–422
  arterial supply to, 418–420, 421*f*
  bones of, 388, 389*f*
  cutaneous nerves of, 418, 420*f*
  deep veins of, 420
  joints of, 394
  lymphatic drainage of, 422, 423*f*
  motor nerves to muscles of, 154
  movements of, 394, 417*t*
  muscles of, 394, 401–414
  nerve supply to, 415
  skeleton of, 388, 389*f*
  superficial veins of, 420–422
  venous return from, 420, 422*f*
Upper motor neurons, 24, 232
Upper subscapular nerve, 418, 419*t*
Ureteral colic, 124
Ureters, 122–123
Urethra, 124, 126
Urinary bladder, 123
Urinary calculi (stones), 124
Urinary system, 121–124, 122*f*
Urogenital diaphragm, 99
Urogenital triangle, 99
Uterine tubes, 128–129
Uterus, 129
  peritoneal coverings and supporting
    ligaments, 129
  round ligament of, 95
  structure and function of, 129
Uvula, 313
Uvular muscle, 316, 318*t*

V

Vagina, 129–130
Vagus nerve (cranial nerve X), 84, 103–104,
    138, 148, 149*f*, 157, 254,
    316–317, 321, 340, 347, 369*t*,
    381–382, 381*f*

branches of, 340, 382
  functional components of, 30, 30*t*,
    381–382
Vallate papillae, 320
Valleculae, 340
Valvular insufficiency, 76
Valvular stenosis, 76
Varicocele, 96
Varicose veins, 454
Vas deferens, 95
Vasa recti, 110
Vascular accidents, 291
Vasectomy, 95
Vastus intermedius muscle, 437–438,
    439*t*
Vastus lateralis muscle, 437–438, 439*t*
Vastus medialis muscle, 437–438, 439*t*
Veins, 17.*See also specific veins*
  of eyeball, 264
  of face, 225–227
  of head and neck, 358, 362*f*
  intercostal, 62
  that accompany cutaneous nerves and
    arteries, 225–227
  of thorax, 82, 83*f*
  varicose veins, 454
Venae cordis minimae, 77
Venipuncture, 421
Ventricles
  brain, 249, 250*f*
  cardiac, 16
Ventricular folds, 342–343
Ventricular ligaments, 342
Venules, 17
Vermiform appendix, 111
Vermilion border, 233, 233*f*, 310
Vertebrae
  cervical, 38–39, 40*f*
  lumbar, 39, 40*f*
  thoracic, 39, 57, 57*f*
  typical features of, 37–38, 39*f*
Vertebral artery, 46–47, 156, 163, 250, 359*f*,
    360*t*, 363*t*
Vertebral column, 37–39, 46*f*
Vertebral muscles, 162–163, 162*t*
Vertebral unit, 133
Vertebral venous plexus, 46–47
Vesicular arteries, 122–123
Vestibular fold, 310
Vestibular gingivae, 310–311, 312*f*, 459
Vestibular mucosa, 459
Vestibular nerve, 353
Vestibular window, 352
Vestibule, 297–299
  buccal, 311, 312*f*
  internal ear, 352
  visual inspection of, 310–311, 312*f*
Vestibulocochlear nerve (cranial nerve VIII),
    30, 30*t*, 253–254, 353, 369*t*,
    378–379, 379*f*
Villi, 110
Viscera
  abdominal, 104
  cervical, 158–159
  retroperitoneal, 99
Visceral (pretracheal) fascia, 136

Visceral (autonomic) nervous system, 23
  afferent (sensory) system, 30
  central nervous system origins of, 25–30
  efferent (motor) system, 25–30
Visceral peritoneum, 99, 104, 106
Visceral pleura, 63–64
Visceral structures, 24
Visceral unit, 133–134
Viscerocranium, 167
Visual inspection
  of lips and cheeks, 310
  of oral cavity, 310–314
Vitamin D, 33
Vitreous humor, 263
Vocal folds, 342–343
  false, 342
  muscles that close, 347
  muscles that control tension of, 347
  muscles that open, 347
  true, 342
Vocal ligaments, 342
Vocal process, 341
Vocalis muscle, 344–346, 344*t*
Vomer, 167, 169*f*, 177, 210, 210*f*

W

Walking, 437
Wernicke's (sensory speech) area,
    245–246
White communicating rami, 27, 28–29
White matter, 23
  brain, 244, 246–247, 247*f*
  spinal cord, 44
Wrist
  bones of, 393, 393*f*
  imaging of, 473, 477*f*
  joints of, 397*f*
  movements at, 399–400, 400*f*
  muscles of, 412*t*
Wrist joint, 399–400
Wry neck (torticollis), 140

X

Xerostomia (dry mouth), 328
Xiphoid process, 54

Z

Zeis, glands of, 236–237
Zygomatic (malar) area, 221
Zygomatic artery, 224–225
Zygomatic bone, 167, 205–206, 205*f*,
    206*f*
Zygomatic canal, 171
Zygomatic nerve, 293, 374
Zygomatic process, 184, 186*f*
Zygomaticofacial artery, 262
Zygomaticofacial foramen, 168, 169*f*, 205,
    214*t*
Zygomaticofacial nerve, 223, 293
Zygomatico-orbital foramen, 205
Zygomaticotemporal artery, 238, 262
Zygomaticotemporal foramen, 205, 214*t*
Zygomaticotemporal nerve, 223, 238,
    293
Zygomaticus major muscle, 227, 229*t*